Pediatric and Neonatal Care

Pediatric and Neonatal Care

Editor: Santiago Alicea

AMERICAN
MEDICAL PUBLISHERS
www.americanmedicalpublishers.com

AMERICAN
MEDICAL PUBLISHERS
www.americanmedicalpublishers.com

Cataloging-in-Publication Data

Pediatric and neonatal care / edited by Santiago Alicea.
p. cm.
Includes bibliographical references and index.
ISBN 979-8-88740-367-0
1. Pediatrics. 2. Neonatology. 3. Newborn infants--Diseases. 4. Newborn infants--Care.
5. Newborn infants--Hospital care. 6. Newborn infants--Medical care. I. Alicea, Santiago.
RJ47 .P43 2023
618.92--dc23

American Medical Publishers,
41 Flatbush Avenue,
1st Floor, New York,
NY 11217, USA

ISBN 979-8-88740-367-0 (Hardback)

Contents

Preface IX

Chapter 1 **End-of-Life Care for Neonates: Assessing and Addressing Pain and Distressing Symptoms** 1
Shelly Haug, Alicia Dye and Sara Durrani

Chapter 2 **Perinatal Palliative Care: Cultural, Spiritual and Religious Considerations for Parents—What Clinicians Need to Know** 9
Victoria J. Kain

Chapter 3 **A "Fundamentals" Train-the- Trainer Approach to Building Pediatric Critical Care Expertise in the Developing World** 19
Sheri S. Crow, Beth A. Ballinger, Mariela Rivera, David Tsibadze, Nino Gakhokidze, Nino Zavrashvili, Matthew J. Ritter and Grace M. Arteaga

Chapter 4 **Perinatal Palliative Care Birth Planning as Advance Care Planning** 26
Donna Maria E. Cortezzo, Kelstan Ellis and Amy Schlegel

Chapter 5 **Fostering Vicarious Resilience for Perinatal Palliative Care Professionals** 35
Kathryn R. Grauerholz, Michaelene Fredenburg, Premala Tara Jones and Kristy N. Jenkins

Chapter 6 **Development of a Perinatal Palliative Care Model at a Level II Perinatal Center Supported by a Pediatric Palliative Care Network** 50
Marco Bolognani, Paola Daniela Morelli, Isabella Scolari, Cristina Dolci, Valentina Fiorito, Francesca Uez, Silvia Graziani, Barbara Stefani, Francesca Zeni, Gino Gobber, Elena Bravi, Saverio Tateo and Massimo Soffiati

Chapter 7 **Challenges and Priorities for Pediatric Critical Care Clinician-Researchers in Low- and Middle-Income Countries** 55
Amelie O. von Saint André-von Arnim, Jonah Attebery, Teresa Bleakly Kortz, Niranjan Kissoon, Elizabeth M. Molyneux, Ndidiamaka L. Musa, Katie R. Nielsen and Ericka L. Fink

Chapter 8 **Moral Distress in the Neonatal Intensive Care Unit: What is it, Why it Happens and How we can Address it** 61
Manisha Mills and Donna Maria E. Cortezzo

Chapter 9 **Assessment of Healthcare Professionals' Self-Perceived Competence in Perinatal/Neonatal Palliative Care After a 3-Day Training Course** 71
Jennifer Hammond, Charlotte Wool and Elvira Parravicini

Chapter 10 **"Percorso Giacomo": An Italian Innovative Service of Perinatal Palliative Care** 78
Chiara Locatelli, Luigi Corvaglia, Giuliana Simonazzi, Maria Bisulli, Lucia Paolini and Giacomo Faldella

Chapter 11 **Advances in Pediatric Critical Care Research in India** 84
Utpal Bhalala, Arun Bansal and Krishan Chugh

Chapter 12 **Teaching the Principles of Pediatric Critical Care to Non-Intensivists in Resource Limited Settings: Challenges and Opportunities** 91
Michael F. Canarie and Asha N. Shenoi

Chapter 13 **The Potential Harm of Cytomegalovirus Infection in Immunocompetent Critically Ill Children** 96
Raidan Alyazidi, Srinivas Murthy, Jennifer A. Slyker and Soren Gantt

Chapter 14 **Clinical Presentation and Outcomes among Children with Sepsis Presenting to a Public Tertiary Hospital in Tanzania** 104
Teresa Bleakly Kortz, Hendry R. Sawe, Brittany Murray, Wayne Enanoria, Michael Anthony Matthay and Teri Reynolds

Chapter 15 **Pediatric Critical Care in Resource-Limited Settings—Overview and Lessons Learned** 113
Tina M. Slusher, Andrew W. Kiragu, Louise T. Day, Ashley R. Bjorklund, Arianna Shirk, Colleen Johannsen and Scott A. Hagen

Chapter 16 **Decisions Parents Make when Faced with Potentially Life-Limiting Fetal Diagnoses and the Importance of Perinatal Palliative Care** 119
Krishelle L. Marc-Aurele

Chapter 17 **Pediatric Critical Care Medicine Training in india: Past, Present and Future** 124
Utpal Bhalala and Praveen Khilnani

Chapter 18 **A Review of the Integrated Model of Care: An Opportunity to Respond to Extensive Palliative Care Needs in Pediatric Intensive Care Units in Under-Resourced Settings** 128
Michelle Grunauer and Caley Mikesell

Chapter 19 **Successful Deployment of High Flow Nasal Cannula in a Peruvian Pediatric Intensive Care Unit Using Implementation Science—Lessons Learned** 137
Katie R. Nielsen, Rosario Becerra, Gabriela Mallma and José Tantaleán da Fieno

Chapter 20 **Pediatric Trauma Care in Low Resource Settings: Challenges, Opportunities and Solutions** 143
Andrew W. Kiragu, Stephen J. Dunlop, Njoki Mwarumba, Sanusi Gidado, Adesope Adesina, Michael Mwachiro, Daniel A. Gbadero and Tina M. Slusher

Chapter 21 **Neonatal End-of-Life Symptom Management** 157
Donna Maria E. Cortezzo and Mark Meyer

Chapter 22 **A Standardized Needs Assessment Tool to Inform the Curriculum Development Process for Pediatric Resuscitation Simulation-Based Education in Resource-Limited Settings** 169
Nicole Shilkofski, Amanda Crichlow, Julie Rice, Leslie Cope, Ye Myint Kyaw, Thazin Mon, Sarah Kiguli and Julianna Jung

Chapter 23 **Considerations for Assessing the Appropriateness of High-Cost Pediatric Care in Low-Income Regions** 180
Andrew C. Argent

Chapter 24 **Clinical and Pathological Correlation in Pediatric Invasive Pulmonary Aspergillosis** 190
Nattachai Anantasit, Noramon Nuntacharruksa, Pimpin Incharoen and Aroonwan Preutthipan

Chapter 25 **Barriers to Perinatal Palliative Care Consultation** 196
Franca Benini, Sabrina Congedi, Francesca Rusalen, Maria Elena Cavicchiolo and Paola Lago

Chapter 26 **The Neonatal Comfort Care Program: Origin and Growth Over 10 Years** 201
Charlotte Wool and Elvira Parravicini

Chapter 27 **Summary of the Key Concepts on How to Develop a Perinatal Palliative Care Program** 209
Paola Lago, Maria Elena Cavicchiolo, Francesca Rusalen and Franca Benini

Chapter 28 **Bibliometric Analysis of Global Research on Perinatal Palliative Care** 218
Yiting Wang, Chunjian Shan, Yingying Tian, Congshan Pu and Zhu Zhu

Chapter 29 **aEEG Use in Pediatric Critical Care—An Online Survey** 227
Nora Bruns, Ursula Felderhoff Müser, Christian Dohna-Schwake, Joachim Woelfle and Hanna Müller

Permissions

List of Contributors

Index

Preface

This book has been an outcome of determined endeavour from a group of educationists in the field. The primary objective was to involve a broad spectrum of professionals from diverse cultural background involved in the field for developing new researches. The book not only targets students but also scholars pursuing higher research for further enhancement of the theoretical and practical applications of the subject.

Pediatrics and neonatal care refers to a type of medical specialty that cares for newborn infants, premature babies, young children and teenagers. It focuses on various fields including pulmonary rehabilitation, child obesity, pediatrics sinusitis, pediatric endocrinology, childhood asthma, and pediatric oncology. It also deals with innate immunity, inborn errors, protein misfolding disorder and interventional cardiac catheterization. Pediatric care provides medical therapy for children who are chronically or acutely ill, and delivers preventative health care for children who are otherwise healthy. The provision of neonatal intensive care has improved the outcomes of high-risk newborns, who were born prematurely, or with severe surgical or medical issues. It encompasses the care of infants who are ill or require specific medical attention because of medical conditions such as intrauterine growth restriction, sepsis, preterm conditions, congenital anomalies, low birth weight, birth asphyxia or pulmonary hypoplasia. This book explores all the important aspects of pediatric and neonatal care in the present day scenario. It contains researches and studies performed by experts across the globe. This book is appropriate for students seeking detailed information in this area as well as for experts.

It was an honour to edit such a profound book and also a challenging task to compile and examine all the relevant data for accuracy and originality. I wish to acknowledge the efforts of the contributors for submitting such brilliant and diverse chapters in the field and for endlessly working for the completion of the book. Last, but not the least; I thank my family for being a constant source of support in all my research endeavours.

Editor

1

End-of-Life Care for Neonates: Assessing and Addressing Pain and Distressing Symptoms

Shelly Haug[1*], Alicia Dye[2] and Sara Durrani[3]

[1] Department of Neonatology, Eastern Idaho Regional Medical Center, Pediatrix Medical Group, Idaho Falls, ID, United States, [2] Department of Pharmacy, Eastern Idaho Regional Medical Center, Idaho Falls, ID, United States, [3] Department of Neonatology, Beth Israel Deaconess Medical Center, Boston, MA, United States

***Correspondence:**
Shelly Haug
haugshelly@gmail.com

One of the most essential components of end-of-life (EOL) care for neonates is assessing and addressing distressing symptoms. There is limited evidence to guide neonatal EOL symptom management and therefore significant variety in treatment (1–4). EOL neonatal palliative care should include identifying and relieving distressing symptoms. Symptoms to manage at neonatal EOL may include pain using both non-pharmacologic and pharmacologic comfort measures, respiratory distress, secretions, agitation and neurologic symptoms, nutrition and gastrointestinal distress, and skin care. Also of equal importance is communication surrounding familial existential distress and psychosocial care (1, 5–7). Institutions should implement a guideline for neonatal EOL care as guidelines have been shown to decrease variability of interventions and increase use of pharmacologic symptom management (4). Providers should consult with palliative care teams if available for added multidisciplinary support for family and staff, which has been shown to enhance EOL care in neonates (8, 9).

Keywords: neonatal, end-of-life care, neonatal hospice, neonatal palliative care, neonatal pain

INTRODUCTION

Neonatal end-of-life (EOL) care includes addressing pain and other distressing symptoms (1, 7, 10, 11). Neonatal intensive care units (NICUs) are generally competent in EOL care of neonates; however, evidence shows there are wide variations in methods for evaluating and addressing symptoms (1, 12). This variation likely stems from limited evidence regarding neonatal EOL symptom management given the lack of on-label neonatal pharmacologic treatments (5, 10). A 2016 survey showed only 55% of NICUs in the United States have a neonatal EOL guideline, and 45% do not have access to a palliative care team, showing there is much room for improvement regarding neonatal EOL care (1). This review aims to incorporate scientific research evidence with clinical expertise to aid in assessing and addressing neonatal EOL symptoms.

Vignette

A 25-week gestation 5-day-old neonate with severe grade 4 bilateral intraventricular hemorrhage and acute pulmonary hemorrhage is currently intubated on high frequency oscillator ventilation. Parents have decided to transition to EOL comfort care. The bedside nurse is concerned regarding increased facial grimacing of the neonate and asks which pain scale to use.

ASSESSMENT OF PAIN IN NEONATES

The most common symptom related to pediatric EOL care is pain, which is often underestimated in neonates (13–15). In comparison to adults, neonates experience pain that is more severe, diffuse, and prolonged (16). Several different pain assessment tools are validated for neonates; however, one has not been found superior over the others (5, 16, 17). These assessment tools do not evaluate for distress from other etiologies such as hunger, and interpretation must be completed in proper clinical context (5).

Pain should be evaluated every 15 min upon initial discovery. Once controlled, we recommend evaluation of pain at least every 3 h. The scale chosen should be part of your institutional guidelines. Your chosen assessment scale should be used consistently, as scenarios allow, and chosen with input from your nursing staff. Assessment scales to consider include but are not limited to the following.

Acute neonatal pain scales to consider:

- Behavioral Indicators of Infant Pain (BIIP) evaluates pain using behavioral state, facial expressions, and hand movements. Validated since 2007 for acute pain in preterm infants 23- to 32-weeks gestation (18).
- Premature Infant Pain Profile (PIPP) uses gestational age, behavior, heart rate, oxygen saturation, brow bulge, eye squeeze, and nasolabial furrow. Validated since 1996 for acute and postoperative neonatal pain (19).

Prolonged neonatal pain scales to consider:

- COMFORTneo Scale uses alertness, calmness, respiratory response, crying, body movement, facial tension, and body muscle tone. It was validated in 2009 for prolonged neonatal pain (20).
- EDIN Scale (Echelle Douler Inconfort Nouveau Né) evaluates facial activity, body movements, quality of sleep, quality of contact with nurses, and consolability. Validated in 2001 for prolonged pain specifically in preterm neonates (21).
- NPASS (Neonatal Pain, Agitation, and Sedation Scale) looks at crying, behavior, facial expression, tone, and vital signs. Validated in 2008 for prolonged postoperative pain as well as pain with mechanical ventilation. It is validated for use down to 23-weeks gestation (22).

Vignette Discussion

Does your unit have a consistent acute pain scale used at EOL? We recommend BIIP, PIPP, or NPASS scale here given the relatively acute nature, prematurity, and use of mechanical ventilation. No one scale has been found superior, though certain scales are validated for particular scenarios such as prolonged pain or gestation.

NON-PHARMACOLOGICAL COMFORT MEASURES

Critically ill neonates frequently undergo painful interventions (16, 23). Care should be given to decrease noxious stimuli. Regularly scheduled procedures, such as bath time, can often be held or deferred; orders for obtaining vitals less often can decrease noxious stimuli (24).

Non-pharmacological neonatal comfort measures include swaddling, facilitated tucking, kangaroo care/skin-to-skin care, non-nutritive sucking with or without oral sucrose, and breastfeeding (16, 25, 26). Each of these methods has been shown to increase comfort or decrease oxidative stress markers of neonates in situations of acute pain. In fact, combining measures enhances comfort over using a single method alone (5, 27).

PHARMACOLOGICAL MANAGEMENT

Non-opioid mediations are recommended for mild pain, while opioid medications with or without adjuvant therapies are used for moderate to severe pain (16, 24). Efficacious administration routes include enteral, intravenous (IV), mucosal (buccal, lingual, or rectal), intranasal, transdermal, and subcutaneous depending on the agent. Agents may need to be combined for optimal comfort (5, 16). See **Table 1** for initial dosing guidelines and **Figure 1** for a general guide to stepwise approach for providers.

The principle of "Double Effect" is an important consideration for clinicians concerned about the use of pharmacologic agents for EOL care. The principle asserts it is morally permissible to unintentionally cause harm as a side effect if the original overarching intent is to bring about a good effect. Extrapolating this principle to EOL care explains the use of medications that might potentially cause respiratory depression given the intent is to relieve pain and suffering (28, 29).

Non-opioid Medications

Sucrose is effective in reduction of pain behavior during acute procedures and noted to have increased efficacy when used in combination with nonnutritive sucking (5, 16, 30).

Although acetaminophen does not show analgesic effectiveness for reducing effects of painful procedures in neonates, it does show an opioid sparing effect (31, 32). Acetaminophen should only be used to treat mild pain or as an opioid sparing agent. Side effects include liver toxicity, although this is less common in neonates than older children (33).

Literature examining nonsteroidal anti-inflammatory agents such as ibuprofen, ketorolac, or indomethacin for neonatal EOL care is lacking and therefore not generally recommended.

Opioids

Opioids should be first-line therapy in management of neonates with moderate to severe pain. Route of administration should take into consideration onset of action, duration of action, and most efficacious route for desired opioid.

Morphine has been shown to be less effectively absorbed when used mucosally due to less lipophilicity than other opioids like fentanyl (34, 35). Side effects include urinary retention, decreased gastrointestinal motility, nausea, vomiting, hypotension, and respiratory depression. Respiratory depression is always preceded by sedation (16, 36).

Benefits of fentanyl include fast onset of action and efficacy of intranasal administration due to high lipophilicity (16, 34).

TABLE 1 | Neonatal pharmacologic agents for end-of-life palliative care with initial doses*.

	Enteral or Mucosal	Intravenous	Other
NON-OPIOIDS			
Sucrose	Buccal/Lingual: 0.1–1 mL/dose every 2 min		
Acetaminophen	PO: 10–15 mg/kg every 6–8 h PR: 15–20 mg/kg every 6–8 h	7.5–15 mg/kg every 6–8 h	
OPIOIDS			
Morphine	PO/PR/Buccal: 0.1–0.2 mg/kg every 3–6 h	Bolus: 0.05–0.1mg/kg every 2–4 h Continuous: 0.01–0.1 mg/kg/h	SC: 0.1–0.2 mg/kg every 3–6 h
Fentanyl	Buccal: 1–2 mcg/kg every 1–4 h	Bolus: 1–3 mcg/kg every 5–15 min Continuous: 0.5–5 mcg/kg/h	Intranasal: 1–2 mcg/kg every 1–4 h
ADJUVANTS			
Midazolam	PO/Lingual/PR: 0.2 mg/kg every 2–4 h	Bolus: 0.05–0.1 mg/kg every 2–4 h Continuous: 0.03–0.06 mg/kg/h Maximum Continuous: 0.3–0.5 mg/kg/h**	Intranasal: 0.1–0.3 mg/kg every 2–4 h
Lorazepam	PO/PR/Buccal: 0.05–0.1 mg/kg every 6–8 h	Continuous: 0.05–0.1 mg kg every 6–8 h	
Dexmedetomidine		Bolus: 0.5–1 mcg/kg/h Continuous: 0.3–1 mcg/kg/h	
Clonidine	PO: 2–4 mcg/kg every 4–6 h	***	
Phenobarbital	PO/PR: 5 mg/kg every 24 h	Bolus: 5 mg/kg every 24 h	

IV, intravenous; PO, by mouth; PR, rectal; SC, subcutaneous.
**Table lists suggested doses, recommend titrating as required for symptom management.*
***Maximum sedation EOL dosing, also with anticonvulsant activity at this level which may allow other anticonvulsants to be discontinued.*
****No IV formulation available, see dexmedetomidine IV.*

Fentanyl also does not cause histamine release; therefore, it has decreased vasomotor center activity causing less hypotension than morphine. It also has a shorter duration of action than morphine. A notable adverse effect is chest wall rigidity, especially with higher doses and rapid IV administration (16).

Benzodiazepines

Benzodiazepines potentiate inhibitory GABA (gamma-aminobutryric acid) neuronal activity of the central nervous system (37). They are potent sedative and anxiolytic medications without analgesic effect, which can decrease need for opioids (16). Midazolam has rapid onset as well as short duration of action, enabling ease of titration (5). Lorazepam has an intermediate onset of action but with longer duration of action facilitating baseline sedation needs (37). Side effects include myoclonic jerking and hypotension (16).

Alpha 2-adrenoreceptor Agonists

Dexmedetomidine and clonidine are alpha2-adrenoreceptor agonists that have sympatholytic, sedative, and analgesic effects. In contrast to opioids, they do not have significant ventilatory effects. The most notable side effects include bradycardia and hypotension (5, 16).

Alternative Sedation Medications

Phenobarbital is a barbiturate that can be an adjunct medication for palliative sedation (38–40). It has sedative and anxiolytic effects without analgesia via its inhibition of the central nervous system through augmenting the GABA system. The preferred route in this context is oral due to slow absorption causing less severe side effects (5). Dosage when used as an adjunct sedative is much less than for seizure control in neonates (see **Table 1**). Clinicians should use caution if combining with opioids or benzodiazepines as this may increase the risk of respiratory depression. Pentobarbital is another barbiturate with shorter half-life than phenobarbital but is not well studied in end-of-life care for neonates (16).

NMDA-Receptor Antagonist

Ketamine is an N-methyl-D-aspartate (NMDA)-receptor antagonist used to decrease central sensitization to painful stimuli and perception of pain. Ketamine has proven effective in neonates for peri-procedural sedation and analgesia with a short duration of action. It should only be used in combination with a sedative medication due to hallucination risk. Adjunct dose to consider is 0.5–2 mg/kg/dose intravenous although use at end of life is not well-studied (16, 41).

Vignette Discussion

What comfort medications you consider depend on distressing symptomatology for infant and family. Is the neonate already on an opioid drip for painful chest tubes, ventilator, or recent surgical procedure? At times you may only need titration for improved effect. In other cases, your main distressing symptom may be respiratory distress or secretion management without any pain issues. See ***Figure 1****.*

RESPIRATORY SYMPTOM MANAGEMENT

Respiratory Distress

EOL respiratory distress may manifest as retractions, tachypnea, grunting, nasal flaring, or gasping. Non-pharmacologic treatment interventions may include positioning modifications such as elevating the head of the bed and positioning side-lying or prone. Use of a fan with air movement toward the patient's face has been shown to relieve dyspnea symptoms in adult hospice

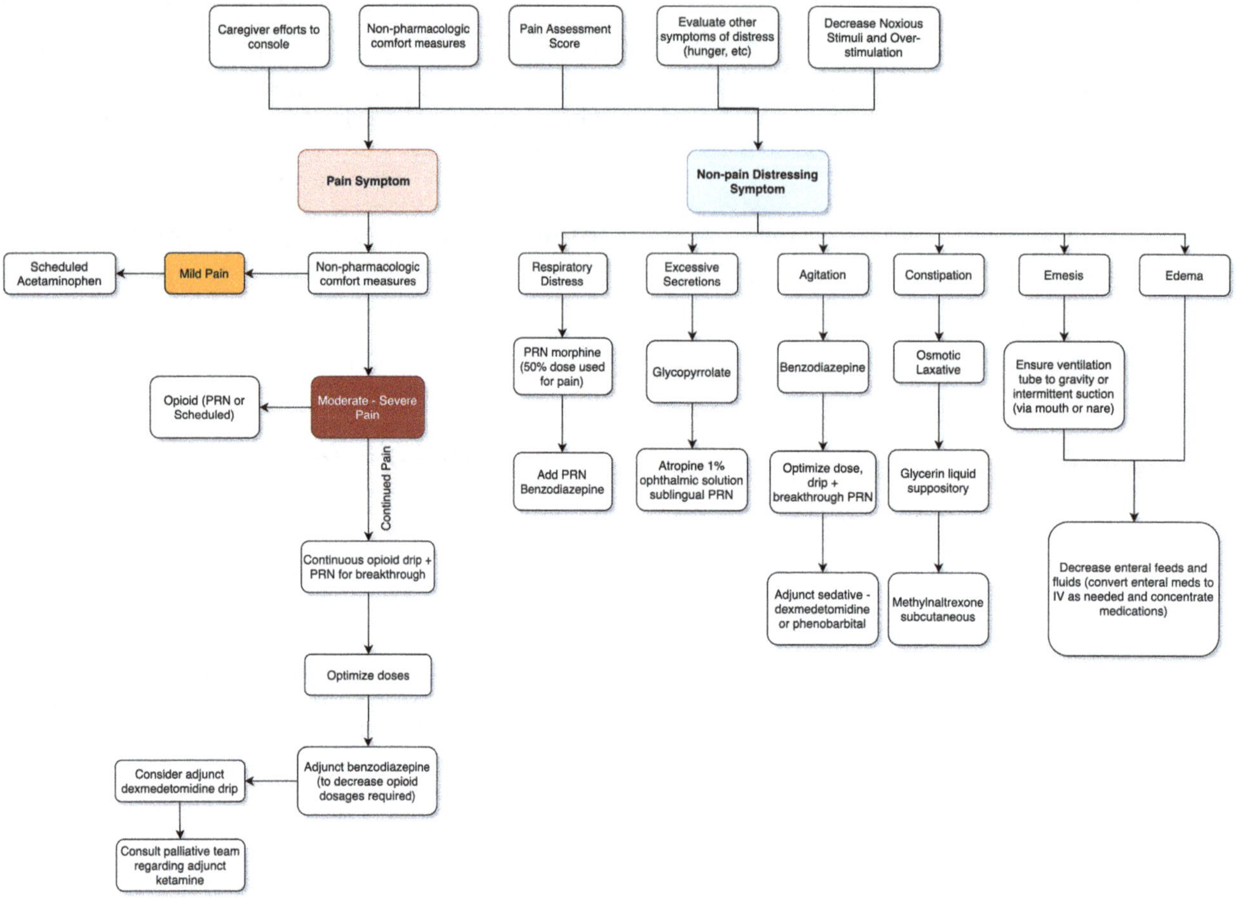

FIGURE 1 | Neonatal EOL Symptom Algorithm.

patients (42). Use of oxygen is not beneficial for respiratory distress for most patients at EOL (43, 44).

Pharmacologic management options include opioids, which can reduce central sensitivity to hypoxia and hypercapnia (45). Morphine is commonly used in neonates and is usually effective at 50% of the dose used for pain (see **Table 1**). Use of an opioid with a benzodiazepine has been shown to significantly reduce respiratory EOL symptomatology (16, 45).

Excessive Secretions

Inability to swallow saliva may lead to pooling in the posterior pharynx and noisy breathing. Anticipatory guidance with the family should be based around treating only if symptoms becomes distressing to the neonate. Least invasive non-pharmacologic treatment would first include decreasing or discontinuing hydrating fluids in an effort to decrease secretion production, positioning the infant to allow gravity to drain secretions (i.e., side-lying or prone), and gentle shallow oral suctioning with soft catheter as needed (46).

Atropine 1% ophthalmic solution may be given sublingually 1–2 drops every 1–6 h as needed (5, 16, 45, 47). Atropine inhibits local salivation via anticholinergic activity. Atropine sublingual drops have shown reasonable effect in reduction of terminal respiratory secretions while not showing cardiac or central nervous system symptoms, though most evidence is adult based at this time (48).

Glycopyrrolate is an anticholinergic that reduces gastric, pharyngeal, tracheal, and bronchial secretions. Dosing PO is 20–100 mcg/kg/dose every 4–8 h as needed. Dosing IV or subcutaneous is 2–10 mcg/kg/dose every 4–8 h as needed. If pharmacologic intervention is needed, glycopyrrolate is generally the preferred pediatric anticholinergic option as it does not cross the blood-brain barrier, so it rarely has central side effects (49). Side effects include mucous plugging due to thickened secretions.

Scopolamine transdermal patches show no increased effectiveness in secretion management and are usually avoided in neonates due to risk of central side effects from crossing the blood brain barrier (50).

Compassionate Extubation

Clinicians must be cautious in the setting of compassionate extubation or discontinuation of respiratory support in neonates. Experts in neonatal EOL care recommend initiating opioids with or without synergistic benzodiazepine and then a slow wean of ventilator settings while monitoring for development of respiratory distress. This allows for titration of medication for symptoms prior to extubation. Parents should be involved with the non-pharmacologic comfort role if able, including holding, swaddling, rocking, and positioning for secretions. Anticipatory guidance should be given to parents in monitoring for pain and respiratory symptoms. Anticipation and prevention of pain, agitation, and dyspnea symptoms is paramount to decrease familial and neonatal discomfort (5, 16).

AGITATION AND NEUROLOGIC SYMPTOM MANAGEMENT

There are multiple etiologies for agitation during EOL care for neonates, which may include brain injury, malformations, seizures, or iatrogenic neonatal abstinence syndrome due to long-term drug exposure from hospitalization. Non-pharmacologic interventions should not be employed first in neurologic scenarios such as seizures.

Pharmacologic interventions for agitation include benzodiazepines as well as opioids as they have a synergistic sedation effect. Barbiturates may also be considered (29). See **Table 1** for agitation medication recommendations. It is important to balance over-sedation and lethargy with desired control of symptoms. Seizure control should include phenobarbital 20 mg/kg/dose up to 40 mg/kg/load IV. Medical consultation with your pediatric neurologist can guide further anticonvulsant recommendations.

NUTRITION AND GASTROINTESTINAL DISTRESS SYMPTOM MANAGEMENT

Nutrition

An important component of neonatal end-of-life care is addressing artificial hydration and nutrition as well as natural hydration/nutrition. There is no reason to preclude breastfeeding or bottle feeding as part of comfort during EOL care if the neonate orally feeds and doing so does not exacerbate distress.

However, discussions around withdrawal of artificial hydration and nutrition present a challenge in neonatal EOL care. Culturally, many parents attach meaning and symbolism of caring for their neonate with nutrition. Using clear language during discussions is of utmost importance (16). Receiving artificial hydration and nutrition may not be in the best interest at EOL as it may worsen symptomatology through fluid overload, respiratory distress, increased abdominal distention, and discomfort or nausea and vomiting (5). Addressing subsequent side effects of dehydration is also important, for example, oral hygiene (see Mouth Care section below) (16).

Constipation

Opioid induced constipation is multifactorial including decreased gastrointestinal motility, inhibition of mucosal transport of electrolytes and fluids, as well as interference with the defecation reflex (16). The risk of opioid-induced constipation increases with duration of opioid therapy. Laxative treatment such as polyethylene glycol is considered first-line with neonatal doses of 0.2–0.8 g/kg/day (51–53). Liquid glycerin suppository 0.2 mL per rectum may be given in addition to scheduled osmotic laxative.

A last resort treatment consideration is methylnaltrexone for reversal of some opioid side effects without precipitating withdrawal. Methylnaltrexone is a peripheral acting mu-opioid receptor antagonist that has emerging data in neonates. Neonatal dosing used is 0.15 mg/kg subcutaneous once daily until bowel movement occurs (54, 55).

SKIN, EYE, AND MOUTH CARE

Physiological changes during EOL may compromise the skin and soft tissues manifesting as changes in skin (color, elasticity, or integrity) or as subjective symptoms such as pain or itching (56). Areas of decreased cutaneous perfusion may exhibit as dusky erythema, mottled discoloration, or areas of localized cooling. Care should include skin assessments and prevention of excessive pressure, friction, moisture, and immobilization during EOL care. Clinicians should monitor for incomplete eyelid closure as this increases risk of exposure keratopathy, which might cause ophthalmic pain and sensitivity (57). Care of mouth xerostomia should also be part of EOL assessment care.

Evidence based treatments for neonatal EOL skin care are lacking; however, pediatric studies show topical emollients may aid in reduction of cutaneous dryness (58). If incomplete eyelid closure is noted, artificial tear ointments have shown to be helpful in multiple intensive care settings (59). Moist sterile water swabs work well for neonatal xerostomia care (60, 61). Topical petroleum jelly to dry lips may be helpful as well (60). Parental involvement in symptom assessment has been shown to be a predictor of quality EOL symptom treatment (62). If counseled appropriately, these skin, eye, and mouth changes can easily be assessed by parents and treated as needed (63).

FAMILIAL EXISTENTIAL DISTRESS AND PSYCHOSOCIAL CARE

Providers should be mindful of the propensity for family members to feel enormous guilt and question their decisions. Many families will be in existential crisis and openly question why this is happening. This part of the grief process should be normalized. Some parents may need reassurance that they are in fact a good advocate for their baby while also being present for their neonate's EOL (11).

Some families have moral distress in believing that withdrawing technological support is not permissible in their cultural or religious customs. Reframing discussions in a way that the family does not have to decide anything may be helpful. For example, the physician may say something like "Additional technological support is inappropriate and will increase the infant's suffering. I recommend we increase the palliative care services and work intensively now to support comfort for your infant" (11).

Helpful discussions for family may include openly asking about religious rituals such as baptism that may be important for closure. Consultations to pastoral care or clergy that align with their religious preference may be of comfort during EOL transition. Consider involvement of social work, child life, and palliative medicine if available at your hospital and circumstances allow. Developing a unit checklist for bedside nurses may aid families in obtaining memories with mementos such as a lock of hair, hospital name bands, crib cards, and photographs (10, 11). Families should also be given bereavement and counselor contact information for the area to aid the grief and healing process after perinatal loss (10, 64, 65).

Anticipatory guidance is an important part of the bereavement process for women who are lactating. Consider consulting your lactation specialist. Helpful methods of care may include the use of medications such as estrogen containing birth control pills, a process of decreasing frequency of milk expression without completely emptying the breast, or milk donation for a time (66, 67).

INSTITUTIONAL NEONATAL EOL CARE GUIDELINES

Most institutions across the United States do not formally address neonatal EOL care in a guideline format (1). However, implementation of clinically practical guidelines increases consistency in patient care as well as education and comfort of staff/trainees (4, 38, 68, 69). Neonatal EOL guidelines should be individualized by institution and case to case as necessary.

DISCUSSION

One of the most difficult parts of neonatal EOL care includes discussion with family. Acknowledgment should be a tool we use with our families, staff, and ourselves. Acknowledge that EOL is sometimes unfair and difficult, and unimaginable even. Acknowledge it is natural to want to lessen the blow of information you have to discuss as the provider, despite research showing this does not help (70). Acknowledge the difficulty of family needing to digest what you discuss. Share with the family how much you wish the situation were different. Speak information as clearly and succinctly as possible. Answer questions, attempt to anticipate questions, and normalize their concerns (71).

EOL care is a multifaceted approach including identifying and treating EOL symptoms while also addressing familial existential distress and psychosocial care (1, 5–7). Implementation of a guideline for neonatal EOL care at your institution can aid in improved EOL processes (4). Consulting with neonatal palliative care teams, if available, can add important multidisciplinary support that enhances neonatal EOL care (8, 9). Increasing neonatal EOL care palliative education with trainees, nursing staff, and colleagues at your institution can increase comfort and competence with EOL care (72). In all, EOL care is a sacred and deeply meaningful part of life around the world. By assessing and addressing symptoms as well as promoting a culture of respect surrounding familial or spiritual traditions, we can help families find closure with a dignified and peaceful neonatal EOL process (73).

AUTHOR CONTRIBUTIONS

SH collected and analyzed data as well as primarily wrote the manuscript. AD and SD critically reviewed and contributed to the final draft of the manuscript. All authors contributed to the article and approved the submitted version.

REFERENCES

1. Haug S, Farooqi S, Wilson CG, Hopper A, Oei G, Carter B. Survey on neonatal end-of-life comfort care guidelines across America. *J Pain Symptom Manage.* (2018) 55:979–84.e2. doi: 10.1016/j.jpainsymman.2017.10.023
2. Fortney CA, Steward DK. A qualitative study of nurse observations of symptoms in infants at end-of-life in the neonatal intensive care unit. *Intensive Crit Care Nurs.* (2017) 40:57–63. doi: 10.1016/j.iccn.2016.10.004
3. Williams C, Munson D, Zupancic J, Kirpalani H. Supporting bereaved parents: practical steps in providing compassionate perinatal and neonatal end-of-life care. A North American perspective. *Semin Fetal Neonatal Med.* (2008) 13:335–340. doi: 10.1016/j.siny.2008.03.005
4. Parravicini E. Neonatal palliative care. *Curr Opin Pediatr.* (2017) 29:135–40. doi: 10.1097/MOP.0000000000000464
5. Garten L, Bührer C. Pain and distress management in palliative neonatal care. *Semin Fetal Neonatal Med.* (2019) 24:101008. doi: 10.1016/j.siny.2019.04.008
6. Shultz EL, Switala M, Winning AM, Keim MC, Baughcum AE, Gerhardt CA, et al. Multiple perspectives of symptoms and suffering at end of life in the NICU. *Adv Neonatal Care.* (2017) 17:175–83. doi: 10.1097/ANC.0000000000000385
7. Carter BS, Hubble C, Weise KL. Palliative medicine in neonatal and pediatric intensive care. *Child Adolesc Psychiatr Clin N Am.* (2006) 15:759–77. doi: 10.1016/j.chc.2006.02.008
8. Pierucci RL, Kirby RS, Leuthner SR. End-of-life care for neonates and infants: the experience and effects of a palliative care consultation service. *Pediatrics.* (2001) 108:653–60. doi: 10.1542/peds.108.3.653
9. Acheson-Silver MJ, Brandt K. The development and implementation of a multidisciplinary perinatal/neonatal palliative care program. *Pediatrics.* (2019) 144:452. doi: 10.1542/peds.2019-3146
10. Carter BS. Comfort care principles for the high-risk newborn. *NeoReviews.* (2004) 5:e484–e90. doi: 10.1542/neo.5-11-e484
11. Catlin A, Carter B. Creation of a neonatal end-of-life palliative care protocol. *Neonatal Netw.* (2002) 21:37–49. doi: 10.1891/0730-0832.21.4.37
12. Soni R, Vasudevan C, English S. National survey on neonatal palliative care in the UK. *Arch Dis Child Fetal Neonatal Ed.* (2011) 96:Fa18. doi: 10.1136/archdischild.2011.300164.7
13. Slater R, Cantarella A, Gallella S, Worley A, Boyd S, Meek J, et al. Cortical pain responses in human infants. *J Neurosci.* (2006) 26:3662–6. doi: 10.1523/JNEUROSCI.0348-06.2006
14. Vinall J, Grunau RE. Impact of repeated procedural pain-related stress in infants born very preterm. *Pediatr Res.* (2014) 75:584–7. doi: 10.1038/pr.2014.16
15. Friedrichsdorf SJ, Collins JJ. Management of non-pain symptoms in pediatric palliative care. *Med Principles Pract.* (2007) 16:3–9. doi: 10.1159/000104540
16. McGrath JM, Wool C, Black BP, Leuthner SR, Jones EL, Muñoz-Blanco S, et al. Chapter 15. Attending to pain and suffering in palliative care. In: Limbo R, Wool C, Carter B, editors. *Handbook of Perinatal and Neonatal Palliative Care, 1st ed.* New York, NY: Springer Publishing Company. (2020) 234–253.
17. Duhn LJ, Medves JM. A systematic integrative review of infant pain assessment tools. *Adv Neonatal Care.* (2004) 4:126–40. doi: 10.1016/j.adnc.2004.04.005

18. Holsti L, Grunau RE. Initial validation of the behavioral indicators of infant pain (BIIP). *PAIN.* (2007) 132:264–72. doi: 10.1016/j.pain.2007.01.033
19. Stevens B, Johnston C, Petryshen P, Taddio A. Premature infant pain profile: development and initial validation. *Clin J Pain.* (1996) 12:13–22. doi: 10.1097/00002508-199603000-00004
20. van Dijk M, Roofthooft DWE, Anand KJS, Guldemond F, de Graaf J, Simons S, et al. Taking up the challenge of measuring prolonged pain in (premature) neonates: the COMFORTneo scale seems promising. *Clin J Pain.* (2009) 25:607–16. doi: 10.1097/AJP.0b013e3181a5b52a
21. Debillon T, Zupan V, Ravault N, Magny J, Dehan M, ABU-SAAD H. Development and initial validation of the EDIN scale, a new tool for assessing prolonged pain in preterm infants. *Arch Dis Child Fetal Neonatal Ed.* (2001) 85:F36–F41. doi: 10.1136/fn.85.1.F36
22. Hummel P, Puchalski M, Creech SD, Weiss MG. Clinical reliability and validity of the N-PASS: neonatal pain, agitation and sedation scale with prolonged pain. *J Perinatol.* (2008) 28:55–60. doi: 10.1038/sj.jp.7211861
23. Carbajal R, Rousset A, Danan C, Coquery S, Nolent P, Ducrocq S, et al. Epidemiology and treatment of painful procedures in neonates in intensive care units. *JAMA.* (2008) 300:60–70. doi: 10.1001/jama.300.1.60
24. Weltgesundheitsorganisation ed. *WHO Guidelines on the Pharmacological Treatment of Persisting Pain in Children with Medical Illnesses.* Geneva: World Health Organization (2012).
25. Forde D, Deming DD, Tan JC, Phillips RM, Fry-Bowers EK, Barger MK, et al. *Oxidative Stress Biomarker Decreased in Preterm Neonates Treated With Kangaroo Mother Care.* Available online at: https://journals.sagepub.com/doi/abs/10.1177/1099800419900231 (accessed February 8, 2020).
26. Hartley K, Miller C, Gephart S. Facilitated tucking to reduce pain in neonates: evidence for best practice. *Adv Neonatal Care.* (2015) 15:201–8. doi: 10.1097/ANC.0000000000000193
27. Bellieni CV, Buonocore G, Nenci A, Franci N, Cordelli DM, Bagnoli F. Sensorial saturation: an effective analgesic tool for heel-prick in preterm infants. *NEO.* (2001) 80:15–8. doi: 10.1159/000047113
28. McIntyre A. Doctrine of double effect. In: Zalta EN, editor. *The Stanford Encyclopedia of Philosophy.*Metaphysics Research Lab, Stanford University. Available online at: https://plato.stanford.edu/archives/spr2019/entries/double-effect/ (accessed June 4, 2020).
29. UCSF Benihoff Children's Hospital. *End of Life Symptom Management Neonatal Intensive Care Unit.* Available online at: https://www.eastbaynewborn.com/docs/End%20of%20Life%20Symptom%20Management-NICU.pdf
30. Cignacco EL, Sellam G, Stoffel L, Gerull R, Nelle M, Anand KJS, et al. Oral sucrose and "facilitated tucking" for repeated pain relief in preterms: a randomized controlled trial. *Pediatrics.* (2012) 129:299–308. doi: 10.1542/peds.2011-1879
31. Littleimages. *Acetaminophen Analgesia in Neonatal Circumcision.* i2 Research Hub (1994) Available online at: https://www.i2researchhub.org/articles/acetaminophen-analgesia-in-neonatal-circumcision/ (accessed June 3, 2020).
32. Ohlsson A, Shah PS. Paracetamol (acetaminophen) for prevention or treatment of pain in newborns. *Cochrane Database Syst Rev.* (2016) 10:CD011219. doi: 10.1002/14651858.CD011219.pub3
33. Jacqz-Aigrain E, Anderson BJ. Pain control: non-steroidal anti-inflammatory agents. *Semin Fetal Neonatal Med.* (2006) 11:251–9. doi: 10.1016/j.siny.2006.02.009
34. Comparison of Fentanyl Oral and Nasal Formulations. Palliative Care Network of Wisconsin. Available online at: https://www.mypcnow.org/fast-fact/comparison-of-fentanyl-oral-and-nasal-formulations/ (accessed June 4, 2020).
35. Noble-Gresty J. Recent and upcoming approaches in the management of cancer breakthrough pain. *Rev Pain.* (2010) 4:2–7. doi: 10.1177/204946371000400202
36. McPherson ML. *Demystifying Opioid Conversion Calculations: A Guide for Effective Dosing, 2nd ed.* Bethesda, MD: ASHP Publications (2018).
37. Kearney TE. Chapter 167: Benzodiazepines (Diazepam, Lorazepam, Midazolam). In: ed. K. R. Olson KR, editor. *Poisoning & Drug Overdose.* New York, NY: The McGraw-Hill Companies. Available online at: accessmedicine.mhmedical.com/content.aspx?aid=55986890 (accessed June 4, 2020).
38. Carter BS, Bhatia J. Comfort/palliative care guidelines for neonatal practice: development and implementation in an academic medical center. *J Perinatol.* (2001) 21:279–83. doi: 10.1038/sj.jp.7210582
39. Setla J, Pasniciuc SV. Home palliative sedation using phenobarbital suppositories: time to death, patient characteristics, and administration protocol. *Am J Hosp Palliat Care.* (2019) 36:871–6. doi: 10.1177/1049909119839695
40. FrizzolaMeg PP, G M. Palliative sedation with oral medicines in an infant with generalized severe junctional epidermolysis bullosa. *J Palliat Med.* (2018) 21:1048–52. doi: 10.1089/jpm.2018.0054
41. Bhutta AT. Ketamine: a controversial drug for neonates. *Semin Perinatol.* (2007) 31:303–8. doi: 10.1053/j.semperi.2007.07.005
42. Kamal AH, Maguire JM, Wheeler JL, Currow DC, Abernethy AP. Dyspnea review for the palliative care professional: treatment goals and therapeutic options. *J Palliat Med.* (2012) 15:106–14. doi: 10.1089/jpm.2011.0110
43. Campbell ML, Yarandi H, Dove-Medows E. Oxygen is nonbeneficial for most patients who are near death. *J Pain Symptom Manage.* (2013) 45:517–23. doi: 10.1016/j.jpainsymman.2012.02.012
44. Davies JD. Noninvasive respiratory support at the end of life. *Respir Care.* (2019) 64:701–11. doi: 10.4187/respcare.06618
45. Basic Symptom Control in Paediatric Palliative Care. Together for Short Lives. Available online at: https://www.togetherforshortlives.org.uk/resource/basic-symptom-control-paediatric-palliative-care/ (accessed June 4, 2020).
46. Clary PL, Lawson P. Pharmacologic pearls for end-of-life care. *Am Fam Physician.* (2009) 79:1059–65.
47. Shinjo T, Okada M. Atropine eyedrops for death rattle in a terminal cancer patient. *J Palliat Med.* (2013) 16:212–3. doi: 10.1089/jpm.2011.0537
48. Protus BM, Grauer PA, Kimbrel JM. Evaluation of atropine 1% ophthalmic solution administered sublingually for the management of terminal respiratory secretions. *Am J Hosp Palliat Care.* (2013) 30:388–92. doi: 10.1177/1049909112453641
49. Kintzel PE, Chase SL, Thomas W, Vancamp DM, Clements EA. Anticholinergic medications for managing noisy respirations in adult hospice patients. *Am J Health Syst Pharm.* (2009) 66:458–64. doi: 10.2146/ajhp080194
50. Wildiers H, Dhaenekint C, Demeulenaere P, Clement PMJ, Desmet M, Van Nuffelen R, et al. Atropine, hyoscine butylbromide, or scopolamine are equally effective for the treatment of death rattle in terminal care. *J Pain Symptom Manage.* (2009) 38:124–33. doi: 10.1016/j.jpainsymman.2008.07.007
51. Opioid Induced Constipation - Part 1: Established Management. Palliative Care Network of Wisconsin. Available online at: https://www.mypcnow.org/fast-fact/opioid-induced-constipation-part-1-established-management/ (accessed June 4, 2020).
52. Michail S, Gendy E, Preud'Homme D, Mezoff A. Polyethylene glycol for constipation in children younger than eighteen months old. *J Pediatr Gastroenterol Nutr.* (2004) 39:197–9. doi: 10.1097/00005176-200408000-00014
53. Tabbers MM, DiLorenzo C, Berger MY, Faure C, Langendam MW, Nurko S, et al. Evaluation and treatment of functional constipation in infants and children: evidence-based recommendations from ESPGHAN and NASPGHAN. *J Pediatr Gastroenterol Nutr.* (2014) 58:265–81. doi: 10.1097/MPG.0000000000000266
54. Rodrigues A, Wong C, Mattiussi A, Alexander S, Lau E, Dupuis LL. Methylnaltrexone for opioid-induced constipation in pediatric oncology patients. *Pediatr Blood Cancer.* (2013) 60:1667–70. doi: 10.1002/pbc.24615
55. Garten L, Degenhardt P, Bührer C. Resolution of opioid-induced postoperative ileus in a newborn infant after methylnaltrexone. *J Pediatr Surg.* (2011) 46:e13–5. doi: 10.1016/j.jpedsurg.2010.10.015
56. Sibbald RG, Krasner DL, Lutz J. SCALE: skin changes at life's Endfinal consensus statement: October 1, 2009©. *Adv Skin Wound Care.* (2010) 23:225–36. doi: 10.1097/01.ASW.0000363537.75328.36
57. Lenart SB, Garrity JA. Eye care for patients receiving neuromuscular blocking agents or propofol during mechanical ventilation. *Am J Crit Care.* (2000) 9:188–91. doi: 10.4037/ajcc2000.9.3.188
58. Cowdell F, Jadotte YT, Ersser SJ, Danby S, Lawton S, Roberts A, et al. Hygiene and emollient interventions for maintaining skin integrity in older people in hospital and residential care settings. *Cochrane Database Syst Rev.* (2020) 1:CD011377. doi: 10.1002/14651858.CD011377.pub2

59. Rosenberg JB, Eisen LA. Eye care in the intensive care unit: narrative review and meta-analysis. *Crit Care Med.* (2008) 36:3151–3155. doi: 10.1097/CCM.0b013e31818f0ee7
60. Palliative Care and Oral Care. Center to Advance Palliative Care. Available online at: https://www.capc.org/seminar/poster-sessions/palliating-palate-making-oral-care-vital-sign/ (accessed March 4, 2020).
61. Hospice Hygiene. Registered Dental Hygienist (RDH) Magazine (2009) Available online at: https://www.rdhmag.com/patient-care/rinses-pastes/article/16404987/hospice-hygiene (accessed March 4, 2020).
62. Vollenbroich R, Borasio GD, Duroux A, Grasser M, Brandstätter M, Führer M. Listening to parents: the role of symptom perception in pediatric palliative home care. *Palliat Support Care.* (2016) 14:13–9. doi: 10.1017/S1478951515000462
63. Classen CF. Pediatric palliative care - the role of the patient's family. *World J Clin Pediatr.* (2012) 1:13–9. doi: 10.5409/wjcp.v1.i3.13
64. Romesberg TL. Understanding grief: a component of neonatal palliative care. *J Hospice Palliat Nurs.* (2004) 6:161–70. doi: 10.1097/00129191-200407000-00012
65. Romesberg TL. Building a case for neonatal palliative care. *Neonatal Netw.* (2007) 26:111–5. doi: 10.1891/0730-0832.26.2.111
66. Moore DB, Catlin A. Lactation suppression: forgotten aspect of care for the mother of a dying child. *Pediatr Nurs.* (2003) 29:383–4.
67. Cole M. Lactation after Perinatal, Neonatal, or Infant Loss. *Clin Lactation.* (2012) 3:94–100. doi: 10.1891/215805312807022897
68. Section on Hospice and Palliative Medicine and Committee on Hospital care. Pediatric Palliative Care and Hospice Care Commitments, Guidelines, and Recommendations. *Pediatrics.* (2013) 132:966–72. doi: 10.1542/peds.2013-2731
69. Camp MW, Barnes JR, Damany M, Donnan LT. Impact of web-based clinical practice guidelines on paediatric fracture clinics. *ANZ J Surg.* (2018) 88:232–5. doi: 10.1111/ans.14260
70. Devine M. *It's OK That You're Not OK: Meeting Grief and Loss in a Culture That Doesn't Understand.* Boulder, CO: Sounds True (2017).
71. Joachim G, Acorn S. Living with chronic illness: the interface of stigma and normalization. *Can J Nurs Res.* (2000) 32:37–48. doi: 10.1046/j.1365-2648.2000.01466.x
72. Wool C. Clinician confidence and comfort in providing perinatal palliative care. *J Obstet Gynecol Neonatal Nurs.* (2013) 42:48–58. doi: 10.1111/j.1552-6909.2012.01432.x
73. Doughty C. *From Here to Eternity: Traveling the World to Find the Good Death.* New York, NY: W. W. Norton (2017).

2

Perinatal Palliative Care: Cultural, Spiritual and Religious Considerations for Parents—What Clinicians Need to Know

*Victoria J. Kain**

Griffith Health, Griffith University, Southport, QLD, Australia

***Correspondence:**
Victoria J. Kain
v.kain@griffith.edu.au

For perinatal palliative care (PPC) to be truly holistic, it is imperative that clinicians are conversant in the cultural, spiritual and religious needs of parents. That cultural, spiritual and religious needs for parents should be sensitively attended to are widely touted in the PPC literature and extant protocols, however there is little guidance available to the clinician as to how to meet these needs. The objective of this review article is to report what is known about the cultural, spiritual and religious practices of parents and how this might impact neonates who are born with a life-limiting fetal diagnosis (LLFD). The following religions will be considered—Islam, Buddhism, Hinduism, Judaism, and Christianity—in terms of what may be helpful for clinicians to consider regarding rituals and doctrine related to PPC. Data Sources include PubMed, Ovid, PsycInfo, CINAHL, and Medline from Jan 2000–June 2020 using the terms "perinatal palliative care," "perinatal hospice," "cultur*," and "religiou*." Inclusion criteria includes all empirical and research studies published in English that focus on the cultural and religious needs of parents who opted to continue a pregnancy in which the fetus had a life-limiting condition or had received perinatal palliative care. Gray literature from religious leaders about the Great Religions were also considered. Results from these sources contributing to the knowledge base of cultural, spiritual and religious dimensions of perinatal palliative care are considered in this paper.

Keywords: perinatal palliative care, parents, religious needs, cultural needs, spiritual needs

INTRODUCTION

Perinatal palliative care (PPC) is a specialized branch of pediatric palliative care that considers an interdisciplinary strategy for the care of newborns with life-limiting or life-threatening conditions. The World Health Organization defines palliative care as the "primary goal for the provision of a good quality of life for those with life-threatening diseases." This expands to palliative care for children and infants as a specialized field that extends to the family of children and infants. The WHO has set up principles of palliative care for children, and it includes the following points: "(a) Complete care of the infant must be taken including mind, soul, and body; (b) Moral support to the family should be provided;

(c) Palliative care should start when the decision for not providing any more intensive care has been made; and (d) Care should be implemented even when resources are limited" (1).

For PPC to be truly holistic, it is imperative that clinicians must be conversant in the cultural, spiritual, and religious needs of parents. The need for cultural, spiritual, and religious considerations to be sensitively attended to is widely touted in the literature on PPC and extant protocols; however, there is little guidance available to the clinician on meeting these needs.

In recent times, most life-limiting fetal diagnoses (LLFD) are made during the prenatal period at a time that should represent hope and joy for parents and families. When faced with an LLFD, however, these hopes and dreams of a healthy child fade. It is at the margins of life and death that people consider the existential questions of life and their spirituality, and, at times, they may even question their religious beliefs. The death of their child will lead to maladaptive grief, long-term diminished quality of life, and symptoms linked to psychological morbidity if parents are unable to reconcile these very personal needs (2). Religious, cultural, and spiritual beliefs can bring profound comfort and healing for parents faced with an LLFD, and the majority of parents want the healthcare team to have the sensitivity and skills to discuss and tend to these needs (2).

While it is not possible for the clinician to be knowledgeable about all religious tenets and cultural norms encountered in practice, having the knowledge of the most common religions and how these religious tenets apply to infants with an LLFD or that are born at the margins of viability can assist parents greatly. Sadeghi et al. (3) identified that belief in the force of the supernatural, the need for comfort of the soul, and human dignity for the newborn were the important dimensions for parents of the infants who were not expected to survive (3).

The large variations in religious practice are known from the outset, and it is beyond the reach of this review to identify and accept all of these variations exhaustively. The objective of this review is to report on what is known about the cultural, spiritual, and religious practices of parents and how this might impact the neonates who are born with an LLFD. The following religions will be considered in terms of what may be helpful for clinicians to consider regarding rituals and doctrine related to PPC: Islam, Buddhism, Hinduism, Judaism, and Christianity.In addition, cultural and spiritual needs will be addressed.

MATERIALS AND METHODS

Data sources for this review included PubMed, Ovid, PsycInfo, CINAHL, and Medline. The data from January 2000 to August 2020 were collected using the terms "perinatal palliative care," "perinatal hospice," "cultur*," "spiritual*," and "religiou*." The inclusion criteria included all empirical and research studies published in English that focused on the cultural, spiritual, and religious needs of parents who opted to continue with their pregnancy, where the fetus had a life-limiting condition or had received PPC. Results from these studies contributing to the knowledge base of cultural and religious dimensions of PPC are considered in this review. **Table 1** provides details of the types of papers included and their level of evidence.

In addition to these published papers, sources discussing the principles of the Great Religions were also included to provide a background about religious doctrine, beliefs, and current global demographics.

DISCUSSION

Religious Considerations for Parents

We live in a multicultural, multi-faith world, where religion is seemingly more important than it has ever been, with four out of five people identifying as belonging to an organized faith (16). Christianity is the fastest growing religion, with Islam and Hinduism also experiencing global growth (16). Medicine, in particular, does not accept religious concepts and practices as part of the medical model (17); however, it is increasingly important in considering how faith intersects with the biomedical and psychosocial model of health. Having one's religious and spiritual beliefs recognized brings comfort and may also promote optimism, even when facing a complex prenatal diagnosis with uncertain outcomes (14).

Religion is somewhat simpler to define than spirituality. It considers beliefs, practices, and rituals and may also include beliefs about spirits, both good (angels) and bad (demons). Religion can be observed either publicly, as part of a community, or privately, and often as both (18). It is estimated that 78% of Americans have belief in God, with another 15% believing in a "higher power" or something "bigger than themselves." In terms of prayer, 84% of Americans believe that their chance of recovery is increased by the act of praying for the sick; 79% believe in the presence of "miracles"; and 72% perceive that God can cure incurable conditions (2). Having religious beliefs can assist people by bringing some order to life when events make life untenable with the offering of rituals, traditions, and guidance. Further, the concept of an "afterlife," or existential heaven, may bring great comfort to parents faced with an infant with an LLFD.

In a discussion paper, McGuirl and Campbell (12) claimed that knowledge of the most common religious beliefs is helpful for clinicians in having end-of-life conversations with parents who are making decisions for their children, including the decision on withholding and/or withdrawing from active involvement in interventions. However, there are also studies that associate religious beliefs with an increased propensity toward life-prolonging care that may prolong the suffering of infants with life-limiting conditions (2).

In the Southeast and East Asian community, religious and spiritual values may also directly affect the pregnancy decisions linked to genetics. Leung et al. (19) stated that while Chinese women in Hong Kong generally support the termination of pregnancy in the early stages for chromosomal defects and non-medical reasons, religious context is a major contributor to the negative attitudes toward termination. Notably, most women in the study also accepted that for an undesired fetal gender, termination should not be performed. Meanwhile, the health values of some strongly traditional Southeast Asian groups concentrate

TABLE 1 | A summary of reviewed studies.

Authors/year	Purpose	Method (study design, sample, and data collection)	Main findings	Level of evidence[1]
Ayed and Ayed (4)	To provide an overview of palliative care and challenges faced by the health care system during treatment of Muslim infants.	Debate paper based in a neonatal unit in Kuwait City.	The questions posed by medical advances related to fetal and newborn palliative care require a degree of interpretation and application of the Quran by authoritative teachers (Imams).	C
Boss et al. (5)	What categorizes parental decision-making regarding delivery room resuscitation in terms of "religion," "spirituality," and "hope."	Qualitative multicenter study; Parents of infants who had died as result of prematurity or congenital anomalies. Interviews and maternal medical charts.	Some parents felt that they had not made any decisions regarding resuscitation and instead "left things in God's hands." These parents typically were documented by staff members to "want everything done." Parents and physicians had different interpretations of what was discussed and what decisions were made.	B
Caulfield et al. (6)	To evaluate trends, outcomes and characteristics of newborn infants of Catholic parents baptized over a 15-year period in an Irish maternity hospital.	Retrospective study. Patients were identified from the "register of baptisms" from the years 2002–2016.	A gradual decline of emergency baptisms over the 15-year period was reported. Maternity hospitals and neonatal units need to have access to emergency baptism service or other equivalent "spiritual blessings" as appropriate to the faiths followed by the family in an emerging multi-faith population.	B
Chichester and Wool (7)	Explores feeding issues for infants who are not expected to survive across a variety of cultures and religions: Amish, Judaism, Hindu, Muslim, African American, Hispanic-Latino and Chinese American.	Discussion paper.	Customs, beliefs and religious laws and ceremonies often involve food and are deeply connected with events, such as birth and death.	C
Das (8)	Belief in reincarnation is widespread amongst Hindus. A newborn is not a new creation, or a by-product of its parents' chemistry—it is an eternal soul continuing its progression of lives within the material world in a new body.	Best-practice guidelines.	Palliative care welcomed for newborns not expected to survive, however Hindus are wary of any intervention that might hasten death or cause it artificially. The Hindu ideal is to remove all active treatments and allow death to come to the baby in its own time.	C
El Sayed et al. (9)	To explore the challenges for trainees when EOL decisions are undertaken and to encourage them to reflect on how they might influence decision-making.	In-depth, semi-structured interview guide developed to address trainees' physician beliefs, attitudes, preferences and expectations regarding discussions of EOL neonatal care.	Dealing with different cultures and an inability to interact effectively with people of different cultures was identified as a barrier.	B
Hawthorne et al. (10)	To examine differences in parents' use of spiritual and religious coping practices by gender, race/ethnicity, and religion at 1 and 3 months after infant/ICU death.	The Spiritual Coping Strategies Scale was used to measure religious and spiritual coping practices, separately. 165 bereaved parents, 78% minority.	Black non-Hispanic mothers used more religious coping practices at 3 months than White non-Hispanic mothers. Protestant and Catholic parents used more religious coping practices than the "no" and "other" religion groups at 1 and 3 months. Within the 30 mother–father dyads, mothers reported significantly greater use of religious coping practices at 1 and 3 months and spiritual coping practices at 3 months than fathers.	B
Kain (11)	To examine the notion of being born dying and karma for Buddhists and non-Buddhists (given that karma is a belief held by both).	Discussion paper.	Spirituality and culture go hand in hand for Buddhists, and Western medicine is beginning to acknowledge the importance of spirituality in healthcare. Spiritual care for dying infants and their families is an essential component of this type of care and is not only the domain of chaplaincy services but of the entire interdisciplinary team.	C

(Continued)

TABLE 1 | Continued

Authors/year	Purpose	Method (study design, sample, and data collection)	Main findings	Level of evidence[1]
McGuirl and Campbell (12)	To provide a foundation about prominent religions so that clinicians can better understand and assess the potential religious/ moral complexities that families face in the process of making treatment decisions for their infants, including decisions regarding withholding and/or withdrawing active intervention.	Discussion paper.	Knowledge of prominent religious beliefs can be helpful as clinicians enter end of life conversations with parents. Clinicians can use this information to better understand a family's perspectives and strongly held views and can foster clerical and other spiritual support to assist families in exploring, detailing and clarifying their beliefs, values and goals.	C
Raingruber and Milstein (13)	To identify which interactions with health care providers were and were not helpful. Parents discussed what it was like to have an infant with a life-threatening illness and what helped them to cope.	Interpretive phenomenological investigation; purposive sample of 7 parents.	Parents indicated that they benefited from identifying "circles of meaning," or ways in which their infant touched another life. They appreciated hearing from health care providers that they felt close to their infant.	B
Rosenbaum et al. (2)	To increase practitioners' awareness of spiritual and existential distress and to provide strategies to address such needs, particularly at the end of life.	Literature review of the spiritual care literature and narratives of parents who have experienced the loss of their baby in our NICU.	It is important to support parents through loss by providing comprehensive care that focuses not only on the infant's physical needs, but also addresses parents' and families' spiritual, religious, and existential needs.	C
Sadeghi et al. (3)	To explore the spiritual needs of families in Iran at the end of life and through bereavement in the NICU.	An exploratory qualitative study using purposeful sampling and semi-structured interviews with 24 participants.	Data analysis revealed three main themes: spiritual belief in a supernatural power, the need for comfort of the soul, and human dignity for the newborn.	B
Seth et al. (14)	To describe the role structured religion and spirituality plays in Latinas' daily lives and to evaluate how religiosity and spirituality influences health care decisions, specifically in prenatal diagnosis.	Cross-sectional qualitative study. Semi-structured interviews with 11 women to describe religious beliefs and thoughts while considering the option of amniocentesis for prenatal diagnosis.	Latino women found their religious and spiritual beliefs comforting, providing validation for their decision regarding prenatal diagnosis, as opposed to a direct influential factor in their decision-making process. Their spiritual faith helped maintain optimism even when faced with the complexity of the amniocentesis decision-making process.	B
Shukla et al. (15)	To identify and formulate recommendations regarding challenges faced while considering redirection of care for Muslim infants based on experiences of neonatologists.	Cross-sectional survey using a web-based questionnaire: Neonatologists practicing in countries with predominantly Muslim population (Kuwait, Oman, Saudi-Arabia and Egypt).	Redirection of care consideration for Muslim infants has many socio-cultural and religious barriers. Comprehensive ethical codes conforming to Islamic and legal standards are required to aid decision-making.	B

[1] *Level of evidence.*
[A] *Body of evidence can be trusted to guide practice.*
[B] *Body of evidence can be trusted to guide practice in most situations.*
[C] *Body of evidence provides some support for recommendation(s), but care should be taken in its application.*
[D] *Body of evidence is weak, and recommendation must be applied with caution.*

on the unity of mind and body and may clash with the biomedical model practiced in the United States. Surgery, for instance, is considered a breach of the "conscience"; blood is considered irreplaceable once drawn; and prenatal treatment is considered unnecessary because pregnancy is not considered a disease (20).

It is critical that clinicians are aware of the importance of inquiring about the social and religious affiliations of a patient, as these do not always correlate with the specified religious affiliation of the patient and these are important guiding principles in perinatal decision-making.

Islam

Islam impacts all aspects of daily living: from eating to clothing to health practices. Islam has been pursued for more than 1,400 years, originating from Mohammad in Mecca, Arabia, who is believed to be the last prophet sent by God (*Allah*, translated literally as "God"). Clinicians should be aware of the Five Pillars

TABLE 2 | Islam—what clinicians need to know.

For the infant	For the parents and family
• Breastfeeding is encouraged: a Muslim child has the right to be breastfed and raised "with kindness and respect." • Anything that hastens the death of the baby, including withholding sustenance is unacceptable because the time of death is predestined by Allah. • Suffering can be interpreted as a test of faith; however, pain relief is considered acceptable. • The dying infant needs to face east, and to die facing east. • Muslims do not like to die in hospitals—the same may be true for infants and this requires discussion with parents. • Muslim adults with terminal illness prefer to stay at home with their families until they die—again, discussion with parents is required for infants. • Muslims may not consider morphine a treatment option and may believe more in Allah's potential to heal and reduce pain then on conservative medicines (i.e., Allah has the power to cure ailments.) • The burial (if the baby is viable) should normally take place as soon as possible. • Upon death, enshroud the baby's body in a white cotton or linen cloth.	• Prayer occurs five times a day: dawn to sunrise, noon, afternoon, sunset, and evening. • Prayers are performed facing east. • Muslim law permits termination of pregnancy only if continuing the pregnancy seriously impacts the mother's life. • After 19 weeks of gestation, Muslim law accepts maternal health as the only reason for terminating the pregnancy. • Muslim parents may lean more toward following the Quran rather than seeking medical advice. • Parents may be less likely to question health care providers about their child because this is interpreted as a sign of mistrust. • Muslim families may not like to be reminded of their child's illness repeatedly, or that their child may die due to a LLFD. • The Quran provides reassurance that the baby will be received into paradise and is increasingly consulted as death approaches.

Ayed and Ayed (4).

of Islam and work with families to understand how this belief may influence their decision-making when having a baby with an LLFD. For Muslims, the Five Pillars are five broad principles that allow them to live a good and responsible life. These include the following: The Declaration of Faith (*Shahada*); praying five times a day (*Salat*); giving charity (*Zakah*); fasting during the month of Ramadan (*Sawm*); and a pilgrimage to Mecca at least once (*Hajj*). It is important that healthcare providers are cognizant and do not confuse Islamic traditions with cultural traditions.

Comprised of 24.1% of the global population (21), Muslims believe that Allah is in control of both the beginning and the end of life. All outcomes, including death, are predetermined by Allah (21). The teachings of their holy book (the Quran) influences healthcare practices and the pivotal moments of life, such as birth, death, and illness (4). **Table 2** provides guidance to clinicians caring for infants of Muslim families.

For practitioners of Islam (Muslims), the pervasive belief is that curative medical interventions come from Allah, and healthcare professionals are the medium for delivering the will of Allah. The Quran provides guidance and is considered the source of healing for psychological and spiritual distress. If family members, including infants and children, require surgical or medical measures, the Quran can be used as an addendum to resolve theological, social, and cultural needs (4).

To facilitate decision-making, rigorous ethical codes are required that adhere to the Islamic social and legal standards (15). When an LLFD is made, the Quran states quite clearly that a pregnancy should not be terminated for reasons that might include financial fears or fears that the parent/s will not be able to care for their infant after birth. However, when considering extremely premature infants born at <25 weeks of gestation (12), the "legal opinion" of the Islamic society is that two specialist physicians need to be involved in the decision-making, and while for some Muslims the sole decision-maker might be the physician who is treating the infant, the parents should always be involved in the decision-making with as much autonomy afforded to them in their decision-making role. The treating physician should, however, freely consult with other pediatricians/neonatologists and caregivers.

The steps of the legal process following the diagnosis of an LLFD according to the Islamic society are as follows: confirmation of lethal malformations by ultrasound and/or chromosomal analysis; approval of the malformation by at least two neonatology and perinatology specialists; documentation of the type of malformation in the medical records of the mother; obtaining the written consent from parents or their delegates; termination of the pregnancy is permitted if the gestational age is longer than 19 weeks, but only if the continuation of the pregnancy is expected to result in the death of the mother and if fetal death *in utero* is confirmed. The infant can receive PPC if born alive (4).

In summary, clinicians need to take care in exploring with families the role of their religion in decision-making and to have some awareness of the teachings and beliefs that guide their daily lives. An understanding of their religious needs provides a framework for discussion and allows the healthcare team to support the parents through difficult decision-making processes (12).

Buddhism

Buddhism is a faith that was established more than 2,500 years ago in India by Siddhartha Gautama ("the Buddha"). Comprised of 6.9% of the global population, Buddhists recognize suffering as central to human existence. Suffering is unavoidable and life-limiting illness serves to prompt reflection on the ultimate meaning of life. Death is associated with rebirth (reincarnation), and having serene surroundings at the time of death and during the dying process is important to the dignity of the person and for their rebirth (21). Although Buddhists believe that death is a part of life, the religion is not somber, but it is full of serenity, hope, and wisdom, but recognizing that suffering is unavoidable, just as death is unavoidable. Central to this is a belief in *karma* (as is also in Hinduism), or the sum of one's actions (and inactions) in their current and previous states of existence. The sum of these karmic actions decides their fate in future existences, influencing how they will be reincarnated and what they will be reincarnated as. Karma, however, is not isolated to Hinduism and Buddhism: in America, 27% of the population were reported to have belief in reincarnation and "some form of karma" (11). In 2014, Kain

TABLE 3 | Buddhism—what clinicians need to know.

For the infant	For the parents and family
• As in Hinduism, the illness of the baby is the result of past and current actions (karma). • At death, Buddhist's believe that the person will go through a process known as "samsara," or reincarnation. Ensuring a serene setting at the time of death will be important. • Buddhists may not practice specific death rituals, however, rituals that do take place focus on helping the baby achieve a better station in their next life. • In Buddhism, burial and cremation are both practiced, so it is important not to make assumptions of this. • When creating an environment of serenity, white or yellow flowers are acceptable; red flowers are to be avoided as they symbolize happiness. • There are no rules or specific timeframe that determines when the burial or cremation of the baby should take place.	• Parent's will believe their baby could be reborn (reincarnated) as a god, demigod, human, animal, "hungry ghost" or "hell creature," depending on the baby's karma and actions during their brief life. • The parents may wish to place images of Buddha and flowers near their infant to maintain a sense of calm in the face of death. • A calm, serene environment helps to maintain the focus on religious thoughts and the "good deeds" performed during the infant's short life. • Parents may also consider the karma of their infant, and their own karma when faced with the death of their infant.

Kain (11) and Lewis and Foley (21).

explored the notion of being born after dying and karma for Buddhists and non-Buddhists, in a discussion paper, reported the dilemma of the karmic "baggage" of being born after dying. Because Buddhist scripture does not delineate at which point death occurs along the continuum, whether at the beginning of life or at the end, Buddhist parents can take comfort by realizing that their infant being reborn as a human suggests that their child already had a degree of untarnished karmic "baggage." Buddhist traditions accept human birth as a beneficial rebirth since the conditions for a sentient being to attain enlightenment are ideal only as a human being, which is the ultimate objective for the Buddhist practitioner (11).

Table 3 summarizes what clinicians need to know in terms of caring for infants of Buddhist families, especially for both the infant and the parents.

Essentially, when the death of their infant becomes imminent, Buddhist parents need to be able to focus on caring for the spiritual state of the infant rather than unnaturally prolonging the life of their child, as this will encourage a good rebirth. It is important for medication to not interfere with consciousness. When caring for Buddhist families, the clinician will benefit from demonstrating the "right understanding" (this is an appreciation of the four noble truths: the truth of suffering; the truth of the cause of suffering; the truth of the end of suffering; and the truth of the course that frees us from suffering) and an understanding of mindfulness (the whole-body-and-mind awareness of the present moment), which in turn creates good karma for the child and encourages the well-being of the child. In both its present state and as a living being, this will benefit the child in the current life and for the next life to come (11).

TABLE 4 | Christianity—what clinicians need to know.

For the infant	For the parents and family
• Baptism by water is considered necessary for salvation using a formulaic prayer, depending upon the sub-denomination. • For infants who die before baptism, the Order of Christian Funerals contains a special rite for these infants.	• Christians of all sub-denominations often have a belief in miracles, especially through prayer. • There is no firm, detailed Dogma regarding consolation of parents, however, parents will find comfort in the simple faith that God wants "what is good" for all His Children. • Emergency baptism can be carried out by staff at the request of parents if the infant is at risk of dying before the arrival of a priest/pastor.

Birgit (22), Caulfield et al. (6), and Lewis and Foley (21).

Christianity

Christianity is a monotheistic Abrahamic faith. Its ideology is based on the life and teachings of Jesus Christ of Nazareth, practiced by over 30% of the global population. Its followers, known as Christians, include many denominations: in the Western world, Roman Catholic; Protestant (Adventist, Anabaptist, Anglican, Baptist, Calvinist, Evangelical, Holiness, Lutheran, Methodist, and Pentecostal); in the East, Eastern Catholic; Eastern Orthodox; Oriental Orthodox Church of the East (Nestorian); and in Nontrinitarian, Jehovah's Witness; Latter Day Saint; and Oneness Pentecostal.

In Christianity, Jesus is considered the savior, and although beliefs vary between sub-denominations, most Christians view illness as a natural process of the body and even as a testing of their faith. While the death of an infant represents profound loss, most Christians view death as being part of the will of God (7). **Table 4** provides guidance for clinicians caring for infants of Christian families, especially for both the infant and the parents.

In a qualitative multicenter study, Boss et al. (5) described some parents whose infants had died due to severe prematurity or congenital defects as being reluctant to make any decisions regarding resuscitation. These parents were described as wanting matters "left … in God's hands," yet typically they were documented to be most likely to "want everything done." In this study, for most parents, faith, spirituality, and hope have influenced the decision-making process.

Prayer is an important component for Christians, regardless of the sub-denomination, and may be directed to one or all the holy trinity: God, the Holy Spirit, and/or Jesus Christ. Baptism, which is a Christian rite of entry into Christianity, almost always through the use of water, is another important ritual, usually performed near the time of birth. According to Birgit (22), the onus is upon parents to seek baptism if their infant dies at birth or is imminently dying as the unbaptized infant cannot "seek truth" or choose to behave in an "ethical way." Christians believe that the baptized child who dies will end up in heaven, but there are reasons for hope that, in the presence of God, children who die without baptism will still feel the joy of everlasting life (i.e., enter Heaven) (22).

Caulfield et al. (6) have recommended that, in order to fulfill the needs of families in an emerging multi-faith community, maternity hospitals and neonatal units need to have access to emergency baptism services or other similar "spiritual blessings." In a study to evaluate trends of infants of Catholic parents baptized over a 15-year period at an Irish maternity hospital, Caulfield et al. (6) reported a gradual decline of emergency baptisms.

Access to emergency baptism services is important, because, in the early stages of grief of parents whose infant had died, 37% of the parents (who were all Christian) said that their religious beliefs were challenged and that they questioned their faith (10). Parents in a study by Hawthorne et al. (10) expressed their anger and betrayal toward God (to whom they had prayed for help) for being cruel and unjust and the perception that they were being punished by His failure to protect their child; 9% said that they had lost their trust in God. While one of the most important early sacraments in Christianity is Baptism (22), it is important for clinicians to be mindful that many Christians may not subscribe to the point of view outlined in the study by Hawthorne et al.

Hinduism

Hinduism, with its origins and traditions dating back more than 4,000 years, is considered the oldest religion in the world. Hinduism is practiced by 15.1% globally and is a broad term that describes many subgroups of the religion, which influence its practice and customs. Most forms of Hinduism are henotheistic, adulating a single deity (*Brahman*), but other gods and goddesses are still acknowledged by their followers. In the scriptures and wisdom heritages of the Vedic tradition, however, all of them have their individual origins (8). Hinduism, irrespective of tradition, offers a systematic explanation of life and death that most Hindus accept. The term "life" translates to "*the atma*," which can be interpreted as the "soul" (8). In Hinduism, achieving a state of *Nirvana* (or "oneness with God") is the primary purpose. Similar to Buddhism, disease and illness are considered the result of karmic actions, and death is simply a passage because the atma has no beginning or end (21). Hindus believe in reincarnation, so a newborn is not a "new" creation but a perpetual being continuing its progression of lives in a new body.

In terms of infants born with an LLFD, the *Bhagavat Purana* (a revered Hindu text) affords personhood to the fetus at 180 days of gestation as the embryo begins to develop awareness and beings to feel pain (8). The *Dharmashastras* (the treatises of Hinduism) view the termination of pregnancy (the "killing" of a human fetus is referred to as "*bhrunahatya*") as a sin; however, in less traditional Hindu families, termination may not be seen this way.

Clinicians should be aware that more importance is placed on the male child in Hinduism, given that they continue the lineage of the family, including the name. Therefore, it is more likely that the death of a male infant will be more acutely felt in traditional Hindu families than the death of a female infant (23). In the Hindu tradition, palliative care is considered appropriate for infants who are not expected to survive. Any interventions that might hasten death are not considered appropriate, and where possible, all active treatments should be ceased and the death of the infant should be allowed to happen in its own time (8). **Table 5** provides guidance for clinicians caring for infants of Hindu families, especially for both the infant and the parents.

TABLE 5 | Hinduism—what clinicians need to know.

For the infant	For the parents and family
• As in Buddhism, the illness of the infant is the result of past and current actions (karma). • Food is viewed as a gift from God and is often part of religious rituals. Not taking nutrition near the time of death is part of the preparation for the end-of-life. • The mother may pump and discard the colostrum, as it's believed to be unsuitable for infants (in Hinduism, most infants are fed sugar water instead.) • Avoid cannulation of the right hand/arm as the right hand is considered holy to promote self-cleaning. • The parents may wish to place holy water (from the Ganges) and basil leaves on the infant's body • Once deceased, the infant's arms should be straightened. • Parents may wish to tie sacred threads around the infant's wrists or neck. • Cremation is the norm in Hinduism. However, this norm generally doesn't apply to children who die within their first year. These infants are usually buried rather than cremated, or their bodies may be consigned to rivers.	• Hindus may place more importance on male children (due to the family name and lineage); the death of a male child may be more acutely felt than the death of a female child. • The father is the head of the household, and decision making is often made at the family leve.l • Hindus believe in reincarnation, believing their child may be reborn in the same family to their children or grandchildren and return to earth. • Death should be a peaceful transition from life to death, ensuring the soul will rest in peace. • Like most, Hindus view death of a child in any family as one of the worst misfortunes imaginable.

Chichester and Wool (7), Jayaram (23), and Lewis and Foley (21).

Judaism

Judaism is practiced by <0.2% of the global population. Judaism is the oldest monotheistic religion, dating back nearly 4,000 years. The followers of Judaism believe in one God who, through ancient prophets, revealed himself. Its primary religious beliefs revolve around a code of ethics with four groupings of Jewish beliefs: reform (largest affiliation [35%] of American Jews), reconstructionist (an evolving civilization of the Jewish people), conservative ("traditional" Judaism outside of North America), and orthodox (adherence to a traditional understanding of Jewish law; this includes Haredi and Hasidic). Jewish clergy are known as *Rabbi*. Psalms, as the last prayer of confession (*vidui*), are conducted at the bedside of the person (21).

Table 6 provides guidance for caring for infants of Jewish families, especially for both the infant and the parents.

A prematurely born infant is referred to as a "*Nefel*": the same word is often applied to an abortus or an infant born with major life-incompatible defects. The word Nefel, in Jewish

TABLE 6 | Judaism—what clinicians need to know.

For the infant	For the parents and family
• Prayer shawls are common and are often passed between generations. • Food and water are considered basic needs. Withholding feeds may not be considered acceptable. However, it is appropriate to remove artificial nutrition and hydration to allow death to take its natural course if death is imminent. • Pain management is acceptable and preferable (and may be mandated) even if death is hastened. • At death, the infant's arms should not be crossed. • Where possible, any clothing or dressings with blood on them should also be prepared for burial with the infant. Jewish people believe it is important that the whole person be buried together. • Encourage the parents to see and touch their infant, photos are appropriate, and it is appropriate to collect mementos. • If the parents have not named their infant, it is appropriate to encourage them to do so. • Autopsy is appropriate (and even encouraged) if it can help determine the future pregnancies for the couple. Remember that the whole person needs to be buried, however. • The infant should be buried as soon as possible, in accordance with Jewish practice.	• All human life has value, principles such as quality of life may not contribute to the decision for curative or palliative care. • It was once thought that if the infant died before 30 days, including the full 30th day the infant is not mourned (Shulchan Aruch Yoreh De'ah 374:8), however nowadays this is mostly untrue. [The Yoreh De'ah is a section of Rabbi Jacob ben Asher's compilation of halakha, Arba'ah Turim]. • If the pregnancy was full-term, parents and other family members are generally obligated to have full bereavement practices, just as for any other child. • The parents will regard the healthcare team as being in a place of authority and may look to their doctors for their opinions regarding treatment options. • Following the death of the term infant, parents will recite Kaddish [hymn of praises about God found in Jewish prayers] for 30 days and may observe yahrzeit [the first anniversary of the death]. • In the case of premature birth, there is still debate within the Jewish community on how to define "viability." Consult with parents and their Rabbi to guide decision making. • No work can be done on the Sabbath (Friday sunset to Saturday sunset). This may result in parents delaying important decisions, including driving to the hospital to speak with the health care team.

Chichester and Wool (7) and Wolfson (24).

culture, refers to an infant who lacks sufficient hair and nail growth; is born in the eighth month of pregnancy; and survives for <30 days. Relevant social rules are different for a Nefel in Judaism compared to a well term infant (12).

It was once thought that if the infant dies, up to and including, on the full 30th day, then the infant is not mourned (Shulchan Aruch Yoreh De'ah 374:8); however, nowadays this is mostly untrue. [The Yoreh De'ah is a section of Rabbi Jacob ben Asher's compilation of halakha, Arba'ah Turim]. It has been reported that Jewish parents still feel a keen sense of loss and grief when an infant dies before the thirty-day benchmark (24).

Spiritual considerations for parents

Though used interchangeably, faith and spirituality are different from each other. Spirituality is more difficult to define because there are no common characteristics that were agreed upon. It is a broader concept that each individual defines for themselves (18). Spiritual care is distinctly different from identifying and resolving specific health problems: It is about being present in the journey of "making meaning" at the pivotal times in one's life.

In an explorative study about relevant sense-making activities, whether through prayer and/or meditation, first-time mothers established two key themes to help them deal with the life-threatening illness of their infants: (a) looking for meaning circles and (b) using intuitive/spiritual experiences to find meaning (13). Similarly, Sadeghi et al. (3) found three spiritual themes identified by parents that had lost an infant following an LLFD: a philosophical belief in the forces of the supernatural; the need for the comfort of the soul; and human dignity for the newborn (3).

To help parents make meaning and meet their spiritual needs when faced with perinatal death, the parents should be encouraged to consider how their infant has touched other lives besides their own; this includes other family members, particularly grandparents, who would have had their own hopes and dreams for the child. Raingruber and Milstein (13) propose that parents imagine the waves that circle around just one pebble tossed into a pool and that this enables parents to recognize how the life and/or death of their child form others. Parents will gain an insight into the life and death of their baby by focusing on these waves (13). These simple practices do not require parents to follow a particular religion, and comfort can be found in simple acts of making meaning. It is important to support parents through their loss by providing care that also addresses the spiritual, religious, and, existential needs of the parents and families (2).

In 2017, Hawthorne et al. explored the disparities between gender, race/ethnicity, and religion in the use of spiritual and religious coping strategies by parents after the death of a child. The study found that non-Hispanic black mothers were more likely to use religious coping strategies than non-Hispanic white mothers. Christian parents used more religious coping practices than the other groups, and mothers reported considerably more use of religious and spiritual coping practices than fathers (10). This study concluded that black mothers were more religious than they were spiritual, and the mothers were more spiritual and religious than the fathers in coping with the loss of an infant, providing some guidance to healthcare professionals on how to support bereaved parents of diverse races/ethnicities and religions. It has been identified in Latino women that their religious and spiritual beliefs were found to be intensely comforting. Their combined beliefs helped them to validate the decisions they had made in response to an LLFD. Their spirituality helped them to maintain a sense of optimism even when faced with difficult decisions following complex amniocentesis findings (14).

Cultural Considerations for Parents

Culture refers to the collective deposit of information, experience, opinions, principles, behaviors, meanings, hierarchies, faith, notions of time, responsibilities, spatial relationships, concepts of the world, and material objects and belongings acquired through person and community by a group of people over different periods of time (25).

In 2008, Davies et al. conducted a survey demonstrating that almost 40% of healthcare professionals cited "cultural differences" as a barrier to providing palliative care. This was particularly so among ethnic minorities whose cultures were poorly understood, including Latino, Indian, and Native and African Americans. Cultural gaps extended to language barriers, religious differences, and mistrust of healthcare providers and care of health practitioners who did not have the same racial or cultural context and who did not recognize these differences (26). In a study that explored the challenges for trainee neonatologists, dealing with different cultures and the inability to interact effectively with people of different cultures were identified as significant when the trainee had different faith and religious beliefs to those of the parents and families. The trainees were more likely to respond with anxiety, wariness, and even anger or fear to unknown cultures or unfamiliar cultures when working with parents that are making the end-of-life decisions about their infant (9).

No matter how committed, highly trained, and dedicated the healthcare team is, when caring for parents and their infant with an LLFD, an expert understanding of how families function, spiritually, cross-culturally, and existentially, presents a considerable challenge in PPC.

CONCLUSIONS

It is not surprising that families rely on their faith and spirituality in times of crisis to help them make sense of the path to the end of life. This analysis revealed why healthcare practitioners need to become familiar with the definitions of the moral and religious ideas that arise in their clinical field or specialization for parents and families. Regardless of the religious, spiritual, or cultural beliefs, all parents facing the death of their infant due to an LLFD require a compassionate, supportive, and knowledgeable healthcare service. Life and death are momentous occasions in the life cycle, and when the two occur in close proximity, beliefs and religious ceremonies become even more profound. All members of the healthcare team providing care to parents from the moment of the diagnosis through the palliation of to death of the infant require a unique skill set, including the ability to pay attention to, and the knowledge of, religious, spiritual, and cultural needs of the parents.

AUTHOR CONTRIBUTIONS

VK conceptualized and designed the review, drafted the manuscript, and is solely responsible for data collection and interpretation of the literature data.

REFERENCES

1. WHO. *WHO Definition of Palliative Care*. (2020). Available online at: https://www.who.int/cancer/palliative/definition/en/ (accessed June 25, 2020).
2. Rosenbaum JL, Smith JR, Zollfrank R. Neonatal end-of-life spiritual support care. *J Perinatal Neonatal Nurs.* (2011) 25:61–9. doi: 10.1097/JPN.0b013e318209e1d2
3. Sadeghi N, Hasanpour M, Heidarzadeh M, Alamolhoda A, Waldman E. Spiritual needs of families with bereavement and loss of an infant in the neonatal intensive care unit: a qualitative study. *J Pain Sympt Manage.* (2016) 52:35–42. doi: 10.1016/j.jpainsymman.2015.12.344
4. Ayed M, Ayed A. Fetal and newborn palliative care in islam-when to be considered. *Case Rep Lit Rev.* (2018) 2:1–8.
5. Boss RD, Hutton N, Sulpar LJ, West AM, Donohue PK. Values parents apply to decision-making regarding delivery room resuscitation for high-risk newborns. *Pediatrics.* (2008) 122:583–9. doi: 10.1542/peds.2007-1972
6. Caulfield FM, Ihidero OA, Carroll M, Dunworth M, Hunt M, McAuliffe D, et al. Spiritual care in neonatology: analysis of emergency baptisms in an Irish neonatal unit over 15 years. *Irish J Med Sci.* (2019) 188:607–12. doi: 10.1007/s11845-018-1894-y
7. Chichester M, Wool C. The meaning of food and multicultural implications for perinatal palliative care. *Nurs Women's Health.* (2015) 19:224–35. doi: 10.1111/1751-486X.12204
8. Das A. Withdrawal of life-sustaining treatment for newborn infants from a Hindu perspective. *Early Hum Dev.* (2012) 88:87–8. doi: 10.1016/j.earlhumdev.2011.12.004
9. El Sayed MF, Chan M, McAllister M, Hellmann J. End-of-life care in Toronto neonatal intensive care units: challenges for physician trainees. *Arch Dis Child Fetal Neonatal Ed.* (2013) 98:F528–33. doi: 10.1136/archdischild-2012-303000
10. Hawthorne DM, Youngblut JM, Brooten D. Use of spiritual coping strategies by gender, race/ethnicity, and religion at 1 and 3 months after infant's/child's intensive care unit death. *J Am Assoc Nurse Pract.* (2017) 29:591–9. doi: 10.1002/2327-6924.12498
11. Kain VJ. Babies born dying: just bad karma? A discussion paper. *J Relig Health.* (2014) 53:1753–8. doi: 10.1007/s10943-013-9779-x
12. McGuirl J, Campbell D. Understanding the role of religious views in the discussion about resuscitation at the threshold of viability. *J Perinatol.* (2016) 36:694–8. doi: 10.1038/jp.2016.104
13. Raingruber B, Milstein J. Searching for circles of meaning and using spiritual experiences to help parents of infants with life-threatening illness cope. *J Holistic Nurs.* (2007) 25:39–49. doi: 10.1177/0898010106289859
14. Seth SG, Goka T, Harbison A, Hollier L, Peterson S, Ramondetta L, et al. Exploring the role of religiosity and spirituality in amniocentesis decision-making among Latinas. *J Genet Couns.* (2011) 20:660–73. doi: 10.1007/s10897-011-9378-5
15. Shukla VV, Ayed AK, Ayed MK. Considerations for redirection of care in muslim neonates: issues and recommendations. *Kuwait Med J.* (2018) 50:417–21.
16. Stark R. *The Triumph of Faith: Why the World Is More Religious Than Ever.* Wilmington, DE: ISI Books (2015).
17. Lüddeckens D, Schrimpf M. *Medicine, Religion, Spirituality: Global Perspectives on Traditional, Complementary, and Alternative Healing.* Bielefeld, NC: Transcript (2018).
18. Koenig HG, McCullough ME, Larson DB. *Handbook of Religion and Health.* New York, NY; Oxford: Oxford University Press (2001).
19. Leung TN, Ching Chau MM, Chang JJ, Leung TY, Fung TY, Lau TK. Attitudes towards termination of pregnancy among Hong Kong Chinese women attending prenatal diagnosis counselling clinic. *Prenat Diagn.* (2004) 24:546–51. doi: 10.1002/pd.950
20. Tsai GJ, Cameron CA, Czerwinski JL, Mendez-Figueroa H, Peterson SK, Noblin SJ. Attitudes towards prenatal genetic counseling, prenatal genetic testing, and termination of pregnancy among southeast and east asian women in the United States. *J Genet Couns.* (2017) 26:1041–58. doi: 10.1007/s10897-017-0084-9
21. Lewis P, Foley D. Assessing spirituality and religious practices. In: *Health Assessment in Nursing Australia and New Zealand Edition.* 2 ed. Wolters Kluwer Health (Sydney) (2014). p. 194–220.

22. Birgit J. *What Happens to Babies Who Die Before Baptism?* (2018). Available online at: http://catholiclifeinourtimescom/babies-die-baptism/ (accessed December 26, 2020).
23. Jayaram V. *Hinduism - Coping With the Death of a Child in the Family.* (2020). Available online at: https://www.hinduwebsite.com/random/chidrendeath.asp (accessed June 26, 2020).
24. Wolfson R. Part 2: neonatal death. In: Federation of Jewish Men's Clubs, editor. *A Time to Mourn, a Time to Comfort: A Guide to Jewish Bereavement (The Art of Jewish Living).* 2nd ed. Jewish Lights (Woodstock) (2005).
25. Hofstede GH, Hofstede GJ, Minkov M. *Cultures and Organizations: Software of the Mind: Intercultural Cooperation and Its Importance for Survival.* New York, NY: McGraw-Hill (2010).
26. Davies B, Sehring S, Partridge J, Cooper B, Hughes A. Barriers to palliative care for children: perceptions of pediatric health care providers. *Pediatrics.* (2008) 121:282–8. doi: 10.1542/peds.2006-3153

3

A "Fundamentals" Train-the-Trainer Approach to Building Pediatric Critical Care Expertise in the Developing World

Sheri S. Crow[1], Beth A. Ballinger[2], Mariela Rivera[2], David Tsibadze[3], Nino Gakhokidze[4], Nino Zavrashvili[4], Matthew J. Ritter[5] and Grace M. Arteaga[1]*

[1] Pediatric Critical Care, Mayo Clinic, Rochester, NY, United States, [2] Department of Surgery, Division of Trauma, Acute Care General Surgery and Surgical Critical Care, Mayo Clinic, Rochester, NY, United States, [3] Head of Maternal and Child Health Department, EVEX Medical Corporation, Tbilisi, Georgia, [4] David Tvildiani Medical University, Tbilisi, Georgia, [5] Department of Anesthesia and Critical Care Medicine, Mayo Clinic, Rochester, NY, United States

***Correspondence:**
Sheri S. Crow
crow.sheri@mayo.edu

Pediatric Fundamental Critical Care Support (PFCCS) is an educational tool for training non-Intensivists, nurses, and critical care practitioners in diverse health-care settings to deal with the acute deterioration of pediatric patients. Our objective was to evaluate the PFCCS course as a tool for developing a uniform, reproducible, and sustainable model for educating local health-care workers in the optimal management of critically ill children in the Republic of Georgia. Over a period of 18 months and four visits to the country, we worked with Georgian pediatric critical care leadership to complete the following tasks: (1) survey health-care needs within the Republic of Georgia, (2) present representative PFCCS lectures and simulation scenarios to evaluate interest and obtain "buy-in" from key stakeholders throughout the Georgian educational infrastructure, and (3) identify PFCCS instructor candidates. Georgian PFCCS instructor training included the following steps: (1) US PFCCS consultant and content experts presented PFCCS course to Georgian instructor candidates. (2) Simulation learning principles were taught and basic equipment was acquired. (3) Instructor candidates presented PFCCS to Georgian learners, mentored by PFCCS course consultants. Objective evaluation and debriefing with instructor candidates concluded each visit. Between training visits Georgian instructors translated PFCCS slides to the Georgian language. Six candidates were identified and completed PFCCS instructor training. These Georgian instructors independently presented the PFCCS course to 15 Georgian medical students. Student test scores improved significantly from pretest results ($n = 14$) (pretest: 38.7 ± 7 vs. posttest 62.7 ± 6, $p < 0.05$). A Likert-type scale of 1 to 5 (1 = not useful or effective, 5 = extremely useful or effective) was used to evaluate each student's perception regarding (1) relevance of course content to clinical work students rated as median (IQR): (a) relevance of PFCCS content to clinical work, 5 (4–5); (b) effectiveness of lecture delivery, 4 (3–4); and (c) value of skill stations for clinical practice, 5 (4–5). Additionally, the mean (±SD) responses were 4.6 (±0.5), 3.7 (±0.6), and 4.5 (±0.6), respectively. Training local PFCCS instructors within an international environment is an effective method for establishing a uniform, reproducible, and sustainable approach to educating health-care providers in the fundamentals of pediatric critical care. Future collaborations will evaluate the clinical impact of PFCCS throughout the Georgian health-care system.

Keywords: education, train-the-trainer, pediatric critical care, training, pediatric fundamental critical care support

INTRODUCTION

The failure to recognize and appropriately intervene in the early presentation of critical illness results in significant morbidity and mortality worldwide (1, 2). Patient outcomes could be dramatically improved through the application of basic resuscitation and stabilization principles (3, 4). Initiatives seeking to successfully spread this high impact medical knowledge to resource-limited health-care settings face significant challenges that are difficult to overcome during short-term visits (5). Overcoming language barriers, relationship building with key local stakeholders, and understanding the intricacies of the cultural environment are critical pre-requisites for implementing and sustaining any educational initiative (6). Recognizing that local providers and leaders are best suited to overcome these challenges (7), we sought an effective tool for teaching acute care management principles to both community and critical care providers within the Republic of Georgia.

Health-care leaders in the Republic of Georgia and the Ministry of Health approached physicians at our institution to explore opportunities for improving Georgian maternal and child health outcomes through education. The Republic of Georgia, through a colleague who completed her professional training at our institution, sought assistance in developing a uniform sustainable approach to educating health-care workers in the acute care management of children throughout the Republic of Georgia.

In 1991, the country's independence from the Soviet Union provided an unprecedented opportunity to transform Georgian health care from the Soviet model (Semashko model) to a new health-care system. The original transition period trialed both free health care to all citizens and privatized medicine, before establishing the current system in 2013 of government funded health care that is distributed through a state agency. Under this model the state finances health care, but the delivery is largely reliant on private medical facilities and personnel. Simultaneous changes in the Georgian political climate, which now permitted unprecedented access to Western medicine, generated growing interest in restructuring the country's health-care education to align with current evidence based practices (8, 9).

The Society of Critical Care Medicine (SCCM) has developed and standardized adult and pediatric courses that teach the fundamentals of critical care management through didactic lectures and hands-on simulation scenarios. The Pediatric Fundamental Critical Care Support (PFCCS) is intended to train non-intensivists, nurses, and critical care providers. The main objective is to provide an educational framework to address recognition and initial management of the clinically unstable pediatric patient and to accurately identify the need for expert consultation and/or transfer to a higher level of care (**Figure 1**) (10). These goals make the PFCCS course an ideal educational tool for advancing critical care expertise in resource-rich and limited areas where training in critical care management is needed (11–13). The course management principles are applicable to all patients, regardless of the resources available within the health-care setting to which they present.

In collaboration with Georgian health-care leaders, a group of multidisciplinary intensivists from the Mayo Clinic utilized a

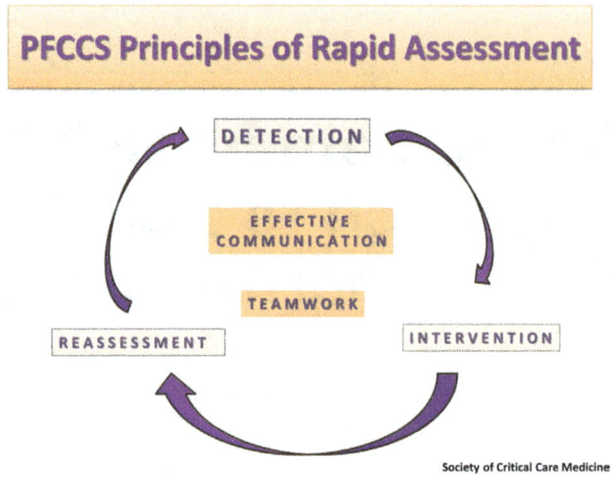

FIGURE 1 | Timeline for instructor training with specific goals for each visit.

"train the trainer" approach to establish a PFCCS course through a series of short-term visits to the Republic of Georgia (14, 15). The main objective was to train Georgian health-care providers as PFCCS instructors to promote the development of a consistent, uniform, and sustainable approach to the management of critically ill children throughout the country.

MATERIALS AND METHODS

Over 18 months and four visits, Mayo Clinic and the Georgian health-care providers collaborated to achieve the following goals: (1) survey the health-care needs within the Republic of Georgia, (2) preview PFCCS lectures and simulation scenarios throughout the Georgian health-care infrastructure to obtain "buy-in" from key stakeholders, and (3) train Georgian health-care workers as PFCCS instructors. Leadership organizations supporting the Georgian PFCCS Development included the Georgian Ministry of Health, United Nations Children's Fund (UNICEF), United Nations Population Fund (UNFPA), United States Agency for International Development (USAID), Centers for Disease Control and Prevention (CDC), and Mayo Clinic Global Health.

The initial needs assessment visit to Georgia included tours of tertiary hospitals providing pediatric critical care and maternal birthing centers. Tours included on-site assessment of equipment resources along with demonstrations of local resuscitation protocols. At each location, Mayo team members presented samples of PFCCS course material to determine interest and relevance of the material to the Georgian health-care system. Meetings were held with the Minister of Health and representatives from UNICEF, UNFPA, and USAID to understand the maternal and child health challenges and the existing efforts to address them.

At the conclusion of the needs assessment visit, through discussions with Georgian health-care leadership the following objective was established: Train local health-care providers as PFCCS instructors to promote the development of a uniform, reproducible, and sustainable approach to the management of acutely ill children throughout Georgia. Once trained, Georgian PFCCS instructors would educate clinicians at every point of care within the health-care system (regional hospitals and clinics, transport teams, and tertiary centers). This approach would have the added benefit of strengthening relationships between health-care providers in tertiary and regional settings thereby enhancing access to critical care expertise across the country.

Instructor Selection and Training

To optimize the success of Georgian PFCCS course development, the initial instructor candidates were selected based on specific criteria. Candidates chosen were established, influential providers within local health-care communities with experience providing critical care. There were no training programs specific to critical care in Georgia, so instructor candidates were physicians practicing in the disciplines of pediatric, neonatal, and emergency medicine. English fluency was required to assure optimal didactic understanding and translation of the PFCCS course materials (textbooks and slide sets) which we could only offer in English.

Training of PFCCS instructor candidates is outlined in **Figure 2** and was accomplished through the following steps consistent with SCCM guidelines for achieving instructor certification (10): (1) US PFCCS consultants presented the PFCCS course in its entirety to the Georgian instructor candidates, (2) US PFCCS consultants and Georgian instructor candidates spent 1 day focused on adult learning principles, practicing hands-on simulated case scenarios, and rehearsing lectures, (3) instructor candidates presented the PFCCS course to Georgian students while mentored by US PFCCS consultants. (4) US consultants provided individual feedback to each instructor candidate based on PFCCS course evaluation forms completed by the students and US PFCCS consultants. (5) Georgian candidates translated the PFCCS slides for their lectures into the Georgian language so that future course presentations could be provided to learners in their native tongue.

At the conclusion of Georgian instructor training, a course director and administrator were identified from the candidate pool. The job description and responsibilities for these positions were outlined and the next steps and expectations were established in collaboration with the Georgian and US leadership. The process for obtaining a Georgian PFCCS course license was reviewed with the newly identified course administrator and director. Prior to this, all training related PFCCS presentations and materials were provided free of charge through the multi-course license purchased by the US consultants home institution. Finally, the appropriate paperwork was completed and submitted to SCCM to obtain official instructor certificates for each Georgian instructor candidate meeting all usual SCCM requirements (10).

Developing Sustainability and Transitioning to Independence

In order to build confidence, optimize instructor retention, and promote dissemination of the course throughout Georgia, US instructors returned to Georgia at 6 month intervals. With each visit, US team members proctored Georgian led PFCCS courses, and dedicated a day during each visit to discuss successes and challenges encountered by Georgian instructors between visits. Additional skill training in simulated learning and educational methods, such as debriefing, were taught and practiced together. Finally, administrative processes were reviewed and goals established for ongoing course maintenance and expansion throughout Georgia.

Nurturing independence and maintaining momentum and enthusiasm for the Georgian PFCCS course between the US provider visits was critical to establishing sustainable infrastructure that would function independently of US collaborators.

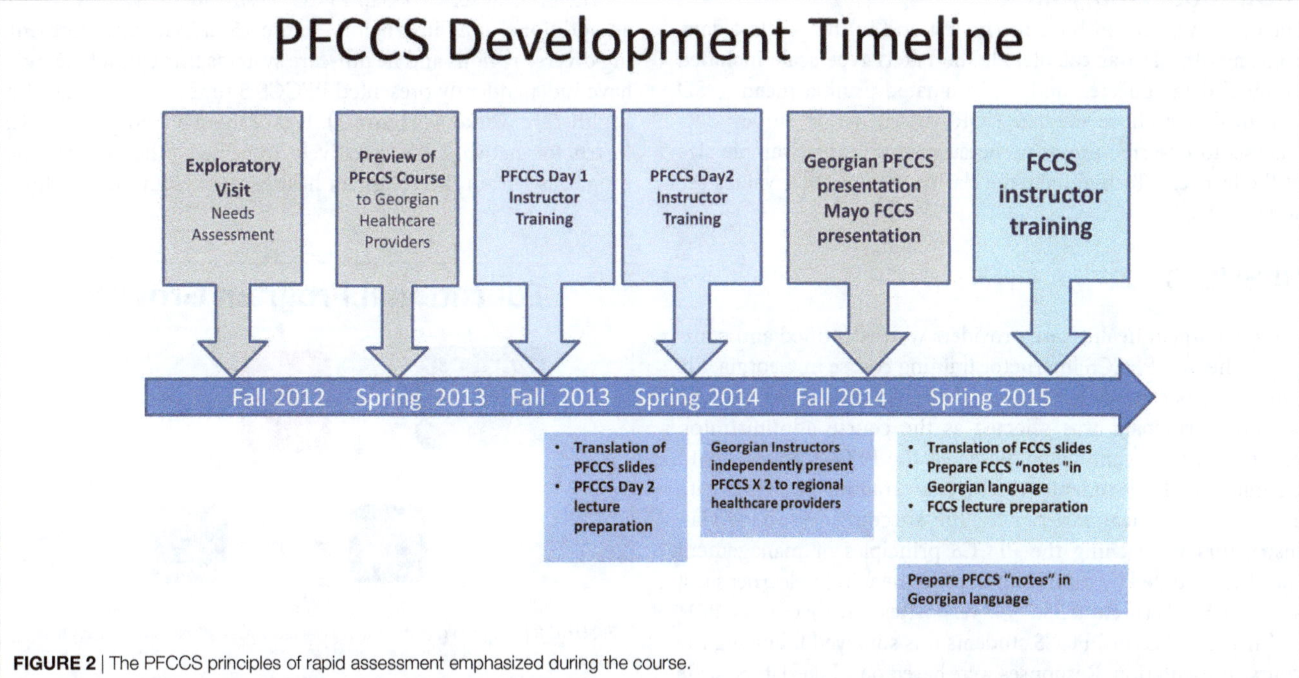

FIGURE 2 | The PFCCS principles of rapid assessment emphasized during the course.

The PFCCS course case-based, interactive, and hands-on approach were novel concepts to the Georgian medical education culture. Therefore, it was important for the Georgian instructors to practice these new presentation and teaching skills. Toward the goal of fostering independence, Georgian instructors were expected to teach a minimum of two courses between US visits, and videotape one presentation to permit remote viewing and feedback.

Regional Dissemination

With the first generation of Georgian instructors established, the collaboration turned to expanding the instructor pool within the country. Regional health-care workers became the next target in order to exponentially increase opportunities for course dissemination and foster adoption of the fundamental principles of patient management across the country. In this phase, at each US visit, Georgian and US instructors presented samples of the PFCCS course within each regional health-care setting. Following each presentation, Georgian leadership identified and invited health-care providers within those regions to pursue instructor training and provided travel and accommodations for candidates to convene at a centralized training site. The Georgian PFCCS instructors then independently trained these new candidates by repeating the steps used in their own training process, under the mentorship of the US consultants. US consultants were paired with an interpreter to observe every aspect of the training process. Specifically, they evaluated the integrity of the course material presented and provided feedback and encouragement to the Georgian instructors as they trained in the new candidates. The interpreters facilitating this process were Georgian physicians educated within both Georgian and United States training programs. The same interpreters were employed for every US visit to assure continuity in the assessment of program development and accuracy in translation of the course material and concepts.

Statistical Analysis

For the test scores in both the pretest and in the posttest data, a mean with SD was calculated. The Likert-type scale included nominal data collected and was evaluated using a mean ± SD statistical. We chose median (IQR) as the set of survey data analysis to describe the value because of the small sample size of the learners. To highlight the clarity, mean (±SD) values are added as well.

RESULTS

Seven Georgian health-care providers were identified and completed the first PFCCS instructor training course in Georgia. Six candidates became SCCM certified PFCCS instructors and the seventh participant was selected as the course administrator. These instructor candidates presented the PFCCS course to 15 Georgian medical students with no prior training in critical care and limited clinical experience. The success of the Georgian instructors in teaching the PFCCS principles of management was demonstrated by significant improvement in the learner's test scores ($n = 14$) (pretest: 38.7 ± 7 vs. posttest 62.7 ± 6, $p < 0.05$).

This first class of PFCCS students was surveyed following the course presentation. Responses were based on a Likert-type scale of 1–5 (1 = not useful; 5 = extremely useful). These 14 students rated as median (IQR): (a) relevance of PFCCS content to clinical work, 5 (4–5); (b) effectiveness of lecture delivery, 4 (3–4); and (c) value of skill stations for clinical practice, 5 (4–5). Additionally, the mean (±SD) responses were 4.6 (±0.5), 3.7 (±0.6), and 4.5 (±0.6), respectively, denoting that relevance of content and value of skills stations were highly rated.

At the completion of their training, the Georgian instructors reported enhanced communication and teamwork surrounding resuscitation events and improved consistency in the application of evidence based principles to clinical management. Furthermore, the instructors believed the course had positively impacted their approach to education within their health-care communities. Specifically, the PFCCS format had improved their presentation skills, ability to increase audience engagement, and introduced them to simulation-based learning methods that were now being utilized for teaching within each instructor's local health-care setting. Finally, instructors reported that PFCCS textbooks were a highly utilized and sought after clinical reference book.

As PFCCS training continued, Georgian instructors began seeking opportunities to establish measurable criteria for hospital performance that would objectively demonstrate the benefit of PFCCS training on patient outcomes. These requests highlighted the need to parallel the PFCCS medical education with an introduction to quality improvement (QI) methods. Thereafter, visits included instruction in QI methodology and identifying relevant applications for QI models such as the Plan-Do-Study-Act cycles. Together, we explored goals and walked through a plan (P) to test the initial goal, introduce the change (D), observe and collect results (S), and identify modifications necessary to achieve the initial goal (A). Specific projects discussed focused on infection prevention, interdisciplinary communication, and protocol compliance.

The original six Georgian PFCCS instructors have now trained an additional nine instructors. These 15 individuals, representing diverse regions and health-care systems throughout Georgia, have independently presented PFCCS 8 times to more than 120 health-care workers (**Figure 3**). Establishing a Georgian PFCCS instructor network has positively impacted other educational programs within the Georgian health-care system. Local efforts

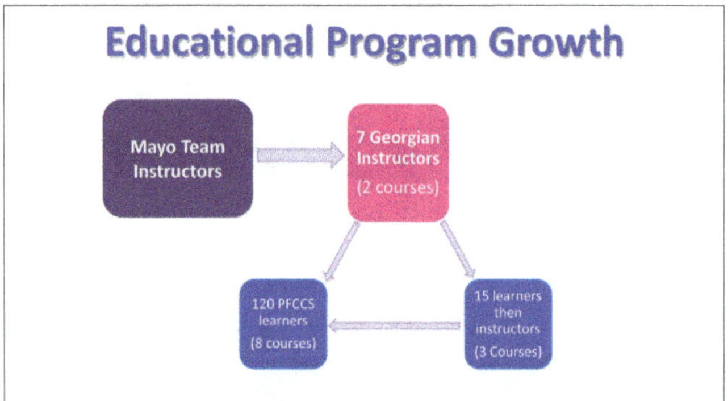

FIGURE 3 | Program growth within local resources at the completion of six visits.

to develop Pediatric Advance Life Support courses within Georgia were already underway when PFCCS was first introduced.

DISCUSSION

There are many advantages to leveraging an educational platform such as PFCCS to support international collaborations. In our experience, PFCCS promoted rapid relationship building between US and Georgian health-care providers. The SCCM sponsorship and oversight of the course provides information deemed important by an internationally recognized organization rather than any one individual or specific institution. The interactive lecture format and case scenarios provide a non-threatening framework for rapidly understanding existing practice patterns, resource limitations, and potential barriers to change within a foreign health-care environment. PFCCS material is presented to learners as being relevant to all health-care settings (resource abundant and resource limited) and therefore unifies international and local collaborators around a common cause.

PFCCS teaches principles that may not only be considered best practices within US systems, but may also represent novel ideas and concepts within certain health-care environments. The course framework facilitates non threatening discussion of these ideas while respectfully highlighting the cultural diversity between the instructor and student's health-care environments. Case discussions unite instructor and student around universal clinical challenges, thereby accelerating relationship building and improving receptiveness to the course objectives. For example, PFCCS development in Georgia introduced interosseous (I/O) needles as a method for gaining rapid intravenous access during resuscitation. The suggestion of an I/O needle during our initial PFCCS presentations was met with shock and dismissed by the Georgian health-care providers in attendance. On future trips, we brought the intraosseous equipment to demonstrate the ease of use and the lifesaving potential of this equipment. The PFCCS instructors were the first Georgians to adopt the idea. Their acceptance of the I/O as a valuable medical tool was the gradual result of continuing to teach about I/O application within the context of the PFCCS case scenarios. Ultimately, one of the PFCCS instructors, the director of Pediatric Emergency Medicine training in Georgia, has decided to implement I/O needles as part of her PhD thesis. The research for her thesis involves the pilot introduction of I/O use in the emergency department and pediatric intensive care unit of a major children's hospital in Georgia.

The PFCCS course approach to addressing common pediatric emergencies creates a platform to promote interdisciplinary communication and team dynamics (**Figure 1**). The simulation-based medical scenarios provide an excellent venue for promoting and practicing positive culture changes to improve collective decision making and ultimately patient care. Health-care delivery in these hands-on sessions is presented as an interdisciplinary team collaboration rather than an individual performance, highlighting the critical role played by both physician and non-physician team members. In Georgia, gradual cultural shifts stemming from these PFCCS teamwork principles, have translated to inviting nurses to join physicians in becoming PFCCS instructor candidates. Inclusion of nursing leadership in the PFCCS instructor network has accelerated adoption of PFCCS principles at the bedside, improved interdisciplinary communication, and led to lifesaving changes in health-care delivery throughout the Georgian health-care system.

Fundamental concepts for enhancing team dynamics include mutual respect and creating a shared mental model. These concepts are explicitly taught and promoted in the debriefing sessions that follow PFCCS simulation scenarios. These discussions play an essential role in establishing a psychologically safe framework where learners can reflect on their actions, identify performance gaps, and discuss areas for personal and process improvements. The opportunity for transparent discussion of patient management was unprecedented in the Georgian medical culture. Following the first introduction to debriefing, Georgian PFCCS instructor candidates expressed immense gratitude for the opportunity to safely ask questions regarding medical decisions the team made during the case scenario, while receiving constructive feedback specific to their management. Eclipsing all this was the opportunity to recognize they were not alone in their feelings of uncertainty or the emotional turmoil that surrounds the care of a critically ill child. The impact of these sessions on our Georgian colleagues impressed upon us the importance of continuing to pursue debriefing opportunities within our own US health-care environment as an effective method for supporting team members and enhancing team dynamics.

Although PFCCS proved to be effective in achieving our educational objectives there are several inherent limitations to this approach that must be addressed. First, it must be acknowledged that PFCCS is one of many courses to utilize the "train the trainer" approach. The American Red Cross and American Heart Association, to name a few, have a long history of educating the world in optimal resuscitation techniques. These forerunners lent support to our idea that this educational model would also be effective for enhancing critical care knowledge in diverse settings. Unfortunately, the most important barrier to developing any of these standardized courses in a developing country is that the cost for training materials and licensing are often prohibitive. These financial barriers limit the feasibility of sustaining the courses over the long run in economically challenged settings. Finally, although trainees found the course useful, we have yet to establish that PFCCS training of health-care providers increases the survival of critically ill children in Georgia. However, the training process led to the country's adoption of QI methodology and implementation of the interosseous needle. The potential for these changes to positively impact patient outcome are well documented in the medical literature.

In addition to the course limitations listed above, we encountered a number of logistic challenges that had to be overcome to successfully achieve our collaborative goals. The language barrier was perhaps the most difficult challenge encountered in the training process. At the time of our first visit, we encountered limited English fluency throughout Georgia. The PFCCS textbook and slides are written in English and time and cost made initial translation of the materials to Georgian infeasible. Instead, we selected PFCCS instructor candidates fluent in English. After gaining permission from the SCCM PFCCS leadership, each instructor translated their lecture into the

Georgian language. This step was an essential work around as English fluency was even less common in the regional areas that have the greatest need for critical care education. Unfortunately, although the course slides have now been translated to Georgian and the course is taught in Georgian, the textbooks are still written in English, thereby limiting this reference as a tool in clinical management for a large percentage of the Georgian health workforce. Efforts are underway to translate the textbook into Georgian. In the interim, English fluency within the Georgian population continues to increase.

The PFCCS course utilizes a combination of case-based lectures and hands-on simulated sessions to reinforce course objectives. The first Georgian instructor candidates had limited experience with simulated case-based learning prior to their PFCCS training. To develop this skill set, extended simulation practice sessions were part of every US visit, and included real-time debrief and training in simulation teaching methods and principles of adult learning. Between visits, instructors were required to lead a minimum of two simulated teaching sessions within their individual place of work. These "practice sessions" raised instructor confidence in simulated teaching and inadvertently changed their approach to training the local medical teams they supervised.

Financing educational programs within low-income countries is always a challenge and often places significant limitations on successful achievement of project goals. Training PFCCS instructors in a foreign health-care system is labor intensive for both the local work force and the international collaborators. The perceived financial cost to developing internationally recognized courses such as PFCCS is often seen as prohibitive for resource-limited locations. PFCCS is not a free educational resource. A license purchased through SCCM is required to access and present the course lectures and training materials. The license cost for a country is determined by a tiered structure and is therefore available at a markedly reduced rate for resource-limited countries (10). However, successful international collaborations that lead to sustainable changes in health-care environments are rare. Recognizing the uncertainty in the feasibility of achieving our objective we sought to minimize the financial cost of this project to our hosts. We asked our Georgian stakeholders and instructor candidates to invest their time and effort in course development without financial risk or obligation. Institutions can purchase a multi-course licenses through SCCM to permit unlimited course presentations in any location they choose. The US PFCCS team under the Mayo Clinic institutional license was able to present the PFCCS course to Georgian instructor candidates free of charge. US instructors covered their own travel costs and donated PFCCS textbooks to reduce the financial cost for development even further. Once the Georgian instructors were certified by SCCM and independently teaching PFCCS in Georgia, they purchased their own multi-course license. At this stage of development, the success of the initiative and value of the program to Georgian health care was well recognized by the Georgian Ministry of Health and the non-government organizational sectors. As a result, Georgian PFCCS leadership was able to secure financial support from local sources and UNICEF, CDC, and UNFPA. Regular meetings with these entities during each US visit to Georgia was critical to maintaining enthusiasm for the project and ultimately financial support. Furthermore, as recognition of the course value grew, opportunities for offering PFCCS to surrounding countries is creating new opportunities for generating revenue to sustain the course and promote the international visibility of the Georgian health-care developments.

Perhaps, the most significant outcome of PFCCS development in Georgia were the relationships developed between US and Georgian health-care teams. Successful certification of Georgian PFCCS instructors increased enthusiasm for considering additional educational courses such as the adult Fundamental of Critical Care Support (FCCS) course and Advanced Trauma and Life Support. Recognizing that the majority of providers in Georgia are treating primarily adults, the efforts to establish FCCS in Georgia proceeded rapidly. The number of clinicians seeking to become FCCS instructors more than doubled that of the original seven PFCCS instructor candidates. FCCS candidates were required to complete the PFCCS course, taught by their pediatric colleagues, who were now certified PFCCS instructors. The PFCCS instructors approached this process with great trepidation. These instructors disclosed to the US consultants that the FCCS instructor candidates were actually their former teachers, each a highly respected anesthesiologist or internist within the Georgian health-care community. Despite their initial concerns, the PFCCS instructors delivered the course seamlessly. At the conclusion, FCCS candidates were overcome with pride in their former students and marveled at the effectiveness of the course format for teaching critical care management and developing instructors into highly competent teachers. To date, there are more than 50 FCCS instructors in Georgia representing every medical discipline and region. The PFCCS and FCCS courses are the first Georgian educational programs to qualify for continuing medical education (CME) credit. The Georgian FCCS director, Dr. Marika Toidze, plans to train an additional 80 FCCS instructors in 2018 to accommodate the new CME requirements in Georgia.

In summary, our experience confirms those reported elsewhere that high impact, sustainable changes in patient management can be accomplished through education that occurs independent of expensive investments in material resources (12, 13). An established and internationally recognized educational program such as PFCCS is a successful method for developing international collaborations with long term benefit through a series of short-term visits. The PFCCS interactive format permits efficient exchange of information to pursue focused needs assessment and understanding of the local infrastructure strengths and challenges. The learning objectives are relevant to all health-care settings (resource abundant and resource limited) and therefore unify international and local collaborators around a common cause. The original request of the US consultants was to help improve maternal and child health-care delivery. We have found PFCCS to be an effective tool for taking the first steps toward that objective. Furthermore, it has helped create a foundational vocabulary amongst stakeholders as we move forward to address other aspects of health-care infrastructure, including medical transport and trauma system development that impact health outcomes for the Georgian population.

CONCLUSION

The SCCM Fundamental's "train the trainer" approach provided a uniform, reproducible, and sustainable framework for educating health-care providers in the fundamentals of pediatric critical care throughout the Republic of Georgia. Developing local PFCCS instructors within an international health-care environment is an effective model for establishing durable educational infrastructure that functions independently of international involvement.

ETHICS STATEMENT

This manuscript describes and educational initiative in another country. Although data are presented regarding the project outcomes, this was not an intervention study or a research project and therefore did not require IRB review. Please let us know if the paper should be submitted under a different format than as an "original research article."

AUTHOR CONTRIBUTIONS

All authors contributed to the conception and design of the study and participated in the training processes described in this manuscript; BB and GA organized the database; GA performed the statistical analysis; SC wrote the first draft of the manuscript with extensive contribution from BB; GA wrote sections of the manuscript. All authors contributed to manuscript revision, read and approved the submitted version.

ACKNOWLEDGMENTS

The authors wish to acknowledge the creators of the Society of Critical Care Medicine's Pediatric Fundamental Critical Care Support (PFCCS) course with special thanks to Dr. Mohan Mysore for his ongoing support of this collaboration. The authors want to acknowledge the support provided to this effort by the EVEX Corporation in the Republic of Georgia, the Georgian Ministry of Health, UNICEF, UNFPA, and the CDC.

REFERENCES

1. Sakr Y, Moreira CL, Rhodes A, Ferguson ND, Kleinpell R, Pickkers P, et al. The impact of hospital and ICU organizational factors on outcome in critically ill patients: results from the extended prevalence of infection in intensive care study. *Crit Care Med* (2015) 43(3):519–26. doi:10.1097/CCM.0000000000000754
2. Turner EL, Nielsen KR, Jamal SM, von Saint André-von Arnim A, Musa NL. A review of pediatric critical care in resource-limited settings: a look at past, present, and future directions. *Front Pediatr* (2016) 4:5. doi:10.3389/fped.2016.00005
3. Tripathi S, Kaur H, Kashyap R, Dong Y, Gajic O, Murthy S. A survey on the resources and practices in pediatric critical care of resource-rich and resource-limited countries. *J Intensive Care* (2015) 3:40. doi:10.1186/s40560-015-0106-3
4. Basnet S, Shrestha S, Ghimire A, Timila D, Gurung J, Karki U, et al. Development of a PICU in Nepal: the experience of the first year. *Pediatr Crit Care Med* (2014) 15(7):e314–20. doi:10.1097/PCC.0000000000000201
5. Lopez-Herce J, Urbano J, Carrillo A, Matamoros M, Red Iberoamericana de Estudio de la Parada Cardiorrespiratoria en la Infancia. Resuscitation training in developing countries: importance of a stable program of formation of instructors. *Resuscitation* (2011) 82(6):780; author reply 780–1. doi:10.1016/j.resuscitation.2010.12.027
6. Dearani JA. Charitable outreach in cardiothoracic surgery: ingredients for success. *World J Pediatr Congenit Heart Surg* (2016) 7(6):732–3. doi:10.1177/2150135116676766
7. Leader A, Cadet C, Lazala D, Roa W, Arroyo O, Jensen L. Collaborative implementation strategy for newborn resuscitation and essential care training in the Dominican Republic. *Front Public Health* (2017) 5:61. doi:10.3389/fpubh.2017.00061
8. Wikipedia. *Healthcare in Georgia (Country)* (2018). Available from: https://en.wikipedia.org/wiki/Healthcare_in_Georgia_(country)#cite_note-georgia-today-5 (Accessed: March 22, 2018).
9. Monica Ellena. *Georgia: Healthcare Costs Making Health Ministry Wheeze.* Eurasianet (2015). Available from: http://www.eurasianet.org/node/75446 (Accessed: October 7, 2015).
10. Society of Critical Care Medicine. *Pediatric Fundamental Critical Care Support* (2001–2018). Available from: http://www.sccm.org/Fundamentals/PFCCS/Pages/default.aspx
11. Atagi K, Nishi S, Fujitani S, Kodama T, Ishikawa J, Shimaoka H. Evaluating the fundamental critical care support course in critical care education in Japan: a survey of Japanese fundamental critical care support course experience. *J Intensive Care* (2013) 1(1):5. doi:10.1186/2052-0492-1-5
12. Macleod JB, Jones T, Aphivantrakul P, Chupp M, Poenaru D. Evaluation of fundamental critical care course in Kenya: knowledge, attitude, and practice. *J Surg Res* (2011) 167(2):223–30. doi:10.1016/j.jss.2009.08.030
13. Schluger NW, Braendli O, Carter EJ, Getaneh A, Sherman CB. Reply: cost and sustainability of respiratory medicine education in low-income countries. *Ann Am Thorac Soc* (2016) 13(9):1665–6. doi:10.1513/AnnalsATS.201606-491LE
14. Lee SWH, Mak VSL. Train-the-trainer program on cardiovascular health for community pharmacists in Malaysia. *Int J Clin Pharm* (2017) 39(6):1166–70. doi:10.1007/s11096-017-0540-5
15. Yu DTY, Gillon JT, Dickson R, Schneider KA, Stevens MW. Developing a sustainable need-based pediatric acute care training curriculum in Solomon Islands. *Front Public Health* (2017) 5:86. doi:10.3389/fpubh.2017.00086

4

Perinatal Palliative Care Birth Planning as Advance Care Planning

DonnaMaria E. Cortezzo [1,2,3,4], Kelstan Ellis [5,6] and Amy Schlegel [7,8]*

[1] Division of Neonatal and Pulmonary Biology, Cincinnati Children's Hospital Medical Center, Cincinnati, OH, United States, [2] Division of Pain and Palliative Medicine, Cincinnati Children's Hospital Medical Center, Cincinnati, OH, United States, [3] Department of Pediatrics, University of Cincinnati College of Medicine, Cincinnati, OH, United States, [4] Department of Anesthesiology, University of Cincinnati College of Medicine, Cincinnati, OH, United States, [5] Department of Pediatrics, University of Missouri Kansas City, Kansas City, MO, United States, [6] Section on Palliative Care, Children's Mercy Kansas City, Kansas City, MO, United States, [7] Division of Neonatology, Nationwide Children's Hospital, Columbus, OH, United States, [8] Department of Pediatrics, Ohio State University of Medicine, Columbus, OH, United States

***Correspondence:**
DonnaMaria E. Cortezzo
donnamaria.cortezzo@cchmc.org

Purpose of Review: A significant number of pregnancies are complicated by a fetus with a life-limiting diagnosis. As diagnoses are made earlier in the pregnancy, families experience anticipatory grief and are faced with navigating goals of care for a baby that has yet to be born. With the support of the care team, families can begin to grieve, plan, and make meaningful memories during the duration of the pregnancy, the birth of their baby, and life of the child. Creating a palliative care birth plan, which expands beyond the traditional concept for delivery planning to include prenatal, perinatal, and neonatal care has become an important method for parents to process the diagnosis, for parents to document their wishes, and for members of the care team to communicate with the goal of supporting and enhancing the experience of the family. This articles reviews recent and relevant literature on the importance of birth planning and the role of perinatal palliative care when a life-limiting fetal diagnosis is made.

Recent Findings: The process of birth planning is an important component of perinatal palliative care. Through this process, families can express their fears, values, hopes, and wishes. It also offers an opportunity for providers to communicate these wishes for the remainder of the pregnancy, the delivery, birth, and time afterwards. This has been demonstrated to decrease maternal stress and promote family centered care.

Summary: Perinatal birth planning is an important component of perinatal palliative care when a fetus has a life-limiting diagnosis. The process of birth planning can be supportive and therapeutic as well as an important communication tool. With multiple practices and designs of perinatal palliative care programs, there are no standard tools even though important components have been identified. Ultimately, the strategies outlined here can be used as advance care planning tools.

Keywords: perinatal palliative care, birth plan, advance care planning, neonatal, life-limiting diagnosis

INTRODUCTION

Advances in prenatal care and diagnostic technologies have allowed for earlier and more frequent identification of life-limiting fetal diagnoses, leading to increased numbers of families seeking support in decision-making surrounding the pregnancy, delivery, and neonatal care of medically complex newborns (1–3). Perinatal palliative care (PnPC) consultation as a part of family-centered fetal care offers opportunities for exploration of goals of care and planning for value-driven medical care for the remainder of the pregnancy, during delivery, and in the neonatal period (4–8). While practices vary and some PnPC teams investigate a spectrum of options that includes interruption of pregnancy, most PnPC consultation occur once a family decides to continue a pregnancy with a potentially life-limiting fetal diagnosis. PnPC teams ensure that families demonstrate sound medical understanding and prognostic awareness. They aid in exploration of unique value-systems from which families may choose various pathways including expectant pregnancy management, close monitoring of the pregnancy, interventions during labor and delivery, comfort-focused newborn care, or subspecialty neonatal evaluation and medical interventions. PnPC providers advocate for clear communication and support each family in vocalizing goals of care and wishes for their child's life (9).

Creation of a palliative care birth plan is an important method of exploring and documenting requests for the remainder of the pregnancy, labor and delivery, and the subsequent care of a newborn with a life-limiting diagnosis (10–12). The process of palliative care birth planning is both functional and therapeutic for families navigating goals of care discussions. Ultimately a care plan, the culmination of the important birth planning process, is developed to document and communicate the family's wishes with the multidisciplinary medical team. In this way, the palliative care birth plan expands beyond the traditional concept of a birth plan, which communicates preferences for the logistics surrounding delivery, to include prenatal, perinatal, and neonatal care. The PnPC birth plan can give families a sense of control in a challenging time and an opportunity to honor the life of their child. This article reviews recent literature on PnPC birth planning in the setting of a life-limiting fetal diagnosis and provides recommendations on developing documents that can be used as effective communication tools in advance care planning.

POTENTIALLY LIFE-LIMITING FETAL DIAGNOSES

In the United States alone, there are over 1 million fetal deaths and over 15,000 neonatal deaths each year (13). The majority of these, with up to 3% of pregnancies complicated by a potentially life-limiting fetal diagnosis, are the result of congenital malformations or chromosomal anomalies (14–16). Expanded early genetic screening or diagnostic options and advances in imaging technology have resulted in earlier and more frequent identification of life-limiting fetal diagnoses. A life-limiting condition is one having a low likelihood of long-term survival without severe morbidity that could impact quality of life. Multidisciplinary fetal care centers have expanded to include perinatal palliative care specialists who assist families facing complicated pregnancies in exploring options for care of the fetus and newborn (1, 3, 17). Some fetuses with life-limiting diagnoses will die *in utero*. Others may die during labor and delivery or in the immediate neonatal period. Others still may survive with varying degrees of interventions for hours, days, or more (1, 10, 18). Within these diagnoses are a wide range of pathology with a high lethal potential where individuals are expected to have varying degrees of survival and life spans. **Table 1** shows a list of common potentially life-limiting fetal diagnoses that perinatal palliative care teams are commonly consulted for.

TABLE 1 | Examples of common potentially life-limiting fetal diagnoses.

Genetic/Metabolic
- Trisomy 13
- Trisomy 18
- Osteogenesis imperfect (severe phenotypes)
- Triploidy
- CPT2 deficiency

Cardiac
- Acardia
- Inoperable lesions
- Lesions with poor prognosis despite palliative surgery options

Central nervous system
- Anencephaly
- Alobar holoprosencephaly
- Pontocerebellar hypoplasia
- Hydrancephaly
- Giant encephaloceles
- Spinal muscular atrophy

Severe pulmonary hypoplasia
- Bilateral renal agenesis with anhydramnios (Potter's sequence)
- Thanatophoric dysplasia and other severe skeletal dysplasias
- Short rib polydactyly syndrome
- Congential diaphragmatic hernia with low O:E lung volumes
- Severe hydrops fetalis

Other
- Severe pentalogy of cantrell
- Limb-body wall complex
- Severe forms of conjoined twins

With opportunities for multidisciplinary evaluation and increased access to perinatal palliative care, more women, between 20 and 40%, are choosing to continue pregnancies with a fetal life-limiting diagnosis (11, 19). Of those choosing to continue the pregnancy, reports of live births range from 60 to 82% (11, 20–23). When a child survives into the neonatal period, families face many decisions surrounding treatment and approaches to care. Some of these options may alter the disease trajectory but are unable to correct the underlying physiology or significantly alter the prognosis of the condition for the child. Earlier and enhanced fetal diagnosis gives families time to receive multidisciplinary fetal care with expert explanation of the suspected or confirmed diagnosis, support in understanding the prognosis and accepting levels of uncertainty, and value-driven shared decision-making in determining appropriate care or treatment options. With this information and support, families can utilize the ongoing prenatal period to create and share hopes, requests, and goals for the remainder of the pregnancy and their child's care after delivery, enhancing opportunities to parent in the face of a life-limiting diagnosis.

Abbreviations: PnPC: Perinatal Palliative Care.

The response to a life-limiting fetal diagnosis is unique to each family and their pregnancy journey. Some families seek comfort-focused medical care for the remainder of the pregnancy and for their child while others seek support in exploring or requesting varying degrees of life-sustaining interventions during the pregnancy and after birth. In a recent evaluation of parental experiences in the face of a life-limiting prenatal diagnosis, 52% of families reported creating birth plans that focused on comfort-care for the remainder of the pregnancy, delivery, and neonatal care, 27% requested some degree of intervention but placed limitations on more extreme levels of life support after delivery, and 25% requested full interventions and monitoring during the remainder of the pregnancy and life-sustaining therapies after delivery (24). Understanding the value system behind parental-decision making, building a supportive longitudinal care relationship, and guiding goals of care discussions are critical roles of the perinatal palliative care team in creating a comprehensive palliative care plan of care encompassing the remainder of prenatal care, perinatal care including preferences about delivery, and post-natal/neonatal care. The authors use the terms palliative care birth planning throughout the article to describe this processes and palliative care birth plan to describe the document created to communicate the wishes to the care team.

PARENTAL DECISION-MAKING EXPERIENCE WITH A PRENATALLY IDENTIFIED LIFE-LIMITING DIAGNOSIS

When a life-limiting diagnosis is made, many variables impact decisions regarding pregnancy continuation and subsequent choices for further care. These factors include maternal age and medical history, religious beliefs, cultural values, severity of anomalies, expected prognosis, gestation at diagnosis, and socioeconomic status (25–28). Additionally, many families consider the worth of their baby, potential quality of life, and personal ethics in the context of the known information (29–31). Several studies have shown the impact of religion on decisions for pregnancy continuation and decisions regarding care after delivery (32, 33). There are times this can lead to feelings of hopefulness, peace, or acceptance. Alternatively parents may experience fatalistic beliefs or fears related to decisions that may be viewed as deviating from their religious beliefs (28). Knowing these factors can help the care team better understand families' decision-making processes as well as help support them through this journey. There are times when personal values and cultural beliefs conflict and families can become lost, experiencing great emotions and turmoil at times leading to ambivalence in the difficult decisions they are asked to make (34).

A qualitative study that described if and how parents decide to proceed with a pregnancy when a diagnosis is made highlighted a three phase process families experience that includes information gathering, assessing implications of multiple uncertainties, and ultimately decision making (35). The manner in which information is presented, as well as parental perception of provider's views, affect the parents' experience and potentially informed decision making (17). During the information gathering phase, providers must be conscious of framing bias and the possibility for this to influence parental choices, as evidenced by the finding that families are more likely to seek interventions if outcomes are portrayed in terms of survival (32). Poor choice architecture and framing bias can be contradictory to the effort to provide non-directive counseling prenatally. Additionally terms such as "lethal," when used for life-limiting conditions, can convey a sense of finality to families, can leave them feeling hopeless, and may alter the decisions made for the remainder of the pregnancy and afterwards (36). Families have shared experiences of hearing insensitive or rushed remarks that cause lasting trauma (8, 37–39). For example, phrases such as "incompatible with life" were found to be insensitive and unhelpful by parents (40). Families take information in the context of their pre-existing views of disability, parenthood, certainty of the information received, their journey to pregnancy, and their support system when making subsequent decisions (41).

Studies of parental experiences show the importance of clear, concise communication at the time of diagnosis. Simultaneously, acknowledging uncertainty and reviewing further plans for testing or follow up in a timely manner is important (42). Families desire support, empathy, and acknowledgment of the difficult situation they are in and the complexity of decision making (43). Parents want information and support as they continue through their pregnancy journey (44). Often, multidisciplinary support and subspecialty care helps families feel that their questions are being addressed and they are receiving comprehensive care that ultimately aids in coping with the diagnosis (43, 45–47).

Unfortunately, many families feel that this information is poorly communicated. Reports indicate families feel discussions are framed based on providers' view of quality of life which may be vastly different from theirs. Families appreciate providers who offer comprehensive care and planning as well as encouragement to embrace the moments and milestones of their pregnancy (40). Providers must utilize reflexive practices so that members of the treatment team are aware of their own views and how information is portrayed during this vulnerable time (17). Families desire continued support while taking time to process the information and do not wish to feel pressured in to making delicate and important decisions. Parents also want providers to learn about them and their baby as individuals which creates the feeling of significance and that their child matters to the medical team (30). Families also appreciate continuity of care and consistency. Pregnant women and their support people are most comfortable when there is a dedicated provider or care team who takes the time to know them and is willing to explore the fears, questions, and uncertainty that lies ahead with them. Families appreciate learning about all support and treatment options from providers as opposed to seeking resources and information on their own (40, 48).

When the decision is made to continue the pregnancy, the parental experience evolves. Recent literature describes parents' experiences and emotional processing with continuing a pregnancy with a lethal fetal diagnosis (44, 49–53). While variation exists in how individuals cope and process information, an overarching theme is not wanting to have regrets for the remainder of the pregnancy and the decisions made. Parents experience a variety of emotions ranging from shock to existential crisis and ultimately life remodeling as they learn about the diagnosis, live with it, experience the birth and at times the death of their child. Across all of these phases, parents have a variety of coping strategies. As they begin to comprehend the implications of the diagnosis, parents seek information, and use that to revise goals for the pregnancy. Then parents may begin to visualize concrete plans for the remainder of the pregnancy, labor and delivery, the birth, and possibly the death of their child. While parents are preparing, they feel as if they are advocating for their baby, one of the most important responsibilities of parenting. During this time, in addition to the support from family, community, and social networks, families rely on the support of the medical providers (44, 50). Psychosocial support enhances their ability to process the information and be active in truly shared decision-making (51–53). As every individual processes information differently and requires different types of support, it is imperative that providers learn about their patient and listen to them so that the medical team can tailor the care to the unique needs of the family. It is likewise important that providers understand the stages and phases parents go through while processing the diagnosis so that they can recognize where their patient is along the journey and as a result provide the appropriate support and anticipate which conversations families are ready or prepared to engage in.

When a woman learns her fetus has a life-limiting diagnosis, she begins to grieve the loss of a baby she is already attached to (54, 55). Some have noted that receiving the diagnosis meets the criteria of a traumatic experience (17, 56). It is important to recognize that this is true for not just the pregnant woman but her partner, if she has one, and family as well. As a result support should be provided to all parties (57). Healthcare providers need to be equipped to provide psychosocial and bereavement support shortly after the diagnosis is made, through the remainder of the pregnancy and afterwards (58, 59). The support and experience the woman and her family receive has impact far beyond the current pregnancy (60). Initial reactions often include a complex dynamic of grief, guilt, hopelessness, and anger (17, 28, 34, 43, 61). At the same time, parents may maintain a feeling of joy and that their baby is a blessing (62). Families are facing having to make difficult and imperfect decisions that impact this current pregnancy and their relationships afterwards (17, 29, 62).

ROLE OF PERINATAL PALLIATIVE CARE-SUPPORTED ADVANCE CARE PLANNING IN ENHANCING OPPORTUNITIES TO PARENT

The importance of quality, collaborative perinatal palliative care is well-recognized (63–65). When parents choose to continue a pregnancy with a life-limiting diagnosis, they have the unique experience of simultaneously grieving the future for which they have hoped, embracing the milestones of the pregnancy, and planning for how they wish to spend the time they will have with their baby. Many will experience a loss of identity and a sense of isolation (39). Parents often seek the support of their medical providers who have familiarity with what is initially foreign and often overwhelming to them (66). Parents also seek opportunities to feel or regain a sense of control. By being able to make decisions about the remainder of the pregnancy and care of their baby, they are given an opportunity to actively parent and may feel a sense of empowerment (50, 66–68). As the pregnancy progresses, parents continue to bond with their baby. They seek respect for the child's life and shared celebration of the pregnancy milestones and mementos such as maternity pictures, heartbeat recordings, detailed ultrasound images, pregnancy journals, or intentional family activities or rituals. By providing guidance, exploring value systems and goals of care, and creating a space for questions and fears, PnPC teams help families feel supported as parents plan for the life and possibly death of their baby (66, 69, 70).

While discussing the birth and expected death of their child can be difficult for families, the process of creating a palliative care birth plan is also therapeutic and grants families a sense of control and confidence in sound communication of their needs, requests, and hopes (67). Exploration of goals of care, assistance in framing limitations of intervention, and advocacy for sound symptom management are best supported by palliative care trained providers. In the process of advance care planning, PnPC team members balance supportive listening and exploration of family value-systems with facilitation of discussion of goals and the translation of those goals in to medical care plans (10–12, 19, 71–73). The therapeutic relationship that develops between the family and providers leads to increased satisfaction and valued experiences during a difficult time. PnPC providers utilize the process of birth planning as a tool to explore meaningful support from the medical team and ideals the family visions for the remainder of the pregnancy and time with their child. When a family knows that their wishes are heard, it validates their parental role (67, 74). Families find joy in the opportunities to love, parent, and make memories with their baby even before the delivery (75). These experiences are chances to celebrate their child's life and to begin to form an enduring memory and legacy.

The experience of parenting and legacy making are included in the concept of the palliative care birth planning and can occur during the prenatal, perinatal and neonatal care phases. PnPC providers should facilitate exploration of how families seek opportunities to parent, make memories, and create a legacy as the PnPC team is well-equipped to anticipate or suggest what opportunities, choices, and options are available and may be important to the family (40). Photography, recordings, sibling involvement, creation of tangible keepsakes, bathing, and family-centered or faith-based rituals are commonly valued memory making opportunities during the remainder of the pregnancy and afterwards (76). Some families also seek to find meaning beyond their interaction with their babies and hope to create a lasting legacy for their child through organ/tissue donation, contributions to research or education, or breast milk donation. As advocates for family well-being, PnPC providers often balance planning for these valuable memory-making and life-honoring opportunities with careful watch for grief and complicated bereavement. This is especially true when carefully planned time with a baby after delivery or the opportunity to donate organs after death does not come to fruition as hoped.

EXPLORING GOALS OF CARE DURING PERINATAL PALLIATIVE CARE CONSULTATION

The perinatal palliative care birth planning process is ideally longitudinal and interdisciplinary. Families benefit from multiple points of contact with care teams. Many PnPC providers advance conversations incrementally through several visits, focusing initially on rapport building and ensuring appropriate medical understanding and prognostic awareness before transitioning to exploration of goals of care and birth planning (10). This allows for manageable amounts of information to be received by families and gives space for reflection and formation of questions. PnPC is interdisciplinary, utilizing care team members with specific training in psychosocial assessment and spirituality as well as communication and medical expertise to optimize a climate of shared decision-making (77). Parents appreciate receiving balanced information about the diagnosis and all treatment options before making decisions. They appreciate being part of the care discussions, having their voices heard, acknowledgment of their difficult situation, and ongoing support (30, 71). They rely on providers to encourage them to express their hopes, fears, and goals (78). Providers and parents collaborate to make decisions and plans, balancing autonomy and parental authority with medical recommendations and prognosis (79).

Discussing goals of care is a key communication skill when caring for patients with a complex or life-limiting illness (69). These conversations generally begin with exploration of parental values, goals, and fears leading to creation of a care plan that honors these views and wishes. When exploring goals of care with the family, it is pertinent providers assess the family's understanding of the diagnosis, prognosis, and range of treatment options. If providers can be present and supportive during these emotional conversations, there is an opportunity to learn more about the family, their views of quality of life, and how they make difficult decisions. This allows the provider to better understand and align with the family and ultimately helps to develop a care plan that is consistent with the family's goals and values. Early discussion of goals of care allows for time to reflect and plan compassionately and thoughtfully (80). For example, wishes for fetal monitoring during labor or newborn medical intervention should be established before families present for the birth of their child (7, 81–83). It is important to acknowledge that goals of care may evolve throughout the course of a pregnancy or after delivery as information available or the family's views and experience may change. For example, if an infant is unable to ventilate despite artificial respiratory support, this could be an opportunity to pause and reevaluate goals of care in the context of the evolving clinical situation. Ongoing perinatal palliative care support provides families with a safe place to explore the uncertainty of life-limiting fetal diagnoses and a team committed to careful communication of goals of care and palliative care birth plans (5, 67). **Table 2** uses a modified REMAP framework to outline key components of exploring goals of care in the setting of life-limiting fetal diagnosis (79).

TABLE 2 | Exploring goals of care for families facing life-limiting fetal diagnoses [modified REMAP framework (80)].

Reframe medical understanding and prognostic awareness
- Help family explore "What does all of this mean?"
- Acknowledge uncertainly and balance of "hope and reality"

Expect emotion
- Ask open ended questions (i.e., what are you most worried about?)
- Validate and respond to emotion. Be okay with silence

Map out value system family uses to makes decisions
- Inquire about faith, spirituality, religion
- Help to put those values in context of child's care (i.e., what is most important to you when thinking about how you want the team to care for your child?)

Align with values and hopes
- Reflect and summarize what we are hearing
- Seek clarification and verification

Propose a plan
- Suggest how identified goals may be achievable
- "I am hearing you ask that we create a plan that focuses on ______ for Baby's care after delivery" (time, comfort, better understanding diagnosis, etc.)

THE PALLIATIVE CARE BIRTH PLAN AS AN ADVANCE CARE PLAN

While the process of palliative care birth planning goes far beyond the tangible specifics of care surrounding delivery, the palliative care birth plan itself is important for families and providers. The palliative care birth plan functions as a communication and advocacy tool among care team providers. Providers caring for the mother often have different perceptions of family's understanding than providers caring for the baby (67). In order to fully support the family and provide seamless care, there must be open communication and shared understanding between all team members. The care team for a family delivering an infant with potentially life-limiting diagnosis will be comprised of both obstetrical and neonatal providers, including physicians, advanced care nurse practitioners, nurses, respiratory therapists, and more. The birth plan reflects the exploration of goals of care, summarizes the pregnancy journey, and shares the voice of the family while simultaneously documenting requests to all potential medical care providers for care during labor, delivery and the neonatal period for both mother and baby.

In order to meet the needs of both the families and providers, the palliative care birth plan should be viewed as an advance care planning document. Advance care planning includes deciding what medical care is desired in the setting of a life-limiting illness, exploring and sharing personal values, and documenting and communicating wishes (84). Each palliative care birth plan is unique to the family that creates it and serves as a tool to share their wishes and medical decisions regarding care of the mother and baby for the remainder of the pregnancy, around the time of delivery, and the subsequent neonatal care. As palliative care birth plans typically reflect discussions with medical care teams, the documents are generally created with the direct support of perinatal palliative care providers.

Palliative care birth plans include a breadth of information pertinent to providers involved in the care of the mother and baby. While many templates exist, key information should be included that will aid in seamless care during the delivery process and afterwards. General information such as the parent's names, the baby's given name (as many EMR's utilize automatic naming conventions based on the mother's name), and the parents' understanding of the diagnosis is important. Likewise, contact information for support persons should be readily available. This allows the care team to delegate tasks such as contacting family to others so that the parents can focus on the labor and delivery process while still having access to the support they desire. The document can include some specifics about goals during the pregnancy including celebrating milestones, memory-making such as pregnancy photography and preferences for follow up and delivery location. Wishes for maternal care during labor and delivery should be addressed ahead of time in the palliative care birth plan. This includes if the mother desires fetal monitoring, if she would want a cesarean delivery, analgesia, who should be present during the time of labor, and any special requests. Some women request music, aromatherapy, dim lights, or time alone with their partner during labor as a way to relax during this potentially stressful, exciting, and anxiety-provoking time. If they baby is live born, the medical care of the baby including specific requests for resuscitation or interventions should be clearly documented. This is an opportunity to express to the care team the wishes based on detailed discussions that have occurred throughout the pregnancy. Common discussions addressed include options for comfort measures only, non-invasive medical interventions, and invasive medical interventions. Beyond those

TABLE 3 | Key components of a palliative care birth plan.

Important information for the care team
- The parents' names
- The baby's name (if known)
- A diagnosis for the baby (if known) and a summary of what the family has been told to expect around/after the time of delivery. Any pertinent medical information should be included
- Names and numbers for important members of the care team (obstetrician, pediatrician, geneticist, other subspecialists)
- Names and numbers for important support persons (family, clergy, friends who should be involved)

Wishes for labor and delivery
- Vaginal or cesarean birth
  - Indications for when they would want a cesarean delivery
- Fetal heart monitoring during labor
- Analgesia for mother
- Special requests during labor
- Who should be present
- Who should cut the umbilical cord
- Preferences for if the baby is stillborn

Wishes for medical care of the baby
- Invasive interventions vs. comfort measures only
  - Any specific interventions they would or would not want
- Wishes for holding the baby
- Wishes for delaying routine procedures or providing them while the baby is in the parent's arms
- Wishes for feeding the baby
- Wishes for medications
- Wishes for additional testing

Wishes for memory-making and support
- Who should be in the room after the baby is born
- If there are siblings/family members, who will talk with them and how do they wish to be involved
- Photographs and videos
- Keepsakes: footprints, handprints, locks of hair, crib card, ID bands, blankets, clothing, heart beat recording
- Wishes for bathing the baby and special outfits
- Spiritual rituals/wishes

Plans for if the baby survives the first day
- If the family would like to take their baby home vs. receive end of life care in the hospital
- If they wish to be discharged home
  - Code status at discharge
  - The name of the hospice/home care that will support them
  - Anticipated care needs at home
  - Information about whom to notify if baby dies at home

Plans for if the baby dies before discharge
- Plans to ensure the baby is comfortable during the dying process
- Wishes to keep the body in their room
- Wishes for organ/tissue donation if eligible
- Wishes for autopsy or further testing
- Funeral home information
- Special wishes about transportation of the body

Any other additional requests the family may have

TABLE 4 | Important components of provider notes on birth planning.

Perinatal palliative care meeting note

Team members present:
Timing and reason for the visit
Family members present at the meeting
The name of the baby
Maternal history
Pertinent OB labs
Results of fetal testing and imaging
Name of the subspecialists involved in the medical care
Social History
    Share with others the important insight you have gained. Talk about the family structure, siblings, jobs, support structures, and faith. It is also helpful to talk about additional stressors and how the individuals involved in the shared decision-making are processing and coping with the diagnosis
Impressions, Counseling, and Plan
  Description of anomalies
  Counseling on prognosis and potential complications
    Who was present and a detailed description of what the family has been told to expect as far as morbidity, mortality, and anticipated medical challenges (including the ranges and both short and long term complications). Discuss what treatment options, care paths, and interventions have been offered and how that is expected to change the disease trajectory.
  Goals of Care
    Discuss the wishes of the family that they have expresses (comfort measures, non-invasive interventions, invasive interventions). Explain the various options and interventions discussed in detail (this is a guide for the providers). Also expand on any uncertainty and things that are important to the family if their goals are conflicting or cannot be met. Discuss labor and delivery wishes in the delivery room, code status, site of newborn care, anticipated procedures, or medications (help the providers who haven't met the family prepare for what to anticipate/expect), memory-making, religious ceremonies, plans for if the baby dies before discharge, and plans for if the baby survives to discharge

goals, parents may have specific requests for feeds, testing, and symptom management. Equally important, if applicable, are wishes for end-of-life care including location of death, symptom management, organ donation, autopsy, and funeral arrangements. One of the most important components of the birth plan to parents is the opportunity for memory-making. Who is included and what keepsakes or rituals are important is unique to each family. **Table 3** outlines details important to a birth plan.

Families identify palliative care birth planning as extremely important in preparing for the medical management of their child (67). It is not uncommon for families to request supportive care, varying degrees of resuscitation/delivery room interventions, and even life-sustaining or life-extending therapies for their child with a life-limiting fetal diagnosis. In creating requests for care, parents balance desires with fears. Common hopes and desires include meeting the child alive, enjoying time together as a family, and even providing a life and home for the child. These are balanced and contrasted with fears of pain, suffering, and extreme medical complexity (24, 79). The PnPC providers consistently utilize goals of care discussions and multidisciplinary birth planning to support families and address this duality resulting in requests for perinatal and post-natal care that is consistent with family values and rooted in medical understanding and prognostic awareness (85).

As much as the palliative care birth plan is a voice for families and communicates their advance care plan to the team, maternal and neonatal medical teams often seek expanded details on the medical care to be provided (67). It is important that all providers understand conversations that having taken place about the diagnosis, prognosis, and treatment options available. This often requires thoughtful and detailed documentation beyond the palliative care birth plan in the medical record. Delivery hospital teams should be directed toward details of collecting post-natal genetic samples or providing further neonatal assessments. Furthermore, documenting a family's decision-making structure and unique needs helps providers to partner with them during labor and delivery and provide optimal family-centered support while minimizing distress and miscommunication. An outline of pertinent information to include in provider notes around advance care planning in the form of birth planning can be found in **Table 4**.

Multidisciplinary fetal care teams have varying formats for discussion and planning upcoming deliveries of complex neonates and babies with life-limiting diagnoses. Discussions including key stakeholders (OB, neonatology, palliative care, etc.) ensure that providers are in agreement and all questions are addressed. Including families, psychosocial and spiritual support staff, and nursing teams may offer the opportunity to ensure interdisciplinary communication, allowing insight in to what is most important to the family and how to collaborate in family-centered-care after delivery. Additionally, palliative care birth plans should be readily available to providers and ideally documented in the electronic medical record before the time of delivery.

DISCUSSION

When a pregnancy is complicated by a life-limiting fetal diagnosis, the remainder of the pregnancy is vastly different from what was hoped for and expected. The grieving process may start well before the family even meets the baby. Often, families seek opportunities to celebrate and honor the life of their child while simultaneously planning for the ongoing pregnancy and navigating decisions surrounding care of the newborn with a life-limiting condition.

Exploration of goals of care, assistance in framing limitations of intervention, and advocacy for sound symptom management are well-supported by palliative care-trained providers. Multidisciplinary fetal care centers are growing to include perinatal palliative care specialists, who support families in processes of exploring value-systems, establishing goals and requests for medical care, and communicate those care plans with the broader multidisciplinary delivery team. Ultimately, perinatal palliative care birth planning and the creation of a palliative care birth plan with the guidance of an interdisciplinary perinatal palliative care team functions as an advance care planning tool for both families and providers. Further research dedicated to perinatal palliative care practices surrounding birth planning and multidisciplinary meetings as well as family experiences related to advance care planning during complicated pregnancies will lead to improved supportive care of families experiencing life-limiting fetal diagnoses.

AUTHOR CONTRIBUTIONS

DC, KE, and AS conceptualized and designed the report, drafted the initial manuscript, and approved the final manuscript as submitted.

REFERENCES

1. Perinatal palliative care: ACOG committee opinion, number 786. *Obstet Gynecol.* (2019) 134:84–9. doi: 10.1097/AOG.0000000000003425
2. Marc-Aurele KL, Hull AD, Jones MC, Pretorius DH. A fetal diagnostic center's referral rate for perinatal palliative care. *Ann Palliat Med.* (2018) 7:177–85. doi: 10.21037/apm.2017.03.12
3. Hui L, Muggli EE, Halliday JL. Population-based trends in prenatal screening and diagnosis for aneuploidy: a retrospective analysis of 38 years of state-wide data. *BJOG.* (2016) 123:90–7. doi: 10.1111/1471-0528.13488
4. Sumner LH, Kavanaugh K, Moro T. Extending palliative care into pregnancy and the immediate newborn period: state of the practice of perinatal palliative care. *J Perinat Neonatal Nurs.* (2006) 20:113–6. doi: 10.1097/00005237-200601000-00032
5. Sidgwick P, Harrop E, Kelly B, Todorovic A, Wilkinson D. Fifteen-minute consultation: perinatal palliative care. *Arch Dis Child Educ Pract Ed.* (2017) 102:114–6. doi: 10.1136/archdischild-2016-310873
6. Tosello B, Haddad G, Gire C, Einaudi MA. Lethal fetal abnormalities: how to approach perinatal palliative care? *J Matern Fetal Neonatal Med.* (2017) 30:755–8. doi: 10.1080/14767058.2016.1186633

7. Balaguer A, Martín-Ancel A, Ortigoza-Escobar D, Escribano J, Argemi J. The model of Palliative Care in the perinatal setting: a review of the literature. *BMC Pediatr.* (2012) 12:25. doi: 10.1186/1471-2431-12-25
8. Wool C. State of the science on perinatal palliative care. *J Obstet Gynecol Neonatal Nurs.* (2013) 42:372–82. doi: 10.1111/1552-6909.12034
9. Penny Simkin P. Birth plans: after 25 years, women still want to be heard. *Birth.* (2007) 34:49–51. doi: 10.1111/j.1523-536X.2006.00126.x
10. Cortezzo DE, Carter B. *Palliative Care. Avery's Disease of the Newborn.* Philadelphia, PA: Elsevier (2018). p. 446–52.
11. Leong Marc-Aurele K, Nelesen R. A five-year review of referrals for perinatal palliative care. *J Palliat Med.* (2013) 16:1232–6. doi: 10.1089/jpm.2013.0098
12. McNamara K, O'Donoghue K, O'Connell O, Greene R. Antenatal and intrapartum care of pregnancy complicated by lethal fetal anomaly. *Obstet Gynecol.* (2013) 15:189–94. doi: 10.1111/tog.12028
13. MacDorman MF, Gregory EC. Fetal and perinatal mortality: United States, 2013. *Natl Vital Stat Rep.* (2015) 64:1–24.
14. Osterman MJ, Martin JA, Curtin SC, Matthews TJ, Wilson EC, Kirmeyer S. Newly released data from the revised U.S. birth certificate, 2011. *Natl Vital Stat Rep.* (2013) 62:1–22.
15. Lorenz JM, Ananth CV, Polin RA, D'Alton ME. Infant mortality in the United States. *J Perinatol.* (2016) 36:797–801. doi: 10.1038/jp.2016.63
16. Heron M. Deaths: leading causes for 2016. *Natl Vital Stat Rep.* (2018) 67:1–77.
17. Hodgson J, McClaren BJ. Parental experiences after prenatal diagnosis of fetal abnormality. *Semin Fetal Neonatal Med.* (2018) 23:150–4. doi: 10.1016/j.siny.2017.11.009
18. Parravicini E. Neonatal palliative care. *Curr Opin Pediatr.* (2017) 29:135–40. doi: 10.1097/MOP.0000000000000464
19. Breeze AC, Lees CC, Kumar A, Missfelder-Lobos HH, Murdoch EM. Palliative care for prenatally diagnosed lethal fetal abnormality. *Arch Dis Child Fetal Neonatal Ed.* (2007) 92:56–8. doi: 10.1136/adc.2005.092122
20. Calhoun BC, Napolitano P, Terry M, Bussey C, Hoeldtke NJ. Perinatal hospice. Comprehensive care for the family of the fetus with a lethal condition. *J Reprod Med.* (2003) 48:343–8. doi: 10.1097/01.OGX.0000093270.97479.A4
21. Madeuf A, Roman H, Verspyck E. Continuation of pregnancy despite a diagnosis of severe fetal anomaly: a retrospective French study. *Acta Obstet Gynecol Scand.* (2016) 95:934–40. doi: 10.1111/aogs.12906
22. Bourdens M, Tadonnet J, Hostalery L, Renesme L, Tosello B. Severe fetal abnormality and outcomes of continued pregnancies: a French multicenter retrospective study. *Matern Child Health J.* (2017) 21:1901–10. doi: 10.1007/s10995-017-2305-0
23. Hostalery L, Tosello B. Outcomes in continuing pregnancies diagnosed with a severe fetal abnormality and implication of antenatal neonatology consultation: a 10-year retrospective study. *Fetal Pediatr Pathol.* (2017) 36:203–12. doi: 10.1080/15513815.2017.1296519
24. Janvier A, Farlow B, Barrington KJ. Parental hopes, interventions, and survival of neonates with trisomy 13 and trisomy 18. *Am J Med Genet C Semin Med Genet.* (2016) 172:279–87. doi: 10.1002/ajmg.c.31526
25. Chenni N, Lacroze V, Pouet C, Fraisse A, Kreitmann B, Gamerre M, et al. Fetal heart disease and interruption of pregnancy: factors influencing the parental decision-making process. *Prenat Diagn.* (2012) 32:168–72. doi: 10.1002/pd.2923
26. Schechtman KB, Gray DL, Baty JD, Rothman SM. Decision-making for termination of pregnancies with fetal anomalies: analysis of 53,000 pregnancies. *Obstet Gynecol.* (2002) 99:216–22. doi: 10.1016/S0029-7844(01)01673-8
27. Michalik A, Preis K. Demographic factors determining termination of pregnancy following the detection of lethal fetal malignancy. *J Matern Fetal Neonatal Med.* (2014) 27:1301–4. doi: 10.3109/14767058.2013.856411
28. Statham H, Solomou W, Chitty L. Prenatal diagnosis of fetal abnormality: psychological effects on women in low-risk pregnancies. *Baillieres Best Pract Res Clin Obstet Gynaecol.* (2000) 14:731–47. doi: 10.1053/beog.2000.0108
29. Redlinger-Grosse K, Bernhardt BA, Berg K, Muenke M, Biesecker BB. The decision to continue: the experiences and needs of parents who receive a prenatal diagnosis of holoprosencephaly. *Am J Med Genet.* (2002) 112:369–78. doi: 10.1002/ajmg.10657
30. Guon J, Wilfond BS, Farlow B, Brazg T, Janvier A. Our children are not a diagnosis: the experience of parents who continue their pregnancy after a prenatal diagnosis of trisomy 13 or 18. *Am J Med Genet A.* (2014) 164A:308–18. doi: 10.1002/ajmg.a.36298
31. Blakeley C, Smith DM, Johnstone ED, Wittkowski A. Parental decision-making following a prenatal diagnosis that is lethal, life-limiting, or has long term implications for the future child and family: a meta-synthesis of qualitative literature. *BMC Med Ethics.* (2019) 20:56. doi: 10.1186/s12910-019-0393-7
32. Haward MF, Murphy RO, Lorenz JM. Message framing and perinatal decisions. *Pediatrics.* (2008) 122:109–18. doi: 10.1542/peds.2007-0620
33. Balkan M, Kalkanli S, Akbas H, Yalinkaya A, Alp MN, Budak T. Parental decisions regarding a prenatally detected fetal chromosomal abnormality and the impact of genetic counseling: an analysis of 38 cases with aneuploidy in Southeast Turkey. *J Genet Couns.* (2010) 19:241–6. doi: 10.1007/s10897-009-9275-3
34. Bijma HH, van der Heide A, Wildschut HI. Decision-making after ultrasound diagnosis of fetal abnormality. *Reprod Health Matters.* (2008) 16:82–9. doi: 10.1016/S0968-8080(08)31372-X
35. Lotto R, Smith LK, Armstrong N. Diagnosis of a severe congenital anomaly: a qualitative analysis of parental decision making and the implications for healthcare encounters. *Health Expect.* (2018) 21:678–84. doi: 10.1111/hex.12664
36. Wilkinson D, de Crespigny L, Xafis V. Ethical language and decision-making for prenatally diagnosed lethal malformations. *Semin Fetal Neonatal Med.* (2014) 19:306–11. doi: 10.1016/j.siny.2014.08.007
37. Saigal S, Tyson J. Measurement of quality of life of survivors of neonatal intensive care: critique and implications. *Semin Perinatol.* (2008) 32:59–66. doi: 10.1053/j.semperi.2007.12.007
38. Saigal S, Feeny D, Rosenbaum P, Furlong W, Burrows E, Stoskopf B. Self-perceived health status and health-related quality of life of extremely low-birth-weight infants at adolescence. *JAMA.* (1996) 276:453–9. doi: 10.1001/jama.276.6.453
39. O'Connell O, Meaney S, O'Donoghue K. Anencephaly; the maternal experience of continuing with the pregnancy. Incompatible with life but not with love. *Midwifery.* (2019) 71:12–8. doi: 10.1016/j.midw.2018.12.016
40. Kamrath HJ, Osterholm E, Stover-Haney R, George T, O'Connor-Von S, Needle J. Lasting legacy: maternal perspectives of perinatal palliative care. *J Palliat Med.* (2019) 22:310–5. doi: 10.1089/jpm.2018.0303
41. Sandelowski M, Barroso J. The travesty of choosing after positive prenatal diagnosis. *J Obstet Gynecol Neonatal Nurs.* (2005) 34:307–18. doi: 10.1177/0884217505276291
42. Mack JW, Joffe S. Communicating about prognosis: ethical responsibilities of pediatricians and parents. *Pediatrics.* (2014) 133:24–30. doi: 10.1542/peds.2013-3608E
43. Hodgson J, Pitt P, Metcalfe S, Halliday J, Menezes M, Fisher J, et al. Experiences of prenatal diagnosis and decision-making about termination of pregnancy: a qualitative study. *Aust N Z J Obstet Gynaecol.* (2016) 56:605–13. doi: 10.1111/ajo.12501
44. Bratt EL, Järvholm S, Ekman-Joelsson BM, Mattson L, Mellander M. Parent's experiences of counselling and their need for support following a prenatal diagnosis of congenital heart disease–a qualitative study in a Swedish context. *BMC Pregnancy Childbirth.* (2015) 15:171. doi: 10.1186/s12884-015-0610-4
45. Kowalcek I. Stress and anxiety associated with prenatal diagnosis. *Best Pract Res Clin Obstet Gynaecol.* (2007) 21:221–8. doi: 10.1016/j.bpobgyn.2006.11.009
46. Kratovil AL, Julion WA. Health-care provider communication with expectant parents during a prenatal diagnosis: an integrative review. *J Perinatol.* (2017) 37:2–12. doi: 10.1038/jp.2016.123
47. Marokakis S, Kasparian NA, Kennedy SE. Parents' perceptions of counselling following prenatal diagnosis of congenital anomalies of the kidney and urinary tract: a qualitative study. *BJU Int.* (2017) 119:474–81. doi: 10.1111/bju.13668
48. Wool C, Repke JT, Woods AB. Parent reported outcomes of quality care and satisfaction in the context of a life-limiting fetal diagnosis. *J Matern Fetal Neonatal Med.* (2017) 30:894–9. doi: 10.1080/14767058.2016.1195362
49. Côté-Arsenault D, Denney-Koelsch E. "Have no regrets:" parents' experiences and developmental tasks in pregnancy with a lethal fetal diagnosis. *Soc Sci Med.* (2016) 154:100–9. doi: 10.1016/j.socscimed.2016.02.033
50. Carlsson T, Starke V, Mattsson E. The emotional process from diagnosis to birth following a prenatal diagnosis of fetal anomaly: a qualitative

study of messages in online discussion boards. *Midwifery.* (2017) 48:53–9. doi: 10.1016/j.midw.2017.02.010
51. Senanayake H, de Silva D, Premaratne S, Kulatunge M. Psychological reactions and coping strategies of Sri Lankan women carrying fetuses with lethal congenital malformations. *Ceylon Med J.* (2006) 51:14–7. doi: 10.4038/cmj.v51i1.1370
52. McCoyd JL. Pregnancy interrupted: loss of a desired pregnancy after diagnosis of fetal anomaly. *J Psychosom Obstet Gynaecol.* (2007) 28:37–48. doi: 10.1080/01674820601096153
53. Lalor JG, Devane D, Begley CM. Unexpected diagnosis of fetal abnormality: women's encounters with caregivers. *Birth.* (2007) 34:80–8. doi: 10.1111/j.1523-536X.2006.00148.x
54. Cjté-Arsenault D, Dombeck MT. Maternal assignment of fetal personhood to a previous pregnancy loss: relationship to anxiety in the current pregnancy. *Health Care Women Int.* (2001) 22:649–65. doi: 10.1080/07399330127171
55. Wool C. Systematic review of the literature: parental outcomes after diagnosis of fetal anomaly. *Adv Neonatal Care.* (2011) 11:182–92. doi: 10.1097/ANC.0b013e31821bd92d
56. Aite L, Zaccara A, Mirante N, Nahom A, Trucchi A, Capolupo I, et al. Antenatal diagnosis of congenital anomaly: a really traumatic experience? *J Perinatol.* (2011) 31:760–3. doi: 10.1038/jp.2011.22
57. McKechnie AC, Pridham K, Tluczek A. Preparing heart and mind for becoming a parent following a diagnosis of fetal anomaly. *Qual Health Res.* (2015) 25:1182–98. doi: 10.1177/1049732314553852
58. Hughes K, Goodall U. Perinatal bereavement care: are we meeting families' needs? *Br J Midwifery.* (2013) 21:248–53. doi: 10.12968/bjom.2013.21.4.248
59. Wool C, Catlin A. Perinatal bereavement and palliative care offered throughout the healthcare system. *Ann Palliat Med.* (2019) 8:22–9. doi: 10.21037/apm.2018.11.03
60. Leithner K, Maar A, Maritsch F. Experiences with a psychological help service for women following a prenatal diagnosis: results of a follow-up study. *J Psychosom Obstet Gynaecol.* (2002) 23:183–92. doi: 10.3109/01674820209074671
61. Leuthner SR, Bolger M, Frommelt M, Nelson R. The impact of abnormal fetal echocardiography on expectant parents' experience of pregnancy: a pilot study. *J Psychosom Obstet Gynaecol.* (2003) 24:121–9. doi: 10.3109/01674820309042809
62. Hickerton CL, Aitken M, Hodgson J, Delatycki MB. "Did you find that out in time?": new life trajectories of parents who choose to continue a pregnancy where a genetic disorder is diagnosed or likely. *Am J Med Genet A.* (2012) 158A:373–83. doi: 10.1002/ajmg.a.34399
63. Duff RS, Campbell AG. Moral and ethical dilemmas in the special-care nursery. *N Engl J Med.* (1973) 289:890–4. doi: 10.1056/NEJM197310252891705
64. Whitfield JM, Siegel RE, Glicken AD, Harmon RJ, Powers LK, Goldson EJ. The application of hospice concepts to neonatal care. *Am J Dis Child.* (1982) 136:421–4. doi: 10.1001/archpedi.1982.03970410039009
65. Landon-Malone KA, Kirkpatrick JM, Stull SP. Incorporating hospice care in a community hospital NICU. *Neonatal Netw.* (1987) 6:13–9.
66. Wool C, Kain VJ, Mendes J, Carter BS. Quality predictors of parental satisfaction after birth of infants with life-limiting conditions. *Acta Paediatr.* (2018) 107:276–82. doi: 10.1111/apa.13980
67. Cortezzo DE, Bowers K, Cameron Meyer M. Birth planning in uncertain or life-limiting fetal diagnoses: perspectives of physicians and parents. *J Palliat Med.* (2019) 22:1337–45. doi: 10.1089/jpm.2018.0596
68. Whitford HM, Entwistle VA, van Teijlingen E, Aitchison PE, Davidson T, Humphrey T, et al. Use of a birth plan within woman-held maternity records: a qualitative study with women and staff in northeast Scotland. *Birth.* (2014) 41:283–9. doi: 10.1111/birt.12109
69. Wool C, Côté-Arsenault D, Perry Black B, Denney-Koelsch E, Kim S, Kavanaugh K. Provision of services in perinatal palliative care: a multicenter survey in the United States. *J Palliat Med.* (2016) 19:279–85. doi: 10.1089/jpm.2015.0266
70. Moore BS, Carter BS, Beaven B, House K, House J. Anticipation, accompaniment, and a good death in perinatal care. *Yale J Biol Med.* (2019) 92:741–5.
71. Lathrop A, Vandevusse L. Affirming motherhood: validation and invalidation in women's perinatal hospice narratives. *Birth.* (2011) 38:256–65. doi: 10.1111/j.1523-536X.2011.00478.x
72. Carter BS. Providing palliative care for newborns. *Pediatr Ann.* (2004) 33:770–7. doi: 10.3928/0090-4481-20041101-12
73. Kobler K, Limbo R. Making a case: creating a perinatal palliative care service using a perinatal bereavement program model. *J Perinat Neonatal Nurs.* (2011) 25:32–41. doi: 10.1097/JPN.0b013e3181fb592e
74. Klaus M, Kennell J, Klaus P. *Bonding: Building the Foundations of Secure Attachment and Independence.* Boston, MA: Da Capo Lifelong Books (1996).
75. Wool C, Limbo R, Denny-Koelsch EM. "I Would Do It All Over Again": cherishing time and the absence of regret in continuing a pregnancy after a life-limiting diagnosis. *J Clin Ethics.* (2018) 29:227–36.
76. Hasegawa SL, Fry JT. Moving toward a shared process: the impact of parent experiences on perinatal palliative care. *Semin Perinatol.* (2017) 41:95–100. doi: 10.1053/j.semperi.2016.11.002
77. Rocha Catania T, Bernardes L, Guerra Benute GR, Bento Cicaroni Gibeli MA, Bertolassi do Nascimento N, Aparecida Barbosa TV, et al. When one knows a fetus is expected to die: palliative care in the context of prenatal diagnosis of fetal malformations. *J Palliat Med.* (2017) 20:1020–31. doi: 10.1089/jpm.2016.0430
78. Carter BS, Brown JB, Brown S, Meyer EC. Four wishes for Aubrey. *J Perinatol.* (2012) 32:10–4. doi: 10.1038/jp.2011.171
79. Kukora SK, Boss RD. Values-based shared decision-making in the antenatal period. *Semin Fetal Neonatal Med.* (2018) 23:17–24. doi: 10.1016/j.siny.2017.09.003
80. Childers JW, Back AL, Tulsky JA, Arnold RM. REMAP: a framework for goals of care conversations. *J Oncol Pract.* (2017) 13:844–50. doi: 10.1200/JOP.2016.018796
81. Engelder S, Davies K, Zeilinger T, Rutledge D. A model program for perinatal palliative services. *Adv Neonatal Care.* (2012) 12:28–36. doi: 10.1097/ANC.0b013e318244031c
82. Kenner C, Press J, Ryan D. Recommendations for palliative and bereavement care in the NICU: a family-centered integrative approach. *J Perinatol.* (2015) 35:19–23. doi: 10.1038/jp.2015.145
83. Catlin A, Carter B. Creation of a neonatal end-of-life palliative care protocol. *J Perinatol.* (2002) 22:184–95. doi: 10.1038/sj.jp.7210687
84. National Hospice and Palliative Care Organization 2020. (2020). Available online at: https://www.nhpco.org/ (accessed May 29, 2020).
85. Denney-Koelsch E, Black BP, Côté-Arsenault D, Wool C, Kim S, Kavanaugh K. A survey of perinatal palliative care programs in the United States: structure, processes, and outcomes. *J Palliat Med.* (2016) 19:1080–6. doi: 10.1089/jpm.2015.0536

5

Fostering Vicarious Resilience for Perinatal Palliative Care Professionals

Kathryn R. Grauerholz[1*], *Michaelene Fredenburg*[1], *Premala Tara Jones*[1,2] *and Kristy N. Jenkins*[1]

[1] *Life Perspectives, San Diego, CA, United States,* [2] *Counseling and Testing Center, University of Akron, Akron, OH, United States*

***Correspondence:**
Kathryn R. Grauerholz
kathryn@lifeperspectives.com

Background: The demands on healthcare professionals caring for families grappling with a life-limiting condition in an unborn or newly born child can be overwhelming. Clinicians working in emergency/trauma, hospice, and pediatric settings are already at high risk for burnout and compassion fatigue, which can leave healthcare institutions increasingly vulnerable to poor retention, absenteeism, and waning quality of care. The provision of exemplary palliative care requires a cohesive interdisciplinary team of seasoned professionals resilient to daily challenges. In September 2019, the American College of Gynecology, in a committee opinion, published standard of care guidelines for perinatal palliative care. This has created an impetus for exceptional caregiving and a greater demand for both physician and interdisciplinary healthcare provider education, training, and ongoing support that promotes truly beneficent care for pregnant patients confronted with life-limiting fetal conditions.

Methods: A scoping review of the research literature was conducted in order to distinguish the barriers and facilitators of professional resiliency in perinatal palliative care. PubMed, Medline, CINAHL, and EBSCO Psychology & Behavioral Sciences Collections were systematically reviewed. Because of the paucity of studies specific to perinatal palliative care, several interviews of nurses and physicians in that field were conducted and analyzed for content distinctly pertaining to personal practices or workplace factors that support or hinder professional resiliency.

Results: The research indicated that medical professionals often cite a lack of knowledge, inexperience using effective communication skills related to perinatal palliative care and bereavement, challenges with interdisciplinary collaboration, misconceptions about the role and function of palliative care in the perinatal or neonatal settings, moral distress, and workload challenges as encumbrances to professional satisfaction. Strategic implementation of facility-wide bereavement care training, effective communication modalities, and evidenced-based practical applications are critical components for a thriving perinatal palliative care team. Authentic formal and informal debriefing, peer mentoring, adequate caseloads, robust provider self-care practices, exceptional relational efficacy, and cultural and spiritual humility can foster personal growth and even vicarious resilience for perinatal palliative care professionals.

Conclusions: Support should be strategic and multifaceted. The onus to implement salient measures to cultivate resilience in the perinatal palliative caregiver should not be only upon the individuals themselves but also upon prevailing regulatory governing bodies and healthcare institutions.

Keywords: perinatal, palliative, compassion, burnout, ethical, self-care, grief, resiliency

INTRODUCTION

Perinatal palliative care professionals have an integral role in the decision making and care delivery for many families encountering uncertain perinatal outcomes, some of which may have a reverberating and lasting impact. Palliative care champion Byock (1), in his 1997 book *Dying Well*, described how the time preceding a death can be a time of personal and spiritual growth for many. Researchers Côté-Arsenault et al. [(2), p. 12] said that "contrary to common societal reaction where focus is on what is wrong with the baby, [the study participants] focused on everything positive about their babies." The parents also said that their participation in the research study was a positive experience and added meaning to their children's short lives (2). Nurses in a study that explored their reactions to perinatal death revealed that when adequately supported, "growth and transformation" emerged from "the anguish and grief" (3). This article will systematically explore ways that professional caregivers can glean a fecundate resilience and vicarious personal growth sojourning with their patients who are enduring a life-limiting fetal diagnosis.

The loss of a child in infancy can be a profoundly traumatic experience. Psychologists Jaffe and Diamond (4) described in their 2011 book, *Reproductive Trauma: Psychotherapy with Infertility and Pregnancy Loss Clients,* the hopes and dreams that individuals envision for their future family long before conception. They also portrayed the trauma that can occur when those hopes and dreams go awry. The psychological ramifications when one's fundamental beliefs about themselves and their offspring are disrupted by a life-limiting antenatal diagnosis can be devastating. Lang et al. (5) demonstrated in their research that the death and dying of unborn or newly born children, though culturally disenfranchised, is as emotionally painful as the loss of an older child or adult family member. The researchers also concluded that because of the lack of social support, intrinsic to disenfranchised losses, parents' emotional reactions to perinatal losses tend to be particularly traumatic compared to more traditional types of losses (5). Doka [(6), p. 5] described disenfranchised grief as an experience that "is not openly acknowledged, socially validated, or publicly observed." The birth and/or untimely death of an infant and the associated grief reaction is outside of typical grieving norms, and parents can find themselves on an unworn path of bereavement.

The emotional impact on families confronted with a life-limiting fetal illness is often complex. At the time of diagnosis, parents may experience a variety of emotions including fear, shock, anger, anxiety, sadness, guilt, and even jealousy of other parents with healthy babies (7). The risk for severe psychological distress including depression, anxiety, and obsessive-compulsive behaviors was shown to be as much as five times higher in parents with a very low birth weight infant in comparison to parents with normal birth weight babies (8). In addition, some families have to cope with financial strain, time away from other family members, long commutes, and travel expenses (8). Furthermore, a couple planning a delivery or termination of a fetus with a life limiting condition is likely to encounter disagreements about their decision from healthcare professionals, family members, and friends. In the absence of multidisciplinary planning and support, the antenatal and postpartum bereavement has the potential to be fraught with ambivalence, shame, secrecy, and isolation. Those involved in the care provision may also find that, in the absence of personal resiliency practices, the persistent emotional strain is unsustainable (9, 10).

Palliative care teams, comprised of multidisciplinary professionals serving inpatient and home environments, are a relatively new concept in medical practice, particularly in pediatrics, and perinatal care. The team usually consists of two or more interdisciplinary professionals with complementary skills who collaborate and move toward common focused goals in the delivery of care (11). Team members often depend on and hold each other accountable for different complex and mutable aspects of palliative care. Perinatal teams are structured like adult and pediatric palliative care teams, which usually include medical care providers, social workers, chaplains, respiratory therapists, and lactation consultants. It is recommended that nurses and physicians in these teams be trained in obstetrics and neonatology (12). Because of improved technology and the earlier diagnoses of genetic anomalies and lethal malformations over the past four decades, expectant couples are now being counseled about the health of their unborn child earlier in the pregnancy. Since the onset of antenatal prognostication, the option of pregnancy termination was initially purported as the only measure to avoid suffering, and comfort-focused alternatives were not developed nor presented as a modality of care (13). Now, couples are being offered a broader spectrum of care that includes palliative and hospice provisions for their unborn (14). Thus, frequent acquiescence of the palliative professional's approach to varied patient care situations is essential, and enduring occupational resiliency is indispensable.

METHODS

A scoping review according to the methods described by (15) was used to explore and amplify the key factors necessary for promoting professional stability in the perinatal palliative setting (**Figure 1**). The scope of practice for perinatal palliative care is still evolving, but for the purposes of this study the field of reference was that outlined by the American College of Gynecology (14). There is a body of research that explores various aspects of self-care and supportive measures to prevent compassion fatigue and burnout in healthcare providers in pediatric and palliative settings, but there is a paucity of studies specific to perinatal palliative care. The search included systematic reviews, qualitative case studies, and quantitative survey studies that had been published in the past 11 years (January 2009–January 2020) (**Figure 1**). Searches were made in PubMed, Medline, CINAHL, and an EBSCO Psychology & Behavioral Sciences Collection. Search words included *perinatal, neonatal,* and/or *palliative* combined with the words *burnout, compassion fatigue,* or *resilience.* Relevant studies were identified from screening summary and abstracts. Full articles were analyzed for components associated with professional caregiver burnout, compassion fatigue, resilience, and satisfaction (**Table 1**). In addition, semi-structured interviews were conducted (**Table 2**). The participants included four registered nurses and two physicians involved in various perinatal palliative and hospice care programs in the following US cities: San Diego, CA; New York, NY; Denver, CO; and Flagstaff, AZ. The interview questions were emailed to the perinatal palliative professionals who had agreed to participate. They either composed and returned written responses or answered the questions in a phone call conducted by the primary author, which were then transcribed. The responses were aggregated and then the content was analyzed for facilitators and barriers to professional resilience by two coders who have graduate level education in nursing or psychology (**Table 3**). There was no specific funding utilized for the conduction of this study.

RESULTS

Database searches revealed 4,247 studies. Initial review and removal of duplicates, unavailable full-text article, marginal relevance to perinatal palliative care, and language barriers reduced to the search to 123 articles. Another 102 were removed because they did not report primary research. Therefore, 21 articles were selected. The literature review process and content analysis of the interviews yielded the following factors that contribute to distress in neonatal and palliative care professionals: challenges associated with both multi- and interdisciplinary collaboration, gaps in training, moral and ethical issues, misconceptions about the role and function of palliative care in the acute setting, and unfeasible workloads. Alternatively, components that supported resilience and career satisfaction included more comprehensive and interdisciplinary bereavement care training, formal and informal debriefing, supportive measures to strengthen teams and care delivery models, individualized self-care measures, and a humble approach to care provision that included both cultural and spiritual humility.

DISCUSSION

Palliative Care Collaboration

Professionals agree that initiating palliative care and education to the family as soon as possible after the devastating diagnosis procures more salient comfort measures, which, in turn, enhances the significance of the care received (16). Care demonstrated to be effective and relevant can improve caregiver satisfaction and resilience. A registered nurse and clinical coordinator of the Neonatal Comfort Care program at New York's Presbyterian Morgan Stanley Children's hospital, Fran McCarthy, recalled a recent case involving a mother who had just received the initial introduction with the comfort care program and staff when she delivered prematurely. A birth plan and end-of-life options and procedures had not yet been reviewed, nor had there been time to develop a trusting alliance. Consequently, the attending medical resident and nurses were distressed about the despondent mother's demands for continued and prolonged resuscitation measures that were not typically indicated for an infant born in the presented condition. The difficult timing issues resulted in a knowledge gap that, in turn, caused parental and staff distress. In contrast, McCarthy recalled that some of the cases she considered to be most optimal had been those in which the staff and the families had adequate time to prepare and nurture a reciprocal relationship prior to the birth of the child. Karen Christie, Registered Nurse Pediatric/Perinatal Case Manager at The Elizabeth Hospice in San Diego, also recalled that more affirming bereavement experiences occurred for families who had received maximum in-depth training and antepartum palliative care planning. In regard to one memorable encounter, Christie said, "I appreciated having continuity and the experience of being part of a spiritually uplifting situation observing the parents' joy in the life, albeit short, of their son."

Bereavement care initiated soon after an ominous prenatal diagnosis can address the anticipatory grief that parents often experience and help them cope with a loss that is typically multifaceted (17, 18). Perinatal palliative care teams aim to mitigate the trauma of disenfranchised grief through supportive modalities, ongoing education, and active care for patients and their families throughout the perinatal and bereavement periods (12, 19). In several studies (2, 20–22), Côté-Arsenault demonstrated how professionals providing effective family-centered palliative support can potentially optimize the parents' adjustment to the painful event. Many parents also reported feeling fulfilled and even joyful to have had the short time to parent and love their severely ill children (2, 21).

Moral, Ethical Issues, and Misconceptions

Palliative, neonatal, and obstetric care teams have had to become increasingly flexible to varying patient values and desires for the trajectory of their pregnancy. The increasing scope in the range of care delivery options has not occurred in the absence of moral distress experienced by those providing the care (23–25). When interviewed about the barriers and challenges to keeping a cohesive and effective palliative care team together, the medical director of the Perinatal/Pediatric Hospice Program at The Elizabeth Hospice and a family practice in San Diego,

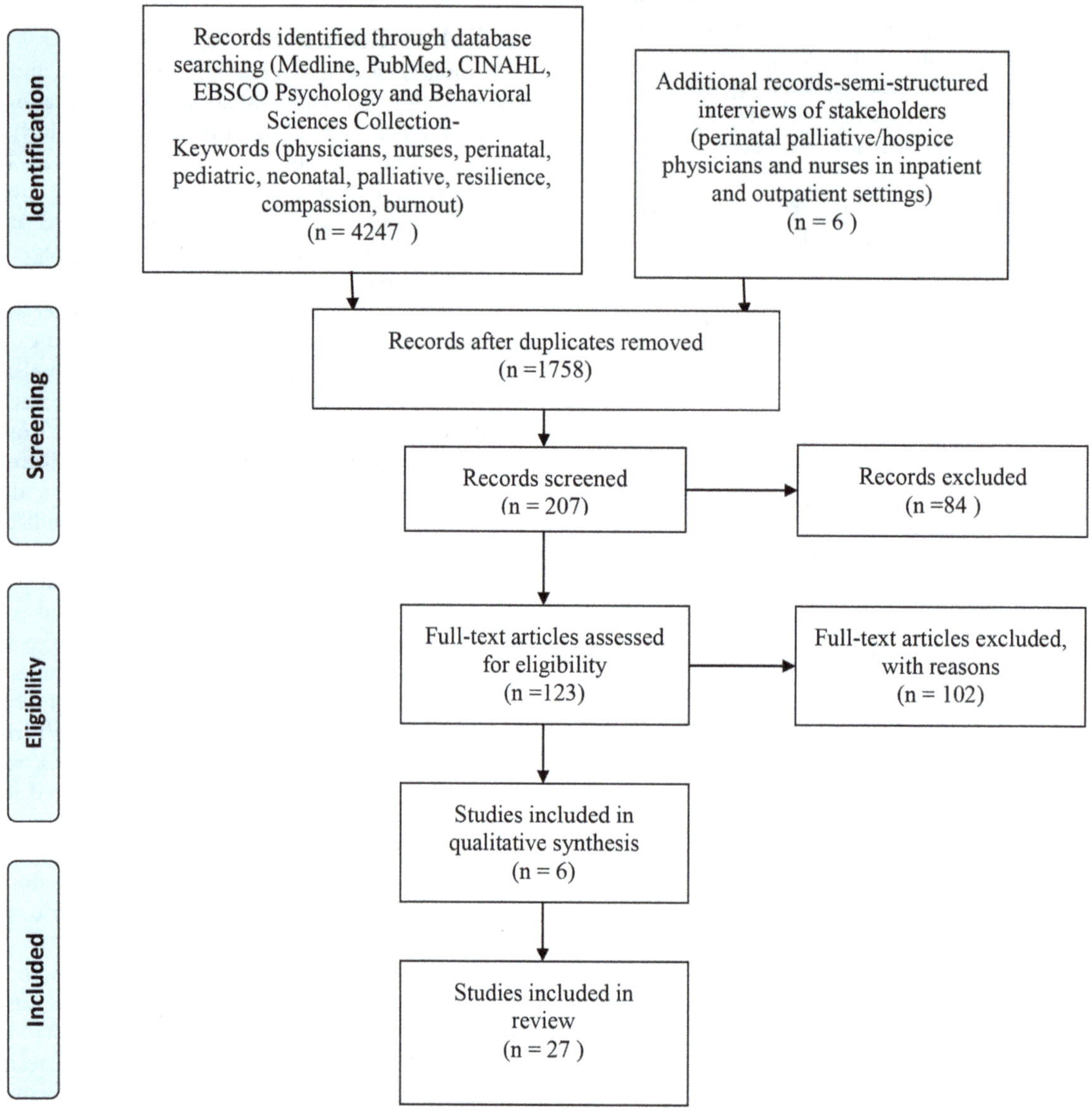

FIGURE 1 | Flow diagram of article section process.

Dr. George Delgado, said the "challenges include emotional stress, compassion fatigue, ethical dilemmas, and cost-cutting across healthcare." From his experience most of the conflicts are ethical, extending from contrasting societal philosophical axioms influencing healthcare, which can leave professionals in an ideological betwixt and between in the delivery of care. Ethical dilemmas not only surround the termination of a live fetus but also accompany the initiation and continuation of life-sustaining treatments that can be perceived as a prolongation of suffering and an exercise in futility for an infant bound to die (24, 26, 27). Both options are indicated as palliative options on the spectrum of services for those diagnosed with life-limiting fetal malformations by the American College of Obstetrics and Gynecology (14). Emerging perinatal palliative care programs are involved in the provision of comfort care to the neonate that neither aims to hasten death nor aggressively prolong life.

Additionally, moral distress can occur when professionals experience reluctance advocating the interests of their patients for fear of discord with the parental prerogative or institutional constraints (28, 29). Practitioners delivering direct patient care in acute situations are more vulnerable to moral distress, which can lead to burnout and staff retention issues (30, 31). Strategies for addressing and alleviating moral distress include frequent communication with the family, clarifying patient understanding of diagnosis/prognosis, engaging in ongoing goal setting, discussing the ethical issues, increasing team collaborative efforts, and using a skilled ethics facilitator for high levels of distress (23, 32).

Misconceptions surrounding the goals and spectrum of palliative care are often the most challenging aspects of its provision and collaboration amid the dominant curative culture of medicine. Caregivers may also deduce that their service

TABLE 1 | Study descriptions and details.

Author(s)	Year of publication	Aim of Study	Methodology	Findings summary
Back et al.	2016	Examine the approaches to building resilience in palliative care physicians—clinician resilience skills & workplace factors	Literature review and stakeholder interviews	Introduced a structural model of individual skills and system construction that support professional resilience
Cortezzo et al.	2019	Study of birth planning for life-limiting fetal diagnosis from both the patient and parents' perspectives	Mixed methods, quantitative-descriptive & univariate analysis; qualitative-thematic analysis	Proposed eliciting parental preferences for greater participation and decision making. Physician comfort levels were adequate, but found that time limitations made communication aspects with birth planning was most unfeasible aspect
Cortezzo et al.	2015	Explore the practices and perceptions of end-of-life care in NICU—examined patient and provider experiences	Survey study- explorative, description cross-sectional evaluation	Found debriefing/closure conferences, bereavement support, and education provision was variable and suboptimal at times. Value of formal palliative care teams rather than individual consultants ascertained.
Forster and Hafiz	2015	Explore the coping strategies and perceptions of support available to professionals encountering pediatric death	Qualitative: multidisciplinary professional interviews	Personal coping strategies, peer support, family support, spiritual beliefs, relational efficacy when caring for the dying child and family all improved coping
Hamric	2014	Illustrate ethical issues and moral distress associated with end-of-life issues that occur in the NICU which impact perinatal palliative care provision.	Case study	Expounded ethical climate building with debriefing, improving communication, multidisciplinary care conferences, and resilience factors
Hutti et al.	2016	Evaluate nurses reactions to caregiving for patient experiencing fetal demise	Recorded group discussions structured by Swanson's Theory of Caring was analyzed	Risks for compassion fatigue were revealed. Coping strategies and interventions based on latest research was presented which included debriefing, mentoring, more perinatal bereavement education, and self-care practices were implicated.
Jonas-Simpson et al.	2016	Explore thematic patterns of obstetrical or neonatal nurse's grief experiences to perinatal death	Qualitative study: interpretive phenomenology	Thematic patterns included: Growth and transformation emerging with anguish and grief, collegial supports, education, aspects of reciprocal mentorship, the intrinsic value of compassionate caregiving
Kamal et al.	2016	Examine the prevalence and predicting factors associated with burnout rates in hospital and palliative care clinicians in the U.S.	Quantitative: Survey study and statistical analysis	Higher rates of burnout correlated with emotional exhaustion and depersonalization, working at smaller organizations, extended work hours, age < 50, and working weekends. Activities related to interpersonal relationships and vacation use were associated with less burnout rates.
Klein	2009	Study issues of ethical dilemma and moral distress in pediatric palliative care—infants born with severe life-limiting anomalies	Case studies	Prognostication challenges, cultural, and social factors can cause moral distress in parents and palliative staff. Beliefs and aspects regarding the suffering of the infant can create emotional dilemma. Ethics and palliative care collaboration can be supportive to staff and caregivers.
Kilcullen and Ireland	2017	Present facilitators and barriers to palliative care provision in an Australian NICU	Qualitative: Thematic analysis of semi-structured interviews	Facilitators of the provision of palliative care included: cultural awareness, experienced and proficient mentors and supportive staff, clinical skills and knowledge, personal knowledge of one's own values, morals, & beliefs, emotional & communication skills, and knowledge of bereavement practices. Barriers to the provision of palliative care included: lack of education/inservices, workspace environment, parents' inaccessibility to infant, nurses' own grief, and included input into development of policies and procedures.
McCloskey and Taggart	2010	Probe the occupational stressors of pediatric palliative care nurses	Qualitative focus group discussions: thematic content analysis	Workload demands included: emotional, ethical, constraints to care delivery, lack of resources, documentation, community misconceptions, maintaining relationships with patient & family, and cultivating autonomy within the profession
Mehta et al.	2016	Study aspects of palliative care teams- pilot study of model for team resilience	Quantitative- Resiliency model testing with physicians	Team building measured a feasible reduction in perceived stress, and improved the perspective taking of the others in the team

(Continued)

TABLE 1 | Continued

Author(s)	Year of publication	Aim of Study	Methodology	Findings summary
Mills et al.	2017	Evaluate perceptions, education, and practices related to self-care in palliative nurses and medical professionals in Australia	Survey studies	Self-care was regarded as important by most. Many had not practiced self-care and also denied having any education on self-care. A large portion of those reported that self-care plans would be considered if training was provided.
Mills et al.	2018	Explore the meaning and practice of self-care in palliative nurses and physicians	Qualitative content analysis of semi-structured interviews	A practice of self-care contributed to a better capacity to care for others. Self-care practices in both occupational and personal settings is necessary. Facilitators of self-care practices included supportive environments, self-assessment, prioritization, and an ongoing planning process. Barriers included overwhelming workload & excessive busyness, stigma against self-care at the workplace, low self-worth or self-criticism, and lack of planning.
Perez et al.	2015	Examine the barriers and facilitators of resiliency in palliative care clinicians	Qualitative: content analysis of semi-structured interviews	Identified stressors, coping strategies, and training needs. Stressors included limited resources & cost-cutting, conflicting interdisciplinary expectations, increased caseloads, intensity of the cases, boundary setting, personal & professional limitations, competing demands from administrative & documentation activities, patients, & staff. Coping strategies included personal self-care, emotional & physical distancing from work off the clock, and social & emotional supports. Training needs included mind-body skills, stress education, cognitive stress management skills, and brief coping strategies to implement in real time.
Profit et al.	2014	Explore aspects of burnout and resilience in NICU	Cross-sectional surveys	NICUs with higher levels of burnout were correlated with a reduced teamwork climate, safety climate, job satisfaction, perceptions of management, and working conditions. A resilient culture was show to enhance safety and quality of care.
Sanso et al.	2015	Determine the relationship between self-care & awareness and development of burnout, compassion fatigue, and coping with death in palliative care professionals	Quantitative- survey study	Self-care and self-awareness improved coping with death and compassion satisfaction, less burnout and compassion fatigue. The data collection after the spiritual training exercises did not have those desired effects.
Dev et al.	2018	Evaluate the relationship between barriers to compassion and burnout in nurses.	Quantitative study: survey	Barriers to compassion, contributors to burnout included workload, clinical barriers, practice of self-compassion, encounters with patient and families
Weitraub et al.	2016	Contrast physician burnout, compassion fatigue, and compassion satisfaction	Quantitative study: linear regression analysis	Overlapping of burnout and compassion fatigue found. Impacts emotional well-being and professional performance of neonatologists. Self-identifying as being Hispanic debriefing and utilization of pediatric palliative care services resulted in compassion satisfaction.
Wright et al.	2011	Examine the facilitators and barriers to the provision of end-of-life care in the NICU settings from the perspectives of neonatal nurses.	Quantitative: Questionnaire survey study	Five barriers were identified as: inability to express values and beliefs regarding palliative care, environmental constraints, engagement in technology, demands from parents, and lack of education. Eight facilitators identified as: staff support, involvement of parents in decision making, support from medical team when palliative care was implemented, parents informed of options, staffing, time allotment with dying baby, policies/guidelines that supported palliative care, and available counseling.
Zwack and Schweitzer	2013	Analyze stakeholder interviews regarding aspects of burnout and resilience	Qualitative study: Concept analysis	Both attitudes and strategies (social, mental, and physical) assisted physicians' success to augment decision making, coping, and promoting resilience in others.

TABLE 2 | Interview questions based on initial research review.

Please avoid including any patient identification information that would violate HIPAA regulations.
1. Tell me about your experience as a healthcare professional involved in caring for pregnant patients confronted with life-limiting fetal conditions?(Certification, length of time, positions)
2. Are there any particularly memorable experiences when you felt the care received by the patient and the child was at its best?
3. Can you recount an experience when you felt that the care and/or prognostication process were less than ideal for the situation?
4. How often does it seem like there is one or more members on the palliative/hospice care team that are in disagreement with the plan of care? (An estimate of average amount of time)
5. Have there been times when you disagreed with the plan of care and felt morally conflicted by the care given? Do these situations occur more often with particular diagnoses rather than others?
6. What types of interdisciplinary issues seem to cause the most conflict in creating and carrying out a plan of care?
7. Does it ever seem like residue of past distress over patient care experiences effects the quality of care that you provide now?
8. Does it seem difficult to keep a cohesive and effective palliative care team together? What do you think are the barriers or challenges?
9. In what way have you changed as a provider than you were when you began providing perinatal palliative care/hospice?
10. Is there someone who was a mentor to you when beginning this type of work? Now?
11. What did the mentor do that was helpful to your professional development?
12. Do you have particular self-care practices that are helpful in managing work related tension or distress? How long have you been practicing these?
13. Does your employer provide any supports to well-being at work or for off-work hours?
14. Do you have any ideas about methods of self-care that could be provided in the work place or by your employer that would be beneficial to employee well-being?

efforts are marginalized when the modality of palliation is disparaged within the healthcare system. Despite decades of research, misunderstandings and erroneous beliefs surrounding the value of palliative care, particularly in the inpatient setting, have been pervasive. Grunauer and Mikesell [(33), p. 3] listed the more prevalent misconceptions regarding the implementation of palliative care in intensive care units as:

> [It] is (1) ineffective and unimportant for most ICU patients, (2) synonymous with hospice and hopeless on the part of the family, patients, and/or clinician, (3) equivalent to the "soft skills" that health-care professionals already innately have, and (4) wasteful in that it absorbs valuable time and resources from intensivists.

However, they went on to state that none of these misconceptions were supported by research. In fact, multiple studies show that initiation of palliative care in a timely manner can improve symptom control, professional communication, the patient's perception of their quality of life, and even lengthen survival times (33). Dispelling the myths about palliative care and holistic care for neonates and infants with life limiting conditions and their families can be accomplished with ongoing education provided to the entire caregiving staff within each unit (18, 33, 34). More research and widespread education can enhance the appreciation of palliative care, which can foster a benevolent environment. Dr. Elvira Parravicini, M.D., neonatologist from Columbia University Irving Medical Center, said that "most obstetricians have come along to supporting us after seeing the benefits and appreciation from the patient of what we have done for them."

Professional Strength

Professional caregivers experiencing distress and high levels of stress have been associated with the development of cynicism, depersonalization of patients, diminished professional satisfaction, impaired decision making, medical errors, increased rates of adverse events, and higher mental and physical morbidities (9, 10, 35). Compassion fatigue or secondary traumatic stress disorder can also occur when empathetic caregivers experience, through a phenomenon known as countertransference, the trauma of their patients. Figley (36) coined the term *compassion fatigue* when he examined his own reaction to caring for military veterans debriefing from their traumatic combat experiences. He (36) said this regarding the personal anguish he encountered: "We feel the feelings of our clients. We experience their fears. We dream their dreams. Eventually, we lose a certain spark of optimism, humor and hope. We tire. We aren't sick, but we are not ourselves."

Palliative and hospice professionals have higher rates of burnout and compassion fatigue than most other specialists with rates averaging as much as 61% in some studies (9, 37). Increased levels of distress and burnout can lead to absenteeism and negatively impact the palliative care team (38). Efforts to mitigate burnout and compassion fatigue are not without significant benefits for both the patient and the caregiver (39). Long-term job satisfaction can also flourish from relational efficacy (40).

Fostering Resilience

Hernandez et al. (41) revealed that vicarious resilience occurs when professional caregivers experience their own growth through the provision of care and witness of patients enduring and recovering from traumatic experiences. Author van Dernoot Lipsky [(42), p. 11] wrote, "Those who support trauma stewardship believe that joy and pain are realities of life, and that suffering can be transformed into meaningful growth and healing when a quality of presence is cultivated and maintained even in the face of great suffering." Therefore, a self-assessment to determine one's level of compassion fatigue or professional satisfaction is essential. The Professional Quality of Life Measure (ProQol) is a tool found to be useful for this appraisal (43). Self-care has been found to be a key aspect in developing resilience and maintaining an instrumental presence in the midst of suffering and loss (10, 35, 44, 45).

Resilience is an individual's ability to cope with adversity and maintain a healthy response to stressors (46). Effective coping and resilience can be nurtured by participation in a variety of

TABLE 3 | Pertinent, categorized quotations from palliative professionals' interviews.

Palliative Care Collaboration

"The family and staff became well acquainted with the [palliative] goals of care and the relationship with the palliative established prior to the delivery."

"A patient with a complex relationship with [her] partner was recently handled well with multi-disciplinary support we had available for her."

"The social worker continued contact and visits with family, providing psychosocial support, birth plan guidance and memory making tools."

"The baby was stillborn, and parents' needs were met, however I felt they would have had more support if they had let the team be more involved."

"We have a great deal of respect for each other. We have extreme trust in each other. We all are in agreement about the mission and vision of our program."

"Most professionals in other disciplines (speech pathology, lactation consultants, chaplains, and child-life therapist) admire the work of our program, moreover there are some who are very comfortable with palliative care and help us a lot facilitating comfort for babies and support for parents. I believe that no professional in our institution has been in conflict with our program. Most obstetricians have come along to supporting us after seeing the benefits and appreciation from the patients of what we have done for them."

Moral, Ethical Issues, and Misconceptions

"The mother was a nurse and asked for oxygen and pain meds to prevent her baby from suffering. Although the healthcare team knew this to be unnecessary nor beneficial, we accommodated the mother's request to empower her during this time. By doing so, she was able to have the motherly control to help her during the grieving process."

"More disagreements occur with other specialties like maternal-fetal medicine physicians or when staff members are not understanding role of perinatal palliative care."

"[Conflict] often occurs because medical professionals feel compelled to suggest abortion whenever there is an anomaly."

"Sometimes the parents choose not to feed the baby, even if feeding might be tolerated."

"Sometimes other professionals have questioned our plan of care because they have a different mindset and are not familiar with a palliative care approach. However, when they see the results, the comfort of the baby and parental satisfaction, they come along and they want to learn more about it."

"Mostly the conflicts are ethical. Many team members are utilitarian in their ethical approaches, not out of malice but due to the prevailing utilitarian ethic in medicine."

"There was one situation where the baby was born severely malformed and the parents had the school age children take pictures with baby who did not have severe brain malformation covered. My concern was the internal difficulties the children may have had with viewing the malformation, although externally they presented as accepting."

"In many institutions, babies with life-limiting conditions are not fed at all, we prefer to offer food for comfort, unless the baby is in end of life stage. The experience of feeding their baby is very important for parents, we had babies who lived for only a couple of days successfully breast-fed. We also strongly believe that is comfortable to end life with a 'full stomach'."

"Sometimes bedside caregivers are morally conflicted and concerned about the futility of care and suffering."

Professional Strength

"I think each patient's experience is different. Their needs are catered differently. Providing that compassion for the families actually allows me to use my vocation as a nurse to my utmost ability. I think that's when my quality of care is the strongest."

"Occasional vacancies are difficult in the neonatal intensive care unit and palliative programs."

"I have become more open minded and attentive. I look at each single patient and look to them to tell me through objective signs and cues as to what to do for them. It is a tremendous gift to learn from my little patients and from their parents."

Educational Strategies

"Field staff are offered presentations and webinars including those on compassion fatigue and burnout."

"Bedside staff [report] not feeling comfortable with nature of palliative care. [It is because of] a lack of training and experience. [They are] used to curative goals."

"The perinatal palliative program was difficult when it was located on the postpartum unit, because the nurses had a hard time transitioning to a palliative approach."

"Babies die differently than other children and the outpatient hospice nurses not always educated to the differences. For instance a baby with trisomy 18 will have a different breathing patterns than typical counterparts."

"My previous experience taking care of hospice patients or elderly as they passed was quite different than taking care of families that lost their babies. The grieving seems to have different, complex elements to it."

Formal and Informal Debriefing

"Our team works very well together and we have discussions, planning, and debriefing as a team. We are friends, a tight, knit group, and are not afraid to express concerns to each other."

"Debriefing is a huge benefit to me. I find that debriefing immediately after a case before going home helps me to relieve that pressure in my heart and mind. It helps me learn from mistakes and set goals for myself for improvement. I also like to call a friend that understands my line of work to debrief with."

"Personally, I think a standardized debriefing practice after unexpected events or difficult situations can promote/be connected to self-care. It is possible that until a situation is debriefed and talked through do healthcare workers really realize how they are feeling about a situation."

"The hospital provides more formal team debriefing on caseloads and challenging cases- increasing and improving these processes."

"In addition, debriefing is essential. It can be a formal debrief or decompressing with a coworker about what happened, how I feel about it, etc. The process of 'talking things through' not only helps me digest the situation, learn from it and grown as a nurse."

Care Delivery Models

"In the world of [maternity care], we are able to provide the time and compassion to help families during these difficult times. Fortunately, fetal demise or palliative care is staffed as a one-to-one care."

"The family expressed their gratefulness afterward that they were able to spend as much time with their baby prior to her death at home, and that her last days were not spent in the hospital. Parents were especially grateful for having avoided the surgery because clearly her death was associated with brain stem anomalies."

Self-Care Initiatives

"This realization can point to the need of self-care and additional supportive interventions."

"They have Reiki, chair massages, hand massages. However, these work best for the people in the office."

"Yes, they provide mental health and debriefing sessions upon request. Also, our clinical manager is very supportive in terms of allowing time to grieve or leave of absence if needed."

"My previous employer and management team were always very supportive and had definitely cared about the overall well-being of the staff. It helps that nurse managers and directors know what it's like as a floor nurse and the difficult situations surrounding [perinatal care] so they know from experience the importance of support, self-care and promoting overall well-being of their staff."

(Continued)

TABLE 3 | Continued

"[My employer] offers plenty of opportunities for employees such as arranged lunches for nurses and physicians, even nicely arranged coffee breaks. They also offer different exercise programs, yoga, and counseling services. I haven't participated in any of these, I believe because I have so much help through my team and my friends."
"[Our routine team] meetings have time for bereavement and support. Additionally, we have an employee assistance program."
"[I] exercise, garden, and do a lot of home maintenance. I am also very involved with family, grandchildren that live nearby."
"Mostly, I enjoy the friendship of many people. My friends care for my psychological needs. I also sing in a choir."
"I have been practicing self-care all of my career. However, am much more organized now in active planning of self-care. Spiritual discussions and personal involvement with an excellent small group of very close friends (most of them work in hospice) and family; owning and interacting with dogs; daily walks and stretching exercises; massage and chiropractic care; keeping up with medical and dental routine care and issues (years ago I delayed these until they became urgent). My belief is that one can only do any type of hospice and palliative care with a wide variety, and regular, self-care activities."
Cultural and Spiritual Humility
"The family was also able to sing praise and worship songs to their lovely daughter and love on her."
"I appreciated having continuity and the experience of being a part of a spiritually uplifting situation observing the parents' joy in the life, albeit short, of their son."
"We also rely on the parents to tell us what they think their child needs. They are more intuitive about their own child's needs."
"Honestly, I pray to Mother Mary a lot during my times of distress. If anyone understands what these patients are going through, it's [Mary]. I pray that she helps and guides me as well."
"[An] anencephalic baby delivered at hospital before I arrived. I baptized the baby, [as the parents were] fearing that a priest or deacon would not arrive in time. We provided comfort to the baby including time on breast."
"I keep in mind that 'I am not God'. I cannot solve everything. Our time is finite, just a drop in the ocean."
"Taking into account their cultural background also is important. Sometimes, the conflicts occur within the partnership of the parents and their cultural differences."

self-care practices such as physical activity, mindful focusing, meditation, breathing exercises, and positive interactions with colleagues and friends (47). Hutti [(48), p. 25] found that "nurses reported strength to cope primarily from three sources: faith, relationships with fellow health care providers, and their own families." Active involvement in a range of personal and employer organized supportive care strategies can augment coping, effective decision-making, and ultimately caregiver resilience in the midst of stressful workplace conditions (40). Dr. Parravinici said in regards to her comfort care team professionals, "We are friends, a tight knit group, and are not afraid to express concerns to each other. My friends care for my psychological needs. For instance, my nurse coordinator tells me things like 'slow down,' 'go home,' or 'be realistic' when I need to hear it."

A cohesive team is essential to the delivery of effective and beneficial palliative care in the perinatal/neonatal setting. Teams that have a well-defined program mission, vision, and goals that are fully embraced by each of the constituents are in an advantageous position to provide the necessary support for both individual and team resilience (11, 49). When the role of each team member is clearly delineated and in agreement with shared aspects of palliative care, the team as a whole benefits (11). Other aspects that can define the efficacy of a team include clear workload or productivity expectations, established lines of accountability, and a constructive evaluation process (49). Fostering respect and appreciation of the individual team members and the team as a whole requires evolving trust, open communication, prompt conflict resolution, and a shared movement toward common goals. Tempering factors that impair team function such as absenteeism, ongoing conflict, poor team structure, insufficient training, fear of conflict, and lack of commitment and accountability can help mitigate team erosion (49).

Studies have shown that caseloads perceived to be manageable by care providers often coincide with professional satisfaction and resilience. Keeton and colleagues [(50), p. 954] said that the "strongest single predictor of emotional resilience and personal accomplishment was control over schedule and hours worked." Burnout and emotional exhaustion have been attributed to an increased workload (31, 51, 52). Specifically, palliative care providers reported more difficulty managing increasing caseloads because of the challenges in estimating the length of time needed for the provision of individual care plans, locating the family members involved in the care, and collaborating with the other team members (47, 53). In order to address issues related to absenteeism, employee retention, and burnout, healthcare institutions and legislative entities should carefully examine staffing polices and reimbursement guidelines (9).

Educational Strategies

Lack of education and training has frequently been cited as a barrier to the provision of consistent and comprehensive palliative and bereavement support in the neonatal setting (7, 54–57). Haug et al. (55) demonstrated, in a nationwide study, that fewer than a third of institutions offer any formal training for physicians or staff on perinatal palliative or comfort care. However, research has shown that professionals exhibit better emotional coping when they have been provided with education related to bereavement and end-of-life issues (56, 58–60). For example, a strong majority (91.8%) of neonatologists involved in that study indicated that increased education in perinatal palliative and end-of-life care would be beneficial (55). Elements of self-care activity, as well as the symptoms and risk factors for both burnout and compassion fatigue, should be included in the education for perinatal palliative care professionals (7, 61). An enhanced knowledge base can increase caregiver confidence when serving patients.

A commitment to continuous learning is key to providing the best possible care for patients (62). "Staff education should be provided during orientation and then periodically throughout the course of every year" [(7), p. S30]. Palliative and bereavement care training with a multifaceted approach improves caregiver communication and confidence. Allyson McCullough, Registered Nurse and Bereavement Care Coordinator at

Bella Natural Women's Care & Family Medicine and former Bereavement Care Coordinator on an inpatient maternity ward, said, "As a new nurse, I was uncomfortable ... and felt that I needed to fill the silence with saying the right thing." She went on to explain that education and experience have improved her confidence in communicating with and comforting patients.

Wilkinson and Roberts (63) demonstrated that it is most beneficial to use a range of teaching methods to nurture effective communication techniques. Utilizing experts for on-site training to facilitate group analyses of case studies, role-playing exercises, and demonstrations is an effective means of teaching professional caregivers techniques that will improve their comfort level in delivering bad news and confidence in supporting the family. According to Sweeney et al. [(64), p. 14], role-play is particularly impactful, stating:

> [It] led to increased understanding of and changes in attitudes toward key palliative care principles, interdisciplinary teamwork, and communication of bad news. There was evidence of increased self-awareness. Findings suggest that the interdisciplinary breaking bad news role-play was a [particularly] rich integrative learning experience valued by students.

Professional caregivers who communicate effectively with parents facing a life-threatening illness in a neonate have been shown to have more professional confidence and better patient rapport. Increasing self-awareness, practicing specific responses via role-play activities, improving eye contact and body language, and learning to mirror a patient's own language are key components of providing quality patient care. Boles [(65), p. 307] asserts that empathy, sensitivity, active listening, a calming presence, and advocacy are essential skills "all nurses and psychosocial staff are called to provide at various points in the patient and family's illness journey." McCullough also said, "[it] is often not what you say, but [in] the things not said—the non-verbal communication [and] body language, sitting with the family, holding their hand, crying with them, sitting in silence, and meeting them where they are." Caregivers can provide an environment conducive to emotional healing by acknowledging the individual's feelings, withholding judgmental comments, reassuring them that they are not alone, and essentially giving them permission to grieve.

Patients and families grappling with the life-limiting diagnosis of an unborn or newly born child often report feeling powerless and marginalized in their involvement of care for their child (18). The provision of practical applications to assist the family bonding with and memorializing their severely ill or deceased neonate can empower both the bereaved and the caregivers. Providing personalized care that is directed in part by the patient or parent also fosters relational efficacy and provider resilience (40). Côté-Arsenault (2) said, "Parents in [her] study chose to focus their love and attention on what they could do at the present moment and on memory making," which included memorialization, photography, and comfort measures. Examples of patient-focused care include recognizing physical cues from the baby and asking the parent to assist in determining their child's needs such as holding, skin-to-skin time, breastfeeding, and assessing for comfort, hunger, thirst, and cold (19).

Formal and Informal Debriefing

Research indicates a beneficial advantage to members of a palliative team when they all participate as a group in scheduled discussions about the plan of care, appropriateness of the interventions, and the need for ongoing intensive support (39, 66, 67). Opportunities for formal debriefing should occur after every death and can be arranged to allow for reflection, quality improvement, shared narrative from the staff, and improved interdisciplinary cohesion (67). Many care teams have found that the utilization of a facilitator at these meetings can enhance the debriefing experience. For employers, it is important to note that stress management modalities and pre-incident education improve effective coping after encountering traumatic events (68).

Informal debriefing to a trusted colleague or mentor immediately or soon after a death or traumatic experience can also assist in mitigating the impact and facilitate personal emotional recovery (50, 69, 70). Also, small groups following a standardized debriefing process can help to ensure that all aspects of the incident were appropriately handled and allow for review from multiple perspectives (68). A nurse educator for the maternal ward at Flagstaff Medical Center reported, "I find that debriefing immediately after a case before going home helps me to relieve that pressure in my heart and in my mind." She also reported that her employer had provided ample formal debriefing and mental health assistance, which she thought was indeed helpful for those caregivers needing more intense or prolonged assistance.

Care Delivery Models

An institution should consider the manner in which perinatal palliative care is integrated with each unit. Currently there are two palliative care models integrated into the healthcare system. One model comprises a core group of professionals who provide consultation and care for families meeting the criteria for palliative care. Another model of care educates and trains the entire staff to provide palliative care (71). Casarett et al. [(71), p. 653] found that "families reported better outcomes when the patient received care in a palliative unit than they did when the patient received a palliative care consultation." A pattern of favorable outcomes can fuel compassion satisfaction and foster resilience in the care provider.

In 2002, Catlin and Carter (28) deciphered that those staff members willing to provide perinatal palliative care should be the ones primarily involved in its provision rather than it being required of all in a given unit. However, Mancini (67) countered that all staff members should receive the training to care for any patient they are presented with including those needing end-of-life care. The physicians and nurses I interviewed reported that they had colleagues who had expressed their discomfort with the provision of palliative and end-of-life support and avoided assignments requiring it. A neonatal nurse from Flagstaff, Arizona, said in an interview, "having dedicated members is a challenge because that's usually not the reason why nurses went into this specialty [maternal/child nursing] in the first place ... [and] it takes a toll [on the nurse] emotionally, physically, and psychologically." Her statements underscore the need for increased training in palliative and end-of-life care early on in each professional education track. Ongoing education provided to the entire staff about palliative and end-of-life care should train and equip all staff with basic communication modalities to be compassionate and comforting in their interactions with patients. In 2019, Wool and Catlin [(34), p. S28] reported that "an integrated system of care increases quality and safety and contributes to patient satisfaction. The goal for respectful caregiving throughout the entire hospital system is achievable." Professionals should feel free to disclose moral distress and receive the debriefing, spiritual, and emotional support necessary for a manageable resolution and promotion of ongoing occupational resilience (67).

In 2018, U.S. reproductive grief care experts Michaelene Fredenburg and Katie Geppert provided training for all staff members of the Ukrainian L'Viv Children's Hospital Perinatal Unit. The nurses who organized the event indicated that a high incidence of neonatal death and the staff's lack of knowledge about reproductive grief were the galvanizing motivations. The entire unit participated in the training including physicians, nurses, medical assistants, and anesthesiologists as well as social workers and a hospital chaplain. Nurses attending to the NICU patients also listened to the presentation on headsets.

Participants were introduced to research and concepts related to the unique nature of reproductive loss (5), disenfranchised grief (6), and the tasks of grieving (72). Evidence-based grief care best practices were shared as well as basic self-care ideas. Frequent staff debriefings were also recommended. After an uncomfortable amount of silence during the time allotted for questions, one of the nurses ventured to admit, "Please don't interpret our silence as disagreement, it's just that we culturally haven't been allowed to discuss this topic. Thank you for giving us the words and for giving us permission to talk to each other and to the parents of our patients." Concertedly affirmed by the rest of the staff with applause and inquiries, the medical director pledged to adopt the recommended reproductive grief care and self-care policies. Months later, the nurses who had organized the in-service confirmed enhanced patient care and improved staff morale after the training.

Self-Care Initiatives

Self-care is an imperative component to abating compassion fatigue (47, 73). One study reported that only 11% of the participating nurses and doctors practiced self-care [(74), p. 628]. Only 6% of that study's participants had an active self-care plan, and of those respondents "100% reported that they found the use of a self-care plan to be an effective self-care strategy" [(74), p. 627]. Koch and Jones [(30), p. 10] reported, "self-care is not only preventative for practitioners but can serve as a model for family caregivers about the critical importance of self-compassion and care." Earnest intention to care for oneself can, in turn, result in an enhanced capacity for empathy and the service of others. Progressive resilience can be cultivated through a concerted and intentional effort to develop, implement, and fulfill a self-care plan.

The care provider should make an inventory of aspects of their personal and work practices that contribute to both distress and wellness (40, 46). The dimensions of holistic-wellness plans are multifactorial requiring attention to the mind, body, spirituality, and emotions (47, 75–77). Initially, a plan that includes pertinent goals and methods of accountability should be strategically developed. The anticipation of potential barriers can help the individual avoid being derailed from their pursuit (78). Diligent attention to potential subversions can foster timely attainment of the desired outcomes (79). Enlisting the assistance of a supportive person(s) to partner in the interventions and process of evaluating goals can improve accountability and overall beneficence (80). Care providers find that the creation of a written plan or contract for themselves is a motivating factor for their intended endeavor.

A cadre of wellness programs are often available at larger institutions. Kase et al. [(76), p. 3] found that only 60% of pediatric physicians had participated in those programs and their reasons for not partaking in them included "inconvenience of scheduling" (45.3%), time constraints (27.2%), the preference of participants to "handle things on my own" (34.1%), and the sentiment that partaking in the activity would not be helpful (21.9%). Studies have found that "one-size-fits-all" wellness programs offered by an institution might not effectively address specific needs of their employees and professional affiliates (76, 78, 79). Parravicini concurred, stating, "What people find to be helpful for self-care is a highly individual matter. Some prefer tennis, some skiing, some a walk in the park, others getting a beer." Individualized discussions regarding the implementation of self-care strategies that include goals to be accomplished outside the work environment and continuing education can be integrated into occupational debriefing and evaluation conversations. Use of a self-administered assessment tool such as the Professional Quality of Life Assessment (43) or the Self-Care Assessment Worksheet (80) in planned intervals can assist in evaluating favorable progression toward the desired benefits (81).

A self-care plan would be ill equipped if it did not involve caring for personal losses. Caregivers cannot adequately assist others when they ignore their own bereavement, and they should not impose nor inject their personal grief experience into the care of others (82). James and Gilliand (82) observed that the palliative care provider can experience bereavement challenges when they encounter multiple meaningful losses in their domestic and occupational environments. They can find themselves overloaded emotionally and need more time to invest in adequate bereavement (82, 83). Obstacles to adequate grieving can occur when the nature of the loss is ambiguous. The absence of physical reminders, shared memories with others, and memorialization of the loss contribute to ambiguity and carrying out of the tasks associated with a typical grieving trajectory (5, 6, 72). When the grieving individual assimilates a healthier pattern of mourning losses through bereavement education and assistance "the knowledge and perspective gained from one's own growth following grief should serve as a quiet reservoir of strength" [(82), p. 461].

Cultural and Spiritual Humility

A humble approach to assess the particular relational, emotional, cultural, and spiritual needs of the patient and family receiving palliative care is essential. In the midst of the suffering inherent to neonatal end-of-life care, healthcare professionals can have a human but irrational tendency to deduce that their clients' anguish could have been avoided with more expert care (11). A reverent but curious approach with not only patients and their families but also with other consulting or attending providers can enhance open, nonjudgmental communication and collaboration (84). Physician and inspirational author Coulehan [(85), p. 206] wrote:

> [An] operational definition of medical humility includes four distinct but closely related personal characteristics that are central to good doctoring: unpretentious openness, honest self-disclosure, avoidance of arrogance, and modulation of self-interest. Humility, like other virtues, is best taught by means of narrative and role modeling. We may rightly be proud of contemporary medical advances, while at the same time experiencing gratitude and humility as healers.

In addition, Sasagawa and Amieux [(86), p. 925], researchers of multidisciplinary care collaboration, found that "both quantitative and qualitative analyses revealed that humility was viewed as an important character trait for successful inter-professional collaboration." Dr. Parravicini exemplified an unassuming approach to patient assessment when she said, "I have to look at each single patient, look to them to tell me through objective signs and cues what to do for them. It is a tremendous gift to learn from my little patients and from their parents."

Culturally sensitive care is necessary for families enduring the loss of an infant. Caregivers need to be alert and respectful to their clients' cultural, racial, ethnic, spiritual, linguistic, educational, and geographical differences. Cultural competency is a process of gathering knowledge about particular cultural groups; cultural humility is a process of inquiry and interpersonal curiosity approached with openness toward another (87). The pervasive nature of multiculturalism in the United States has made basing cultural competency on knowledge alone increasingly challenging (88). Yancu and Farmer [(89), p. e1–e2] said:

> In practice, cultural diversity is manifested in a broad range of ever-changing behaviors, beliefs, rituals, restrictions, traditions, norms, institutions, and relationships that form the basis of cultural knowledge. This makes cultural mastery something akin to trying to grab onto a cloud.

In response to the change, cultural humility is quickly becoming the preferred style to assessing and addressing the cultural needs of patients (90).

Cultural and spiritual humility are conducive to superlative interpersonal communication and relational efficacy contributing to provider compassion satisfaction (88). Nurse researcher Kalu (91) concluded that religious and spiritual beliefs can support and promote better coping for individuals experiencing a reproductive loss. In her study done in Africa, one woman said, "The midwife sat and listened to me. She was very knowledgeable, spiritual and caring. She asked me if I wanted to see the baby. I said yes and spent time with [her]. I have a good memory of [my baby]. That helped me to find ways to adjust and move on knowing that the baby will always be part of my family" [(91), p. 6]. The inference from this patient exemplifies how a provider's reserved but open communication style can support a patient's spiritual beliefs without imposing any religious maxims.

Awareness of one's personal cultural and spiritual values enhances the caregiver's ability to accommodate multicultural and multiracial differences in the patients they serve (90, 92). Appreciation and practice of one's spirituality can promote professional resilience (40, 47, 93, 94). Belcher and Griffiths [(95), p. 271] said that:

> Personal spirituality and a knowledge base to support spiritual caregiving were significant factors in hospice nursing staff members' competence and confidence in providing this intimate level of care. Respondents related a commitment to, and the ability to achieve, a level of spiritual care that was highly consistent with the spiritual needs of patients: the need for meaning and purpose in life, the need to give love, the need to receive love, and the need for hope and creativity.

Exploration of one's own cultural and spiritual background, particularly in aspects of family, childbearing, and grieving, can be a journey that enhances receptivity and caregiving satisfaction.

Research and Practice Implications

Larger scale qualitative studies would make a valuable contribution to explicit needs of perinatal palliative care providers particularly in the aspects of occupational misconceptions, moral distress, aspects of humility, and professional resiliency. Quantitative studies on the effectiveness of more widespread bereavement education on patient and professional satisfaction indicators throughout a hospital system could potentially help healthcare systems to mitigate caregiver burnout and turnover. Qualitative and quantitative studies utilized to explore the efficacy of team enhancing interventions and structured debriefing processes may also yield benefits for institutions.

Perinatal palliative care is greatly valued in the lives of those grappling with life-limiting neonatal conditions. Support for those gifted and compassionate professionals who provide the caregiving needs to be strategic and multifaceted. The onus to implement salient measures to cultivate resilience in the perinatal palliative caregiver should not be only upon the individuals themselves, but also upon prevailing regulatory governing bodies and healthcare institutions as well. The implementation of efficacious staffing, debriefing protocols, and ongoing bereavement and self-care education are also vital components to resiliency.

There is a societal trend to minimize the impact of death for those that occur within the perinatal period. It is often erroneously believed that suffering and grieving is obsolete because the unborn or newly born child has not lived long enough to establish themselves. The assumption and commentary that one can "just move on and try to have another one" is incredibly hurtful to those mourning the loss of their child. Perinatal palliative care providers support and become that benevolent community necessary for families to endure and mourn. Parravicini said (96) in an interview, "I'm most proud of the babies because they are so abandoned to our care. In fact, what is unique in our program is that we always put ourselves in the babies' shoes." She incites a professional humility that can assist perinatal palliative care providers to flourish within the setting of illness and death. "In its relational aspect, humility includes reverence or awe for the grace and strength of patients and their care-givers, a sense that the care-provider is not self-sufficient but needs the care-receiver" [(97), p. 291].

Byock [(98), p. 10] was posed the question from a woman with a terminal diagnosis, "Do I need to die well?" He went on to clarify that by promoting palliative care he had "hoped to dispel the notion that life ends the moment you receive a lousy diagnosis" [(98), p. 11]. He also profoundly concluded that, "it is possible to feel well within oneself and right with the world, even as one dies" and "that therein lies the hope for us all." [(98), p. 13] The profession of caregiving has traditionally been a trajectory of hope for the future that involves a relationship between the patient and provider. However, in palliative care the aim of care provision is not focused on curing the ailment but on bettering the course of the illness. Professional and personal strengths rise to accommodate the vulnerabilities inherent to perinatal palliative care, but that relational efficacy requires concerted fortification.

AUTHOR'S NOTE

Professionals working in perinatal palliative care are at risk for burnout and compassion fatigue because of the emotional, collaborative, and ethical demands associated with the birth and death of infants with life-limiting illnesses. Consequently, healthcare institutions with perinatal palliative programs may be more vulnerable to poor retention, absenteeism, and waning quality of care. Medical professionals often report a lack of knowledge, inexperience in using effective communication skills (i.e., fear of saying the wrong thing), and emotional anguish concurrent with compassion fatigue as reasons for their emotionally avoidant or even irreverent behaviors in bereavement care delivery. Existential suffering and moral distress are common challenges inherent to the provision of care for life limiting neonatal conditions. There is an increased need for physician and interdisciplinary healthcare provider education, training, and ongoing support that promotes beneficial palliative care in the perinatal setting. Support should be to be strategic and multifaceted. The implementation of bereavement care training, effective communication modalities, and evidenced based practical applications are critical components for a thriving perinatal palliative care team. Authentic formal and informal debriefing, peer mentoring, adequate caseloads, robust provider self-care practices, cultural and spiritual humility can foster personal growth and vicarious resilience for perinatal palliative care professionals.

AUTHOR CONTRIBUTIONS

All authors listed have made a substantial, direct and intellectual contribution to the work, and approved it for publication.

REFERENCES

1. Byock I. *Dying Well: Peace and Possibilities at the End of Life*. New York, NY: The Berkley Publishing Group. (1997).
2. Côté-Arsenault D, Krowchuk H, Hall WJ, Denney-Koelsch E. We want what's best for our baby: prenatal parenting of babies with lethal conditions. *J Prenat Perinat Psychol Health*. (2015) 29:157–76.
3. Jonas-Simpson C, Pilkington FB, MacDonald C, McMahon E. Nurses' experiences of grieving when there is a perinatal death. *Sage Open*. (2013) 3. doi: 10.1177/2158244013486116
4. Jaffe J, Diamond MO. *Reproductive Trauma: Psychotherapy with Infertility and Pregnancy Loss Clients*. Washington, DC: American Psychological Association. (2010).
5. Lang A, Fleiszer A, Huhammel F, Sword W, Gilbert K, Corsini-Munt S. Perinatal loss and parental grief: the challenge of ambiguity and disenfranchised grief. *Omega*. (2011) 63:183–96. doi: 10.2190/OM.63.2.e
6. Doka K, editor. *Disenfranchised Grief: New Directions, Challenges, and Strategies for Practice*. Champaign, IL: Research Press (2002).
7. Hall SL, Cross J, Selix NW, Patterson C, Segre L, Chuffo-Siewert R, et al. Recommendations for enhancing psychosocial support of NICU parents through staff education and support. *J Perinatol*. (2015) 35:S29–36. doi: 10.1038/jp.2015.147
8. Singer LT, Salvator A, Guo S, Collin M, Lilien L, Baley J. Maternal psychological distress and parenting stress after the birth of a very low-birth-weight infant. *JAMA*. (1999) 281:799–805. doi: 10.1001/jama.281.9.799
9. Kamal AH, Bull JH, Wolf SP, Swetz KM, Shanafelt TD, Ast K, et al. Prevalence and predictors of burnout among hospice and palliative care clinicians in the U.S. *J Pain Symptom Manage*. (2016) 51:690–6. doi: 10.1016/j.jpainsymman.2015.10.020
10. Sansó N, Galiana L, Oliver A, Pascual A, Sinclair S, Benito E. Palliative care professionals' inner life: exploring the relationships among awareness, self-care, and compassion satisfaction and fatigue, burnout, and coping with death. *J Pain Symptom Manage*. (2015) 50:200–7. doi: 10.1016/j.jpainsymman.2015.02.013
11. Cherny NI, Fallon MT, Kaasa S, Portenoy, RK, Currow, et al. *Oxford Textbook of Palliative Medicine*. 5th Edn. New York, NY: Oxford University Press. (2015).
12. Carter BS. Pediatric palliative care in infants and neonates. *Children (Basel)*. (2018) 5:21. doi: 10.3390/children5020021
13. Hoeldtke NJ, Calhoun BC. Perinatal hospice. *Am J Obstetr Gynecol*. (2001) 185:525–8. doi: 10.1067/mob.2001.116093
14. Perinatal palliative care: ACOG committee opinion, number 786. *Obstetr Gynecol*. (2019) 134:e84–9. doi: 10.1097/AOG.0000000000003425
15. Arksey H, O'Malley L. Scoping studies: towards a methodological framework. *Int J Soc Res Meth*. (2005) 8:19–32. doi: 10.1080/1364557032000119616
16. Taplak AS, Gurol A, Polat S. Nurses' perceptions of the palliative care need of neonates with multiple congenital anomalies. *J Hos Pall Nurs*. (2020) 22:137–44. doi: 10.1097/NJH.0000000000000628
17. Balaguer A, Martín-Ancel A, Ortigoza-Escobar D, Escribano J, Argemi J. The model of palliative care in the perinatal setting: a review of the literature. *BMC Pediatr*. (2012) 12:1–6. doi: 10.1186/1471-2431-12-25
18. Kenner C, Press J, Ryan D. Recommendations for palliative and bereavement care in the NICU: a family-centered integrative approach. *J Perinatol*. (2015) 35 (Suppl. 1):S19-S23. doi: 10.1038/jp.2015.145
19. Parravicini E, Daho' M, Foe G, Steinwurtzel R, Byrne M. Parental assessment of comfort in newborns affected by life-limiting conditions treated by a standardized neonatal comfort care program. *J Perinatol*. (2018) 38:142–7. doi: 10.1038/jp.2017.160
20. Côté-Arsenault D, Denney-Koelsch E. "My baby is a person": parents' experiences with life-threatening fetal diagnosis. *J Palliat Med*. (2011) 14:1302–8. doi: 10.1089/jpm.2011.0165

21. Côté-Arsenault D, Denney-Koelsch E. "Have no regrets:" Parents' experiences and developmental tasks in pregnancy with a lethal fetal diagnosis. *Soc Sci Med.* (2016) 154:100–9. doi: 10.1016/j.socscimed.2016.02.033
22. Côté-Arsenault D, Donato K. Emotional cushioning in pregnancy after perinatal loss. *J Reprod Infant Psychol.* (2011) 29:81–92. doi: 10.1080/02646838.2010.513115
23. Hamric AB. A case study of moral distress. *J Hosp Palliat Nur.* (2014) 16:457–63. doi: 10.1097/NJH.0000000000000104
24. Klein SM. Moral distress in pediatric palliative care: a case study. *J Pain Symptom Manage.* (2009) 38:157–60. doi: 10.1016/j.jpainsymman.2009.04.014
25. Wool C. State of the science on perinatal palliative care. *J Obstet Gynecol Neonatal Nurs.* (2013) 42:372–E55. doi: 10.1111/1552-6909.12035
26. Chervenak F, McCullough LB. Responsibly counselling women about the clinical management of pregnancies complicated by severe fetal anomalies. *J Med Ethics.* (2012) 38:397–8. doi: 10.1136/medethics-2012-100491
27. Blakeley C, Smith DM, Johnstone ED, Wittkowski A. Parental decision-making following a prenatal diagnosis that is lethal, life-limiting, or has long term implications for the future child and family: a meta-synthesis of qualitative literature. *BMC Med Ethics.* (2019) 20:19. doi: 10.1186/s12910-019-0393-7
28. Catlin A, Carter B. Creation of a neonatal end-of-life palliative care protocol. *J Perinatol.* (2002) 22:184–95. doi: 10.1038/sj.jp.7210687
29. Garros D. Moral distress in the everyday life of an intensivist. *Front Pediatr.* (2016) 4:4. doi: 10.3389/fped.2016.00091
30. Koch KD, Jones BL. Support parent caregivers of children with life-limiting illness. *Children (Basel).* (2018) 5:85. doi: 10.3390/children5070085
31. McCloskey S, Taggart L. How much compassion have I left? an exploration of occupational stress among children's palliative care nurses. *Int J Palliat Nurs.* (2010) 16:233–40. doi: 10.12968/ijpn.2010.16.5.48144
32. Epstein EG, Hamric AB. Moral distress, moral residue, and the crescendo effect. *J Clin Ethics.* (2009) 20:330–42.
33. Grunauer M, Mikesell C. A review of the integrated model of care: an opportunity to respond to extensive palliative care needs in pediatric intensive care units in under-resourced settings. *Front Pediatr.* (2018) 6:9. doi: 10.3389/fped.2018.00003
34. Wool C, Catlin A. Perinatal bereavement and palliative care offered throughout the healthcare system. *Ann Palliat Med.* (2019) 8 (Suppl. 1):S22–9. doi: 10.21037/apm.2018.11.03
35. Profit J, Sharek PJ, Amspoker AB, Kowalkowski MA, Nisbet CC, Thomas EJ, et al. Burnout in the NICU setting and its relation to safety culture. *BMJ Qual Saf.* (2014) 23:806–13. doi: 10.1136/bmjqs-2014-002831
36. Figley C. *Compassion Fatigue: Coping with Secondary Traumatic Stress Disorder in Those Who Treat the Traumatized.* New York, NY: Brunner/Mazel. (1995).
37. Kamal A, Bull J, Wolf S, Samsa G, Ast K, Swetz KM et al. Burnout among palliative care clinicians in the United States: results of a national survey. *J Clin Oncol.* (2014) 32 (Suppl. 35):e20530. doi: 10.1200/jco.2014.32.15_suppl.e20530
38. Barrett L, Yates P. Oncology/haematology nurses: a study of job satisfaction, burnout, and intention to leave specialty. *Aust Heatlh Rev.* (2002) 25:109–21. doi: 10.1071/AH020109
39. Weintraub AS, Geithner EM, Stroustrup A, Waldman ED. Compassion fatigue, burnout and compassion satisfaction in neonatologists in the US. *J Perinatol.* (2016) 36:1021–6. doi: 10.1038/jp.2016.121
40. Zwack J, Schweitzer J. If every fifth physician is affected by burnout, what about the other four? Resilience strategies of experienced physicians. *Acad Med.* (2013) 88:382–9. doi: 10.1097/ACM.0b013e318281696b
41. Hernández P, Gangsei D, Engstrom D. Vicarious resilience: a new concept in work with those who survive trauma. *Fam Process.* (2007) 46:229–41. doi: 10.1111/j.1545-5300.2007.00206.x
42. van Dernoot Lipsky L. *Trauma Stewardship.* San Fransisco, CA: Berrett-Koehler Publishers. Inc. (2009).
43. Stamm BH. *The Concise ProQOL Manual.* 2nd Edn. Pocatello: Beth Hudnall (2010).
44. Mehta DH, Perez GK, Traeger L, Park ER, Goldmn RE, Haime, et al. Building resiliency in a palliative care team: a pilot study. *J Pain Symptom Manage.* (2016) 51:604–8. doi: 10.1016/j.jpainsymman.2015.10.013
45. Montgomery AJ. The inevitability of physician burnout: implications for interventions. *Burnout Res.* (2014) 1:50–6. doi: 10.1016/j.burn.2014.04.002
46. Epstein RM, Krasner MS. Physician resilience: what it means, why it matters, and how to promote it. *Acad Med.* (2013) 88:301–3. doi: 10.1097/ACM.0b013e318280cff0
47. Perez GK, Haime V, Jackson V, Chittenden E, Mehta DH, Park ER. Promoting resiliency among palliative care clinicians: stressors, coping strategies, and training needs. *J Palliat Med.* (2015) 18:332–7. doi: 10.1089/jpm.2014.0221
48. Hutti MH, Polvka B, White S, Hill J, Clark P, Cooke C, et al. Experiences of nurses who care for women after fetal loss. *J Obstetr Gynecol Neonat Nurs.* (2016) 45:17–27. doi: 10.1016/j.jogn.2015.10.010
49. Altilio T, Dahlin C, Tucker R, Remke SS, Weissman DE. *Strategies for Maximizing the Health/Function of Palliative Care Teams: A Resource Monograph for the Center to Advance Palliative Care.* New York, NY: Center to Advance Palliative Care (2019). Available online at: https://www.capc.org/documents/98/ (accessed on February 18, 2020).
50. Keeton K, Fenner DE, Johnson TR, Hayward RA. Predictors of physician career satisfaction, work-life balance, and burnout. *Obstet Gynecol.* (2007) 109:949–55. doi: 10.1097/01.AOG.0000258299.45979.37
51. Dev V, Fernando AT 3rd, Lim AG, Consedine NS. Does self-compassion mitigate the relationship between burnout and barriers to compassion? a cross-sectional quantitative study of 799 nurses. *Int J Nurs Stud.* (2018) 81:81–8. doi: 10.1016/j.ijnurstu.2018.02.003
52. Leiter MP, Maslach C. Six areas of worklife: a model of the organizational context of burnout. *J Health Hum Serv Adm.* (1999) 21:472–89.
53. Cortezzo DE, Bowers K, Meyer MC. Birth planning in uncertain or life-limiting fetal diagnoses: perspectives of physicians and parents. *J of Pall Med.* (2019) 22:1337–45. doi: 10.1089/jpm.2018.0596
54. Cortezzo DE, Sanders MR, Brownell EA, Moss K. End-of-life care in the neonatal intensive care unit: experiences of staff and parents. *Am J Perinatol.* (2015) 32:713–24. doi: 10.1055/s-0034-1395475
55. Haug S, Farooqi S, Wilson CG, Hopper A, Oei G, Carter B. Survey on neonatal end-of-life comfort care guidelines across America. *J Pain Symptom Manage.* (2018) 55:979–84.e2. doi: 10.1016/j.jpainsymman.2017.10.023
56. Hughes KH, Goodall UA. Perinatal bereavement care: are we meeting families' needs? *Br J Midwif.* (2013) 21:248–53. doi: 10.12968/bjom.2013.21.4.248
57. Wright V, Prasun MA, Hilgenberg C. Why is end-of-life care delivery sporadic? A quantitative look at the barriers to and facilitators of providing end-of-life care in the neonatal intensive care unit. *Adv Neonatal Care.* (2011) 11:29–36. doi: 10.1097/ANC.0b013e3182085642
58. Chan MF, Lou FL, Arthur DG, Cao FL, Wu LH, Li P et al. Investigating factors associate to nurses' attitudes towards perinatal bereavement care. *J Clin Nurs.* (2008) 17:509–18. doi: 10.1111/j.1365-2702.2007.02007.x
59. Leinweber J, Rowe HJ. The costs of 'being with the woman': secondary traumatic stress in midwifery. *Midwifery.* (2010) 26:76–87. doi: 10.1016/j.midw.2008.04.003
60. McCreight BS. Perinatal grief and emotional labour: a study of nurses' experiences in gynae wards. *Int J Nurs Stud.* (2005) 42:439–48. doi: 10.1016/j.ijnurstu.2004.07.004
61. Braithwaite M. Nurse burnout and stress in the NICU. *Adv Neonatal Care.* (2008) 8:343–7. doi: 10.1097/01.ANC.0000342767.17606.d1
62. Moore DE, Green JS, Gallis HA. Achieving desired results and improved outcomes: Integrating planning and assessment throughout learning activities. *J Contin Educ Health Prof.* (2009) 29:1–15. doi: 10.1002/chp.20001
63. Wilkinson S, Roberts A, Aldridge J. Nurse-patient communication in palliative care: an evaluation of a communication skills programme. *Palliat Med.* (1998) 12:13–22. doi: 10.1191/026921698675034697
64. Sweeney C, O'Sullivan E, McCarthy M. Keeping it real: exploring an interdisciplinary breaking bad news role-play as an integrative learning opportunity. *J Scholarsh Teach Learn.* (2015) 15:14–32. doi: 10.14434/josotl.v15i2.13262
65. Boles J. Bearing bad news: supporting patients and families through difficult conversations. *Pediatr Nurs.* (2015) 41:306–8.
66. Hazebroek FW, Smeets RM, Bos AP, Ouwens C, Tibboel D, Molenaar JC. Staff attitudes towards continuation of life-support in newborns with major congenital anomalies. *Eur J Pediatr.* (1996) 155:783–6. doi: 10.1007/BF02002907

67. Mancini A, Uthaya S, Beardsley C, Wood N, Modi D. *Practical Guidance for The Management of Palliative Care on Neonatal Units*. London: Chelsea and Westminster Hospital (2014).
68. Vaithilingam N, Jain S, Davies D. Clinical governance, helping the helpers: debriefing following an adverse incident. *Obstatr Gynaecol.* (2008) 10:251–6. doi: 10.1576/toag.10.4.251.27442
69. Mitchell AM, Sakraida TJ, Kameg K. Critical incident stress debriefing: implications for best practice. *Disaster Manag Response.* (2003) 1:46–51. doi: 10.1016/S1540-2487(03)00008-7
70. Pratt SD, Jachna BR. Care of the clinician after an adverse event. *Int J Obstet Anesth.* (2015) 24:54–63. doi: 10.1016/j.ijoa.2014.10.001
71. Casarett D, Johnson M, Smith D, Richardson D. The optimal delivery of palliative care: a national comparison of the outcomes of consultation teams vs inpatient units. *Arch Intern Med.* (2011) 171:649–55. doi: 10.1001/archinternmed.2011.87
72. Worden JW. *Grief Counseling and Grief Therapy: A Handbook for the Mental Health Practitioner*, 5th Edn. New York, NY: Springer Publishing Company. (2018).
73. Boyle DA. Countering compassion fatigue: a requisite nursing agenda. *Online J Issues Nurs.* (2011) 16:2. doi: 10.3912/OJIN.Vol16No01Man02
74. Mills J, Wand T, Fraser JA. Self-care in palliative care nursing and medical professionals: a cross-sectional survey. *J Palliat Med.* (2017) 20:625–30. doi: 10.1089/jpm.2016.0470
75. Jones SH. A delicate balance: self-care for the hospice professional. *Aging Well.* (2008) 1:38. Available online at: https://www.todaysgeriatricmedicine.com/archive/spring08p38.shtml
76. Kase SM, Gribben JL, Waldman ED, Weintraub AS. A pilot study exploring interventions for physician distress in pediatric subspecialists. *Pediatr Res.* (2020) 88:1–6. doi: 10.1038/s41390-020-0805-x
77. Sanchez-Reilly S, Morrison LJ, Carey E, Bernacki R, O'Neill L, Kapo J, et al. Caring for oneself to care for others: physicians and their self-care. *J Support Oncol.* (2013) 11:75–81. doi: 10.12788/j.suponc.0003
78. Back AL, Steinhauser KE, Kamal AH, Jackson VA. Building resilience for palliative care clinicians: an approach to burnout prevention based on individual skills and workplace factors. *J Pain Symptom Manage.* (2016) 52:284–91. doi: 10.1016/j.jpainsymman.2016.02.002
79. Mills J, Wand T, Fraser JA. Exploring the meaning and practice of self-care among palliative care nurses and doctors: a qualitative study. *BMC Palliat Care.* (2018) 17:63. doi: 10.1186/s12904-018-0318-0
80. Saakvitne KW, Pearlman LA, Staff of TSI/CAAP. *Transforming the Pain: A Workbook on Vicarious Traumatization.* New York, NY: Norton (1996).
81. Alkema K, Linton JM, Davies R. A study of the relationship between self-care, compassion satisfaction, compassion fatigue, and burnout among hospice professionals. *J Soc Work End Life Palliat Care.* (2008) 4:101–19. doi: 10.1080/15524250802353934
82. James RK, Gilliland BE. *Crisis Intervention Strategies*, 7th Edn. Belmont, CA: Brooks/Cole (2013).
83. Kilcullen M, Ireland S. Palliative care in the neonatal unit: neonatal nursing staff perceptions of facilitators and barriers in a regional tertiary nursery. *BMC Palliat Care.* (2017) 16:32. doi: 10.1186/s12904-017-0202-3
84. Back AL, Arnold RM, Baile WF, Fryer-Edwards KA, Alexander SC, Barley GE, et al. Efficacy of communication skills training for giving bad news and discussing transitions to palliative care. *Arch Intern Med.* (2007) 167:453–60. doi: 10.1001/archinte.167.5.453
85. Coulehan J. "A gentle and humane temper": humility in medicine. *Perspect Biol Med.* (2011) 54:206–16. doi: 10.1353/pbm.2011.0017
86. Sasagawa M, Amieux PS. Dispositional humility of clinicians in an interprofessional primary care environment: a mixed methods study. *J Multidiscip Healthc.* (2019) 12:925–34. doi: 10.2147/JMDH.S226631
87. Hook JN, Davis DE, Owen J, Worthington Jr. EL, Utsey SO. Cultural humility: measuring openness to culturally diverse clients. *J Counsel Psychol.* (2013) 60:353–66. doi: 10.1037/a0032595
88. Hughes V, Delva S, Nkimeng M, Spaulding E, Turkson-Ocran R, Cudjoe J, et al. Not missing the opportunity: strategies to promote cultural humility among future nursing faculty. *J Profession Nurs.* (2020) 36:28–33. doi: 10.1016/j.profnurs.2019.06.005
89. Yancu CN, Farmer DF. Product or process: cultural competence or cultural humility? *Palliat Med Hosp Care Open J.* (2017) 3:e1–4. doi: 10.17140/PMHCOJ-3-e005
90. Waters A, Asbill L. *Reflections on Cultural Humility: Given the Complexity of Multiculturalism, it Is Beneficial to Understand Cultural Competency as a Process Rather Than an End Product.* American Psychological Association (2013). Available online at: https://www.apa.org/pi/families/resources/newsletter (accessed on February 19, 2020).
91. Kalu AF. Women's experiences of utilizing religious and spiritual beliefs as coping resources after miscarriage. *Religions.* (2019) 10:185. doi: 10.3390/rel10030185
92. Richardson P. Spirituality, religion and palliative care. *Ann Palliat Med.* (2014) 3:150–9. doi: 10.3978/j.issn.2224-5820.2014.07.05
93. Maytum JC, Heiman MB, Garwick AW. Compassion fatigue and burnout in nurses who work with children with chronic conditions and their families. *J Pediatr Health Care.* (2004) 18:171–9. doi: 10.1016/j.pedhc.2003.12.005
94. Forster E, Hafiz A. Paediatric death and dying: exploring coping strategies of health professionals and perceptions of support provision. *Int J Palliat Nurs.* (2015) 21:294–301. doi: 10.12968/ijpn.2015.21.6.294
95. Belcher A, Griffiths M. The spiritual care perspectives and practices of hospice nurses. *J Hosp Palliat Nur.* (2005) 7:271–79. doi: 10.1097/00129191-200509000-00014
96. Mariani L. Before death there is life. *Communion and Liberation.* (2019). Available online at: https://english.clonline.org/stories/encounters/2019/01/12/before-death-there-is-life
97. Lebacqz K. Humility in health care. *J Med Philosophy.* (1992) 17:291–307. doi: 10.1093/jmp/17.3.291
98. Byock I. Do I need to die well? sharing a personal growth experience. *Touching lives.* (2010) 2:10–3. Available online at: https://www.todaysgeratricmedicine.com/archive/spring08p38.shtml

6

Development of a Perinatal Palliative Care Model at a Level II Perinatal Center Supported by a Pediatric Palliative Care Network

Marco Bolognani [1,2], Paola Daniela Morelli [2], Isabella Scolari [2], Cristina Dolci [2], Valentina Fiorito [2], Francesca Uez [2], Silvia Graziani [1], Barbara Stefani [1,2], Francesca Zeni [1,2], Gino Gobber [2], Elena Bravi [2], Saverio Tateo [2] and Massimo Soffiati [1]*

[1] *Department of Neonatology, Santa Chiara Hospital, Trento, Italy,* [2] *Azienda Provinciale per i Servizi Sanitari (APSS), Trento, Italy*

***Correspondence:**
Marco Bolognani
marco.bolognani@gmail.com

Objective: To describe the model build up to take care of fetuses and newborns eligible to perinatal palliative care (PnPC) followed in an Italian II level perinatal center.

Methods: Retrospective chart review of all fetuses and newborn infants eligible to PnPC admitted to level II perinatal center within a 4 years period.

Results: Forty-five of 848 infants (0.5%) referred to II level NICU were eligible to PnPC. Twenty-seven percentage had fetal diagnosis. Twenty percentage were preterm infants at the limit of viability, 35% were newborns with life limiting or life threatening disease diagnosed *in utero* or at the postnatal ward, 45% were newborns not responding to intensive care intervention with high health care needs or medical complexity. Fifty-seven percentage of neonates admitted to NICU died before discharge, while 16 (35% of population considered) were discharged home. Median age at death was 4 days after birth, and delivery room death immediately after birth occurred in six patients (13%).

Conclusions: Despite the paucity of our population and the high variability in disease trajectories the perinatal palliative care program build up in our region provides a reproducible method for a structured taking in charge of fetuses and neonates eligible to PnPC and their families, from the time of diagnosis to bereavement, in both outpatient and inpatient settings.

Keywords: life limiting conditions, pediatric palliative care, perinatal palliative care, life threatening conditions, fetal diagnosis

INTRODUCTION

Perinatal palliative care (PnPC) focuses on coordinated care strategies for babies born at the edge of viability, fetuses and neonates with confirmed or potential diagnosis of life-limiting and life-threatening conditions, neonates who become critically ill during a neonatal intensive care unit (NICU) stay and are not responding to aggressive medical management (1). PnPC implies multidisciplinary, global and continuous care of the family from the time of diagnosis to the end-of-life. Initial combination of life-prolonging and disease-modifying treatment with palliative care could afterwards turn to exclusive attention to quality of life and comfort care because of inappropriateness and futility of previous treatments (2).

Lack of evidence-based empirical studies to identify the best model for PnPC (2) and the insufficient diffusion of structured PnPC programs leaves many aspects challenging in an otherwise growing field of evidence. A recent national survey reports that only 30% of Italian NICUs offer a structured PnPC program (3) despite a national law of 2010 which protects the citizen's right to access palliative care (4).

The pediatric palliative care (PPC) Network in our region, since 2016 has started to develop a program for PnPC in collaboration with level II perinatal center, considering national and international suggestions and experiences (5–10). Palliative care is disposable at any time in the pregnancy cycle: when the fetus is *in utero*, when the pregnancy is ended, when there is an early induction, after a live birth and transition to palliative care in the NICU or upon discharge home (5). PnPC planning and care is provided at the time of diagnoses on through the whole trajectory of life, and is applied indifferently in hospital settings and at home. PPC team coordinates care with hospital and local staff in a collaborative, community-based and family centered frame.

OBJECTIVE

The aim of this study was to describe the model build up to take care of fetuses and newborns eligible to perinatal palliative care and followed in an Italian II level perinatal center.

METHODS

The study population consisted of all fetuses and neonates eligible to PnPC who were cared for in the Trentino II level perinatal center from January 1, 2016 to May 31, 2020. All eligible participants were identified by examining retrospectively hospital documentation and were subsequently distributed in three groups according to current literature about eligibility to PnPC (1, 10, 11).

Group 1: newborns at the threshold of viability (birth weight <500 g or gestational age under 24 weeks).

Group 2: newborns with life limiting or life threatening disease diagnosed *in utero* or at the postnatal ward.

Group 3: newborns not responding to intensive care intervention with high health care needs or medical complexity.

PnPC Model Description

The PPC team can be activated at any time from diagnosis of a fetal or neonatal condition eligible to palliative care (**Figure 1**). This first contact serves to meet the parents, describe PPC network, establish a therapeutic alliance and focus on exploring parental goals.

Thereafter a multidisciplinary assessment of problems and needs takes place involving: parent(s) and members of their support system, obstetrician, neonatologist, PPC team (pediatrician, nurse, and psychologist), other specialists (neuropsychiatrist, pediatric cardiologist, and geneticist) if appropriate. Problems, needs and goals are reassessed through a model utilized in PPC (12), exploring also specific perinatal needs and tailored on each family, considering every available resource in order to achieve the endorsed goals.

The PPC team elaborates subsequently an individualized advanced birth and care plan which contains anticipatory management (**Table 1**).

A family conference is than arranged to review the individualized birth and care plan and introduce PPC network team members. Parents are given the opportunity to re-express their goals of care and they are told that the plan will be continuously reassessed. These meetings range in length from 1 to 3 h.

The plan is finally discussed with all the health care providers involved and targeted training on PPC is offered and provided to all the nodes of the network involved (obstetrician, neonatologist, nurses, psychologist, emergency services, social service, and home care service).

During prenatal, birth and postnatal periods the PPC team has repeated interactions with parents and the health care providers involved. Psychological support is provided for parents, siblings and other family members and the team caring for the fetus or neonate. This support proved to be particularly valuable in providing age-appropriate, honest and concrete explanations to young children to help them understand.

At time of delivery one of the members of the PPC team is present or available for consultation.

After delivery for neonates who survive the immediate newborn period rooming-in–if appropriate and desired–is ensured. Infants who survive long enough to be discharged from the hospital are taken care of at home, were planned physician visits take place once a fortnight and planned nurse visits twice a week. Visits of psychologists, social workers, physiotherapists are planned according to individual needs of each family. Patients and parents have a round-the-clock access to telephone consultation service, and intervention visits are a standard procedure in case of a patient's health deterioration. PPC team takes care of bereavement counseling and provides support for health workers involved who are dealing with emotional distress. PPC is free of charge and all medical equipment is loaned to the families free of charge.

RESULTS

Between January 2016 and May 2020, 9.849 neonates were born at the Trentino II level perinatal center "S Chiara" and 848 neonates were cared for at the II level NICU. The center counts an annual working volume of 2,200 prenatal diagnostic ultrasound investigations, 1,400 screening techniques for chromosomal abnormalities, 80 villocentesis and 40 amniocentesis. During the period in exam 62 voluntary interruptions of pregnancy, 60 spontaneous abortions and 15 fetal deaths took place.

Forty-five neonates (0.5% of all NICU admissions and 0.05% of all newborns) eligible to PnPC were retrospectively identified, 12 (27%) of them had fetal diagnoses, two stillbirths and 43 livebirths. Median (range) gestation at delivery was 31 (23–41) weeks. Babies survived for 1 h to 565 days (median 4 days). Deaths in the delivery room shortly after birth accounted for

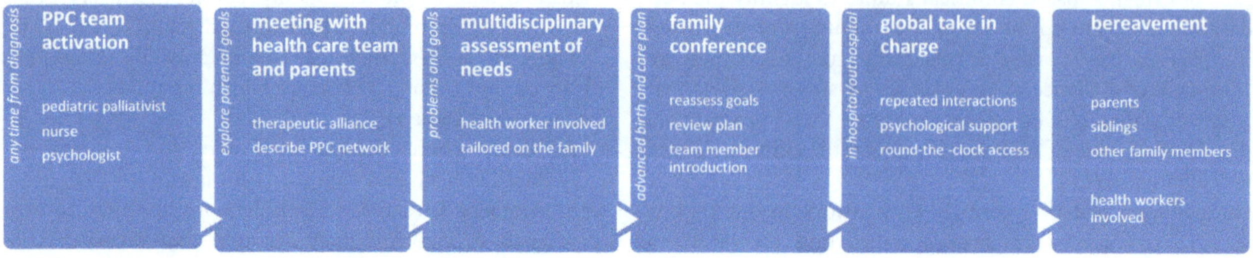

FIGURE 1 | PnPC model description.

TABLE 1 | Content of advanced birth and care plan.

Birth care plan	• Place • Timing • Mode • Monitoring in labour • People to be present at delivery • Care provided at delivery • Which (if any) diagnostic interventions to be done • Postnatal care • Skin to skin
Palliative care plan	• Pain • Medical system access and quality • Family oriented care • Dignity and respect • Decision making • Psychosocial • Spiritual symptoms treatment plan • Family support (siblings and grandparents)
Bereavement care plan	• Arranging for spiritual/cultural care • Psychosocial support • Supporting memories

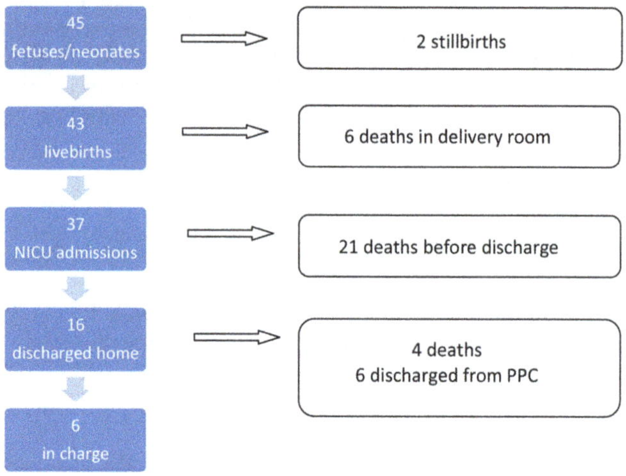

FIGURE 2 | Outcome of 45 neonates.

13%. Twenty one out of 37 neonates (57%) admitted to the NICU died before discharge (median age at death was 4 days). Of the 21 patients who died, 12 (57%) died while receiving maximal support measures (including cardiopulmonary resuscitation), and 9 (44%) died under primary comfort care or after withholding or withdrawal of life support measures. 16 (35%) were discharged home. Outcome is reassumed in **Figure 2** and main characteristics of the 45 fetuses and neonates analyzed in the study are summarized in **Table 2**.

In group 1, two out of nine newborns died in delivery room, while seven died in intensive care unit receiving support measures (median age at death was 3 days). Only in one case PPC team has been involved.

In group 2, besides two stillborns, four out of 16 newborns died in delivery room, two in NICU and eight were discharged home. Four of these eight infants died in hospital (place of death chosen by the parents) receiving comfort care at a median age at death of 111 days. Four to date are in charge of CPP network.

Group 3 includes 20 neonates, 12 of them died in NICU and eight were discharged home and taken care of by the PPC network. For six of these it has been possible to discharge them from PPC network and entrust them to the family pediatrician because of the improvement of clinical conditions and the reduction of complexity of care. Two to date are in charge of CPP network.

Altogether for 30 of the 45 fetuses and newborns eligible to PPC (67%) PPC team has been involved. The involvement grew during the period analyzed (from 50% in 2016 to 88% in 2019) and differed between group 1 and 2–3, respectively (11 vs. 80%).

The duration of PPC among all fetuses/neonates varied from 1 to 853 days with a median duration of 99 days. For those discharged home instead from 18 to 853 days with a median duration of 316 days. In this group of 16 infants the most frequent clinical problems included neurological symptoms (69%) and dysphagia (81%). A high percentage of the infants (62%) had a feeding tube (naso-orogastric) inserted, 20% percutaneous endoscopic gastrostomy and 12% tracheostomy, 40% of patients needed mechanical ventilation at discharge one patient had a central venous catheter inserted. Fifteen of all the 30 families

TABLE 2 | Distribution of neonates eligible to PnPC.

Group	1		2		3	
	Newborns at the threshold of viability (birth weight < 500 g or gestational age under 24 weeks)		**Newborns with life limiting or life threatening disease diagnosed *in utero* or at the postnatal ward**		**Newborns not responding to intensive care intervention with high health care needs or medical complexity**	
nr (%)	9 (20)		16 (35)		20 (45)	
Died before discharge						
nr (%)	9 (100)		8 (50)		12 (60)	
Age at death	*4.5 ± 4.6 (3) 0.04–13 days		*0.8 ± 1.5 (4) 0.04–4 days		*5 ± 7 (2.5) 0.4–21 days	
In charge of PPC						
nr (%)	1 (11)		13 (80)		16 (80)	
Duration	1day		*257 ± 205 (316) 18–494 days		*163 ± 240 (47) 1–853 days	
After discharge						
Died at home	0		0		0	
Died in hospital	0		4		0	
Discharged from PPC	0		0		6	
In charge to PPC	0		4		2	
	BW 490 (415–522)		Trisomy 13, 18	$n = 4$	HIE	$n = 8$
	GA 23 (23–25)		Thanatophoric dwarfism	$n = 1$	Severe brain injury	$n = 3$
			Potter's syndrome	$n = 2$	MOF	$n = 2$
			Metabolic disease	$n = 2$	Dysphagia and CLD	$n = 7$
			Multiple malformations	$n = 4$		
			Epidermolysis bullosa	$n = 1$		
			Cardiomyopathies	$n = 2$		

BW, birth weight; GA, gestational age; HIE, hypossic-ischemic encephalopathy; MOF, multiorgan failure; CLD, chronic lung disease.
**Mean ± standard deviation (median) min-max.*

taken in charge agreed and received permanent psychological care and every family received social supports needed.

Eight of the 45 pathways begun at prenatal diagnosis of a life limiting or life threatening condition, three out of eight were achieved beyond 20 weeks of gestational age (13), whereas the other five diagnoses were obtained within 22 weeks of gestation but parents decided to continue pregnancy.

DISCUSSION

This study retrospectively analyzes data of all fetuses and neonates cared for in the II level perinatal center of Trento during a 4 year period from January 2016 to May 2020. Regional PPC network began to elaborate a PnPC program since 2016.

In our experience newborns belonging to group 1 rarely were notified to PPC team thus reproducing results of other experiences (11). Reasons for this may be the difficulty in acknowledging prognosis in this subgroup of patients and the reduced exposure of treating team to this kind of patient (one every 5–6 months), moreover there is to consider lack of palliative care education in medical and nursing school in our country.

Whereas, the involvement of the PPC network is growing in regard of fetuses and infants of group 2 because health professionals were previously unfamiliar with alternative management such as PnPC and the growing evidence of the importance of early referral to PnPC has been shared and recognized. Even if lethal fetal abnormalities are uncommon and most couple request termination after a diagnosis of lethal abnormality, late diagnoses will continue to arise as incidental discoveries and many of these babies will be life born with a variable and unpredictable life course (14) thus requiring adequate and comprehensive care.

Outcome of group 3 results very heterogeneous but takes in account a group of patients which can take advantage of an early referral to PnPC because of the clinical complexity of their condition. Health care providers are faced with the difficult task to revise treatment from aggressive cure-oriented intervention to palliative care goals coping with personal values and feelings.

Since the implementation of the model described, an improvement has been noted by health workers involved in terms of facilitated decision making and consensus building, improvement of therapeutic alliance, better flow of information in a framework characterized by difficult and complex matters and many "gray zones."

Taking inspiration from this first years of networking a formal education plan for possible staff members involved is in a planning stage and team support in order to manage properly communication management and emotional containment has been completed (15, 16).

NICU may not be the optimal place for provision of palliative care, but according to the evidence that location is not as important as the "mind set" of persons involved (1) and considering our experience appropriate levels of PnPC can be accomplished through attitudes, appropriate skills training and shared birth and advanced care plans.

CONCLUSIONS

At a first glance our data depict the broad variability health workers have to face in managing patients and families in need of PnPC. The vast clinical conditions with different and unpredictable trajectories of life in terms of length and burden of care requires multidisciplinarity, communication between services, forecasting of problems, flexibility and adaptation to different settings. Despite our small population and the high variability in disease trajectories the perinatal palliative care program developed in our region provides a replicable method for a structured responsibility of fetuses and neonates eligible to PnPC and their families, from the time of diagnosis to bereavement, in both outpatient and inpatient settings. Outcomes from our program support development of similar programs to meet the needs of the families who do not wish to terminate pregnancies or who do not wish to use intensive care services for babies, if born alive and as near to their home as possible.

ETHICS STATEMENT

Ethical review and approval was not required for the study on human participants in accordance with the local legislation and institutional requirements. Written informed consent from the participants' legal guardian/next of kin was not required to participate in this study in accordance with the national legislation and the institutional requirements.

AUTHOR CONTRIBUTIONS

MB, PM, and IS contributed in collecting data. CD, VF, and FU contributed in building the PnPC program. SG, BS, and FZ participated in defining the pathways. EB, GG, ST, and MS participated in manuscript review. All authors contributed to the article and approved the submitted version.

REFERENCES

1. Catlin A, Carter B. Creation of a neonatal end-of-life palliative care protocol. *J Perinatol.* (2002) 22:184–95. doi: 10.1038/sj.jp.7210687
2. Balaguer A, Martín-Ancel A, Ortigoza-Escobar D, Escribano J, Argemi J. The model of palliative care in the perinatal setting: a review of the literature. *BMC Pediatrics.* (2012) 12:25. doi: 10.1186/1471-2431-12-25
3. Cavicchiolo ME, Rusalen F, Benini F, Baraldi E Lago P. Perinatal palliative care: a national survey in Italy. *Arch Dis Child Fetal Neonatal Ed.* (2019) 104:F567–8. doi: 10.1136/archdischild-2018-316327
4. Italian Law 38/2010, art 1 "Disposizioni per garantire l'accesso alle cure palliative e alla terapia del dolore". Gazzetta Ufficiale n 65, 19 marzo 2010.
5. British Association of Perinatal Medicine: (2009). Available online at: http://www.bapm.org/publications/documents/guidelines/Palliative_Care_
6. American Academy of Pediatrics Committee on Fetus and Newborn. Noninitiation or withdrawal of intensive care for high-risk newborns. *Pediatrics.* (2007) 119:401–3. doi: 10.1542/peds.2006-3180
7. Kenner C, Press J, Ryan D. Recommendations for palliative and bereavement care in the NICU: a family-centered integrative approach. *J Perinatol.* (2015) 35:S19–S23. doi: 10.1038/jp.2015.145
8. Parravicin E. Neonatal palliative care. *Curr Opin Pediatr.* (2017) 29:135–40. doi: 10.1097/MOP.0000000000000464
9. Perinatal Palliative Care. ACOG committee opinion. *Obstetrics Gynecol.* (2019) 134:e84–9. doi: 10.1097/AOG.0000000000003425
10. Rusalen F, Cavicchiolo ME, Lago P, Salvadori S, Benini F. Perinatal palliative care: the need of a dedicate care pathway. *BMJ Support Palliat Care.* (2019) 1–6. doi: 10.1136/bmjspcare-2019-001849
11. Garten L, Ohlig S, Metze B, Buhrer C. Prevalence and characteristics of neonatal comfort care patients: a single-center, 5 - year, retrospective, observational study. *Front Pediatr.* (2018) 6:221 doi: 10.3389/fped.2018.00221
12. Donnelly JP, Huff, SH, Lindsey ML, McMahon KA, Schumacher JD. The needs of children with life-limiting conditions: a healthcare-provider-based model. *Am J Hosp Palliat Care.* (2005) 22:259. doi: 10.1177/104990910502200406
13. Italian Law 194/1978, art 7. Gazzetta Ufficiale n 140, 22 maggio 1978.
14. Breeze ACG, Lees CC, Kumar H, Miss-Felder Lobos HH, Murdoch EM. Palliative care for prenatally diagnosed lethal fetal abnormality. *Arch Dis Child Fetal Neonatal Ed.* (2007) 92:F56–F58. doi: 10.1136/adc.2005.092122
15. Hoeldtke NJ Calhoun BC. Perinatal hospice. *Am J Obstet Gynecol.* (2001) 185:525–9. doi: 10.1067/mob.2001.116093
16. Howard ED. Family-centered care in the context of fetal abnormality. *J Perinat Neonatal Nurs.* (2006) 20:237–42. doi: 10.1097/00005237-200607000-00011

7

Challenges and Priorities for Pediatric Critical Care Clinician-Researchers in Low- and Middle-Income Countries

Amelie O. von Saint André-von Arnim[1,2], Jonah Attebery[3], Teresa Bleakly Kortz[4,5], Niranjan Kissoon[6], Elizabeth M. Molyneux[7], Ndidiamaka L. Musa[1], Katie R. Nielsen[1,2], Ericka L. Fink[8] and The Pediatric Acute Lung Injury and Sepsis Investigators (PALISI) Network on Behalf of the PALISI Global Health Subgroup*

[1] Department of Pediatrics, Division of Pediatric Critical Care, Seattle Children's Hospital, University of Washington, Seattle, WA, United States, [2] Department of Global Health, University of Washington, Seattle, WA, United States, [3] Department of Pediatrics, Division of Critical Care, Washington University, St. Louis, MO, United States, [4] Department of Pediatrics, Division of Pediatric Critical Care, University of California, San Francisco, San Francisco, CA, United States, [5] Institute of Global Health Sciences, University of California, San Francisco, San Francisco, CA, United States, [6] Department of Pediatrics and Emergency Medicine, University of British Columbia and British Columbia Children's Hospital, Vancouver, Canada, [7] College of Medicine, University of Malawi, Blantyre, Malawi, [8] Division of Pediatric Critical Care Medicine, Children's Hospital of Pittsburgh of UPMC, Pittsburgh, PA, United States

***Correspondence:**
Amelie O. von Saint André-von Arnim
ameliev@uw.edu

Introduction: There is need for more data on critical care outcomes and interventions from low- and middle-income countries (LMIC). Global research collaborations could help improve health-care delivery for critically ill children in LMIC where child mortality rates remain high.

Materials and methods: To inform the role of collaborative research in health-care delivery for critically ill children in LMIC, an anonymous online survey of pediatric critical care (PCC) physicians from LMIC was conducted to assess priorities, major challenges, and potential solutions to PCC research. A convenience sample of 56 clinician-researchers taking care of critically ill children in LMIC was targeted. In addition, the survey was made available on a Latin American PCC website. Descriptive statistics were used for data analysis.

Results: The majority of the 47 survey respondents worked at urban, public teaching hospitals in LMIC. Respondents stated their primary PCC research motivations were to improve clinical care and establish guidelines to standardize care. Top challenges to conducting research were lack of funding, high clinical workload, and limited research support staff. Respondent-proposed solutions to these challenges included increasing research funding options for LMIC, better access to mentors from high-income countries, research training and networks, and higher quality medical record documentation.

Conclusion: LMIC clinician-researchers must be better empowered and resourced to lead and influence the local and global health research agenda for critically ill children. Increased funding options, access to training and mentorship in research methodology, and improved data collection systems for LMIC PCC researchers were recognized as key needs for success.

Keywords: low- and middle-income countries, low resource settings, researchers, pediatric critical care, support of research, surveys and questionnaires, intensive care unit

INTRODUCTION

The United Nations established Millennium Development Goal 4 aimed to reduce the under-five mortality rate by 2/3 between 1990 and 2015 based on the United Nations Millennium Declaration (1). Although overall progress was realized, only 58 of 138 countries achieved these targets with highest rates of childhood deaths concentrated primarily in low- and middle-income countries (LMIC) (2–4). For example, despite a 67% decrease in under 5 mortality rates (U5MR) in Latin America (LA) over the last 25 years, U5MR on average are still 10% higher in LA than in high-income countries (HIC) (5). Investment in resuscitation and critical care improves patient outcomes in LMIC (6–9). However, this health disparity is exacerbated by the "10–90 gap": only 10% of health-care research expenditures worldwide address diseases that primarily affect the poorest 90% of the world's population (10).

The high burden of child mortality in LMIC is egregious considering that many lives could be saved by proven, simple resuscitative, and critical care interventions despite austere environments and fewer pediatric critical care (PCC) resources compared with HIC (11–15). There is need for LMIC institutions and researchers to conduct critical care research according to local resources and disease spectra, to disseminate results in-country, and influence policymakers, program managers and medical/public health practice (15, 16). Recent data from LMIC showed very clearly that we cannot translate critical care guidelines from HIC to LMIC, and in fact this practice, especially for sepsis, can be harmful (17–19). As such, the World Health Report 2013 called for LMIC to be not only users, but also producers of health research (16). Such health research requires study of leading regional causes of death and disability, which will provide data necessary to inform allocation, determine health-care delivery strategy, and assess quality standards required for effective critical care (15, 20, 21). Therefore, we conducted a survey with the following objectives: (1) to assess major challenges and potential solutions to PCC research in LMIC; (2) to foster worldwide research collaborations; and (3) to begin building a global research network to promote high quality research focused on improving outcomes for critically ill children.

MATERIALS AND METHODS

The Pediatric Acute Lung Injury and Sepsis Investigators (PALISI) Global Health (GH) subgroup (http://www.palisiglobalhealth.org), which includes PCC investigators from Canada and the United States (US), developed an online survey with input from leaders in PCC research in LMIC (Table S1 in Supplementary Material). Survey data were collected and managed using Research Electronic Data Capture (REDCap), an electronic data capture tool, hosted at the University of Washington in Seattle, United States (22). The survey was determined exempt by the Seattle Children's Institutional Review Board (IRB). The anonymous survey was emailed four times between January and June 2016 to a convenience sample of 56 clinician scientists in LMICs. These clinician scientists were identified by leading PCC researchers from LMIC, and through the PALISI GH subgroup's network. In addition, survey recipients were asked to forward the survey to LMIC colleagues in the field, and a survey recipient from LA placed this survey on the PCC website "Sociedad Latino Americana de Cuidados Intensivos Pediatricos." Given that responses were anonymous, we cannot determine between responders from the original convenience sample and responses to the survey posted on the above website. A response rate can therefore not be determined. Descriptive statistics were used for data analysis with subgrouping into respondents' geographic areas using STATA12.

RESULTS

Survey Respondent Characteristics

Forty-seven clinician-researchers from LMIC responded to the survey, the majority from LA (62%) (**Table 1**). Sixty-six percent of respondents were trained pediatric intensivists, and 23%

TABLE 1 | Survey respondents' demographics, research background, and involvement.

Survey respondents' information	Total	SE Asia	Africa	Latin America	Eastern Europe
	n = 47 (%)	*n* = 5 (%)	*n* = 12 (%)	*n* = 29 (%)	*n* = 1 (%)
Credentials					
Pediatric intensivist	31 (66)	4 (80)	4 (33)	22 (76)	1 (100)
Pediatrician with ICU experience	11 (23)	1 (20)	5 (42)	5 (17)	0 (0)
Other	5 (11)	0 (0)	3 (25)	2 (7)	0 (0)
ICU beds					
Less than 7	12 (25)	0 (0)	5 (41)	7 (24)	0 (0)
7–12	16 (34)	3 (60)	4 (33)	8 (28)	1 (100)
More than 12	19 (40)	2 (40)	3 (25)	14 (48)	0 (0)
Protected research time[a]					
None	18 (53)	3 (60)	4 (50)	11 (55)	0 (0)
<10 h/week	10 (29)	1 (20)	0 (0)	8 (40)	1 (100)
>10 h/week	5 (15)	1 (20)	3 (38)	1 (5)	0 (0)
Research training					
Research degree	5 (15)	0 (0)	0 (0)	4 (20)	1 (100)
University-level coursework	14 (41)	2 (40)	1 (13)	11 (55)	0 (0)
Research seminar	15 (44)	4 (80)	3 (38)	8 (40)	0 (0)
Research project	25 (74)	5 (100)	4 (50)	16 (80)	0 (0)
Potential research funding sources					
International collaboration	9 (19)	0 (0)	5 (42)	4 (14)	0 (0)
Local hospital/foundation	19 (40)	3 (60)	2 (17)	14 (48)	0 (0)
Government	2 (4)	1 (20)	1 (8)	0 (0)	0 (0)
International grant	6 (13)	1 (20)	5 (42)	0 (0)	0 (0)
None	18 (38)	2 (40)	3 (25)	12 (41)	1 (100)
Currently funded research	7 (21)	1 (20)	3 (40)	3 (15)	0 (0)
Current research involvement	34 (72)	5 (100)	8 (67)	20 (69)	1 (100)
Clinical observational	27 (79)	5 (100)	6 (75)	15 (75)	1 (100)
Randomized controlled trial	14 (41)	2 (40)	3 (38)	9 (45)	0 (0)
Quality improvement	15 (44)	3 (60)	4 (50)	8 (40)	0 (0)
Research publication	18 (53)	3 (60)	5 (63)	10 (50)	0 (0)
Research role					
Principal investigator	20 (59)	4 (80)	6 (75)	9 (45)	1 (100)
Coinvestigator	10 (29)	1 (20)	2 (25)	7 (35)	0 (0)
Data collector	2 (6)	0 (0)	0 (0)	2 (10)	0 (0)
Local research network	12 (26)	2 (40)	4 (33)	6 (21)	0 (0)

SE, South East; ICU, intensive care unit.

[a]Nine respondents were not actively involved in a research project at the time of survey participation and did not respond to this question.

were intensivists by experience gained through practice. The proportion of trained pediatric intensivists was lowest in Africa (33%). Most respondents worked in combined adult–pediatric intensive care units at urban, public teaching hospitals.

Respondents' Research Involvement and Resources

Active research involvement was reported by 34 (72%) respondents, all of whom had completed variable amounts of training in research methodology (**Table 1**). Fifty-eight percent were principal investigators (PIs) and 29% Co-PIs. Most respondents classified their research focus as clinical (82%), as compared with basic science (2%) and quality improvement (QI) (3%). Forty-seven percent had protected research time, and of those, 29% reported no more than 10 h of dedicated research time per week (**Table 1**). Twenty-one percent of active researchers, mostly from Africa, had research funding, and 53% reported publishing their results in a peer-reviewed journal.

Current Research Priorities, Challenges, and Potential Solutions

Most respondents considered research of high importance (**Table 2**). Generating data that improved clinical care (51%) and establishing guidelines to standardize care (28%) were the most important reasons to perform research involving critically ill children. The main personal benefits cited were opportunities for research collaboration (70%), peer recognition (62%), and career advancement (40%).

Sepsis was the most common research area (38%), followed by invasive/non-invasive mechanical ventilation management (30%), trauma/traumatic brain injury (26%), and QI/patient safety (23%). Key research topics varied by region, with African respondents emphasizing cost-effectiveness, while South East (SE) Asian and LA respondents favored sepsis.

The highest-rated challenges to performing PCC research in LMIC were lack of funding (60%), few research support staff (47%), and high clinical workload (47%). A higher proportion of African researchers found it challenging to find mentors (42%); whereas LA researchers lacked statistical support (31%). The highest-rated solutions to these challenges were increasing research funding options for LMIC (70%), better access to mentors from HIC (51%), improved access to research training (45%), and better medical record keeping (34%).

Research networks were available to 26% of responders, to which LA researchers had the least access. Over half of the respondents collaborated with HIC researchers. These relationships were critically important for 9%, very important or important for 26 and 13% of LMIC clinician-researchers, respectively. The benefits of HIC collaborations included obtaining formal research training and experience (45%); gaining experience in manuscript preparation and publication (40%); and using established guidelines, protocols, and pathways to guide protocol development (34%). The top-rated benefits varied slightly by geographic region (**Table 2**). The primary challenges of HIC research collaboration were a lack of understanding of local settings (38%), communication limitations (26%), and the inability to sustain benefits over time (26%). Overall, 62% of researchers

TABLE 2 | Importance of challenges and solutions to pediatric critical care (PCC) research in LMIC.

Research description, challenges and solutions	Total	SE Asia	Africa	Latin America	Eastern Europe
	n = 47 (%)	n = 5 (%)	n = 12 (%)	n = 29 (%)	n = 1 (%)
Importance of PCC research in LMIC					
Critical	18 (38)	3 (60)	5 (42)	9 (31)	1 (100)
Very important	20 (43)	1 (20)	4 (33)	15 (52)	0 (0)
Important	9 (19)	1 (20)	3 (25)	5 (17)	0 (0)
Most important reason to do research					
Affect positive change in clinical care	24 (51)	3 (60)	6 (50)	14 (48)	1 (100)
Establish guidelines/protocols	13 (28)	2 (40)	3 (25)	8 (28)	0 (0)
Greater understanding of disease	2 (4)	0 (0)	0 (0)	1 (3)	0 (0)
Increase resource availability	3 (6)	0 (0)	2 (17)	1 (3)	0 (0)
Quality and safety	4 (9)	0 (0)	1 (8)	3 (10)	0 (0)
Key areas of research in LMIC					
Sepsis	18 (38)	2 (40)	3 (25)	12 (41)	1 (100)
Trauma	12 (26)	0 (0)	1 (8)	10 (34)	1 (100)
Invasive and non-invasive positive pressure ventilation	14 (30)	0 (0)	3 (25)	11 (38)	0 (0)
Quality improvement and patient safety	11 (23)	2 (40)	2 (17)	7 (24)	0 (0)
Health-care associated infections	9 (19)	3 (60)	2 (17)	4 (14)	0 (0)
ARDS/ALI	7 (15)	1 (20)	0 (0)	6 (21)	0 (0)
Cost-effectiveness	7 (15)	1 (20)	5 (42)	1 (3)	0 (0)
Education/capacity building	6 (13)	1 (20)	2 (17)	3 (10)	0 (0)
Nutrition	6 (13)	2 (40)	0 (0)	4 (14)	0 (0)
Mortality risk/severity of illness scores	5 (11)	1 (20)	0 (0)	4 (14)	0 (0)
Ethics and palliative care	5 (11)	0 (0)	1 (8)	4 (14)	0 (0)
Personal benefits of research					
Research collaboration	33 (70)	3 (60)	6 (50)	23 (79)	1 (100)
Peer recognition	29 (62)	3 (60)	7 (58)	18 (62)	1 (100)
Career advancement	19 (40)	3 (60)	6 (50)	9 (31)	1 (100)
Salary	6 (13)	0 (0)	4 (44)	2 (7)	0 (0)
Other	4 (9)	2 (40)	1 (8)	1 (3)	0 (0)
Research challenges					
Lack of funding	28 (60)	4 (80)	8 (67)	16 (55)	0 (0)
High clinical burden	22 (47)	3 (60)	3 (25)	15 (52)	1 (100)
Limited research support staff	22 (47)	3 (60)	3 (25)	16 (55)	0 (0)
IRB issues	12 (26)	0 (0)	4 (33)	7 (24)	1 (100)
Lack of statistical support	12 (26)	2 (40)	0 (0)	9 (31)	1 (100)
Limited research training opportunities	10 (21)	1 (20)	3 (25)	6 (21)	0 (0)
Finding research mentor(s)	7 (15)	0 (0)	5 (42)	2 (7)	0 (0)
Difficulty with publications	8 (17)	1 (20)	2 (17)	5 (17)	0 (0)
Lack of reliable medical records	4 (9)	0 (0)	3 (25)	1 (3)	0 (0)
Study subject recruitment	4 (9)	0 (0)	1 (8)	3 (10)	0 (0)
Research solutions					
More funding for low resource settings	33 (70)	5 (100)	8 (67)	19 (66)	1 (100)
Access to mentors in HIC	24 (51)	3 (60)	8 (67)	13 (45)	0 (0)
Access to research training	21 (45)	0 (0)	4 (33)	16 (55)	1 (100)
Access to research network	18 (38)	2 (40)	3 (25)	13 (45)	0 (0)
Improved medical records	16 (34)	2 (40)	3 (25)	10 (34)	1 (100)
Opportunities to present	9 (19)	1 (20)	3 (25)	5 (17)	0 (0)
Streamlined IRB review	6 (13)	0 (0)	3 (25)	3 (10)	0 (0)
Protected research time	4 (9)	2 (40)	0 (0)	2 (7)	0 (0)
HIC research collaborations	27 (57)	4 (80)	8 (67)	14 (48)	1 (100)
Importance of collaboration					
Critical	4 (9)	0 (0)	3 (25)	0 (0)	1 (100)
Very	12 (26)	3 (60)	3 (25)	6 (21)	0 (0)

(Continued)

TABLE 2 | Continued

Research description, challenges and solutions	Total	SE Asia	Africa	Latin America	Eastern Europe
	n = 47 (%)	n = 5 (%)	n = 12 (%)	n = 29 (%)	n = 1 (%)
Important	6 (13)	0 (0)	1 (8)	5 (17)	0 (0)
Less	3 (6)	1 (20)	0 (0)	2 (7)	0 (0)
Not	1 (2)	0 (0)	0 (0)	1 (3)	0 (0)
Benefits of collaboration					
Research training	21 (45)	0 (0)	6 (50)	14 (48)	1 (100)
Experience in manuscript preparation	19 (40)	2 (40)	4 (33)	12 (41)	1 (100)
Established guidelines	16 (34)	3 (60)	3 (25)	9 (31)	1 (100)
Financial support	13 (28)	0 (0)	5 (42)	8 (28)	0 (0)
Medical supplies	9 (19)	0 (0)	6 (50)	3 (10)	0 (0)
Other	5 (11)	1 (20)	2 (17)	2 (7)	0 (0)
Problems with collaboration					
Lack of understanding of local setting	18 (38)	1 (20)	6 (50)	11 (38)	0 (0)
Lack of sustainable benefit	12 (26)	0 (0)	6 (50)	6 (21)	0 (0)
Communication limitations	12 (26)	0 (0)	3 (25)	1 (3)	0 (0)
Lack of data sharing	9 (19)	1 (20)	1 (8)	6 (21)	1 (100)
Lack of local research administration	7 (15)	2 (40)	3 (25)	2 (7)	0 (0)
Lack of proper acknowledgment	7 (15)	1 (20)	1 (8)	4 (14)	1 (100)
Dissimilar vision and goals	7 (15)	0 (0)	1 (8)	6 (21)	0 (0)
Ethical conflict	4 (9)	1 (20)	0 (0)	3 (10)	0 (0)
Political barriers	4 (9)	0 (0)	3 (25)	1 (3)	0 (0)
Lack of high tech equipment	1 (2)	0 (0)	1 (8)	0 (0)	0 (0)
Benefits of collaboration outweigh problems	29 (62)	4 (80)	8 (67)	16 (55)	1 (100)

LMIC, low- and middle-income counties; HIC, high-income countries; SE, South East; ARDS/ALI, acute respiratory distress syndrome/acute lung injury; IRB, Institutional Review Board.

in LMICs thought the benefits of collaboration outweighed the difficulties.

DISCUSSION

This study provides information on the vast needs and enormous challenges facing PCC clinician-researchers in LMIC. Most respondents rated the importance of research in PCC to improving health outcomes very highly, but cited lack of funding, heavy clinical workload, and limited research staff as major disincentives. Highest-rated solutions included increased funding opportunities and access to HIC mentors and research training.

Currently, no LMIC invests >1% of its gross domestic product on research and development, as compared with 2–4% in Korea, Japan, the US, and the United Kingdom (17, 23). HIC funders may insist that principal recipients of grants are based in donor countries, thus excluding LMIC institutions from receiving overhead support. It is not surprising then that only 21% of respondents were able to obtain funding and 60% lacked the financial support to conduct research. Lack of trained personnel is also a barrier; however, some solutions exist, such as the US National Institute of Health Fogarty Emerging Global Leader Award program, the NHLBI-UnitedHealth Global Health Centers of Excellence Program, and the World Health Organization/Special Programme for Research and Training in Tropical Diseases Career Development Fellowship, which support scientists from LMIC (24). These programs are promising and are partly facilitated in LMIC, but successful applicants need established mentorship and if locally not available, mentors will come from HIC. Global networking should not be daunting because frugal technology is ubiquitous, hence building research communities, and linking like-minded scientists is relatively easy and highly beneficial. Improving record keeping was also rated as one of the main solutions to research challenges. In low-income settings, there is considerable pressure to contain the cost of data acquisition and still implement effective data management frameworks that produce quality data while research staff and physician time are limited. Introduction of the data capture tool REDCap, a non-commercial software solution designed for rapid development and deployment of electronic data, to a multi-site clinical information and research network in Kenya is now delivering quality pediatric data for clinical improvement and research use (25). This low-cost, sustainable and scalable program could be a solution for other resource-limited settings.

Physician-investigators in HIC face similar challenges as faculty in LMIC, which include securing funding for research programs; promotion or tenure systems not being responsive to the different needs of faculty working in both research and clinical care; and the increasing burdens of clinical care (26, 27). Problems with workload and burnout have been described for intensivists in HIC (28). Equivalent literature is lacking from LMIC, but given that most of sub-Saharan Africa has less than 0.5 doctors, and a large portion of LA less than 1.5 doctors per 1,000 population, compared with 2.5 and 3–4 per 1,000 in North America and Western Europe, respectively (29), clinician-researchers in LMIC are likely more stretched than in HIC. The contrast for numbers of PCC providers between LMIC and HIC is even more stark and likely plays into a PCC clinician-researchers workload dilemma: in LA the number of PCC physicians ranges between 2 in Honduras and 318 in Mexico, respectively; Kenya has a total of 3 PCC physicians serving more than 21 million people less than 18 years of age; compared with 1,805 PCC doctors in the US for 78 million children and adolescents (30–32).

The vast majority of LMIC researchers involved in collaborations with HIC rated these relationships as important for their research, emphasizing the value of nurturing and sustaining these partnerships. The main benefit of collaborations was the opportunity to be trained and gain experience in research, protocol, and guideline development. Mentoring was important, as well as the need for equal, mutually beneficial partnerships. Recent qualitative studies from LMIC highlight common themes of poorly distributed benefits from research involvement, and poor translation of research into local settings (21, 23).

Researchers in LMIC should have opportunities to obtain research funding to provide protected time for research. Research partnerships are often unequal; LMIC researchers should be included in research protocol development, grant applications, and investigation leadership. Funding often depends on successful research track records; if LMIC researchers are not given the opportunity to be PIs or gain acknowledgment for their work, they will continue to be disenfranchised. Mentorship should be complementary of expertise, experience, and understanding, and foster symbiotic relationships. Previous high-impact studies have proven that HIC–LMIC collaboration can successfully improve clinical care, directly benefit the participating communities and give career opportunities to local researchers (17, 33, 34). This should be the paradigm for PCC research study design in LMIC.

Association with experienced PALISI researchers and mentorship in grant writing could help address the funding problems of LMIC PCC researchers. To help address barriers to research in LMIC identified in this survey, the PALISI GH subgroup has begun outreach to PCC researchers in LMIC. Specifically, some PCC researchers have presented research proposals (in-person and *via* webinar) for purposes of feedback and/or recruitment of sites, while others have identified mentors and collaborators. The PALISI-GH subgroup supports the development of PALISI-like groups in LMIC to increase growth of research collaborations and research investigator development. PALISI provides annual research training opportunities for North American PCC fellows, which could be modeled by LMIC countries or potentially be offered to LMIC researchers *via* remote participation or subsidized for in-person attendance by grants.

Although this survey generated interesting data regarding PCC research in LMIC, it had several limitations. The low total number of survey responses limits the generalizability of the results, especially for SE Asia and Eastern Europe. Responses from LA were higher likely due to better local survey publicizing. A response rate cannot be determined given that respondents *via* original invitation versus website survey cannot be distinguished. Given some of the survey recipients were acquired through the PALISI GH subgroup's network, responses may be biased. The term "local research network" was not specifically defined in the survey and could have been interpreted differently by responders, such as hospital, regional, country or continent-wide networks.

CONCLUSION

Since over 95% of the global under-five mortality still occurs in LMIC, researchers from these regions must play a role in setting research priorities, developing clinical guidelines for their settings, informing national policy and improving care for their communities. Increased funding options; access to training and mentorship in research methodology, to research networks, and improved data collection systems are paramount for the success of LMIC PCC researchers. Even in the absence of independent funding mechanisms, HIC–LMIC collaborations as well as regional and international research networks such as PALISI GH can provide important support to colleagues around the world.

ETHICS STATEMENT

This study was carried out in accordance with the recommendations of the Seattle Children's Institutional Review Board, which determined the study to be exempt from IRB approval, since the human subject research involved the use of survey procedures; and the survey did not record information in such a manner that human subjects could be identified, directly or through identifiers linked to the subjects; and any disclosure of the human subjects' responses outside the research could not reasonably place the subjects at risk of criminal or civil liability or be damaging to the subjects' financial standing, employability, or reputation.

AUTHOR CONTRIBUTIONS

AA was involved in survey design, obtained IRB approval, distributed the survey, and participated in data analysis and manuscript writing. EF was involved in survey design, assisted in survey distribution, and participated in data interpretation and in manuscript writing. JA, NK, and EM were involved in survey design, data interpretation, and manuscript writing. NM was involved in manuscript writing. KN completed the data analysis and was involved data interpretation and manuscript writing. TK was involved in data interpretation and manuscript writing.

REFERENCES

1. UN General Assembly. *United Nations Millennium Declaration*. New York: UN General Assembly (2000). p. 1–9.
2. Liu L, Oza S, Hogan D, Chu Y, Perin J, Zhu J, et al. Global, regional, and national causes of under-5 mortality in 2000–15: an updated systematic analysis with implications for the sustainable development goals. *Lancet* (2017) 388(10063):3027–35. doi:10.1016/S0140-6736(16)31593-8
3. Global Burden of Disease Study 2013 Collaborators. Global, regional, and national incidence, prevalence, and years lived with disability for 301 acute and chronic diseases and injuries in 188 countries, 1990–2013: a systematic analysis for the global burden of disease study 2013. *Lancet* (2015) 386(9995):743–800. doi:10.1016/S0140-6736(15)60692-4
4. Bhutta ZA, Das JK, Walker N, Rizvi A, Campbell H, Rudan I, et al. Interventions to address deaths from childhood pneumonia and diarrhoea equitably: what works and at what cost? *Lancet* (2013) 381(9875):1417–29. doi:10.1016/S0140-6736(13)60648-0
5. You D, Hug L, Ejdemyr S, Idele P, Hogan D, Mathers C, et al. Global, regional, and national levels and trends in under-5 mortality between 1990 and 2015, with scenario-based projections to 2030: a systematic analysis by the UN inter-agency group for child mortality estimation. *Lancet* (2015) 386(10010):2275–86. doi:10.1016/S0140-6736(15)00120-8
6. Kesinger MR, Nagy LR, Sequeira DJ, Charry JD, Puyana JC, Rubiano AM. A standardized trauma care protocol decreased in-hospital mortality of patients with severe traumatic brain injury at a teaching hospital in a middle-income country. *Injury* (2014) 45(9):1350–4. doi:10.1016/j.injury.2014.04.037

7. Reynolds TA, Stewart B, Drewett I, Salerno S, Sawe HR, Toroyan T, et al. The impact of trauma care systems in low- and middle-income countries. *Annu Rev Public Health* (2017) 38:507–32. doi:10.1146/annurev-publhealth-032315-021412
8. Baker T, Schell CO, Lugazia E, Blixt J, Mulungu M, Castegren M, et al. Vital signs directed therapy: improving care in an intensive care unit in a low-income country. *PLoS One* (2015) 10(12):e0144801. doi:10.1371/journal.pone.0144801
9. Molyneux E, Ahmad S, Robertson A. Improved triage and emergency care for children reduces inpatient mortality in a resource-constrained setting. *Bull World Health Organ* (2006) 84(4):314–9. doi:10.2471/BLT.04.019505
10. Research GFfH. *The 10/90 Report on Health Research 2003–2004*. Geneva: Global Forum for Health Research (2004).
11. Cheah IG, Soosai AP, Wong SL, Lim TO; Cost-Effectiveness NICU Study Group. Cost-effectiveness analysis of Malaysian neonatal intensive care units. *J Perinatol* (2005) 25(1):47–53. doi:10.1038/sj.jp.7211254
12. Cubro H, Somun-Kapetanovic R, Thiery G, Talmor D, Gajic O. Cost effectiveness of intensive care in a low resource setting: a prospective cohort of medical critically ill patients. *World J Crit Care Med* (2016) 5(2):150–64. doi:10.5492/wjccm.v5.i2.150
13. Profit J, Lee D, Zupancic JA, Papile L, Gutierrez C, Goldie SJ, et al. Clinical benefits, costs, and cost-effectiveness of neonatal intensive care in Mexico. *PLoS Med* (2010) 7(12):e1000379. doi:10.1371/journal.pmed.1000379
14. Tripathi S, Kaur H, Kashyap R, Dong Y, Gajic O, Murthy S. A survey on the resources and practices in pediatric critical care of resource-rich and resource-limited countries. *J Intensive Care* (2015) 3:40. doi:10.1186/s40560-015-0106-3
15. Fowler RA, Adhikari NK, Bhagwanjee S. Clinical review: critical care in the global context – disparities in burden of illness, access, and economics. *Crit Care* (2008) 12(5):225. doi:10.1186/cc6984
16. WHO. *World Health Report 2013: Research for Universal Health Coverage*. Geneva: WHO press (2013).
17. Maitland K, Kiguli S, Opoka RO, Engoru C, Olupot-Olupot P, Akech SO, et al. Mortality after fluid bolus in African children with severe infection. *N Engl J Med* (2011) 364(26):2483–95. doi:10.1056/NEJMoa1101549
18. Andrews B, Semler MW, Muchemwa L, Kelly P, Lakhi S, Heimburger DC, et al. Effect of an early resuscitation protocol on in-hospital mortality among adults with sepsis and hypotension: a randomized clinical trial. *JAMA* (2017) 318(13):1233–40. doi:10.1001/jama.2017.10913
19. Sankar J, Ismail J, Sankar MJ, Suresh CP, Meena RS. Fluid bolus over 15–20 versus 5–10 minutes each in the first hour of resuscitation in children with septic shock: a randomized controlled trial. *Pediatr Crit Care Med* (2017) 18(10):e435–45. doi:10.1097/PCC.0000000000001269
20. Adhikari NK, Fowler RA, Bhagwanjee S, Rubenfeld GD. Critical care and the global burden of critical illness in adults. *Lancet* (2010) 376(9749):1339–46. doi:10.1016/S0140-6736(10)60446-1
21. Joseph PD, Caldwell PH, Tong A, Hanson CS, Craig JC. Stakeholder views of clinical trials in low- and middle-income countries: a systematic review. *Pediatrics* (2016) 137(2):e20152800. doi:10.1542/peds.2015-2800
22. Harris PA, Taylor R, Thielke R, Payne J, Gonzalez N, Conde JG. Research electronic data capture (REDCap) – a metadata-driven methodology and workflow process for providing translational research informatics support. *J Biomed Inform* (2009) 42(2):377–81. doi:10.1016/j.jbi.2008.08.010
23. United Nations Educational, Scientific, and Cultural Organization (UNESCO) Institute for Statistics. *Research and Development Expenditure (% of GDP)* (2015). Available from: http://databank.worldbank.org/data/reports.aspx?source=2&series=GB.XPD.RSDV.GD.ZS&country=#
24. Bloomfield GS, Xavier D, Belis D, Alam D, Davis P, Dorairaj P, et al. Training and capacity building in LMIC for research in heart and lung diseases: the NHLBI-United Health Global Health Centers of Excellence Program. *Glob Heart* (2016) 11(1):17–25. doi:10.1016/j.gheart.2016.01.004
25. Tuti T, Bitok M, Paton C, Makone B, Malla L, Muinga N, et al. Innovating to enhance clinical data management using non-commercial and open source solutions across a multi-center network supporting inpatient pediatric care and research in Kenya. *J Am Med Inform Assoc* (2016) 23(1):184–92. doi:10.1093/jamia/ocv028
26. Hall AK, Mills SL, Lund PK. Clinician-investigator training and the need to pilot new approaches to recruiting and retaining this workforce. *Acad Med* (2017) 92(10):1382–9. doi:10.1097/ACM.0000000000001859
27. Lingard L, Zhang P, Strong M, Steele M, Yoo J, Lewis J. Strategies for supporting physician-scientists in faculty roles: a narrative review with key informant consultations. *Acad Med* (2017) 92(10):1421–8. doi:10.1097/ACM.0000000000001868
28. Embriaco N, Papazian L, Kentish-Barnes N, Pochard F, Azoulay E. Burnout syndrome among critical care healthcare workers. *Curr Opin Crit Care* (2007) 13(5):482–8. doi:10.1097/MCC.0b013e3282efd28a
29. World Health Organization. *Global Health Observatory – Density of Physicians* (2017). Available from: http://www.who.int/gho/health_workforce/physicians_density/en
30. Campos-Mino S, Sasbon JS, von Dessauer B. [Pediatric intensive care in Latin America]. *Med Intensiva* (2012) 36(1):3–10. doi:10.1016/j.medin.2011.07.004
31. UNICEF. *UNICEF Statistics* (2015). Available from: https://www.unicef.org/infobycountry/kenya_statistics.html
32. Pediatrics ABo. *Pediatric Physicians Workforce Data Book, 2016–2017*. Chapel Hill, NC: American Board of Pediatrics (2017).
33. Fink EL, Kochanek PM, Tasker RC, Beca J, Bell MJ, Clark RS, et al. International survey of critically ill children with acute neurologic insults: the prevalence of acute critical neurological disease in children: a global epidemiological assessment study. *Pediatr Crit Care Med* (2017) 18(4):330–42. doi:10.1097/PCC.0000000000001093
34. Molyneux E, Mathanga D, Witte D, Molyneux M. Practical issues in relation to clinical trials in children in low-income countries: experience from the front line. *Arch Dis Child* (2012) 97(9):848–51. doi:10.1136/archdischild-2011-301476

8

Moral Distress in the Neonatal Intensive Care Unit: What is it, Why it Happens and How we can Address It

Manisha Mills [1*] *and DonnaMaria E. Cortezzo* [1,2,3,4]

[1] *Division of Neonatal and Pulmonary Biology, Cincinnati Children's Hospital Medical Center, Cincinnati, OH, United States,*
[2] *Division of Pain and Palliative Medicine, Cincinnati Children's Hospital Medical Center, Cincinnati, OH, United States,*
[3] *Department of Pediatrics, University of Cincinnati College of Medicine, Cincinnati, OH, United States,* [4] *Department of Anesthesiology, University of Cincinnati College of Medicine, Cincinnati, OH, United States*

Correspondence:
Manisha Mills
Manisha.mills@cchmc.org

Moral distress is prevalent in the neonatal intensive care unit (NICU), where decisions regarding end-of-life care, periviable resuscitation, and medical futility are common. Due to its origins in the nursing literature, moral distress has primarily been reported among bedside nurses in relation to the hierarchy of the medical team. However, it is increasingly recognized that moral distress may exist in different forms than initially described and that healthcare professions outside of nursing experience it. Advances in medical technology have allowed the smallest, sickest neonates to survive. The treatment for critically ill infants is no longer simply limited by the capability of medical technology but also by moral and ethical boundaries of what is right for a given child and family. Shared decision-making and the zone of parental discretion can inform and challenge the medical team to balance the complexities of patient autonomy against harm and suffering. Limited ability to prognosticate and uncertainty in outcomes add to the challenges faced with ethical dilemmas. While this does not necessarily equate to moral distress, subjective views of quality of life and personal values in these situations can lead to moral distress if the plans of care and the validity of each path are not fully explored. Differences in opinions and approaches between members of the medical team can strain relationships and affect each individual differently. It is unclear how the various types of moral distress uniquely impact each profession and their role in the distinctively challenging decisions made in the NICU environment. The purpose of this review is to describe moral distress and the situations that give rise to it in the NICU, ways in which various members of the medical team experience it, how it impacts care delivery, and approaches to address it.

Keywords: moral distress, decision-making, neonatal intensive care, ethical confrontation, periviability, end-of-life care, medical futility

INTRODUCTION

American philosopher Martha Nussbaum writes "in all situations of choice, we face a question that I call 'the obvious question': what shall we do? But sometimes we also face, or should face, a different question, which I call 'the tragic question:' is any of the alternatives open to us free from serious moral wrongdoing?"(1) In Nussbaum's "tragic question" lies the crux of moral distress. This concept in relation to the field of medicine was first described and defined by Jameton in 1984 as "the psychological distress of being in a situation in which one is constrained from acting on what one knows to be right"(2). Though its first applications were primarily limited to nursing practice, the concept has since been broadened to include other groups of healthcare professionals.

The concept of constraint is central to the essence of the original definition moral distress and is a predominant theme in nursing literature. Moral dilemma or conflict, on the other hand, is more often reported as being experienced by physicians (3). In circumstances where there is moral conflict, values systems or duties relating to multiple treatment options are incompatible with one another and lead to psychological distress (4). The provider feels he must act in a way or provide care that is contrary to what he believes is the appropriate care plan (5). This discrepancy inherently challenges one's ethical principles. As a result, the term ethical confrontation has also been used to describe the associated distress (6). In an effort to provide the most inclusive review possible, moral constraint, moral conflict, and ethical confrontation will be considered in the discussion of moral distress.

While it is necessary to expand the definition of moral distress beyond the idea of moral constraint as providers are rarely faced with one definitive action on which to make a moral or ethical judgement, there must be a clear distinction between separate albeit related concepts of uncertainty, ethical dilemmas, and moral distress. In the neonatal intensive care unit (NICU), there is seldom absolute assurance in the outcome for a baby with the choices or treatment options available. There is always an element of uncertainty in outcomes that can lend itself to varying degrees of distress when discussing treatment options and decision-making with families. In addition, the NICU is wrought with ethically ambiguous clinical circumstances and complex decisions for a vulnerable population. This innately leads to feelings of internal discord, powerlessness, and uncertainty in physicians, nurses, and other healthcare professionals. This type of uncertainty, while undoubtedly causing stress and discomfort, should not be confused with moral distress. While there are times when these situations lead to distress if values are challenged, the presence of uncertainty or ethical dilemmas do not automatically equate to moral distress.

Frequently, though, decisions regarding end-of-life care and life-sustaining measures provoke moral distress, requiring a closer look at how this ultimately influences the care that is provided. Providers may feel constrained by the uncertainty in these decisions and having to counsel parents with limited information about the possible outcomes. Regardless of the etiology, moral distress can impact patient care and provider longevity (5, 7–9). If addressed, though, providers can minimize the negative affects while supporting each other and fostering personal growth (10, 11). The purpose of this review is to describe the role of moral distress in the NICU, reasons it occurs, how it presents unique challenges to different healthcare professions, and how providers can address it.

THE SCOPE OF THE PROBLEM

While it is accepted that moral distress is ubiquitous for those who work in healthcare, the true prevalence in the NICU is not well-established (12). Some historical challenges in assessing the prevalence include a focus in the literature on parental moral distress and adult patients, multiple definitions of moral distress, and an emphasis on the nursing profession (13, 14). While moral distress can affect any member of the healthcare team, it is most prevalent in those who provide direct care, such as physicians and nurses. This is likely due to the close relationships formed with patients and their families and the sense of responsibility in providing care (15). As such, it is increasingly recognized that moral distress can affect any member of the medical team regardless of profession.

For nurses, common causes of moral distress can be patient-focused or nursing-focused (16). Patient factors largely focus on quality of life, advocacy for the patient, and communication challenges with the families and care team. Nursing factors may include not having a voice within the care team, unclear roles, personal or team conflict, and feeling their integrity is being compromised. Historically, it was thought that the factors leading to moral distress were rooted in paternalistic approaches to medicine where nurses were instructed by physicians to provide care they did not always feel was appropriate (5).

With newer multidisciplinary care models, a recent focus on understanding healthcare provider moral distress has given more insight to the scope of this issue. In a recent qualitative analysis of attitudes around moral distress of NICU physicians and nurses, it was reported that up to 72% of providers experience moral distress at least once a month (10). Other studies show similar findings with up to 58% of nurses and physicians reporting specific work related moral distress (8). While it presents differently for each profession, all members of the medical team are vulnerable to this phenomenon.

Despite the prevalence, there is significant variability around the degree and frequency at which providers experience moral distress or ethical confrontation. This is likely due in part to the characteristics of the individuals included in studies. One study evaluating the impact of experience and knowledge of providers on the frequency of ethical confrontation reported that 35% of experienced NICU nurses and 19% of pediatric or obstetric residents experienced this challenge frequently at work. Overall, in the presence of ethical confrontation, greater experience and a higher level of understanding were associated with lower rates of moral distress. Perhaps with experience providers are able to process and cope with ethically challenging situations in a

Abbreviations: NICU, Neonatal Intensive Care Unit.

manner that they do not feel moral constraint. On the other hand, increased knowledge about particular medical situations can open the possibility of experiencing moral distress. Individuals at medical centers that reported lower rates of moral distress around periviable resuscitation were less knowledgeable about outcomes for extremely preterm infants and were less likely to offer resuscitation at the lowest gestational ages. Those with more experience in the consequences of extreme prematurity, especially nursing staff, tend to overestimate poor outcomes and have higher rates of moral distress around offering resuscitation. Overall, the culture of a given center had the greatest impact on levels of moral distress, with the lowest frequencies of moral distress reported at centers that were the most homogenous with respect to language spoken and religious affiliation (6). This is in contrast to the longstanding notion that moral distress primarily originates from medical team hierarchy and suggests that heterogeneous values and background may contribute more to moral distress than was originally thought. Results of this and similar studies varied considerably with respect to the frequency and intensity of moral distress experienced by varying members of the medical team (6, 8, 12, 17).

Interestingly despite the challenges associated with moral distress, up to 76% of healthcare professionals feel it is a necessary part of caring for critically ill neonates (10). They view this feeling as a byproduct of being a caring, compassionate provider who is invested in the well-being of their patient and providing the best possible care. It is also viewed as a sign of innovation and progress in patient care (11). The internal struggle created by a difficult situation can, at times, be necessary. It challenges providers to acknowledge their own distress and biases in caring for patients and talking with families. This is important because the information communicated to families and the manner in which it is communicated can impact decisions made and ultimately lead to transference of distress (5). Simply because the medical team and/or parents agree upon a specific treatment course does not guarantee the accuracy or benefit of the treatment. Without the challenge of differing opinions, the ethical, moral, and medical appropriateness of such a decision goes unscrutinized (11). Discussions that emerge from moral distress promote exploration of multiple courses of action and encourage the most informed decision possible.

While providers feel that moral distress is an innate part of caring for NICU patients, it is accompanied by some degree of burden. Physician trainees in the NICU reported, through longitudinal narrative writing, that they experienced conflict in multiple situations that caused them distress and led them to question their own morals (18). The unique position of trainees in the medical team hierarchy places them at risk for constraint distress. They may feel obligated to provide care they do not agree with and are unable to voice these disagreements due to lack of confidence, fear of unfavorable evaluation, or concern for retaliation. As a result, they may feel numb and cope through detachment and desensitization, which can lead to compassion fatigue and burnout over time (18, 19). The emotional toll, which transcends beyond trainees, can lead to disengagement and ultimately effect patient care with avoidance behaviors amongst staff, increase length of patients' hospital stays, adverse patient outcomes, and increased pain levels in patients (12, 20). In addition, moral distress can contribute to increased burnout, decreased job retention by the healthcare provider, decreased staff retention by institutions, career transitions, threatened moral integrity, and a sense of failure to perform a professional and moral duty (5, 7–9). In order to provide optimal patient care and a safe environment for providers to thrive, when moral distress is prevalent providers are faced with a balancing act of minimizing the negative impact and leveraging the potential for progress (9).

WHY IS MORAL DISTRESS SO PREVALENT IN THE NICU?

Many factors can contribute to moral distress. Intensive care settings, staffing shortages, the need for timeliness/efficiency, and situations involving perceived futile care or different perspectives on end-of-life decisions place individuals at higher risk for moral distress (12). Structural aspects of the NICU, including lack of a consistent care team, poor communication, and understaffing lead to moral distress due to feelings of providing substandard care (21). Beyond the structure itself, variation in providers' own views and values within an institution can lead to reports of greater moral distress (6). Perhaps there are factors innate to the providers themselves and the culture of the institution that play a role in the presence of moral distress. When providers on the same care team have different values and moral compasses, there is a higher likelihood of some team members feeling moral constraint and subsequently moral distress based on the care provided.

The vulnerability of the NICU population, combined with the need for decision-making by proxy further compounds this risk. In the face of advancing medical knowledge and increasing reliance on technology and life sustaining measures, parents and healthcare providers struggle to find balance and determine what is truly in the best interest of the child (22). The frequency of end-of-life situations and the complex nature of NICU care lends itself to moral distress. One study found that a higher number of deaths and issues surrounding end-of-life care and resuscitations are associated with the highest levels of moral distress (8, 17). Interactions between team members and with parents and family can ease or amplify these feelings (17). Similarly, the degree to which medical team members agree with one another and with the parents' decisions can influence perceptions of constraint or control. It is far more common for healthcare providers to feel they are "doing too much" rather than too little. While this can be seen as an ethical dilemma, the resulting concern for inflicting undue harm and suffering results in a greater degree of moral distress (23). Interestingly, while physicians were more likely to disagree with the level of care a patient was receiving than nurses were, their reported levels of moral distress were lower than those of nurses. This may relate to the notion that increased education and experience with these challenging clinical scenarios allows physicians to better delineate ethical questions from moral distress. It also may relate to the fact that nurses are the individuals actively carry out the care plan.

While many factors contribute to how decisions are made for a vulnerable patient who cannot convey their own wishes, as with a neonate, there are external constraints beyond provider judgement that can impact and alter the care plan. Some factors that influence decisions include limitations put forth by laws and regulations, institutional policy, parental wishes and views of quality of life, hierarchy of the healthcare system, or ethics committee rulings. If these factors are in opposition to provider beliefs, it can lead to significant moral distress (25). Similarly, if there is a perception that medical interventions are causing unnecessary suffering, it can lead to feelings of helplessness (26).

Just as important to consider are factors internal and innate to the provider. If there is uncertainty or doubt about the diagnosis, prognosis, or most effective treatment course, it can lead to feelings of powerlessness, fear, lack of knowledge, or hesitation to advocate for their patient (8). These internal constraints are commonly described in the literature but less frequently recognized as sources of moral distress (9, 13, 27, 28). While some have advocated to expand the definition of moral distress to encompass situations beyond where there is moral constraint, these circumstances of uncertainty, even with a broader definition of moral distress are more appropriately described as moral sensitivity or ambiguity rather than moral distress (3, 4).

While moral distress can arise from any complex situation, most common scenarios that give rise to moral distress in the NICU involve end-of-life care, medical utility and futility, periviability, and disagreements about care plans (24). Each of these challenging clinical scenarios, which are described in greater detail below, involve medically complex decision-making.

End-Of-Life-Care and Palliative Care

There are over 15,000 neonatal deaths each year in the United States and the majority of these occur in the NICU (29). As a result, end-of-life care is routinely tasked to providers who take care of babies in an intensive care setting. Transitions to end-of-life care are never easy and are fraught with grief and uncertainties at a time of heightened emotions for all involved. More than 80% of the time, deaths in the NICU are preceded by a decision to limit, withdraw, or withhold life-sustaining treatments (30). This requires difficult conversations about the prognosis and multiple treatment options and approaches to care available. Once a decision to redirect care is made or it is evident that a patient is dying despite invasive medical interventions, subsequent care can greatly influence parental coping and medical team attitudes surrounding the death.

How providers define or personally view aggressive care, redirection of care, and the reasons for pursuing these care paths can contribute to feelings of moral distress. Singh et al. claim that when an actively dying patient is extubated so the mother may hold the infant as he or she passes, it is ethically different than compassionate withdrawal of care in the setting of a severe neurologic insult with likely poor long-term outcomes. The study also noted that timing of death did not significantly differ for infants who received full support vs. those for whom care was withdrawn (31). Both resulted in the infant's passing, but perhaps, the authors suggest, the former situation offers a clearer assessment of futility and allows moral judgement of providers to align with the actions taken.

The timing of when options such comfort measures, redirection of care, or pursuing invasive medical interventions are discussed is important as it can also impact feelings of moral distress. It may feel different to parents or healthcare providers to withhold care and refrain from initiating a particular care path than to withdraw or redirect care after invasive interventions are initiated. With increasing medical capabilities to care for the tiniest, sickest infants, trials of therapy are not uncommon. Parents may need time to process the information and prognosis, especially with unanticipated events or diagnoses and providers must balance the need to minimize suffering to the patient and utilize resources appropriately. Parents and providers utilize a shared decision-making approach to determine the boundaries of care plans, based not only on prognostic factors, but parental values and goals of care (32). Concern for prolonging suffering while awaiting parental decisions may intensify the medical team's feelings of failure to prevent undue suffering or harm to the patient. Likewise, due to provider discomfort with having these difficult conversations or their own perceptions about the appropriateness of such care plans, discussions often occur late in the hospital course. This can lead to distress and constraint of other providers or the families (32). Moral distress may result from the choice to provide invasive medical interventions, withhold therapies, or withdraw invasive medical interventions especially in circumstances in which there is little data to drive the decision that is in opposition to what the provider believes to be morally right.

Consider a former premature child corrected past term with bronchopulmonary dysplasia who thrives on continuous positive airway pressure and awaits parental decision regarding a tracheostomy to aid in development and facilitate transition to home. Despite declining redirection of care when the baby was critically ill, parents have consistently expressed the desire for an acceptable quality of life over quantity of life. In their eyes, dependence on any medical technology long-term is not an acceptable quality of life. They are increasingly distressed and often in disagreement with the medical team over the amount of invasive care the child is receiving. They express they would not want their child to be dependent on a tracheostomy or gastrointestinal tube feeds for an extended period of time. Ultimately, they elect to redirect care and remove the continuous positive airway pressure mask. The baby dies over the course of a several days. Some of the medical team expresses anguish over withdrawing non-invasive support on a baby with a favorable neurodevelopmental prognosis. They are faced with the constraint of parental desires and request to redirect care despite their own beliefs and views. In the zone of parental discretion, one may choose to honor such a request with appropriate counseling and risk assessment. While there is a level of moral judgement that this treatment course exposes the child to risk and ultimately death, the decision of the parents does not constitute medical neglect as there are also significant risks and burdens associated with the alternate care paths. A child with a tracheostomy who is ventilator dependent requires around-the-clock care and vigilance. They may have significant medical complications including death related to the tracheostomy and long-term ventilator support. In this challenging scenario, the involvement of palliative care and ethics is important. Through their involvement, the care team can better understand the complex factors that went in to the difficult decision made by the parents. This also allows for an avenue for staff to express their concerns, better understand the ethical questions at hand, and process their personal views in relation to the case.

Medical Utility and Futility

Consideration of medical futility when pursuing life-sustaining measures is important but difficult to apply to a clinical setting. Given the present degree of uncertainty in neonatal outcomes and continual advances in therapies and medical technology available, it is challenging to determine if interventions being provided have a reasonable likelihood of success and what defines success for any particular baby/family. Futility can be defined as a treatment that fails to provide discernable benefit (33). It innately requires delineation of goals as it is a term relative to the desired outcome. This is a challenging concept as many interventions provide some benefit and invasive interventions may allow an individual to live for a period of time. Due to the increasing use of technology and medical innovations, providers may feel that care is at times overly aggressive, without clear or definitive benefit. This can lead to distress and concern that they are causing undue suffering to their patient. It is reported that over half of attending neonatologists and over one-third of nurses have provided care they view as "overly burdensome." Similarly, 80% of physicians and 69% of nurses felt they had saved a child who "should not be saved," despite personal and moral objections to doing so (34). The decision of whether or not to continue aggressive care in the setting of a poor prognosis can be morally distressing. In particular, neurodevelopmental outcomes and the impact on long-term perceived quality of life is of great concern when weighing benefit against risk. Simply enabling survival is no longer the goal. A delicate balance between preserved quality of life, incorporating family goals, and minimizing suffering complicates the decision of the most appropriate treatment plan.

Quality of life is inherently personal as what is considered acceptable for one person may not be for another. While physicians overwhelmingly support parental involvement in decisions regarding end-of-life and palliative care, there is a tendency to anchor in the statistical majority with respect to outcomes (35). This can greatly influence how healthcare providers counsel a family and the degree of moral distress following a parental decision that does not align with their own views. In these situations, providers are asking themselves if a life with profound disabilities is a life worth living and if providing life-sustaining measures is worth the cost (36). While weighing these costs, they view what that life could potentially look like. Physicians tend to place a much higher value on cognitive function and independence than families do (37). This is likely, in part, due to the limited context and surroundings in which they interact with children with severe impairments. It can cause moral distress when a provider is challenged to accept different values and provide balanced counseling and at times provide interventions with goals in opposition to their personal values.

Regardless of the underlying diagnosis, when the medical team is asked to provide care that will extend a child's life, they often do so with the best interest of the baby in mind. However, when this is in the context of a child who will have a profound cognitive disability, the best interest standard often comes in to question (38). This is largely based on weighing the burdens and benefits of various treatment pathways for the child in the context of their family. While providers may have personal views, they cannot presume to know if the child would prefer death to a life with profound impairments especially when the child would have no other comparison (39). Often times the treatments available will extend the child's life and potentially facilitate leaving a hospital setting. The interventions themselves do not place the child at risk for imminent, preventable harm. As a result, it is difficult for providers to use ethical principles of best interest and non-maleficence as justification for advocating against such interventions. While there will likely be burdens for the child and family with the pursuit of invasive interventions, some feel these burdens are miniscule in comparison to the life the child is able to have and the potential relationship the baby is able to develop with their family and surroundings (40). With this notion, some advocate for providers to focus on the moral value of that relationship and the capacity for a caring relationship as opposed to neurodevelopmental outcomes when determining if invasive interventions are appropriate. The relational potential for which some advocate is morally meaningful regardless of others ability to see the reciprocity of the relationship (40). It is only with the help of the providers that these potentials can be realized. By acknowledging the significance of this relationship, providers can support their patients' families and potentially feel more comfortable with the interventions they are being asked to provide.

Often, providers find themselves in the zone of parental discretion when the risk of an option does not clearly outweigh the benefit. In such circumstances, parents are assumed to have their child's best interest at heart and know what is best for their family. As a result they are encouraged to be the decision-makers for their child unless the decision will cause express harm (41). When parental decisions ultimately differ from what providers believe is the right or most appropriate treatment course, either professionally or personally, the uncertainty of the outcome coupled with constraint of parental preference may produce profound moral distress for providers (42). This can be exacerbated by significantly differing beliefs and views on which these decisions are based. If a physician or nurse experiences moral distress as a result of disagreement with parental wishes, communication may become filtered through their own views and values, such that it offers more or less hope for achievement of parental goals than truly exists. This has been described as "ethically indefensible" and amounting to "deception" (43).

Consider a child with a long and arduous clinical course fraught with multiple bouts of severe clinical instability. He has undergone several invasive surgical procedures with refractory hypotension and hypoxia leading to irreversible end-organ damage. There has been no progress for months. Despite frequent counseling on the poor prognosis and lack of ability to wean ventilator support, parents continue to advocate for interventions with the goal of extending his life. They request that the medical team minimize discussions around redirection of care as they have expressed their wishes for their child. Physicians rounding on the child find themselves at a loss for contributions to his care plan that will lead to improvement in his clinical status and bedside nurses feel increasingly distressed by the invasive care they must provide. For months, he remains on the ventilator with no evidence of interacting with his surroundings in a meaningful or purposeful manner. When parents are available, they participate in his care. Otherwise, the nursing staff are his primary care-takers. He develops an infection and acutely decompensates. Despite interventions to treat the infection, he ultimately dies. Staff struggled with continuing to provide invasive medical care. Initially there was great distress over the perception that he was suffering. After discussions with the ethics committee and a better understanding of the degree of his neurological injury and appropriate administration of medications, most providers believed inventions were prolonging a short life in the hospital but no longer felt he was suffering. Ultimately, some reported less moral distress after understanding that he was not suffering, that parents needed more time with him, and that his parents needed to see him die under those circumstances to feel that they advocated for him and gave him every chance to survive.

Periviability

Periviable deliveries and resuscitation remain a controversial topic. Different institutions have various thresholds for resuscitation based on patient-specific factors, local data and outcomes, physician attitudes and maternal characteristics (44). Population-based estimation of outcomes lacks the precision necessary to make decisions on an individual level. The extreme uncertainty and lack of clear evidence or definitive clinical guidelines on periviable resuscitation can make counseling parents and caregivers challenging. In addition, knowledge and experience of the medical team members are recognized as factors that influence providers' personal views and greatly impact thresholds for resuscitation, estimation of mortality risk, and assessment of long-term outcomes they convey to parents (6).

Discussions around resuscitation often occur at a time with high emotions and stress where outcomes are uncertain and decisions are often made quickly. Providers are tasked with guiding parents through the recognition of their own values while providing available evidence to aid in a shared decision-making approach to care. However, the decisions that are ultimately made can remain a moral and ethical challenge for providers when their personal views and values are in opposition to the care plan they are developing (45). The vast majority of the time, neonatologists and parents are able to come to a mutually agreed upon course of action through discussion and goal sharing. In fact, in a cross-sectional study surveying neonatologists about their preferences surrounding periviable resuscitation, physicians chose options that aligned with parental wishes 66% percent of the time, as compared with options supported by institutional guidelines just 34% of the time (46). The agreeable nature of acting in accordance with parental wishes supports previous findings that understanding parental values and aiding in developing a care plan based on those values results in a lower frequency of moral distress. Further, defaulting to parental wishes and realizing there is no clear right or wrong option despite variation in personal views could partially remove the burden of decision-making from the neonatologist and reduce the moral dilemma he or she would otherwise face. There may also be an element of constraint from institutional guidelines that parental preference helps to override. Rather than strict criteria, guidelines may incorporate parental discretion and offer options that can be tailored to a particular patient. In this way, uncertainty is acknowledged, and shared decision-making can proceed with less impact from medical team bias or distress. A better understanding of the complexities involved in prognostication and decision-making can foster discussions and address discomfort or questions individuals may have (45).

Conflict and Disagreement

While differing views and opinions can result in discussions that encourage progress and novel ideas, it can also serve as a nidus for moral distress and residue that degrades the relationship between members of the care team and with the family (13, 47). Differences in the application of the zone of parental discretion may lend itself to variability in the amount of parental latitude given in determining interventions and treatment goals. Physicians may be viewed as overindulgent to seemingly unreasonable requests or too inflexible in incorporating parental perspectives. Physicians may agree to parents' wishes if those wishes do not constitute medical neglect while nurses feel distressed at having to carry out interventions that they feel cause more harm than good (48). Consultants may struggle to find helpful recommendations for a case they feel is futile. Different teams caring for the same patient may have opposing recommendations that can erode confidence and trust of the family and care team (13, 47, 49). In these situations, achievement of consensus despite initial disagreement may ultimately allow parents and caregivers to justify their decisions internally and serve to assuage discomfort associated with such ethical dilemmas.

ADDRESSING MORAL DISTRESS

As moral distress can have a significant impact on providers, patients, their families, and the care management plans that are derived, it is imperative that providers go beyond recognizing moral distress and develop effective ways to address it (50). This can lead to improved moral resilience, the capacity to tolerate moral distress and effectively function while mitigating the negative effects (49). While improving moral resilience is greatly dependent upon an individual's internal resources and ability to navigate ethically challenging situations, mindful and intentional reflection of the situation is pertinent to help providers process their emotions. There needs to be training around emotional support and coping for healthcare providers (18).

One of the most important initial steps is recognizing moral subjectivity. This can promote open discussions about the different views and perspectives of others that are driving their opinions and lead to a feeling of comradery. As a result, a shared sense of burden and responsibility for the decisions that are made can develop (5). Specific to end-of-life settings, studies suggest that higher levels of emotional intelligence may temper the negative effects of moral distress (20). By being able to recognize and reflect on emotions and incorporate them with cognitive reasoning, one can more productively manage and cope with morally challenging situations rather than having them lead to moral distress. Ultimately, this leads to improved interactions with patients and decreased levels of stress and anxiety (20). An important factor in this practice is improved and effective communication skills amongst all team members.

There have been many suggestions to support recognizing and addressing moral distress. Included in these suggestions are workshops, debriefings, ethics training, and practices such as reflective writing (20, 51, 52). These methods all have a uniting theme of bringing to the forefront the emotional impact of various situations and events. Writing, specifically, tasks an individual with critically examining the experience as a way of processing and coping. Narrative medicine can aid with coping and enhance physician empathy (18). While studies in other avenues have shown a positive effect in this type of interventions, a small study for NICU nurses in Iran failed to show a difference in moral distress intensity or frequency after 8 weeks of narrative writing (53). This may suggest that there are more complex factors than the act of writing about traumatic events that must occur in order for the practice to be effective. Beyond these measures of personal reflections, the way in which an individual approachs conversations and arrives at or navigates through challenging decisions can have a positive impact on moral distress.

Counseling and Decision-Making

Since the early 2000's, decision-making in neonatology has seen a shift in practice from providing information to parents and recommending a course of treatment based on evidence alone to a shared decision-making process. In this collaborative approach, factors such as parental values, emotions, trust in the care being provided, life experiences, goals of care, and other personal considerations are taken in to account when developing a care plan (54). The medical team and family must balance the often competing principles of autonomy, beneficence, and non-maleficence. This model of care allows for various stakeholders to express their personal views and values that help them determine a care plan. Values that predominate among healthcare professionals are intertwined with their own personal values. They often emphasize concepts such as patient dignity, quality of care, integrity, a duty to "do no harm," and alleviate suffering. There are times when their personal views of quality of life vastly differ from that of the parents. As a result, while a shared decision-making approach ensures that all members invested in the care of the baby have input, there are still situations where providers enact a treatment plan they do not feel is optimal for their patient (5). The highest level of distress reported by nurses occurs when following family's wishes when the medical team perceived they were doing "too much" (55). Regardless of the providers' personal views, through the processes of shared decisions-making, he can better understand the views and values of the family. Through recognizing important factors for them in determining quality of life or an appropriate care plan, the provider can make recommendations that align with those views rather than their own personal views. This understanding and approach to navigating goals of care or treatment plans can lead to confidence that the care plan established is a collaborative approach to care that is most appropriate for the individual baby and family regardless of the providers' personal views. As a result, this approach to counseling and decision-making can lead to decreased moral distress.

Continuity of Care

Inherent in successful shared decision-making is the cultivation of a relationship between the neonatologist, other members of the medical team, the patient, and their parents or other surrogate decision makers. Due to the nature of prematurity and critical illness in newborns, it is not uncommon for a child and their family to encounter multiple care teams throughout their NICU stay, with physician teams rotating approximately every 1–4 weeks. While nursing care teams are typically more consistent, they also involve some degree of variability. Though the same team members may come and go throughout the hospitalization, they participate in different parts of a given patient's care. This can make it difficult for parents to develop consistent relationships that foster trust and an understanding of values.

Despite efforts at standardization and adherence to evidence-based guidelines, there are often differences in the care provided due to the relative paucity of definitive data and algorithms for treatment in neonates. Constraint distress may be experienced due to a plan set in place by another physician or care team and in turn, bedside nurses or other staff members may be faced with the dilemma of aligning with the changing recommendations of the medical team while advocating for frustrated parents and original care plans (5, 16). Their personal views on the best course of action may also make counseling families or communicating with other staff more difficult, thus impacting overall the team's decision-making ability.

Watching a patient suffer due to poor communication and lack of continuity of care leads to high levels of self-reported moral distress (14, 23, 49). It is important with the multiple hand-offs and transitions in care that there are detailed conversations between care providers about the conversations that have taken place and that the unit has a collaborative approach to care. This will allow the providers to better understand how families make decisions, what information has been conveyed to them, and what the expectations for the care plan and treatment options are. Standardizing this approach can lead to seamless care despite changing providers. All providers should be engaged in methods to promote teamwork and to work collaboratively. It is important to ensure all members of the multidisciplinary team have an opportunity to share their thoughts and information to truly promote an environment of shared understanding and community (8). There should be clear methods in place to address conflict or disagreements that may arise among team members (12). It will also allow the family to feel more confident that the providers know their child and decreases the chances of abrupt changes in the care plan.

Education and Communication

An integrative review examining moral distress in NICU nurses around palliative care found that experiences of moral distress were variable (56). Factors associated with a higher level of moral distress included conflicts among care providers, lack of continuity of care, perceived futile care, false hope, and fluctuation in patients' clinical status. In response to recognizing moral distress, many centers have developed formal and informal educational opportunities to attempt to address causes of distress (18). While the etiology of moral distress appear multifactorial, certain interventions appear to alleviate moral distress. Education around end-of-life care, formation of a care team with the focus of establishing goals of care, and a protocol with a clear plan to address the dying process tend to decrease moral distress.

One center developed comprehensive educational interventions with modules to address nursing moral distress around end-of-life care (57). Overall comfort level with dying patients increased after participating in the educational program. After the educational sessions, nurses reported less compassion fatigue and noted that learning about self-care was important. They also benefited significantly from educations around legal and ethical issues surrounding neonatal end-of-life care. The importance of communication and the many emotions surrounding these situations was also highlighted. Through educational sessions, the importance of the desire for support was recognized. Regardless of the format, having avenues to discuss situations and allow staff to feel supported and heard is critical. Providing support through shared experience is beneficial and a way to foster meaningful relationships (18).

Specific training around communication and environments conducive to meetings and support for staff beyond traditional debriefings is crucial (12). It is known that that those who are less informed about outcomes may make a moral judgement based on misinformation or lack of information and experience moral distress as a result of treatment decisions that challenge their judgment (6). Clear and consistent communication with all members of the team regarding rationale, expected outcomes and options provided to the parents may help to alleviate distress that occurs as a result of simply "not knowing." To facilitate communications in an educational environment, some centers have introduced rounds or designated sessions for multidisciplinary teams to discuss challenging patients. One center described their approach to a multidisciplinary conference with the goal of promoting communication and consensus building (58). In a structured setting, all members of the NICU staff were invited to attend a discussion about a patient where there was distress or concerns related to the patient care. Input is sought from all team members as well as invited ethicists with the hope of navigating through the complex issues with the goal of improving communication and collaboration to reach a consensus about the case at hand. It appeared that participants felt these conferences took place later than they should in the course of care. Comfort with expressing distress directly correlated to the perceived support of the institution. While communication was cited as a cause of distress, the sessions were attended predominately by those who already felt comfortable recognizing and addressing distress. As a result it was suggested that with education around communication there may be an improved comfort level with crucial conversations that would lead to improved comfort in attending such sessions with the intent of improving patient care and decreasing moral distress.

Role of Ethics Consultation

With the frequency of ethically challenging situations in the NICU, the utilization of ethics consultations is common. These consultations can serve as forum to promote discussions on moral subjectivity and clarifying ethical challenges that arise (5, 59). This can aid in supporting moral resilience and alleviating compassion fatigue. Recommendations may vary from one institution to the other and laws vary from state to state. Lack of futility clauses and vague language regarding definitions of benefit and harm further complicate many complex clinical situations. In most cases, physicians and nurses feel the ethics committee role is to give advice and help promote a better understanding of the situation. In cases where parents and physicians disagree despite open communication an education, team members feel the ethics committee should make the decision on the most appropriate care plan. A small minority of providers would allow courts and the legal system to make the final decision in the case of clear disagreement (60).

Without clear disagreement, despite moral dilemma physicians and nurses would rather be involved with making the decisions. An ethics committee can help facilitate thoughtful discussions and open communication to better understand the issues that are leading to distress. Through these discussions, the important distinction between an ethical dilemma and moral distress can be made. There can be multiple treatment options that are acceptable while personal views on the most appropriate path may differ. By allowing thoughtful discussions about these options and why they are ethically acceptable, providers may have less moral distress as they have a better understanding in the complexity behind such decisions and also have an opportunity to express their views and concerns (49). Beyond that, ethics committees can help the team navigate communication with parents while understanding that the parents have ultimate responsibility of acting as moral agents for their baby (61). It is only with the recognition of the moral and ethical dilemmas unique to the NICU that organizational support for establishing ethical framework to support complex decision-making can truly come to fruition (62). With this support and structure in place, there can be improved quality of care through less conflict and distress amongst team members.

DISCUSSION

Moral distress is far more prevalent than even the current literature describes. It transcends healthcare professions and affects the entire healthcare team, the family, and most importantly the patient. While historically described as a negative emotion resulting from poor communication, discrepant values, and paternalistic hierarchy, it can be a source of growth and progress if leveraged correctly. However, if left unaddressed, it can contribute to burnout, job dissatisfaction and, ultimately, a lower quality of care provided.

The multitude of circumstances that can lead to moral distress require a thoughtful and tailored approach to patient care. Ethics rounds, debriefing after deaths, codes, or other challenging situations, and exceptional communication among team members and with caregivers are the cornerstones of minimizing the negative impact of moral distress while leveraging its role in progress. Understanding that different team members will feel moral distress to varying degrees is imperative. Offering options, such as the choice to abstain from care with which they disagree, may be one way to combat constraint in those who are most at risk to feel powerless or "without a voice." Simulation or case-based discussion can provoke thought and acknowledgment of one's own feelings in various situations so that providers feel confident in their approach to care. In addition, not delaying difficult conversations with parents can minimize the trauma associated with aggressive medical interventions or end-of-life care and will encourage open, deliberate communication. This will allow providers and families to feel that they made the most informed decision.

Most importantly, perhaps, is the recognition of moral distress as an entity, its impact on care provided, and helping staff identify its presence. By acknowledging the influence and implications of moral distress, providers are better equipped to minimize the negative effects and provide safer, more resilient care. Utilization of behavioral medicine resources, team discussions, mentorship and buddy systems for emotional and moral support can encourage self-awareness and a focus on addressing moral distress. Fostering a culture of openness, ethical sincerity and support for those who are struggling can reduce consequences such as burnout and job dissatisfaction. Communication with team members can offer insight in to other perspectives and guide future actions. Guidance from seasoned mentors and reassurance from colleagues regarding the normalcy of moral distress and advice for managing it provides the tools for personal and professional growth.

The impact of moral distress on decisions made in the NICU is under-recognized and represents a potential area for improvement in communication among staff members and with parents. Future areas of investigation should focus on the zone of parental discretion and its boundaries. In addition, given that physicians are most often involved in the medical decision-making for a child, further research on optimal interventions for moral distress tailored to address the specific challenges of different professions would aid in providing additional tools to combat moral distress.

AUTHOR CONTRIBUTIONS

MM conceptualized and drafted the initial manuscript. DC aided in conceptualizing, designing, and editing the manuscript. All authors approved the final manuscript as submitted.

REFERENCES

1. Nussbaum M. The costs of tragedy: some moral limits of cost-benefit analysis. *J Legal Stud.* (2000) 29:1005–36. doi: 10.1086/468103
2. Jameton A. *Nursing Practice: The Ethical Issues.* Glenview, NJ: Prentice-Hall (1984). p. 1–331.
3. Fourie C. Who is experiencing what kind of moral distress? distinctions for moving from a narrow to a broad definition of moral distress. *AMA J Ethics.* (2017) 19:578–84. doi: 10.1001/journalofethics.2017.19.6.nlit1-1706
4. Fourie C. Moral distress and moral conflict in clinical ethics. *Bioethics.* (2015) 29:91–7. doi: 10.1111/bioe.12064
5. Prentice TM, Gillam L, Davis PG, Janvier A. The use and misuse of moral distress in neonatology. *Semin Fetal Neonatal Med.* (2018) 23:39–43. doi: 10.1016/j.siny.2017.09.007
6. Janvier A, Nadeau S, Deschênes M, Couture E, Barrington KJ. Moral distress in the neonatal intensive care unit: caregiver's experience. *J Perinatol.* (2007) 27:203–8. doi: 10.1038/sj.jp.7211658
7. Barr P. Burnout in neonatal intensive care unit nurses: relationships with moral distress, adult attachment insecurities, and proneness to guilt and shame. *J Perinat Med.* (2020). doi: 10.1515/jpm-2019-0323. [Epub ahead of print].
8. Sannino P, Giannì ML, Carini M, Madeo M, Lusignani M, Bezze E, et al. Moral distress in the pediatric intensive care unit: an Italian study. *Front Pediatr.* (2019) 7:338. doi: 10.3389/fped.2019.00338
9. Sundin-Huard D, Fahy K. Moral distress, advocacy and burnout: theorizing the relationships. *Int J Nurs Pract.* (1999) 5:8–13. doi: 10.1046/j.1440-172x.1999.00143.x
10. Prentice TM, Gillam L, Davis PG, Janvier A. Always a burden? Healthcare providers' perspectives on moral distress. *Arch Dis Child Fetal Neonatal Ed.* (2018) 103:F441–5. doi: 10.1136/archdischild-2017-313539
11. Lantos JD. Moral distress and ethical confrontation: problem or progress? *J Perinatol.* (2007) 27:201–2. doi: 10.1038/sj.jp.7211679
12. Thorne S, Konikoff L, Brown H, Albersheim S. Navigating the dangerous terrain of moral distress: understanding response patterns in the NICU. *Qual Health Res.* (2018) 28:683–701. doi: 10.1177/1049732317753585
13. Prentice T, Janvier A, Gillam L, Davis PG. Moral distress within neonatal and paediatric intensive care units: a systematic review. *Arch Dis Child.* (2016) 101:701–8. doi: 10.1136/archdischild-2015-309410
14. Whitehead PB, Herbertson RK, Hamric AB, Epstein EG, Fisher JM. Moral distress among healthcare professionals: report of an institution-wide survey. *J Nurs Scholarsh.* (2015) 47:117–25. doi: 10.1111/jnu.12115
15. Musto L, Rodney P. What we know about moral distress. In: Ulrich C, Grady C, editors. *Moral Distress in the Health Professions.* Springer International Publishing (2018). p. 9–20. doi: 10.1007/978-3-319-64626-8_2
16. Burton M, Caswell H, Porter C, Mott S, DeGrazia M. Moral distress: defined and described by neonatal and pediatric critical care nurses in a quaternary care free-standing pediatric hospital. *Dimens Crit Care Nurs.* (2020) 39:101–9. doi: 10.1097/DCC.0000000000000403
17. Larson CP, Dryden-Palmer KD, Gibbons C, Parshuram CS. Moral distress in PICU and neonatal ICU practitioners: a cross-sectional evaluation. *Pediatr Crit Care Med.* (2017) 18:e318–26. doi: 10.1097/PCC.0000000000001219
18. Boss RD, Geller G, Donohue PK. Conflicts in learning to care for critically ill newborns: "It Makes Me Question My Own Morals." *J Bioeth Inq.* (2015) 12:437–48. doi: 10.1007/s11673-015-9609-9
19. Dzeng E, Colaianni A, Roland M, Levine D, Kelly MP, Barclay S, et al. Moral distress amongst American physician trainees regarding futile treatments at the end of life: a qualitative study. *J Gen Intern Med.* (2016) 31:93–9. doi: 10.1007/s11606-015-3505-1
20. Lewis SL. Emotional intelligence in neonatal intensive care unit nurses: decreasing moral distress in end-of-life care and laying a foundation for improved outcomes: an integrative review. *J Hosp Palliat Nurs.* (2019) 21:250–6. doi: 10.1097/NJH.0000000000000561
21. Sauerland J, Marotta K, Peinemann MA, Berndt A, Robichaux C. Assessing and addressing moral distress and ethical climate Part II:

neonatal and pediatric perspectives. *Dimens Crit Care Nurs.* (2015) 34:33-46. doi: 10.1097/DCC.0000000000000083
22. Walters A, Grosse J. Is this my home? a palliative care journey through life and death in the NICU: a case report. *Adv Neonatal Care.* (2020) 20:127-35. doi: 10.1097/ANC.0000000000000697
23. de Boer JC, van Rosmalen J, Bakker AB, van Dijk M. Appropriateness of care and moral distress among neonatal intensive care unit staff: repeated measurements. *Nurs Crit Care.* (2016) 21:e19–27. doi: 10.1111/nicc.12206
24. Field D, Deeming J, Smith LK. Moral distress: an inevitable part of neonatal and paediatric intensive care? *Arch Dis Child.* (2016) 101:686-7. doi: 10.1136/archdischild-2015-310268
25. Allen R, Judkins-Cohn T, deVelasco R, Forges E, Lee R, Clark L, et al. Moral distress among healthcare professionals at a health system. *JONAS Healthc Law Ethics Regul.* (2013) 15:111–8. doi: 10.1097/NHL.0b013e3182a1bf33
26. Ford NJ, Austin W. Conflicts of conscience in the neonatal intensive care unit: Perspectives of Alberta. *Nurs Ethics.* (2018) 25:992–1003. doi: 10.1177/0969733016684547
27. McCarthy J, Deady R. Moral distress reconsidered. *Nurs Ethics.* (2008) 15:254-62. doi: 10.1177/0969733007086023
28. Hefferman P, Heilig S. Giving "moral distress" a voice: ethical concerns among neonatal intensive care unit personnel. *Camb Q Healthc Ethics.* (1999) 8:173–8. doi: 10.1017/S0963180199802060
29. MacDorman MF, Gregory EC. Fetal and perinatal mortality: United States, 2013. *Natl Vital Stat Rep.* (2015) 64:1–24.
30. Cook LA, Watchko JF. Decision making for the critically ill neonate near the end of life. *J Perinatol.* (1996) 16:133–6.
31. Singh J, Lantos J, Meadow W. End-of-life after birth: death and dying in a neonatal intensive care unit. *Pediatrics.* (2004) 114:1620-6. doi: 10.1542/peds.2004-0447
32. Niehaus J, Maurer S. NICU communication: the many disguises of opportunity. *NeoReviews.* (2018) 19:e526. doi: 10.1542/neo.19-9-e526
33. Schneiderman LJ. Defining medical futility and improving medical care. *J Bioeth Inq.* (2011) 8:123–31. doi: 10.1007/s11673-011-9293-3
34. Solomon MZ, Sellers DE, Heller KS, Dokken DL, Levetown M, Rushton C, et al. New and lingering controversies in pediatric end-of-life care. *Pediatrics.* (2005) 116:872–83. doi: 10.1542/peds.2004-0905
35. Thiele P, Berg SF, Farlow B. More than a diagnosis. *Acta Paediatr.* (2013) 102:1127–9. doi: 10.1111/apa.12411
36. Wilfond BS. Tracheostomies and assisted ventilation in children with profound disabilities: navigating family and professional values. *Pediatrics.* (2014) 133(Suppl.1):S44–9. doi: 10.1542/peds.2013-3608H
37. Janvier A, Farlow B, Wilfond BS. The experience of families with children with trisomy 13 and 18 in social networks. *Pediatrics.* (2012) 130:293-8. doi: 10.1542/peds.2012-0151
38. Lantos JD. Trisomy 13 and 18–treatment decisions in a stable gray zone. *JAMA.* (2016) 316:396–8. doi: 10.1001/jama.2016.9470
39. Robertson JA. Involuntary euthanasia of defective newborns: a legal analysis. *Stanford Law Rev.* (1975) 27:213–69. doi: 10.2307/1228265
40. Wightman A, Kett J, Campelia G, Wilfond BS. The relational potential standard: rethinking the ethical justification for life-sustaining treatment for children with profound cognitive disabilities. *Hastings Cent Rep.* (2019) 49:18–25. doi: 10.1002/hast.1003
41. Gillam L. The zone of parental discretion: An ethical tool for dealing with disagreement between parents and doctors about medical treatment for a child. *Clinical Ethics.* (2016) 11:1–8. doi: 10.1177/1477750915622033
42. Janvier A. I would never want this for my baby. *Pediatr Crit Care Med.* (2009) 10:113–4. doi: 10.1097/PCC.0b013e3181937adf
43. Kluge EH. Hope in the neonatal intensive care nursery: values, ethics, and the injury of continued existence. *MedGenMed.* (2006) 8:74.
44. Cavolo A, Dierckx de Casterlé B, Naulaers G, Gastmans C. Physicians' attitudes on resuscitation of extremely premature infants: a systematic review. *Pediatrics.* (2019) 143:3972. doi: 10.1542/peds.2018-3972
45. Janvier A, Prentice T, Wallace J, Robson K, Mann P, Lantos JD. Does it matter if this baby is 22 or 23 weeks? *Pediatrics.* (2019) 144:113. doi: 10.1542/peds.2019-0113
46. Krick JA, Feltman DM. Neonatologists' preferences regarding guidelines for periviable deliveries: do we really know what we want? *J Perinatol.* (2019) 39:445–52. doi: 10.1038/s41372-019-0313-1
47. Carnevale FA. Moral distress in the ICU: it's time to do something about it! *Minerva Anestesiol.* (2020) 86:455–60. doi: 10.23736/S0375-9393.19.14021-7
48. Prentice TM, Gillam L, Janvier A, Davis PG. How should neonatal clinicians act in the presence of moral distress? *Arch Dis Child Fetal Neonatal Ed.* (2020) 105:348–9. doi: 10.1136/archdischild-2019-317895
49. Santos RPD, Garros D, Carnevale F. Difficult decisions in pediatric practice and moral distress in the intensive care unit. *Rev Bras Ter Intensiva.* (2018) 30:226–32. doi: 10.5935/0103-507X.20180039
50. Chehab M. Moral distress: what is next? *Pediatr Crit Care Med.* (2017) 18:814–5. doi: 10.1097/PCC.0000000000001243
51. Beumer CM. Innovative solutions: the effect of a workshop on reducing the experience of moral distress in an intensive care unit setting. *Dimens Crit Care Nurs.* (2008) 27:263–7. doi: 10.1097/01.DCC.0000338871.77658.03
52. Lawrence LA. Work engagement, moral distress, education level, and critical reflective practice in intensive care nurses. *Nurs Forum.* (2011) 46:256-68. doi: 10.1111/j.1744-6198.2011.00237.x
53. Saeedi S, Jouybari L, Sanagoo A, Vakili MA. The effectiveness of narrative writing on the moral distress of intensive care nurses. *Nurs Ethics.* (2019) 26:2195–203. doi: 10.1177/0969733018806342
54. Lantos JD. Ethical problems in decision making in the neonatal ICU. *N Engl J Med.* (2018) 379:1851–60. doi: 10.1056/NEJMra1801063
55. Cavaliere TA, Daly B, Dowling D, Montgomery K. Moral distress in neonatal intensive care unit RNs. *Adv Neonatal Care.* (2010) 10:145-56. doi: 10.1097/ANC.0b013e3181dd6c48
56. Cavinder C. The relationship between providing neonatal palliative care and nurses' moral distress: an integrative review. *Adv Neonatal Care.* (2014) 14:322–8. doi: 10.1097/ANC.0000000000000100
57. Rogers S, Babgi A, Gomez C. Educational interventions in end-of-life care: part I: an educational intervention responding to the moral distress of NICU nurses provided by an ethics consultation team. *Adv Neonatal Care.* (2008) 8:56–65. doi: 10.1097/01.ANC.0000311017.02005.20
58. Okah FA, Wolff DM, Boos VD, Haney BM, Oshodi AA. Perceptions of a strategy to prevent and relieve care provider distress in the neonatal intensive care unit. *Am J Perinatol.* (2012) 29:687–92. doi: 10.1055/s-0032-1314889
59. Mercurio MR. The role of a pediatric ethics committee in the newborn intensive care unit. *J Perinatol.* (2011) 31:1–9. doi: 10.1038/jp.2010.39
60. Bucher HU, Klein SD, Hendriks MJ, Baumann-Hölzle R, Berger TM, Streuli JC, et al. Decision-making at the limit of viability: differing perceptions and opinions between neonatal physicians and nurses. *BMC Pediatr.* (2018) 18:81. doi: 10.1186/s12887-018-1204-x
61. Wocial L. Moral distress–the role of ethics consultation in the NICU. *Bioethics Forum.* (2002) 18:15–23.
62. Stanak M. Professional ethics: the case of neonatology. *Med Health Care Philos.* (2019) 22:231–8. doi: 10.1007/s11019-018-9863-9

9

Assessment of Healthcare Professionals' Self-Perceived Competence in Perinatal/ Neonatal Palliative Care After a 3-Day Training Course

Jennifer Hammond [1], Charlotte Wool [2] and Elvira Parravicini [1]*

[1] Division of Neonatology, Department of Pediatrics, Columbia University Irving Medical Center, New York, NY, United States,
[2] Department of Nursing, York College of Pennsylvania, York, PA, United States

Correspondence:
Elvira Parravicini
ep127@cumc.columbia.edu

Background: Perinatal/neonatal palliative care (PNPC) offers a plan of care for improving the quality of life of infants when the prolongation of life is no longer the goal of care. The number of PNPC programs has increased in recent years, but training for clinicians has not kept pace. Therefore, an interdisciplinary team developed a 3-day intensive PNPC training course for physicians, nurses, and other healthcare professionals at Columbia University Irving Medical Center (CUIMC).

Objective: The aim of this study was to assess the efficacy of a PNPC training course in improving the self-reported competence of participants.

Study Design: A cross-sectional survey design was used to obtain data from 88 healthcare professionals who attended the PNPC training course. Data was collected using a validated questionnaire. The questionnaire included 32 items that queried participants about their self-assessed competence using a forced 1–4 Likert scale. The 32 items, which served as the outcome variables, were clustered into the eight domains of palliative care. The survey was administered through a web-based tool at the beginning and the conclusion of the course.

Results: Results from two-sample *t*-tests comparing pre-test and post-test self-assessed competence were statistically significant for each item across disciplines. Additional analysis revealed that after participation in the training course, the statistically significant differences between physicians' and nurses' pre-course self-reported competence disappeared.

Conclusion: The development of an evidence-based curriculum improved the self-reported competence of participants across disciplines, filled a specific gap in nurses' self-reported competence and addressed a global training need.

Keywords: perinatal, neonatal, palliative care, competence, training course

INTRODUCTION

Perinatal/neonatal palliative care (PNPC) offers a plan of care for improving the quality of life of infants when the prolongation of life is no longer the goal of care or the complexity of the medical condition is associated with an uncertain prognosis. Palliative care in the perinatal period is a coordinated, interdisciplinary approach to obstetric and newborn care that includes a focus on maximizing the quality of life and comfort of newborns with life-limiting conditions (LLC) (1). This focus extends to supportive, coordinated care for parents and family members by providing anticipatory guidance, honoring parents' values, providing targeted consultations, formulating birth and treatment plans for the infant, and offering bereavement counseling.

The number of perinatal palliative care programs has increased in recent years (2, 3), but training and education for clinicians has not kept pace. There remains a gap in knowledge and competence regarding the management of parents expecting an infant with a LLC during pregnancy and birth and after delivery (4, 5). Furthermore, healthcare professionals from different backgrounds and disciplines have varying experiences, training, and confidence with regards to the delivery of PNPC (6–8). While suggestions for education and training have been proposed (9), formal professional coursework for PNPC is still very limited (10).

A policy statement from the American Academy of Pediatrics (11) on pediatric palliative and hospice care recommends that palliative care should be a part of all pediatric education, training curricula, and quality improvement. In addition, the National Consensus Project (NCP) Clinical Practice Guidelines for Quality Palliative Care states that all clinicians in direct care of seriously ill patients should have the necessary training and experience to complete palliative assessments and address common sources of suffering (12).

In response to clinicians' educational needs and recommendations from national organizations, an interdisciplinary team developed a 3-day intensive training course at Columbia University Irving Medical Center (CUIMC).

TABLE 1 | Items assessing self-reported competence grouped by palliative care domain (12).

Domain	Survey Items
Domain 1: Structure and Process	1. Offering the parent(s) the option of palliative care when they are making decisions about a fetus with a life-limiting condition 2. Talking to parent(s) about the range of options including palliative care after their fetus/infant has been diagnosed with a serious medical condition and potential adverse outcome 3. Talking to parent(s) about the range of possible outcomes after their fetus/infant has been diagnosed with a life-limiting condition 4. Engaging in shared decision-making after a life-limiting diagnosis is confirmed 5. Including parent(s) to create a plan of care for the pregnancy and birth 6. Including parent(s) to create a plan of care for the infant after birth 7. Providing prenatal care in a consistent way 8. Communicating with families about priorities of care 9. Understanding the role of palliative care and its integration into intensive care in the NICU 10. Accessing palliative care expertise and support when needed
Domain 2: Physical	11. Attending the delivery and providing palliative care to an infant with a life-limiting condition 12. Assessing the basic needs of infants with life-limiting conditions 13. Making a comprehensive care plan to address an infant's basic needs 14. Developing a nutrition plan for an infant with a life-limiting condition who is breathing and stable on room air 15. Providing interventions to achieve an infant's comfort 16. Assessing pain/discomfort in infants 17. Managing pain/discomfort in infants 18. Assessing other symptoms in infants (respiratory distress, irritability) 19. Managing other symptoms in infants (respiratory, irritability) 20. Following through with documentation of goals of care for an infant with a serious condition and potential adverse outcomes
Domain 3: Psychological and Psychiatric	21. Addressing the unborn child by name 22. Giving parent(s) a sense of normalcy during pregnancy and birth 23. Providing emotional support to parent(s) expecting an infant with a life-limiting condition 24. Exploring with families how they talk with their other children about the infant who is not expected to live
Domain 4: Social	25. Creating a comfortable, caring environment for parent(s) 26. Accessing resources related to perinatal palliative care (clinical resource materials, continuing education) 27. Knowing the community resources available for palliative care and how to access these resources
Domain 5: Religious, Spiritual, Existential	28. Sensitivity to spiritual needs
Domain 6: Cultural	29. Sensitivity to cultural values
Domain 7: Care of the Imminently Dying	30. Having conversations with families about the possibility of their infant dying 31. Recognizing signs of impending death in an infant
Domain 8: Legal and Ethical	32. Identifying and understanding ethical issues related to end of life care for infants

This study had two specific aims. First, the study aimed to evaluate the efficacy of the PNPC training course in improving the self-reported competence of course participants in perinatal and neonatal palliative care. Second, the study aimed to examine differences between physicians' and nurses' self-reported competence.

MATERIALS AND METHODS

Training Course

A 3-day course entitled *Next-Level Perinatal/Neonatal Comfort Care Training Course: Developing a Medical and Interdisciplinary Plan for Each Baby and Support for Their Family* was offered at CUIMC in June 2019. The program was designed by a team of medical experts to cover all aspects of PNPC (13). The target audience included the entire perinatal team: physicians, nurses, nurse practitioners, and other allied health professionals practicing in the perinatal arena (i.e., obstetrics, neonatology) who were interested in improving the practice of PNPC both nationally and internationally. Participants were provided with educational resources including a syllabus with objectives and literature references for each session. The course included presentations from an interdisciplinary team of clinicians including physicians, nurses, and researchers from neonatology and obstetrics as well as other professionals (a social worker, psychologist, speech-language pathologist, child life professional, and chaplain) involved in perinatal care and parent interviews. Faculty presented evidence-based rationale and strategies, offered interactive learning opportunities, modeled elements of effective communication, and practiced hands-on activities with participants. These educational strategies were administered to demonstrate and teach family-centric support and the attainment of a state of comfort for newborns with LLC. The eight domains of palliative care published by the NCP (12) were woven into the course curriculum, which included the following topics:

(1) The current state of the science on perinatal palliative care
(2) Strategies to assist families during decision-making processes
(3) Definition and roles of the members of the interdisciplinary team
(4) Essential elements of the perinatal palliative consult
(5) Advance care planning
(6) Evidence-based interventions in the prenatal, intrapartum, and postnatal periods that promote the health of the mother and family
(7) Essential elements of a neonatal palliative care plan
(8) Identification of potential barriers to institutional uptake of perinatal palliative care.

Study Survey

A survey was developed to assess participants' self-reported competence before and after the course and included 50 items with three sections. Section one included demographic data. Section two contained the outcome variables, which were 32 items addressing self-reported competence (**Table 1**). Participants were asked to rate their competence on a forced Likert scale of one (not competent), two (somewhat competent), three (competent), and four (highly competent). Participants could select "not applicable" if they did not feel as though they could assess their competence for a specific item. Competence was defined as the "habitual and judicious use of communication, knowledge, technical skills, clinical reasoning, emotions, values and reflection in daily practice for the benefits of the individual and the community being served" (14). The 32 items addressing competence were derived using a two-pronged approach. First, the literature was reviewed and a validated questionnaire by Stekenes and colleagues (15) was modified with permission to create the 32 outcome variables in the survey. The items were examined by two neonatologists and a researcher, reworded where needed, and agreement was reached regarding the inclusion of the final items. Next, the NCP's eight domains of quality palliative care were used to organize items and ensure that each domain was represented with at least one item. Section three queried participants' previous education in palliative care.

Study Design

The study was approved by the Institutional Review Board at CUIMC (AAAS4060) and informed consent was obtained from

TABLE 2 | Demographic characteristics of participants.

Demographic Characteristics	Number of Participants (%)
Profession	
Nurse	34/76 (45)
Midwife	2/76 (3)
Physician	31/76 (41)
Other	9/76 (11)
Area of Practice	
Neonatology	49/76 (65)
Obstetrics	9/76 (12)
Palliative Care	8/76 (10)
Pediatrics	3/76 (4)
Other	7/76 (9)
Highest Level of Education	
High School Diploma	2/76 (3)
Undergraduate Degree	24/76 (31)
Master's Degree	21/76 (28)
Doctorate	29/76 (38)
Age	
<30 years	13/76 (17)
31–40 years	32/76 (42)
41–50 years	11/76 (14.5)
51–60 years	11/76 (14.5)
61–70 years	9/76 (12)
Gender	
Male	16/76 (22)
Female	60/76 (78)
Country of Origin	
USA	62/76 (82)
Other	14/76 (18)

TABLE 3 | Pre-course and post-course self-assessed competency for all participants.

Item number	*N* (Pre-test)	*N* (Post-test)	Pre-test M (sd)	Post-test M (sd)	*t*-test (df); sig.
1	63	44	2.86 (0.99)	3.50 (0.35)	−4.17 (103); $p < 0.001$
2	63	46	2.95 (1.01)	3.48 (0.34)	−3.43 (103); $p < 0.001$
3	64	43	2.81 (0.95)	3.44 (0.40)	−4.06 (105); $p < 0.001$
4	64	44	3.00 (0.86)	3.55 (0.35)	−3.74 (105); $p < 0.001$
5	57	44	2.49 (1.22)	3.57 (0.48)	−5.99 (96); $p < 0.001$
6	61	43	2.77 (1.15)	3.70 (0.26)	−5.88 (92); $p < 0.001$
7	53	45	2.57 (1.10)	3.40 (0.65)	−4.44 (95); $p < 0.001$
8	68	42	2.96 (0.88)	3.57 (0.40)	−4.11 (107); $p < 0.001$
9	72	42	2.97 (0.90)	3.76 (0.23)	−5.87 (110); $p < 0.001$
10	68	40	2.88 (0.97)	3.63 (0.29)	−5.05 (106); $p < 0.001$
11	64	41	2.95 (0.93)	3.61 (0.44)	−4.11 (102); $p < 0.001$
12	70	41	2.97 (0.98)	3.56 (0.40)	−3.81 (108); $p < 0.001$
13	69	38	2.86 (0.86)	3.61 (0.30)	−5.26 (104); $p < 0.001$
14	66	40	2.38 (1.07)	3.43 (0.51)	−6.16 (102); $p < 0.001$
15	69	39	2.91 (1.08)	3.64 (0.24)	−4.94 (103); $p < 0.001$
16	67	39	3.09 (0.96)	3.56 (0.30)	−3.19 (104); $p = 0.001$
17	66	37	3.05 (0.97)	3.54 (0.26)	−3.37 (100); $p = 0.001$
18	67	42	3.19 (0.92)	3.67 (0.28)	−3.32 (105); $p = 0.001$
19	63	39	3.16 (0.88)	3.59 (0.30)	−2.93 (100); $p = 0.004$
20	70	43	2.77 (0.93)	3.58 (0.30)	−5.70 (110); $p < 0.001$
21	53	38	3.32 (0.99)	3.84 (0.30)	−3.20 (84); $p = 0.001$
22	57	42	2.92 (1.00)	3.60 (0.39)	−4.06 (95); $p < 0.001$
23	56	43	2.91 (0.88)	3.56 (0.44)	−4.01 (96); $p = 0.001$
24	72	46	2.33 (0.87)	3.46 (0.48)	−7.49 (113); $p < 0.001$
25	65	41	3.31 (0.75)	3.73 (0.25)	−3.19 (103); $p = 0.001$
26	71	47	2.69 (0.87)	3.60 (0.33)	−6.50 (116); $p < 0.001$
27	73	48	2.55 (0.81)	3.29 (0.51)	−5.05 (115); $p < 0.001$
28	65	43	3.12 (0.58)	3.67 (0.22)	−4.64 (106); $p < 0.01$
29	67	44	3.09 (0.60)	3.68 (0.22)	−5.01 (108); $p < 0.01$
30	68	43	3.01 (0.91)	3.53 (0.45)	−3.38 (108); $p < 0.001$
31	66	41	3.02 (0.94)	3.63 (0.33)	−4.13 (105); $p < 0.001$
32	72	46	2.96 (0.69)	3.68 (0.22)	−5.01 (108); $p < 0.01$

(Continued)

TABLE 3 | Continued

participants at the start of data collection. In order to assess the course outcomes, a pre-test, post-test study was developed. The pre-test, post-test design was cross-sectional and data were collected at two discrete points in time: before the training course commenced and after the course was completed. At the start of the course, a link to the pre-test survey was sent to each participant's electronic inbox using the web-based tool Qualtrics. An introduction to the survey and informed consent were provided on the first page. The training course was considered the intervention and lasted a total of 3 days. At the close of the training course, a link to the survey was emailed to participants. Follow-up emails to solicit completion of the post-test survey were sent 1 and 3 weeks after the conclusion of the course.

Statistical Analysis

Prior to performing the analyses, "not applicable" responses for each item were removed from the dataset and therefore not included in the final analyses. In order to examine differences between pre-test and post-test self-reported competence, each of the thirty-two items were compared using a two-sample *t*-test assuming unequal variance. Next, the items were clustered into their respective palliative care domains. The means for each item in each clustered domain were compared using a two-sample *t*-test assuming unequal variance. In addition, an independent sample *t*-test was completed to examine the difference in the self-reported competence between physicians and nurses at the start of and end of the training course.

RESULTS

A total of 88 professionals from nineteen US states and six countries (Australia, Burundi, Canada, England, Italy, and Russia) attended the course; however, only 76 attended the complete 3-day course and qualified for participation in the study. The pre-test survey response rate was 100% and the post-test survey response rate was 67%. Most participants were physicians or nurses and mainly represented the fields of neonatology and obstetrics. One third of participants had limited clinical palliative care experience (cared for

TABLE 4 | Comparison of physician and nurse differences in self-reported competency in pre-test and post-test items.

	Nurses			Physicians			
	Mean	SD	*N*	Mean	SD	*N*	*t*-test (df); sig.
Pre-test Items							
Offering parents options	2.53	1.00	30	3.07	0.92	29	−2.12 (57), $p = 0.03$
Talking about options	2.61	1.05	31	3.18	0.94	28	−2.16 (57), $p = 0.03$
Talk about outcomes	2.39	0.98	31	3.21	0.77	29	−3.55 (58), $p = 0.001$
Engaging in shared decision-making	2.65	1.01	31	3.28	0.79	29	−2.65 (58), $p = 0.01$
Consistent prenatal care	2.17	1.07	23	2.85	0.96	26	−2.30 (47), $p = 0.02$
Access palliative expertise/support	2.50	0.99	34	3.18	0.90	28	−2.78 (60), $p = 0.007$
Nutrition plan for infant	2.09	1.05	32	2.70	0.95	31	−2.36 (60), $p = 0.02$
Follow through with documentation	2.51	1.01	35	3.00	0.78	30	−2.17 (62), $p = 0.03$
Conversations about dying	2.68	1.03	34	3.28	0.79	29	−2.59 (60), $p = 0.01$
Post-test Items							
Offering parents options	3.45	0.67	22	3.53	0.61	19	−0.35 (39), $p = 0.72$
Talking about options	3.45	0.67	22	3.48	0.60	21	−0.11 (41), $p = 0.91$
Talk about outcomes	3.40	0.68	20	3.52	0.60	21	−0.61 (39), $p = 0.54$
Engaging in shared decision-making	3.40	0.68	20	3.67	0.58	21	−1.35 (39), $p = 0.18$
Consistent prenatal care	3.30	0.80	20	3.55	0.80	22	−0.99 (40), $p = 0.32$
Access palliative expertise/support	3.47	0.69	19	3.71	0.47	17	−1.18 (32), $p = 0.24$
Nutrition plan for infant	3.42	0.69	19	3.32	0.82	19	0.42 (36), $p = 0.67$
Follow through with documentation	3.47	0.69	19	3.65	0.48	20	−0.91 (32), $p = 0.36$
Conversations about dying	3.33	0.84	18	3.71	0.56	21	−1.63 (29), $p = 0.11$

fewer than five dying infants in their career), while 47% of participants reported having some previous exposure to palliative care education. Demographic data are presented in **Table 2**.

Analysis of the 32 items assessing self-reported competency showed that pre-course and post-course self-reported competence scores were statistically different for all professionals for each of the 32 items with higher scores on the post-course survey (**Table 3**). Comparisons remained statistically significant when the items were clustered into their respective palliative care domains.

Self-reported competency was then analyzed by discipline. The post-course self-reported competence scores for nurses were statistically higher than their pre-course scores for each of the 32 items. Physicians' post-course self-reported competence scores were higher than their pre-course scores and reached statistical significance for 20 of the 32 items including items 1 ($p = 0.03$), 5 ($p = 0.03$), 6 ($p = 0.01$), 8 ($p = 0.02$), 9 ($p < 0.001$), 10 ($p = 0.005$), 11 ($p = 0.04$), 12 ($p = 0.03$), 13 ($p < 0.001$), 14 ($p = 0.001$), 15 ($p < 0.001$), 16 ($p = 0.004$), 20 ($p = 0.004$), 24 ($p < 0.001$), 26 ($p < 0.001$), 27 ($p = 0.008$), 28 ($p = 0.002$), 29 ($p = 0.001$), 30 ($p < 0.001$), 32 ($p = 0.002$).

Scores for nurses and physicians were also directly compared. Prior to the start of the course physicians' mean scores for self-reported competence were higher than the nurses' mean scores for nine items. In post-course analyses, the nine self-reported competence items were again compared between nurses and physicians and were no longer statistically significant (**Table 4**).

DISCUSSION

This study found that the development and implementation of an evidence-based PNPC training course improves the self-reported competence of its participants across disciplines and in each domain of palliative care. Moreover, participation in the course filled a specific gap in nurses' self-reported competence.

The improvement in the self-reported competence in each item and in each domain of palliative care demonstrates the breadth of the material presented in the training course. The comprehensive training program addressed not only the medical aspects of perinatal palliative care but also the psychological, spiritual, cultural, and ethical aspects of care. The pre-course mean self-reported competence scores were particularly low for participants across disciplines on several items related to the psychological and social aspects of care. Participants reported the lowest self-reported competency scores in the areas of developing a nutrition plan and communication with the siblings of infants with a life-limiting condition. The creation of a nutrition plan is rarely included in PNPC education because most infants with a life-limiting condition have a short life expectancy. However, some infants may be stable at birth and continue to live for days, weeks, or months. Therefore, hunger and thirst must be addressed (16). Furthermore, colostrum care and non-nutritive sucking are recommended by the American Academy of Pediatrics as non-pharmacological interventions to alleviate pain and discomfort in neonates, including at the end of life (11, 17). Although PNPC emphasizes the care and support of the entire family, training is often lacking in this specific area, which was highlighted by the scores in the "somewhat competent" range for communication with siblings. Participation in this PNPC training course adequately addressed these topics as demonstrated by the marked improvement in the post-course self-reported competence scores.

Additional analyses revealed that nurses improved their self-reported competency scores on each item, while physicians improved their scores in 20 of the 32 items. The domains of palliative care most impacted by course participation were related to the integration of palliative care into NICU practices, addressing infants' basic needs, providing interventions to achieve infants' comfort, accessing resources for PNPC and initiating conversations about dying. Future training programs should continue to incorporate these findings to address the specific educational needs of physicians.

Prior to the start of the course, a statistically significant difference between physicians and nurses self-reported competence was calculated for nine items. These items were in three of the eight domains including the structure and process of care, physical aspects of care, and care of the imminently dying and reflect areas of PNPC that physicians often have more experience with. These findings were not surprising since previous work has suggested that physicians are often more confident than nurses in the practice of perinatal and neonatal palliative care (18, 19). After participation in the training course, these differences disappeared. This suggests that an intensive training course can fill a gap in nurses' self-reported competence in the practice of PNPC.

The training course included participants from different disciplines including neonatology, obstetrics, and palliative care. This is particularly important because PNPC practices require an interdisciplinary team of practitioners. Neonatologists are often at the forefront of neonatal palliative care initiatives and obstetricians' interest in acquiring competence in this field is growing (1). This growth is important since obstetricians are often on the front line of delivering news of a fetal diagnosis of a LLC to parents and providing recommendations.

The implementation of this training course addressed an international need. A recent study found that nearly half of the neonatal intensive care units surveyed did not have neonatal comfort care guidelines and 91% of respondents stated that their institution would benefit from PNPC education (20). Previous work suggests that appropriate PNPC education can increase knowledge, self-perceived confidence, and clinical skills (21). Insufficient knowledge about PNPC is a known barrier to its uptake (6). Furthermore, comprehensive training may alleviate some of the distress, helplessness, and discomfort clinicians have reported in previous studies (8). Finally, numerous nationally recognized organizations including the NCP, ACOG and the Worldwide Palliative Care Alliance have recommendations encouraging clinicians and institutions to develop PNPC programs, which can only be done well when there is ample training for clinicians (1, 12, 22). The CUIMC course attracted individuals from several countries. Importantly, despite the vast and diverse demographic origins of the participants, the course content universally improved professionals' self-reported competence in PNPC management.

The present study has several strengths. First, participants represented several disciplines and specialties which contrasts with previous work. Knighting and colleagues evaluated the impact of a training course on self-perceived knowledge and clinical practice in 73 professionals. However, 82% of participants had a nursing background and only three participants were from the field of obstetrics (21). A second strength of the study includes the timing of the administration of the post-course survey. Since participants completed the post-test survey within 1–3 weeks of course completion, it is unlikely that the improvement in self-reported competence can be explained by additional education or experiences outside of the training course.

There are several limitations of the study. In contrast to the study by Knighting and colleagues, participants' pre-course and post-course responses were not matched and fewer participants completed the post-course survey. In addition, the study focused on measures of self-perceived confidence but did not directly assess knowledge and skills. Finally, since this is a cross-sectional study, it does not measure participants' experiences after return to their healthcare systems. It is unknown if the course materials provided professionals with the ability to develop or improve PNPC programs. Therefore, longitudinal research is recommended to measure outcomes in clinical practice environments.

The development and implementation of an evidence-based PNPC course improved the self-reported competence of participants across disciplines and addressed specific self-reported competence gaps of nurses. This study provides a framework for the establishment of a PNPC curriculum, which addresses a global need.

ETHICS STATEMENT

The studies involving human participants were reviewed and approved by Columbia University Irving Medical Center Institutional Review Board. The patients/participants provided their written informed consent to participate in this study.

AUTHOR CONTRIBUTIONS

JH, CW, and EP developed the survey, analyzed the data, and wrote the manuscript. All authors contributed to the article and approved the submitted version.

ACKNOWLEDGMENTS

The authors thank the attendees of the training course for their participation in this study.

REFERENCES

1. Committee Opinion No. 786: Perinatal Palliative Care. American College of Obstetricians and Gynecologists Committee on Obstetric Practice, Committee on Ethics. *Obstet Gynecol.* (2019) 134:e84–9. doi: 10.1097/AOG.0000000000003425
2. Richards CA, Staonnor MR, Bourget E, Lindhorst T, Hays R, Doorenbos AZ. When and why do neonatal and pediatric critical care physicians consult palliative care? *Am J Hosp Palliat Care.* (2018) 35:840–6. doi: 10.1177/1049909117739853
3. Kukora S, Gollehon N, Lavental N. Antenatal palliative care consultation: implications for decision-making and perinatal outcomes in a single-center experience. *Arch Dis Child Neonatal Ed.* (2017) 102:F12–6. doi: 10.1136/archdischild-2016-311027
4. Parravicini E. Neonatal palliative care. *Curr Opin Pediatr.* (2017) 29:135–40. doi: 10.1097/MOP.0000000000000464
5. Carter BS. Pediatric palliative care in infants and neonates. *Children.* (2018) 5:21. doi: 10.3390/children5020021
6. Korzeniewska-Eksterowicz A, Respondek-Liberska M, Przysło Ł, Fendler W, Młynarski W, Gulczyńska E. Perinatal palliative care: barriers and attitudes of neonatologists and nurses in Poland. *Sci World J.* (2013) 2013:168060. doi: 10.1155/2013/168060
7. Wool C. State of the science on perinatal palliative care. *J Obstet Gynecol Neonatal Nurs.* (2013) 42:372–82. doi: 10.1111/1552-6909.12034
8. Wool C. Clinician perspectives of barriers in perinatal palliative care. *MCN Am J Matern Child Nurs.* (2015) 40:44–50. doi: 10.1097/NMC.0000000000000093
9. Mancini A, Kelly P, Bluebond Langner M. Training neonatal staff for the future in neonatal palliative care. *Semin Fetal Neonatal Med.* (2013) 18:111–5. doi: 10.1016/j.siny.2012.10.009
10. Wool C, Côté-Arsenault D, Perry Black B, Denney-Koelsch E, Kim S, Kavanaugh K. Provision of services in perinatal palliative care: a multicenter survey in the United States. *J Palliat Med.* (2016) 19:279–85. doi: 10.1089/jpm.2015.0266
11. Pediatric Palliative Care and Hospice Care Commitments, Guidelines, and Recommendations, American Academy of Pediatrics Policy Statement. *Pediatrics.* (2013) 132:966–72. doi: 10.1542/peds.2013-2731
12. National Consensus Project for Quality Palliative Care. *Clinical Practice Guidelines for Quality Palliative Care*, 4th ed. Richmond, VA: National Coalition for Hospice and Palliative Care (2018).
13. *Next-Level Perinatal/Neonatal Comfort Care Training: Creating an Interdisciplinary Palliative Care Plan for Each Baby and Their Family.* (2019). Available online at: https://www.publichealth.columbia.edu/comfort-care (accessed July 2019).
14. Epstein R, Hundert E. Defining and assessing professional competence. *JAMA.* (2002) 287:226–35. doi: 10.1001/jama.287.2.226
15. Stenekes S, Penner JL, Harlos M, Proulx MC, Shepherd E, Liben S, et al. Development and implementation of a survey to assess health-care provider's competency, attitudes, and knowledge about perinatal palliative care. *J Palliat Care.* (2019) 34:151–9. doi: 10.1177/0825859718790627
16. Limbo R, Wool C, Carter B. *Handbook of Perinatal and Neonatal Palliative Care.* New York, NY: Springer Publishing Company (2020). p. 50–65.
17. Committee on Fetus and Newborn, Section on Anesthesiology and Pain Medicine. Prevention and management of procedural pain in the neonate: an update. *Pediatrics.* (2016) 137:e201. doi: 10.1542/peds.2015-4271
18. Wool C. Clinician confidence and comfort in providing perinatal palliative care. *J Obstet Gynecol Neonatal Nurs.* (2013) 42:48–58. doi: 10.1111/j.1552-6909.2012.01432.x
19. Peng NH, Liu HF, Wang TM, Chang YC, Lee HY, Liang HF. Evaluation of comfort and confidence of neonatal clinicians in providing palliative care. *J Palliat Med.* (2018) 21:1558–65. doi: 10.1089/jpm.2018.0102
20. Haug S, Farooqi S, Wilson CG, Hopper A, Oei G, Carter B. Survey on neonatal end-of-life comfort care guidelines across America. *J Pain Symptom Manage.* (2018) 55:979–84. doi: 10.1016/j.jpainsymman.2017.10.023
21. Knighting K, Kirton J, Silverio SA, Shaw BN. A network approach to neonatal palliative care education: impact on knowledge, efficacy, and clinical practice. *J Perinat Neonatal Nurs.* (2019) 33:350–60. doi: 10.1097/JPN.0000000000000437
22. Connor SR, Sepulveda Bermedo MC. *Global Atlas of Palliative Care at the End of Life.* London: Worldwide Palliative Care Alliance and World Health Organization (2014).

10

"Percorso Giacomo": An Italian Innovative Service of Perinatal Palliative Care

Chiara Locatelli [1], Luigi Corvaglia [1,2], Giuliana Simonazzi [3], Maria Bisulli [3], Lucia Paolini [4] and Giacomo Faldella [1,2]*

[1] Neonatal Intensive Care Unit, S.Orsola-Malpighi University Hospital, Bologna, Italy, [2] Department of Medical and Surgical Sciences (DIMEC), University of Bologna, Bologna, Italy, [3] Obstetric Unit, Department of Medical and Surgical Sciences, Policlinico Sant'Orsola-Malpighi, University of Bologna, Bologna, Italy, [4] University of Bologna, Bologna, Italy

***Correspondence:**
Chiara Locatelli
chiara.locatelli@aosp.bo.it

The perspective proposed by this article will focus on perinatal palliative care as a strategy for improving the quality of life of neonates with life-limiting conditions when extending the patient's life is no longer the goal of care. This manuscript reports the creation of an innovative program of perinatal palliative care called "Percorso Giacomo" (Giacomo's Pathway) at Sant'Orsola Hospital in Bologna, Italy in 2013. Key features include interdisciplinary collaboration between professionals from obstetrics, neonatology and other specialties aiming to reach the most detailed fetal and neonatal diagnosis and prognosis; communication and engagement with the family to discuss goals of care and prepare a birthing plan that follows the family's desires and expectations; and personalized care to achieve comfort for each newborn and support for families according to their social, cultural, and religious backgrounds.

Keywords: perinatal palliative care, neonatal palliative care, life-limiting conditions, comfort care, interdisciplinary team

INTRODUCTION

Perinatal palliative care (PPC) is offered in the settings of fetal or neonatal diagnoses of life-limiting conditions (LLCs) as a plan to achieve comfort of the neonate and to support the family. Given the complexity of the medical and non-medical needs of these neonates and the emotional challenges for parents, PPC is a necessarily holistic and interdisciplinary approach to care. PPC is a journey with families that begins at the moment of diagnosis, whether prenatal or postnatal, and involves a collaboration among maternal-fetal medicine specialists, neonatologists, and other professionals with the goal of establishing an individualized plan of care for the mother-baby dyad.

The American College of Obstetricians and Gynecologists (ACOG) considers PPC one of the options of care that should be offered to patients facing pregnancies complicated by fetal LLC (1). Yet, PPC is not yet routinely integrated in prenatal counseling in the United States (2, 3). This also holds true for Italy. A recent Italian national survey of neonatal intensive care unit (NICU) practitioners demonstrated that only 30% of the institutions represented offer a structured PPC program. Of these, 34% have only one program coordinator, and fewer than 30% organize PPC training for health care providers (4).

Despite technological advances in the ability to detect severe fetal anomalies, infants with LLCs are occasionally diagnosed only after birth. Moreover, critically ill neonates admitted to the NICU can face a potentially adverse prognosis or reach the end-of-life stage, at which point a redirection of goals of care is required. According to the World Health Organization (WHO), palliative care and intensive care should be provided concurrently to critically ill infants with potentially adverse prognoses (5). The American Academy of Pediatrics (AAP) and the Italian Society of Neonatology (SIN) provide recommendations for achieving comfort of terminally ill neonates and of those affected by an LLC (6–9).

The urgent need to provide the option of PPC to families with neonates prenatally or postnatally diagnosed with an LLC prompted the creation and implementation of an innovative PPC program at Sant'Orsola Hospital (SOH) in Bologna in 2013. The program was named "Percorso Giacomo" (Giacomo's Pathway) in honor of the first infant to whom SOH provided such care. This paper describes the origin and the development of the program over its first 7 years.

CLINICAL CASE

Giacomo was prenatally diagnosed with anencephaly. His parents, although aware of his short life expectancy, chose to carry the pregnancy to term. The mother was a G4 P3 woman with two healthy children and another baby with anencephaly whose delivery was complicated by failure to progress and stillbirth. As she again received an anencephaly diagnosis, she asked her provider to manage her care with the goal of having some precious time with her baby after birth. At that time there were no guidelines for PPC at SOH, so the obstetrician involved a neonatologist and a midwife to plan the delivery and the infant's postnatal care according to the mother's desire. Giacomo was delivered by cesarean section (transverse position) with Apgar scores of 9 and 9. After his scalp wound was carefully dressed, he was given to his family to hold. Per parental wish, he was baptized by the hospital chaplain. Following the family desire for bonding, Giacomo was allowed to room-in with his mother in a private postpartum room. At SOH, this was the first time that a baby with LLC was not admitted to the NICU. Comfort measures, including skin-to-skin care and holding to facilitate bonding and warmth, were offered. The infant had no sucking reflex; thus, he was given small feeds via an orogastric tube to relieve hunger and thirst. Discomfort and pain were assessed but Giacomo had no signs of distress and did not need any pharmacological treatment. Giacomo lived for only 19 hours, but he had the opportunity to meet his parents, siblings, and relatives, and he was comfortable throughout his entire life.

Written informed consent was obtained from Giacomo's parents for the publication of any potentially identifiable images or data included in this article.

PERCORSO GIACOMO

Origin

The experience with Giacomo made our perinatal team aware of the urgency to formalize a systematic approach to families who received a fetal or neonatal diagnosis of LLC, and a collaborative journey began. Another key factor that triggered the initiation of a PPC program, was that the neonatologist who provided care to Giacomo received training in PPC in 2009–2011 by participating in the Neonatal Comfort Care Program (NCCP) (10) at Columbia University Medical Center (CUMC) in New York, NY, US. Upon her return to Italy she began to investigate the feasibility of a similar program at SOH, and the meeting with Giacomo's family was the occasion to start the project.

During the debreafing of Giacomo's case, each of the professionals involved in the care expressed interest in developing a service for similar cases and the planning began. The group decided to name the program "Percorso Giacomo" (PG) in honor of Baby Giacomo.

The experience with this family was not only the trigger for the planning of a new service, but also a milestone in the understanding of the complex medical and non-medical needs of these infants and their families.

The group then opened to other professionals interested in the same goal, and a working group of champions called the "Percorso Giacomo Team" (PGT) was established. Two main objectives were identified: (1) assemble an interdisciplinary team, and (2) define guidelines and eventually establish a new hospital policy for PPC.

Gathering an Interdisciplinary Team

SOH is a large academic institution with a busy maternal-fetal medicine service that has approximately 3,500 deliveries each year. The level 3 NICU takes care of some 300 critically ill neonates annually, including infants prenatally or postnatally diagnosed with an LLC. The two services work collaboratively, but until 2013 there was limited knowledge and no direct experience of PPC.

The PGT is an interdisciplinary team that includes nine clinicians from obstetrics and neonatology who identify themselves as champions for the care of mothers and infants with a fetal or neonatal diagnosis of LLC. The program is not funded, and the team members make themselves available as primary providers for the mother-baby dyad and facilitate the execution of the plan of care in collaboration with medical staff involved in the care. Professionals from a variety of other specialties (cardiology, neurology, surgey, nephrology, genetics, etc.) are also available for consultation.

Establishing Guidelines

After carefully reviewing PPC literature, including recommendation from the ACOG (11), the AAP (6), and the SIN (8), and through networking with other national and international academic centers, local guidelines were created and implemented to standardize interventions. The essential elements are summarized in **Tables 1, 2.**

As the focus of care is the satisfaction of neonates' basic needs for bonding, maintanance of body temperature, and relief of hunger and thirst, our guidelines reflected these recommendations. Pain and distress are assessed and treated with pharmacological interventions (12). The Neonatal Infant Pain Scale (NIPS) (13) and Echelle Douleur Inconfort Nouveau-né' (EDIN) (14) are the preferred pain assessment tools because they are based on the infant's behavior and do not require vital signs detection, which could disrupt the bonding experience. Each neonate has unique medical and non-medical

TABLE 1 | Guidelines to provide comfort to neonates prenatally diagnosed with life-limiting conditions.

At prenatal counseling

- Discuss comfort measures in detail and assure parents that a state of comfort for their baby can always be achieved, regardless of his/her condition
- Fill out a birthplan with the family according to their preferences and cultural/social/religious background and give a copy to family
- Obtain pictures/videos of fetal ultrasounds as per family's wishes
- Discuss administration of Vitamin K, eye prophylaxis

Before delivery

- Review birthplan with family
- Collect items for special dressing if needed (anencephaly, limb-body-wall complex, etc.) and clothing appropriate for the baby's clinical condition and size
- In case a blood test is needed to confirm the diagnosis, plan for cord sample

After delivery

- Evaluation of baby's clinical status, provide gentle suction if needed
- Place hat, place dressing as needed and wrap in clean warm blanket
- Allow mother and/or father for skin-to-skin or holding
- Facilitate bonding with siblings and extended family as per family's wishes
- Involve chaplain as per family's wishes
- Obtain pictures, videos and memories as per family's wishes
- Transfer mother and baby to post-pastum for rooming-in in a private room

Neonatal plan of care

- Vital signs: heart rate, respiratory rate, temperature and pain score (NIPS or EDIN) every 3 h or as needed according to the baby's status
- No blood or other tests should be obptained, unless needed for confirmation diagnosis
- Encourage breastfeeding or gavage feeds as appropriate. Establish a minimum intake to guarantee relief of hunger/thirst (breast milk or formula). Consider colostrum care for babies at end of life
- Assessment of respiratory distress (air hunger, agitation, increased work of breathing, gasping) and use of non-pharmacological strategies (gentle suctioning upper airways, positioning) or pharmacological treatment (morphine sulfate PO, lorazepam PO)

NIPS, Neonatal Infant Pain Scale; EDIN, Echelle Douleur Inconfort Nouveau-né; PO, per os.

TABLE 2 | Guidelines to provide comfort to neonates with life-threatening or terminal conditions in the NICU.

Neonates critically ill but still receiving full intensive care

- Discuss baby's clinical status and potential comfort interventions with medical/nursing team
- Discuss with parents a plan of comfort interventions to improve quality of life
- Provide privacy in the NICU
- Facilitate baby/parents bonding by holding, gentle touch, massage
- Encourage breast pumping if mother desires to give her baby breast milk
- Provide parents the opportunity to take care of their baby's needs (colostrum care, non nutritive sucking, diaper change, sponge bath, dressing, etc.)
- Involve siblings and extended family as per family's wishes
- Involved chaplain as per family's wishes
- Obtain pictures, videos and memories as per family's wishes

Neonates at end-of-life stage after redirection from intensive to palliative care

- Discuss plan for weaning of life-sustaining support with parents
- Assure parents that a state of comfort for their baby can always be achieved, regardless of his/her condition
- Encourage parents to stay/hold the baby
- Involve chaplain as per family's wishes
- Involve siblings and extended family as per family's wishes
- Obtain pictures, videos and memories as per family's wishes
- Provide private settings with intermittent supervision of medical/nursing team
- Wean life-sustaining support, silence monitors'alarm, remove unnecessary devices and IV/arterial lines in appropriate fashion
- Maintain an IV access, if present, for pain management
- Facilitate bonding and warmth by skin-to-skin, holding, colostrum care
- Assess signs of respiratory distress (air hunger, agitation, increased work of breathing, gasping) and assess pain by validated clinical scores (NIPS or EDIN)
- Use non-pharmacological strategies (gentle suctioning upper airways, positioning) or pharmacological treatment (acetaminophen PO; morphine sulfate PO/IV; fentanyl IV; lorazepam PO/IV; midazolam PO/IV)
- After the baby dies, help parents to sponge bath and dress their baby
- Discuss with family in regard to autopsy consent

IV, intravenous; NIPS, Neonatal Infant Pain Scale; EDIN, Echelle Douleur Inconfort Nouveau-né; PO, per os.

needs; thus, we personalized the care plan in consideration of diagnosis, prognosis, gestational age, and family preferences. Additionally, as a result of a policy change in our hospital, when a neonate, prenatally diagnosed with an LLC, is not admitted to the NICU, is directly transitioned from delivery room to a post-partum for rooming-in with the mother in private setting. The midwife in charge of the mother-baby dyad provides support and care in collaboration with NICU nurses and neonatologist is available for medical evaluation and interventions.

Criteria for Enrollment

PG offers PPC to neonates prenatally or postnatally diagnosed with an LLC that is expected to render their life brief, such as renal agenesis, anencephaly or extreme prematurity. PPC is also offered to neonates diagnosed with severe genetic, metabolic, skeletal, cardiac, neurological or oncological conditions and life-limiting syndromes. The provision of intensive care can prolong the life of these neonates, but when the burden of invasive and aggressive treatment might exceed the benefit in terms of length of life, an option of PPC is offered.

Perinatal Counseling

The PGT can be accessed in different ways. If a mother receives a diagnosis of fetal LLC at SOH, the obstetric provider offers available options, including consultation with the PGT. Patients might also be referred by outside institutions. After consultation, the mother has the option to transfer her care to SOH, or to continue care with her current provider, with the PGT functioning as consultant.

Members of the PGT—including a neonatologist, an obstetrician, and a midwife—are involved in the encounter with the family. Before meeting the family, team members meet to review available information about the fetal diagnosis, discuss the need to obtain further tests and/or to involve more specialists, and identify care options to be presented to the family. It is essential that the family receives clear and honest information from both obstetricians and neonatologists.

The conversation with the family focuses on communicating of detailed information about the presumed or certain diagnosis and prognosis and, if needed, any further medical investigations. Team members listen attentively to the family to identify concerns, hopes, and expectations that will help them prepare a comprehensive plan for the reminder of the pregnancy, labor and delivery, and postnatal birthing plan. At the end of the meeting the parents are also given the option to meet a psychologist to assess mental health and to provide grief support, resources, and referrals for the family at large. Depending on the complexity of the diagnosis and the gestational age, one or more meetings are needed to complete a comprehensive plan.

The outcome of the conversation/s is documented on the mother's health record to facilitate communication with all clinicians involved in mother-baby care. Moreover, providers and family complete a document -the "birthing plain"- that is kept by the family and presented upon hospital admission.

Members of the PGT follow labor and delivery, and the neonatologist present at birth either confirms the neonate's diagnosis or obtains further tests for confirmation. The team ensures that the birth plan formulated during prenatal counseling is included in the overall management care plan.

When neonates admitted to the NICU are postnatally diagnosed with an LLC or a potentially adverse prognosis, the medical team attentively evaluates each case and may involve the PGT as an extra layer of support to families. Different options can be proposed including the continuation of intensive care with focus on quality of life, or the redirection of goals of care with transition to palliative care.

Pregnancy and Neonatal Outcomes

The PGT cared for 24 cases in its first 7 years. The team followed 20 pregnancies, the outcome of which included two intrauterine fetal deaths, two second trimester spontaneous abortions, and 16 live births. Three of these infants are currently alive and stable, and PPC was not considered medically appropriate for these infants because their postnatal diagnoses were more favorable than had been expected. The PGT also facilitated palliative care plans for four neonates admitted to the NICU with severe brain injury secondary to severe metabolic conditions or hypoxic-ischemic insults, all of whom died.

Education and Program Development

Teaching and training are essential to fostering a mindset that includes palliative care as an essential component of medical practice in perinatology. Over time the PGT built several initiatives for PPC training at SOH. Formal teaching, including a curriculum of six lessons for pediatric residents and fellows, was established in 2017. Bedside training and clinical case discussion for physicians, midwives, and nurses also have been introduced over the past 7 years.

In 2014, the concern for education and program development inspired the PGT to organize a National Workshop featuring national and international experts in PPC. The workshop goals included presentation of cutting-edge experiences of PPC and network development. The workshop was attended by some 300 clinicians from all across Italy and laid the foundation for collaboration with several academic institutions. The meeting was also attended by the Maternal Infant Department leadership and administrators. They expressed their interest and encouraged development of a PPC service at SOH. The PGT then worked tirelessly with administrators and leadership to establish a new hospital policy for PPC, which was approved in 2019.

In our region of Italy, Emilia-Romagna, a new project for the organization of a regional palliative care network has begun (15). This pediatric hospice network offers inpatient care and home care for children with complex medical conditions and chronic health problems. PG has been included in this network by the project committee. This is an essential step to build a continuity of care for neonates born with LLC or for those with complex diseases and potentially adverse prognoses. After hospital discharge, infants can be supported either at home or in a rehabilitation facility by specialists in palliative care. This project is also an opportunity to promote the palliative care mindset in our region and, hopefully, in the entire nation.

DISCUSSION

Over the past years, PPC has been gaining interest in Italy, and clinicians involved in perinatology have been working to define the best care practice (16) and to establish adequate pathways to care for neonates diagnosed with LLCs (17). Moreover, the SIN has offered suggestions for PPC in a document focused on guidelines for prevention and treatment of neonatal pain (8, 9) and Italy has enacted legislation promoting the use of palliative care (18).

PG has positioned itself as an innovative pathway for PPC origins and guidelines.

What triggered the actualization of this program was the desire of a family (Giacomo's parents) to be accompanied along the perinatal journey. The professionals involved in the care were inspired to create a standardized program for families with similar needs. The experience of PG show that a strong motivation is pivotal to the birth of a new program.

PG was modeled after the NCCP in New York. In the planning process the PGT utilized evidence-based recommendations (6, 8, 9, 11); however, the innovative aspects of the PG guidelines came largely from direct experience and ongoing collaboration with the NCCP. An important step for "culture change" at SOH is the transition of neonates with LLC from delivery room directly to post-partum to room-in with the mother, instead of admission to the NICU (**Table 1**).

Another innovative element includes the introduction of early palliative care interventions to improve quality of life of babies still receiving full intensive care (**Table 2**). Both innovations have been supported by studies of parental satisfaction (19) and stress evaluation (20) published by the NCCP.

In pregnancy care, two patients are at stake. Thus, tight collaboration of specialists in obstetrics and neonatology is essential to propose available options (1), to plan a safe pregnancy and delivery, and to provide a personalized care for each neonate in accord with the family's preference (21). Pregnancy is a time of hope and expectation, but with the discovery of severe anomalies, fear can quickly overcome hope as expectations are no longer the norm. The option of PPC supports the family and helps in the decision-making process (22, 23). Moreover, the 7-years experience of PG shows that families felt welcomed and embraced along the perinatal journey. Parents expressed of PG gratitude and praise for the program, as clearly illustrated by parental feed-back messages. *"PG was the light at the end of the tunnel, PG was the hope that our baby would have been able to be embraced by mom, dad an her siblings"*; *"PG taught us that our life cannot be measured by its lenght, rather by the mark we leave"*; *"The program filled somehow the void we experienced and we felt serene."*

The greatest desire of parents of neonates with LLC is not wanting them to suffer. Thus, pain and distress must be attentively assessed and treated (12). In the population we served any degree of discomfort was successfully managed with the use of non-pharmacological strategies, such as skin-to-skin holding, and colostrum care (24) or proper medications. This observation has been validated by studies of parental perception of their infants' state of comfort, when infants were treated with standardized comfort measures (19).

PPC not only addresses the population of neonates expected to have early perinatal demise, but also can be integrated with the intensive care of critically ill neonates at any stage of the illness (20, 25). In its first years, PG focuses largely on the care of mothers with fetal life-limiting diagnoses and followed neonates with short life expectancy however, in time the PGT began to be consulted regarding the plan of care of critically ill neonates with unexpected life-threatening diagnoses. Thus the PGT developed guidelines to facilitate quality of life during the NICU admission and/or to redirect goals of care at end of life (**Table 2**).

FUTURE DIRECTION

PG has been offering perinatologists the opportunity to improve their confidence in this growing field in medicine. Within 1 year of the program's establishment, the PGT organized a national conference. Since that time many other educational initiatives have been proposed to guide and educate providers. When PPC knowledge is lacking, clinicians are uncomfortable and reluctant to offer this much-needed care (26). Thus, PG is planning to continue to offer training courses for medical and nursing professionals built on the knowledge and experience acquired over the past 7 years.

Throughout the years, PG has followed infants with a variety of severe life-threatening conditions, including rare and complex diseases. Collaboration with other academic centers has been essential to share experiences, to discuss challenging cases, and to provide the best possible care to each infant. Further networking opportunities will support the implementation of new programs in tertiary NICUs and will provide the necessary tools to professionals working in small institutions where programs cannot be implemented.

PG intends to facilitate the spreading of a mindset that integrates palliative care in the medical plan for neonates with LLC or critically ill. Being aware that further studies measuring outcomes and quality of care are needed, our group is in the process of analyzing the efficacy of this program.

As recommended by national and international organizations (1, 6, 27), PPC is a crucial option to be offered to families facing a fetal or neonatal diagnosis of LLC. Essential components include early involvement with families at the time of diagnosis, interdisciplinary collaboration of perinatologists, and promotion of education to facilitate a culture change.

ETHICS STATEMENT

Written informed consent was obtained from the participant's parents for the publication of any potentially identifiable images or data included in this article.

AUTHOR CONTRIBUTIONS

CL conceptualized and designed the report. MB, LC, GF, LP, and GS drafted the initial manuscript and approved the final manuscript as submitted. All authors contributed to the article and approved the submitted version.

ACKNOWLEDGMENTS

The authors express their profound gratitude to the members of the Percorso Giacomo Team (Patrizio Calderoni, Santo Merlini, Maria Antonietta Graziano, Silvia Savini, Marika Friguglietti, Caterina Voli, Marta Bucchi) and to the babies and their families, from whom they have learned so much about perinatal palliative care.

REFERENCES

1. Perinatal Palliative Care. Committee Opinion No. 786. American College of Obstetricians and Gynecologists Committee on Obstetric Practice, Committee on Ethics. *Obstet Gynecol.* (2019) 134:e84–9. doi: 10.1097/AOG.0000000000003425
2. Tosello B, Haddad G, Gire C, Einaudi M. Lethal fetal abnormalities: how to approach perinatal palliative care? *J Matern Fetal Neonatal Med.* (2017) 30:755–8. doi: 10.1080/14767058.2016.1186633
3. Kukora S, Gollehon N, Laventhal N. Antenatal palliative care consultation: implications for decision-making and perinatal outcomes in a single-centre experience. *Arch Dis Child Fetal Neonatal Ed.* (2017) 102:F12–16. doi: 10.1136/archdischild-2016-311027
4. Cavicchiolo ME, Rusalen F, Benini F, Baraldi E, Lago P. Perinatal palliative care: a national survey in Italy. *Arch Dis Child Fetal Neonatal Ed.* (2019) 104:F567–8. doi: 10.1136/archdischild-2018-316327
5. World Health Organization. *WHO Definition of Palliative Care.* (2018). Available online at: https://www.who.int/health-topics/palliative-care
6. Section on Hospice and Palliative Medicine and Committee on Hospital Care. Pediatric palliative care and hospice care commitments, guidelines, and recommendations. *Pediatrics.* (2013) 132:966–72. doi: 10.1542/peds.2013-2731
7. Committee on Fetus Newborn, Section on Anesthesiology Pain Medicine, Keels E, Sethna N, Watterberg KL, Cummings JJ, et al. Prevention and management of procedural pain in the neonate: an update. *Pediatrics.* (2016) 137:e20154271. doi: 10.1542/peds.2015-4271

8. Società Italiana di Neonatologia, Gruppo di Studio di Analgesia e Sedazione. *Linee guida per la prevenzione ed il Trattamento del Dolore nel neonato.* Padova: Cooperativa Libraria Editrice Università di Padova (2008).
9. Società Italiana di Neonatologia, Gruppo di Studio di Analgesia e Sedazione nel Neonato. *Linee guida per la prevenzione ed il Trattamento del Dolore nel neonato.* Milano: Biomedia (2016).
10. *Neonatal Comfort Care Program.* Available online at: www.neonatalcomfortcare.com (accessed 21 July 2020).
11. American College of Obstetrician and Gynecologists, Committee on Ethics, American Academy of Pediatrics, Committe on Bioethics. Maternal-fetal intervention and fetal care centers. *Pediatrics.* (2011) 128:e473–8. doi: 10.1542/peds.2011-1570
12. Carter BS, Jones PM. Evidence-based comfort care for neonates towards the end of life. *Semin Fetal Neonatal Med.* (2013) 18:88–92. doi: 10.1016/j.siny.2012.10.012
13. Lawrence J, Alcock D, McGrath P, Kay J, MacMurray SB, Dulberg C. The development of a tool to assess neonatal pain. *Neonatal Netw.* (1993) 12:59–66.
14. Debillion T, Zupan V, Ravault N, Magny JF, Dehan M. Development and initial validation of the EDIN scale, a new tool for assessing prolonged pain preterm infants. *Arch Dis Child Fetal Neonatal Ed.* (2001) 85:F36–41. doi: 10.1136/fn.85.1.F36
15. DRG 1131/2015. *Recepimento dell'accordo tra Governo, Regioni e Province autonome del documento 'Individuazione delle figure professionali competenti nel campo delle cure palliative e della terapia del dolore, nonchè delle strutture sanitarie, ospedaliere e territoriali, coinvolte nelle reti delle cure palliative.* Bologna: Atti della Giunta della Regione Emilia Romagna. (2015).
16. Rusalen F, Cavicchiolo ME, Lago P, Salvadori S, Benini F. Perinatal palliative care: is palliative care really available to everyone? *Ann Palliat Med.* (2018) 7:487–8. doi: 10.21037/apm.2018.07.09
17. Rusalen F, Cavicchiolo ME, Lago P, Salvadori S, Benini F. Perinatal palliative care: a dedicated care pathway. *BMJ Support Palliat Care.* (2019). doi: 10.1136/bmjspcare-2019-001849. [Epub ahead of print].
18. Legge 15 marzo, 2010, n 38. *Disposizioni per Garantire L'accesso alle Cure Palliative e alla terapia del Dolore.* Roma: Gazzetta Ufficiale della Repubblica Italiana (2010).
19. Parravicini E, Daho M, Foe G, Steinwurtzel R, Byrne M. Parental assessment of comfort in newborns affected by life-limiting conditions treated by a standardized neonatal comfort care program. *J Perinatol.* (2018) 38:142–7. doi: 10.1038/jp.2017.160
20. Callahan K, Steinwurtzel R, Bruaire L, Schechter S, Parravicini E. Early palliative care reduces stress in parents of neonates with congenital heart disease: validation of the "Baby, Attachment, Comfort Interventions." *J Perinatol.* (2019) 39:1640–7. doi: 10.1038/s41372-019-0490-y
21. Carter BS. More than medication: perinatal palliative care. *Acta Paediatr.* (2016) 105:1255–6. doi: 10.1111/apa.13529
22. Cote-Arsenault D, Denney-Koelsch E. "Have no regrets:" parents' experiences and developmental tasks in pregnancy with a lethal fetal diagnosis. *Soc Sci Med.* (2016) 154:100–9. doi: 10.1016/j.socscimed.2016.02.033
23. Janvier A, Farlow B, Barrington KJ. Parental hopes, interventions, and survival of neonates with trisomy 13 and trisomy 18. *Am J Med Genet C Semin Med Genet.* (2016) 172:279–87. doi: 10.1002/ajmg.c.31526
24. Parravicini E, McCarthy F. Comfort in perinatal and neonatal palliative care: an innovative plan of care focused on relational elements. In: Limbo R, Wool C, Carter BS, editors. *Handbook of Perinatal and Neonatal Palliative Care: A Guide for Nurses, Physicians, and Other Health Professionals. Chapter 4.* New York, NY: Springer Company, LLC (2020).
25. Parravicini E. Neonatal palliative care. *Curr Opin Pediatr.* (2017) 29:135–40. doi: 10.1097/MOP.0000000000000464
26. Wool C. Clinician confidence and comfort in providing perinatal palliative care. *J Obstet Gynecol Neonatal Nurs.* (2013) 42:48–58. doi: 10.1111/j.1552-6909.2012.01432.x
27. National Consensus Project for Quality Palliative Care. *Clinical practice guidelines for quality palliative care.* 4th ed. Richmond, VA: National Coalition for Hospice and Palliative Care (2018). Available online at: https://www.nationalcoalitionhpc.org/ncp

11

Advances in Pediatric Critical Care Research in India

Utpal Bhalala[1]*****, *Arun Bansal*[2] *and Krishan Chugh*[3]

[1] *Baylor College of Medicine at The Children's Hospital of San Antonio, San Antonio, TX, United States,* [2] *Postgraduate Institute of Medical Education and Research, Chandigarh, India,* [3] *Fortis Hospital, New Delhi, India*

***Correspondence:**
Utpal Bhalala
utpal.bhalala@bcm.edu

Over last 2 decades, there has been a significant progress made in the field of pediatric critical care in India. There has been complementary and parallel growth in the pediatric critical care services in India and the number of pediatric critical care providers who are either formally trained in India or who have returned to India after their formal training abroad. The pediatric critical care community in India has recognized obvious differences in profiles of critical illnesses and patients between Indian subcontinent and the West. Therefore there is a growing interest in generating scientific evidence through local research which would be applicable to critically ill children in Indian subcontinent. This article focuses on advances in pediatric critical care research in India and its future directions.

Keywords: research, pediatric critical care, India, scientific evidence, advances

INTRODUCTION

Pediatric Critical Care Medicine (PCCM) is a relatively new but a rapidly growing pediatric specialty in resource-limited countries. Pediatric Intensive Care Units (PICUs) were introduced into the lower- and middle-income countries (LMICs) somewhere in late 1980's or early 1990's. Few countries in Africa and south-east Asia still do not have a dedicated PICU. Though pediatric intensive care practices were introduced into India in the 1980's, early units were simply located in a special "treatment room" and lacked the constant monitoring of vital sign, respiratory or hemodynamic support characteristic of a PICU. One author (KC) recalls his first exposure to a PICU at Kalawati Saran Children's Hospital, Lady Hardinge Medical College in 1983 in New Delhi, although the first organized PICU was reportedly established in 1991 at Kanchi Kamakoti Childs Trust Hospital in Chennai, India with seven beds, a separate team of doctors and nurses, and with a pediatric anaesthesiologist as the director of the unit (1). Currently, there are more than 100 dedicated PICUs in the private and public sectors in India. With growth in pediatric critical care services in India, there has been a parallel growth in academic medicine in pediatric criticalc care in India. This article describes advances in critical care research in the west and in India, particularly in PCCM and future of pediatric critical care research in India.

Advances in Pediatric Critical Care Research in the West

For any specialty in medicine, research is key to understanding the epidemiology and pathophysiology of disease processes, exploring potential new therapies and measuring response to therapies. With rapidly growing specialty of pediatric critical care, there have been parallel advances in research in pediatric critical care in the West. The first collaborative pediatric critical care study group (PCCSG) was founded by Gregory Stidham and associates in the early 1990s. Approximately 60 pediatric ICUs, mostly from the United States worked together to generate a number of studies related to PICU outcomes (2–7). The Pediatric Acute Lung Injury and Sepsis Investigators (PALISI)

Network, was founded by Adrienne Randolph at Children's Hospital of Boston in the late 1990s. Around 48 pediatric ICUs throughout North America participated to study therapies for acute lung injury, sepsis and multi-organ failure (8–11). Randall Wetzel at Children's Hospital Los Angeles founded the first electronic database, the Virtual PICU (vPICU) in 2000, to create a shared patient database for outcomes analysis and improve critical care practices (12). In 2004, National Institutes of Health, founded the Collaborative Pediatric Critical Care Research Network (CPCCRN) to study the pathophysiological bases of critical illness and safety and efficacy of treatment of critically ill children (12). The pediatric interest group of Canadian Critical Care Trial Group (CCCTG) has conducted large, multicenter trials such as TRIPICU and HypHIT (13). Similarly, European Society of Pediatric and Neonatal Intensive Care (ESPNIC) has been active in multi-center evaluation of respiratory distress syndrome (14) and in collaboration with European Extracorporeal Life Support (EuroELSO), it has created a working group to evaluate actual and future trends about neonatal and pediatric ECMO in Europe (15). The ANZICS (Australian and New Zealand Intensive Care Society) Pediatric Group has fostered and promoted meaningful research within the Australian and New Zealand pediatric intensive care communities (16).

There are now innumerable, ongoing single-site and multi-site clinical trials and large database studies in America and Europe which are substantially contributing to our understanding of science of PCCM. Some examples of recent key studies are—therapeutic hypothermia after pediatric cardiac arrest (THAPCA), heart and lung failure—pediatric insulin titration (HALF-PINT) and randomized evaluation of sedation titration for respiratory failure (RESTORE) trials (17–19).

Advances in Adult Critical Care Medicine Research in India

Before the turn of the century, critical care medicine in India was practiced in a few hospitals, either by those interested in the field and learning on the job, or by physicians returning to India after training overseas. Establishment of the Indian Society of Critical Care Medicine (ISCCM) in 1993 was a turning point in the history of critical care medicine in India. ISCCM has grown to become one of the largest professionl organizations and serves as the premier organization supporting the training and research in critical care medicine in India (20). In 2012, the Medical Council of India (MCI) recognized critical care medicine as an independent speciality, enabling 3-year training programmes, which have facilitated the development of academic departments of intensive care medicine with greater emphasis on research (21). Adult critical care community in India has made significant contributions to large multicenter randomized controlled trials such as the PROWESS-SHOCK (22) and OSCILLATE studies (23) and to a number of international, multicenter observational studies (24–28). Over last decade, several multicenter, adult critical care studies conducted in ICUs in India have contributed to a body of literature relevant to the Indian population (21). Though, Divatia and co-authors reported a 35% increase in the number of abstracts submitted to the annual conference of the ISCCM in 2013 as compared to the 2012 conference, their publication rate in international journals has been low (21, 29). Time constraints and lack of motivation to publish could be important contributing factors to the low publication rate. Overall, the advances in adult critical care medicine research in India have encouraged the pediatric critical care community to make forward steps toward pediatric critical research relevant to the unique diseases and child populations in India.

Advances in Pediatric Critical Care Research in India

The initiative to upgrade neonatal and pediatric critical care facilities has come primarily from major teaching institutions (30). India has shown tremendous growth in the practice of pediatric critical care. From a single PICU in 1991 to a young dynamic speciality in 2017, it has come a long way. India, foremost amongst the resource-limited countries has been a leader in that. The intensive care chapter of the Indian Academy of Pediatrics (IAP) started a formal fellowship training program in 2002 and they now have 22 accredited centers that are running this program successfully. More than 250 students have been trained through this program (31).

Similarly, research in neonatal and pediatric critical care has also picked up in India. The early published reports on outcomes of intensive care units in India were related to neonatal intensive care unit (NICU) graduates (32). Subsequently, Singhi and co-authors published the first report on electrolyte abnormalities in pediatric pneumonia in 1992 (33). As listed in PubMed, pediatric critical care research has grown from only 31 published clinical trials, 19 randomized controlled trials (RCTs) and 2 multicenter studies in 1990 to an impressive 198 RCTs and 92 multicenter studies in 2016. This progress shows that the growth of research in Pediatric Critical Care in India has come a long way. As the interest in research grew, the Government of India also tried to streamline it by setting up the Clinical Trial Registry of India (CTRI) in 2007. Registration of trial in CTRI is now mandatory and is also an important factor for publication in various journals. As on 30th June 2017, 8950 trials are registered with the CTRI (34).

Retrospective and prospective pediatric critical care studies conducted in India and their subsequent publication in regional and international journals have grown steadily in the past two decades (35–41). A handful of studies conducted by pediatric critical care researchers in India have impacted PICU care not only in the region but also outside the region—for example, original studies published from India on monitoring of intracranial and cerebral perfusion pressures in patients with acute meningoencephalitis have reinvigorated the field of neurocritical care (42–44). Recently, newer developments in collaborative, multicenter research initiatives in pediatric critical care have occurred in India. The Postgraduate Institute of Medical Education and Research (PGIMER) in Chandigarh, India has initiated the first, national, multi-institutional database for pediatric cardiac arrest and cardiopulmonary resuscitation. Currently, large, government-run, teaching institutions are

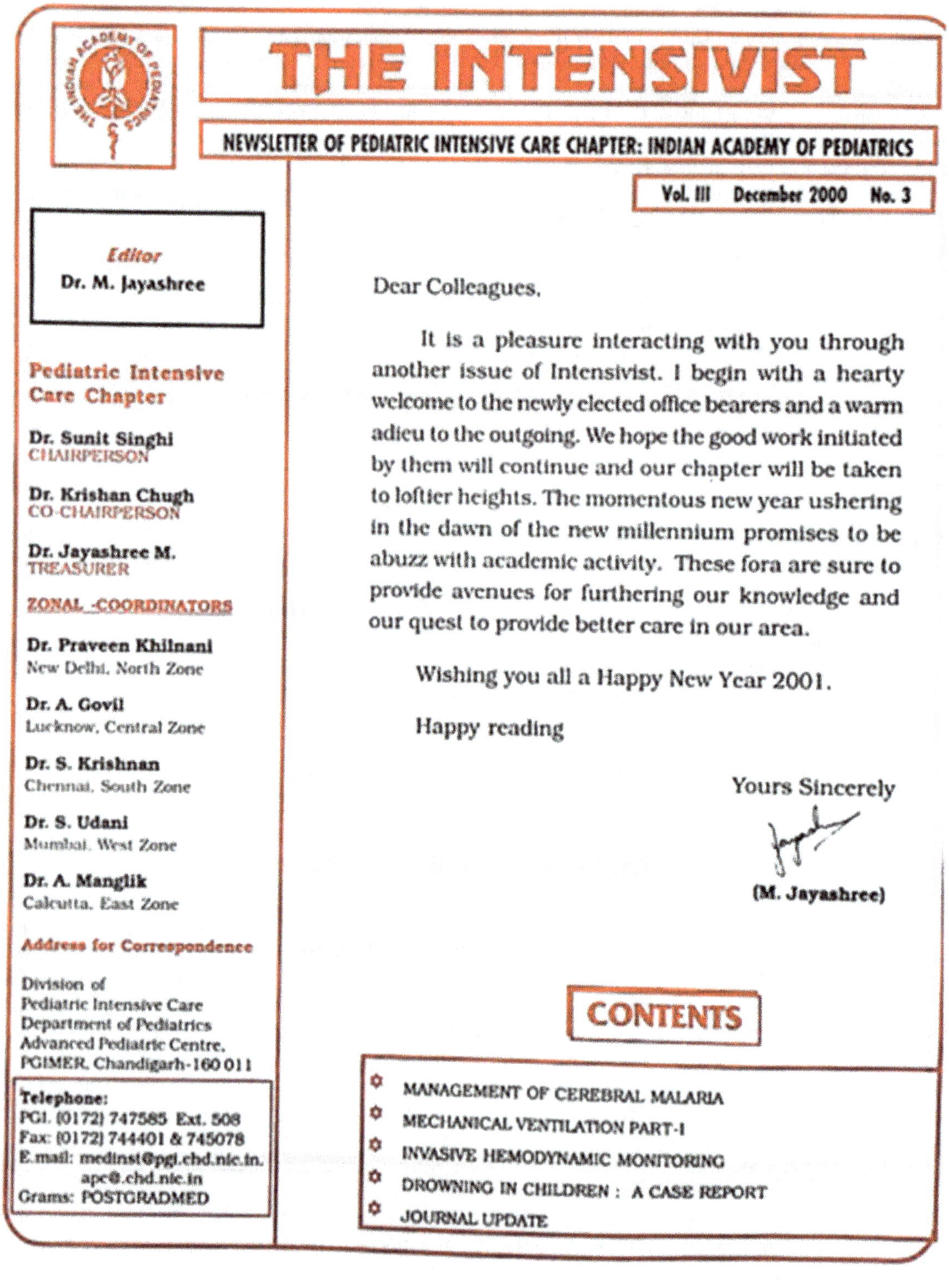

THE INTENSIVIST

NEWSLETTER OF PEDIATRIC INTENSIVE CARE CHAPTER: INDIAN ACADEMY OF PEDIATRICS

Vol. III December 2000 No. 3

Editor
Dr. M. Jayashree

Pediatric Intensive Care Chapter

Dr. Sunit Singhi
CHAIRPERSON

Dr. Krishan Chugh
CO-CHAIRPERSON

Dr. Jayashree M.
TREASURER

ZONAL -COORDINATORS

Dr. Praveen Khilnani
New Delhi, North Zone

Dr. A. Govil
Lucknow, Central Zone

Dr. S. Krishnan
Chennai, South Zone

Dr. S. Udani
Mumbai, West Zone

Dr. A. Manglik
Calcutta, East Zone

Address for Correspondence

Division of
Pediatric Intensive Care
Department of Pediatrics
Advanced Pediatric Centre,
PGIMER, Chandigarh-160 011

Telephone:
PGI. (0172) 747585 Ext. 508
Fax: (0172) 744401 & 745078
E.mail: medinst@pgi.chd.nic.in,
apc@.chd.nic.in
Grams: POSTGRADMED

Dear Colleagues,

It is a pleasure interacting with you through another issue of Intensivist. I begin with a hearty welcome to the newly elected office bearers and a warm adieu to the outgoing. We hope the good work initiated by them will continue and our chapter will be taken to loftier heights. The momentous new year ushering in the dawn of the new millennium promises to be abuzz with academic activity. These fora are sure to provide avenues for furthering our knowledge and our quest to provide better care in our area.

Wishing you all a Happy New Year 2001.

Happy reading

Yours Sincerely

(M. Jayashree)

CONTENTS

- MANAGEMENT OF CEREBRAL MALARIA
- MECHANICAL VENTILATION PART-I
- INVASIVE HEMODYNAMIC MONITORING
- DROWNING IN CHILDREN : A CASE REPORT
- JOURNAL UPDATE

FIGURE 1 | The picture of the periodical "The Intensivist" which was started by Indian Academy of Pediatrics Intensive Care Chapter, which ultimately culminated into launching of the official journal of pediatric critical care of the intensive care chapter of the Indian Academy of Pediatrics.

putting collaborative efforts to launch similar multicenter collaborative studies.

Under the auspices of ISCCM, several pediatric critical care leaders in India have started a multicenter PICU data registry called INSPIRED (personal communication). Also, several institutions in India are now contributing to multicenter, international, pediatric critical care studies such as point prevalence studies, or quality improvement studies led by western institutions (45, 46). The Intensive Care Chapter of IAP started the quarterly periodical called "The Intensivist" (**Figure 1**), which grew in popularity over time and culminated into launching the Journal of Pediatric Critical Care in 2014, which is the official journal of the chapter (**Figure 2**) (47).

Factors Influencing Advancement of Pediatric Critical Care Research in India

India is a large country and continues to be second most populated country in the world. The healthcare in India has been constantly challenged with issues of manpower, resources, infrastructure and financial support. Though the number of pediatric intensivists trained either within or outside India has grown significantly in India over last 15 years, current manpower is not sufficient to cope with the number of critically ill children in India. Due to heavy clinical commitments and burn-out issues, pediatric critical care professionals in India lack sufficient protected time for research. Also, unlike western countries, India has very limited government funds allocated to research. This further restricts the support needed for research data gathering, statistical analyses, research coordination and dissemination of research findings. Several research institutes, research task forces, and grants-in-aid developed by Indian Council of Medical Research (ICMR) have led to improved research support in India (48). The pediatric critical care faculty at large, government-run, teaching institutes have tapped into these resources for investigator-initiated clinical trials in PCCM. Also, some of the industry funds have also become available for PCCM research in India (49).

The initiation of PCCM fellowship training programs by the Intensive Care Chapter of IAP have not only promoted clinical training in pediatric critical care but also fueled research enthusiasm among young and budding pediatric intensivists in India (31). A formal 3-year post-doctoral training program

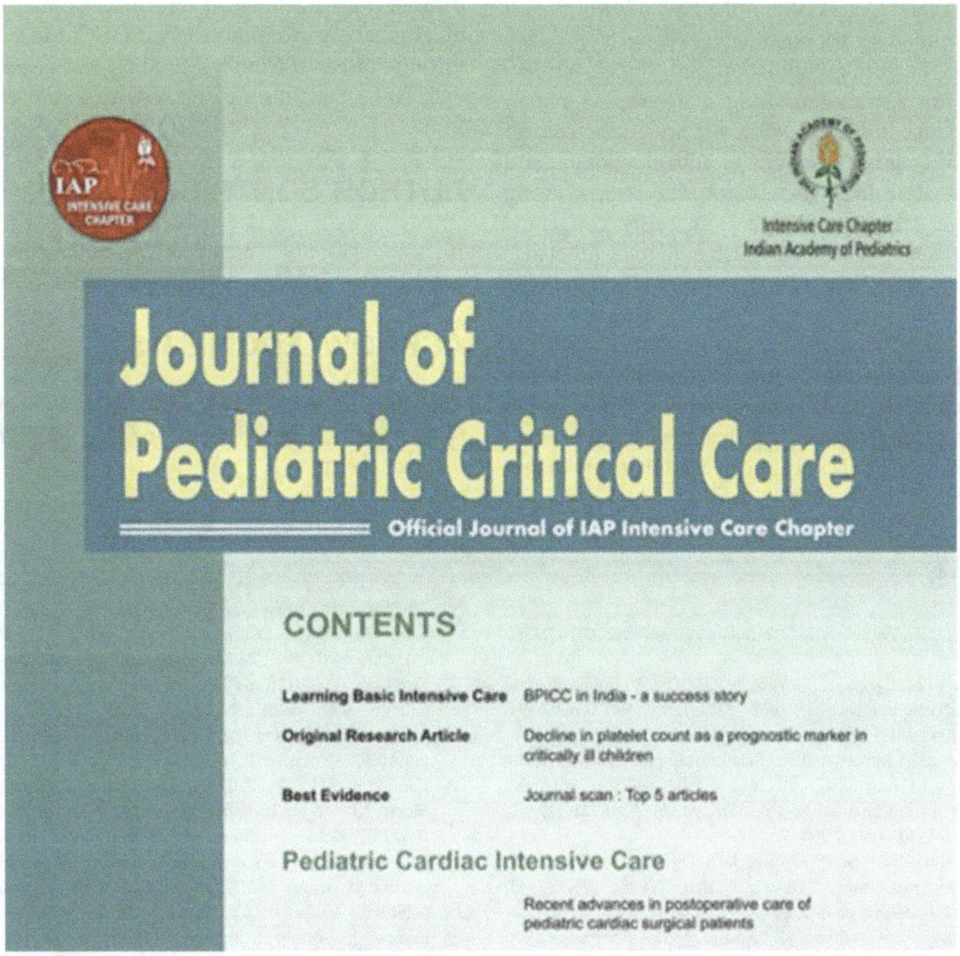

FIGURE 2 | The picture of journal of pediatric critical care—the official journal of the intensive care chapter of the Indian Academy of Pediatrics.

in PCCM, started by the PGIMER in Chandigarh, India and subsequently adopted by two other premier institutes in India has paved the pathway for protected research time and formal research training of PICU fellows.

The national conference of pediatric critical care (NCPCC) organized annually by IAP intensive care chapter has provided tremendous opportunities to PCCM community in India to showcase and discuss their research findings and collaborate on research (50). Similarly, the annual conferences organized by World Federation of Pediatric Intensive and Critical Care Societies and Society of Critical Care Medicine have allowed networking of pediatric intensivists from India with those from other countries and improved research collaborations (51). Several global health institutions of leading universities and hospitals in the West have collaborated with institutes in India and conducted research related to neonatal and pediatric critical care (52).

Future of Pediatric Critical Care Medicine Research in India

India is a country with the world's second largest population, a relatively low median age, and a demographic trend that is very different from developed countries. Also India is a fast growing emerging market, especially in the field of information technology. This signifies a great potential for research especially in pediatrics given the young population and disease burden. It is likely that with a transition from a developing nation to a developed nation, India will witness a wide spectrum of healthcare issues of children common to both developing and developed nations. It is likely that there will be a growing population of longer-term survivors of prematurity, congenital heart disease and genetic syndromes, which used to be otherwise deemed fatal in the past. These future trends will affect PICU research in India.

As the PCCM specialty continues to grow, more research is likely to occur at both government-run, teaching institutions as well as corporate hospitals. Due to several obvious differences in disease profiles, host characteristics (e.g., malnutrition), access to medical care, or resource availability and allocation, the pediatric critical care community understands that scientific evidence generated through studies done in the West cannot always be extrapolated to patients in the Indian context. Among the pediatric intensivists, there is a growing awareness of the need of generating scientific evidence locally through studies within India. This is likely to culminate into an increase in investigator-initiated, single-center studies and also improved collaboration among a larger number of PCCM programs to create data registries and multicenter clinical trials in India.

The strengths of critical care medicine community in India include a huge knowledge-base for tropical and infectious diseases (53, 54), large patient burden, cost-effective strategies and the development of low-cost technology solutions through frugal innovation (55). As the investigator-initiated single-center and multicenters studies in PCCM grow in India, parallel efforts need to be made by government and corporate healthcare systems to improve the research infrastructure. Also, It will be equally important for institutions and professional organizations such as the ISCCM and IAP to establish structured research training for PCCM in India. A quality improvement research project and/or research thesis done during fellowship and an opportunity to present research work at a national and international conferences might encourage the pediatric critical care fellows to pursue academic careers. Finally, the contributions of national organizations such as ISCCM in supporting research through research reources, funding and research collaborations will define the future of the pediatric critical care research in India.

AUTHOR CONTRIBUTIONS

All authors listed have made a substantial, direct and intellectual contribution to the work, and approved it for publication.

ACKNOWLEDGMENTS

The authors wish to acknowledge vital contributions of Dr. Kanwaljeet S Anand for his guidance with writing and editing this manuscript.

REFERENCES

1. Ramesh S. Paediatri intensive care - update. *Indian J Anaesth.* (2003) **47**:338–44.
2. Tilford JM, Simpson PM, Green JW, Lensing S, Fiser DH. Volume-outcome relationships in pediatric intensive care units. *Pediatrics* (2000) **106**:289–94. doi: 10.1542/peds.106.2.289
3. Fiser DH, Tilford JM, Roberson PK. Relationship of illness severity and length of stay to functional outcomes in the pediatric intensive care unit: a multi institutional study. *Crit Care Med.* (2000) **28**:1173–9. doi: 10.1097/00003246-200004000-00043
4. Tilford JM, Roberson PK, Lensing S, Fiser DH. Differences in pediatric ICU mortality risk over time. *Crit Care Med.* (1998) **26**:1737–43. doi: 10.1097/00003246-199810000-00032
5. Moler FW, Steinhart CM, Ohmit SE, Stidham GL. Effectiveness of ribavirin in otherwise well infants with respiratory syncytial virus-associated respiratory failure. Pediatric Critical Study Group. *J Pediatr.* (1996) **128**:422–8. doi: 10.1016/S0022-3476(96)70294-9
6. Green TP, Timmons OD, Fackler JC, Moler FW, Thompson AE, Sweeney MF. The impact of extracorporeal membrane oxygenation on survival in pediatric patients with acute respiratory failure. Pediatric Critical Care Study Group. *Crit Care Med* (1996) **24**:323–9. doi: 10.1097/00003246-199602000-00023
7. Timmons OD, Havens PL, Fackler JC. Predicting death in pediatric patients with acute respiratory failure. Pediatric critical care study group. extracorporeal life support organization. *Chest* (1995) **108**:789–97. doi: 10.1378/chest.108.3.789
8. Randolph AG, Wypij D, Venkataraman ST, Hanson JH, Gedeit RG, Meert KL, et al. Pediatric Acute Lung Injury and Sepsis Investigators (PALISI) Network. Effect of mechanical ventilator weaning protocols on respiratory outcomes in infants and children: a randomized controlled trial. *JAMA* (2002) **288**:2561–8. doi: 10.1001/jama.288.20.2561
9. Lacroix J, Cotting J for the Pediatric Acute Lung Injury and Sepsis Investigators (PALISI) Network. Severity of illness and organ dysfunction scoring in children. *Pediatr Crit Care Med.* (2005) **6**:S126–34. doi: 10.1097/01.PCC.0000161287.61028.D4

10. Curley MA, Thompson JE, Arnold JH. The effects of early and repeated prone positioning in pediatric patients with acute lung injury. *Chest* (2000) **118**:156–63. doi: 10.1378/chest.118.1.156
11. Willson DF, Thomas NJ, Markovitz BP, Bauman LA, DiCarlo JV, Pon S, et al. Pediatric acute lung injury and sepsis investigators. effect of exogenous surfactant (calfactant) in pediatric acute lung injury: a randomized controlled trial. *JAMA* (2005) **293**:470–6. doi: 10.1001/jama.293.4.470
12. Epstein D, Brill J. A history of pediatric critical care medicine. *Pediatr Res.* (2005) **58**: 987–96. doi: 10.1203/01.PDR.0000182822.16263.3D
13. Available online at: https://www.ccctg.ca/Groups-Committees/Pediatric-Interest-Group.aspx (Accessed December 19, 2017).
14. De Luca D, Piastra M, Chidini G, Tissieres P, Calderini E, Essouri S, et al. The use of the Berlin definition for acute respiratory distress syndrome during infancy and early childhood: multicenter evaluation and expert consensus. *Intensive Care Med.* (2013) **39**:2083–91. doi: 10.1007/s00134-013-3110-x
15. Available online at: http://espnic-online.org/SCIENTIFIC-AFFAIRS/Working-Groups (Accessed December 19, 2017).
16. Available online at: http://anzics.com.au/www.anzics.com.au/Pages/Paediatrics.html (Accessed May 15, 2018).
17. Moler FW, Silverstein FS, Holubkov R, Slomine BS, Christensen JR, Nadkarni VM, et al. THAPCA trial investigators. therapeutic hypothermia after in-hospital cardiac arrest in children. *N Engl J Med.* (2017) **376**:318–29. doi: 10.1056/NEJMoa1610493
18. Moler FW, Silverstein FS, Holubkov R, Slomine BS, Christensen JR, Nadkarni VM, et al. (2015). THAPCA trial investigators. therapeutic hypothermia after out-of-hospital cardiac arrest in children. *N Engl J Med.* **372**:1898–908. doi: 10.1056/NEJMoa1411480
19. Agus MS, Wypij D, Hirshberg EL, Srinivasan V, Faustino EV, Luckett PM, et al. HALF-PINT study investigators and the PALISI network. tight glycemic control in critically Ill children. *N Engl J Med.* (2017) **376**:729–41. doi: 10.1056/NEJMoa1612348
20. Available online at: http://www.isccm.org (Accessed December 19, 2017).
21. Divatia JV, Jog S. Intensive care research and publication in India: quo vadis? *Intensive Care Med.* (2014) **40**:445–7. doi: 10.1007/s00134-013-3199-y
22. Ranieri VM, Thompson BT, Barie PS, Dhainaut JF, Douglas IS, Finfer S, et al. Drotrecogin alfa (activated) in adults with septic shock. *N Engl J Med.* (2012) **366**:2055–64. doi: 10.1056/NEJMoa1202290
23. Vincent JL, Rello J, Marshall J, Silva E, Anzueto A, Martin CD, et al. International study of the prevalence and outcomes of infection in intensive care units. *JAMA* (2009) **302**:2323–9. doi: 10.1001/jama.2009.1754
24. Mehta Y, Jaggi N, Rosenthal VD, Rodrigues C, Todi SK, Saini N, et al. Effectiveness of a multidimensional approach for prevention of ventilator-associated pneumonia in 21 adult intensive-care units from 10 cities in India: findings of the International Nosocomial Infection Control Consortium (INICC). *Epidemiol Infect.* (2013) **141**:2483–91. doi: 10.1017/S0950268813000381
25. Phua J, Koh Y, Du B, Tang YQ, Divatia JV, Tan CC, et al. Management of severe sepsis in patients admitted to Asian intensive care units: prospective cohort study. *BMJ* (2011) **342**:d324. doi:10.1136/bmj.d3245
26. Esteban A, Frutos-Vivar F, Muriel A, Ferguson ND, Peñuelas O, Abraira V, et al. Evolution of mortality over time in patients receiving mechanical ventilation. *Am J Respir Crit Care Med.* (2013) **188**:220–30. doi: 10.1164/rccm.201212-2169OC
27. Vincent JL, Sakr Y. The intensive care over nations (ICON) audit: epidemiology of sepsis. *Intensive Care Med.* (2013) **39**:S229.
28. Ferguson ND, Cook DJ, Guyatt GH, Mehta S, Hand L, Austin P, et al. High-frequency oscillation in early acute respiratory distress syndrome. *N Engl J Med.* (2013) **368**:795–805. doi: 10.1056/NEJMoa1215554
29. Tyagi A, Chugh V, Kumar S, Sethi AK. Presentation of research in anesthesia: culmination into publication? *J Anaesthesiol Clin Pharmacol.* (2013). **29**:216–20. doi: 10.4103/0970-9185.111727
30. Vidyasagar D, Singh M, Bhakoo ON, Paul VK, Narang A, Bhutani V, et al. Evolution of neonatal and pediatric critical care in India. *Crit Care Clin.* (1997) **13**:331–46. doi: 10.1016/S0749-0704(05)70313-4
31. Bhalala, U, Khilnani, P. Pediatric critical care medicine training in India: past, present, and future. *Front. Pediatr.* (2018) **6**:34. doi: 10.3389/fped.2018.00034
32. Paul VK, Radhika S, Deorari AK, Singh M. Neurodevelopmental outcome of 'at risk' nursery graduates. *Indian J Pediatr.* (1998) **65**:857–62.
33. Singhi S, Dhawan A. Frequency and significance of electrolyte abnormalities in pneumonia. *Indian Pediatr.* (1992) **29**:735–40.
34. Available online at: http://ctri.nic.in/Clinicaltrials/login.php (Accessed November 30, 2017).
35. Kamath SR, Ranjit S. Clinical features, complications and atypical manifestations of children with severe forms of dengue hemorrhagic fever in South India. *Indian J Pediatr.* (2006) **73**:889–95. doi: 10.1007/BF02859281
36. Ranjit S, Kissoon N, Gandhi D, Dayal A, Rajeshwari N, Kamath SR. Early differentiation between dengue and septic shock by comparison of admission hemodynamic, clinical, and laboratory variables: a pilot study. *Pediatr Emerg Care.* (2007) **23**:368–75. doi: 10.1097/01.pec.0000278403.22450.a2
37. Singhi S, Murthy A, Singhi P, Jayashree M. Continuous midazolam versus diazepam infusion for refractory convulsive status epilepticus. *J Child Neurol.* (2002) **17**:106–10. doi: 10.1177/088307380201700203
38. Mondal RK, Singhi SC, Chakrabarti A, M J. Randomized comparison between fluconazole and itraconazole for the treatment of candidemia in a pediatric intensive care unit: a preliminary study. *Pediatr Crit Care Med.* (2004) **5**:561–5. doi: 10.1097/01.PCC.0000144712.29127.81
39. Singhi SC, Bansal A. Serum cortisol levels in children with acute bacterial and aseptic meningitis. *Pediatr Crit Care Med.* (2006) **7**:74–8. doi: 10.1097/01.PCC.0000192317.90862.44
40. Bansal A, Singhi SC, Jayashree M. Penicillin and gentamicin therapy vs. amoxicillin/clavulanate in severe hypoxemic pneumonia. *Indian J Pediatr.* (2006) **73**:305–9. doi: 10.1007/BF02825824
41. Nallasamy K, Jayashree M, Singhi S, Bansal A. Low-dose vs. standard-dose insulin in pediatric diabetic ketoacidosis: a randomized clinical trial. *JAMA Pediatr.* (2014) **168**:999–1005. doi: 10.1001/jamapediatrics.2014.1211
42. Singhi S, Kumar R, Singhi P, Jayashree M, Bansal A. Bedside burr hole for intracranial pressure monitoring performed by pediatric intensivists in children with CNS infections in a resource-limited setting: 10-year experience at a single center. *Pediatr Crit Care Med.* (2015) **16**:453–60. doi: 10.1097/PCC.0000000000000353
43. Kumar R, Singhi S, Singhi P, Jayashree M, Bansal A, Bhatti A. Randomized controlled trial comparing cerebral perfusion pressure-targeted therapy versus intracranial pressure-targeted therapy for raised intracranial pressure due to acute CNS infections in children. *Crit Care Med.* (2014) **42**:1775–87. doi: 10.1097/CCM.0000000000000298
44. Tasker RC. Raised intracranial pressure during central nervous system infection: what should we do about it? *Crit Care Med.* (2014) **42**:1936–8. doi: 10.1097/CCM.0000000000000419
45. Kojima T, Laverriere EK, Owen EB, Harwayne-Gidansky I, Shenoi AN, Napolitano N, et al. Clinical impact of external laryngeal manipulation during laryngoscopy on tracheal intubation success in critically Ill children. *Pediatr Crit Care Med.* (2017) **19**:106–14. doi: 10.1097/PCC.0000000000001373
46. Weiss SL, Fitzgerald JC, Pappachan J, Wheeler D, Jaramillo-Bustamante JC, Salloo A, et al. Global epidemiology of pediatric severe sepsis: the sepsis prevalence, outcomes, and therapies study. *Am J Respir Crit Care Med.* (2015) **191**:1147–57. doi: 10.1164/rccm.201412-2323OC
47. Available online at: http://www.journalofpediatriccriticalcare.com (Accessed December 19, 2017).
48. Available online at: http://www.icmr.nic.in/About_Us/About_Us.html (Accessed November 30, 2017).
49. Kumar S, Singhi S, Chakrabarti A, Bansal A, Jayashree M. Probiotic use and prevalence of candidemia and candiduria in a PICU. Pediatr Crit Care Med. (2013) 14, e409-15. doi: 10.1097/PCC.0b013e31829f5d88
50. Available online at: http://www.tribuneindia.com/news/chandigarh/national-meet-on-paediatric-intensive-care-from-nov-2/490659.html (Accessed May 15, 2018).
51. Available online at: http://www.wfpiccs.org (Accessed December 19, 2017).
52. Available online at: https://globalhealth.stanford.edu (Accessed December 19, 2017).

53. Jog S, Patel D, Dravid T, Rajhans P, Akole P, Pawar B, et al. Early application of high frequency oscillatory ventilation in 'H1N1 influenza' related ARDS is associated with better outcome: a retrospective study. *Intensive Care Med.* (2013) **39**:1146–47. doi: 10.1007/s00134-013-2878-z
54. Khilnani P, Sarma D, Zimmerman J. Epidemiology and peculiarities of pediatric multiple organ dysfunction syndrome in New Delhi, India. *Intensive Care Med.* (2006) **32**:1856–62. doi: 10.1007/s00134-006-0373-5
55. Chacko J, Nikahat J, Gagan B, Umesh K, and Ramanathan M. Real-time ultrasound-guided percutaneous dilatational tracheostomy. *Intensive Care Med.* (2012) **38**:920–21. doi: 10.1007/s00134-012-2514-3

12

Teaching the Principles of Pediatric Critical Care to Non-Intensivists in Resource Limited Settings: Challenges and Opportunities

Michael F. Canarie[1] *and Asha N. Shenoi*[2]*

[1] *Department of Pediatrics, Yale University School of Medicine, New Haven, CT, United States,* [2] *Department of Pediatrics, University of Kentucky, Lexington, KY, United States*

Keywords: critical care, resource limited, training programs, pediatric, challenges

Correspondence:
Asha N. Shenoi
asha.shenoi@uky.edu

INTRODUCTION

It is a dismal reality of global health that the vast majority of critically ill or injured children are found in regions of the world least equipped to care for them. Most of these severely ill or injured children are cared for in clinics, hospital wards, or, when available, adult intensive care units (ICUs) by providers with variable amounts of training. This lack of training may, in fact, play a significant role in the premature demise of children <5 years old, since millions of these deaths are felt to be preventable with the resources available (1). Evidence shows that even in a setting with constrained resources, early recognition, and prompt, decisive intervention may reduce mortality (2–4). It seems intuitive, therefore, that training of non-intensivists that focuses on these principles might improve the outcomes in critically ill children. How can this instruction be best achieved in areas where it is most needed? In this article, we review the benefits and challenges of implementing short-term curricula to teach the basic principles and practice of critical care medicine in resource limited settings (RLS).

CURRENT STATE OF THE CARE OF THE CRITICALLY ILL CHILD

The essential role of community and preventative healthcare in promoting the well-being of children in RLS is well established and assumed here. Yet, improvements in primary and preventive care do not eliminate need for hospital-based care. A high percentage of children (an estimated 12–34%) seen in ambulatory settings, for example, are felt to require hospital assessment and/or admission (5). Multiple studies have shown mortality inversely related to distance from a hospital and that prehospital/emergent or advanced care resources are most limited where the majority of children die (6–8). In addition, we know that a growing percentage of preventable deaths result from the "neglected burden" of trauma; approximately 90% global trauma deaths occur in low- and middle-income countries (LMICs) and road deaths alone kill more than 200,000 children per year in RLS (9–11). All these ill or injured children require some (and perhaps an increasing) degree of medical care and demise is, in many cases, related to an inability to deliver timely or appropriate care (12).

Yet for those patients who require and receive hospital-level care, mortality remains high, with infection and sepsis often the common final pathway (13). A study from Guinea–Bissau observed that 25% of childhood deaths occurred after admission to a regional hospital (14). In general, the sparse available data cite a pediatric inpatient mortality rate between 12 and 50% in RLS, with a high percentage of those occurring during the first 24 h following admission (9, 15). This latter observation underscores the belief that treatment is often delayed in these settings for children arriving at care facilities after the onset of critical illness. It is not a foregone conclusion, however, that mortality for these hospitalized patients has improved over time. For instance, a large, retrospective study on pediatric sepsis admissions to Brazilian hospitals from 1992 to 2006 showed an overall reduction in cases of sepsis, but no improvement in the mortality rate of 19% (16, 17).

What is clear is that most critically ill children who survive to inpatient care facilities are treated in clinics, hospital wards, and infrequently in mixed ICUs by caregivers with variable amount of pediatric or advanced care training. In Nigeria, for example, there are only 380 ICU trained nurses in a country of 140 million people (17). In reality, critical care is just the continuum of care provided to any child with a life-threatening illness or injury beginning with the time of presentation to a health care facility (18). Where and by whom care is provided may go a long way in determining outcome.

THE ROLE OF CRITICAL CARE TRAINING

There is evidence that the presence of pediatric intensive care units (PICUs) and trained critical care physicians (intensivists) improves patient care and saves lives in both high resource and RLS (19–22). It is likely that the mortality benefit from intensive care is attributable to an integration of multiple elements including basic infrastructure, essential supplies, and equipment, training, and staffing. In practical terms, however, "intensive care" can only be provided where these substantial resources and trained, multidisciplinary personnel are in place. The mere presence of an "intensive care unit" does not guarantee the presence of intensive, integrated care, or good outcomes, as the mortality rates in mixed and exclusively pediatric ICUs in LMICs can be as high as 50–58% (22, 23). In any case, ICUs are uncommon in many parts of the world and, with rare exception, most of the world's sickest children are cared for outside of conventional ICUs (pediatric or mixed) by caregivers without pediatric or critical care training.

How can the critical care of these children be improved? To begin, in RLS, critical care capacity is "developed" not "created" (24–26). This is not just a matter of semantics, but underlines the importance of a gradual cultivation and blending of training and technical capacity over time, rather than the creation of a physical space. Ultimately, there are two intertwining aspects of this undertaking: training and educational enrichment, and developing physical/technological ICU capacity to facilitate care. This is a delicate balance because most would agree that the introduction of material assets without concomitant thoughtful, systemic training is a futile endeavor. In fact, the lack of trained personnel in sufficient numbers is routinely cited as a weakness of healthcare delivery—often even more than inadequate supplies and equipment (26–28). Accordingly, training programs/courses that include a range of health care providers and focus on principles of early recognition and management of severe illness could play an important role in combatting healthcare-associated mortality.

STANDARDIZED CRITICAL CARE COURSE: WHY? WHAT, AND WHERE ARE THEY?

Standardized emergency and pediatric critical care curricula such as emergency, triage, assessment and treatment (ETAT), pediatric basic assessment and support intensive care (BASIC), and pediatric fundamentals of critical care study (PFCCS) are among of the educational initiatives used for supporting training in RLS (29). These courses provide a number of advantages even if they require some degree of "recalibration" to be effective in RLS (30). Standardized teaching modules are readily deployable, consistent, and comprehensive. They can also be shared and implemented for various training levels in a range of settings, reducing needless, and wasteful redundancy (31, 32). Tools such as the pediatric, emergency, assessment, recognition and stabilization (PEARS), and pediatric advanced life support (PALS) have even been bundled and used on system-wide levels to improve the care of sick children in Botswana and India (33).

Pediatric BASIC and PFCCS, both modeled on adult courses, have been specifically designed to teach non-intensivists the essential principles of care for the critically ill (32). The aim of these courses is to serve as a resource for those interested in learning to recognize critical illness and initiate care in the absence of an intensivist. As such, the courses focus on early identification of the critically ill child, initial steps in timely resuscitation, and organ support, and includes the rudiments of mechanical ventilation. Typically 2–3 days in duration, the sessions mix formal didactics, lectures, simulations, and practical sessions. Pretests are administered and the formal assessments at the end of the courses determine whether certificates are awarded to participants.

Pediatric fundamentals of critical care study is licensed by Society of Critical Care Medicine (SCCM). It can be administered either through a traditional live, instructor-led course, directed by a certified PFCCS director, or online. There is a well-defined process and oversight for certification of instructors and directors and periodic revision of content by an appointed task force. Although the course material covered can vary (based on the setting or participants' needs), the contents of particular lectures are not modifiable. There has been a significant increase in international PFCCS courses recently, and between 2013 and 2016, more than 30 courses per year have been conducted around the world. There are currently 32 counties that have international PFCCS sites. SCCM has made significant effort to make the course affordable by having an option for tiered pricing based on a country's gross domestic product at Purchasing Power Parity Per Capita but still the minimum cost is $630. However, in the absence of consistent external funding, even this subsidized rate can make access in RLS prohibitive.

Pediatric BASIC is another standardized critical care course created by pediatric critical care educational leaders during the 2011 World Congress of Pediatric Intensive and Critical Care Societies (WFPICCS). Its creators sought to design a course to teach the fundamentals of critical care in a format that was flexible and affordable and thus suitable for both high-income countries and RLS. This course, endorsed by WFPICCS, is run by volunteer pediatric critical care faculty from around the world in select places with strong local support. Target audience include mainly non-intensivist physicians and pediatric trainees (many with limited PICU experience), emergency medicine physicians, and senior PICU nurses. The development of Pediatric BASIC is overseen by a steering committee with expertise in pediatric critical care. No member of the steering committee, the original writers of the course, the instructors, or their families receive any financial benefit from the use of the course material and no individual owns intellectual property. Since there are no proprietorial fees associated with the course, it is always offered free of charge.

In addition, to meet local needs, the BASIC course allows flexibility to adapt not only the shape and content of the overall course but also individual lectures. Within the course, there is also an effort to do needs assessment at the training facility, soliciting input, and feedback from local faculty. While BASIC also has separate foundation courses for training nurses, in some institutions, nurses can also cotrained in the standard course. Since its inception in 2011, this course has been conducted in 63 different sites across 17 countries on 5 continents and a total of 1,617 providers have been trained. Pediatric BASIC has also shown success in building sustainable local critical care capacity through a "train the trainer" model in select institutions in countries such as India, Trinidad and Tobago, and Barbados. The first course in India was conducted in January 2014 and over next 4 years several local trainers (mostly Pediatricians with ICU experience) were trained as trainers using the model.

STANDARDIZED COURSE: EVIDENCE AND CHALLENGES

There is little research on the utility of short-term training programs, a deficiency not unique to RLS. Such programs, even in high-income countries, have a thin evidentiary underpinning, trying to answer three fundamental questions: Are the courses an effective way to transfer knowledge? Is this knowledge retained for any meaningful period? Finally, does this retained knowledge, in the end, translate into clinical benefit (34). Often data on "softer" or surrogate measures or outcomes are all that are available. Data on a decade of PALS courses in Israel, for example, revealed only participant satisfaction with the course and satisfactory completion by a high percentage of participants (35). Residents in Canada performed well on the PALS posttest, but not on the technical skills assessment, and showed poor retention at 12 months (36).

The lack of data bases in RLS makes it difficult to assess training programs of any kind. However, several studies have looked at various parameters in short-term courses. For instance, there is evidence that short training courses improve short-term knowledge in emergency and critical care (37, 38). Short courses teaching trauma care have been shown to identify deficiencies, increase provider skills, and improve trauma outcomes—including mortality—in developing countries like Trinidad, India, Ecuador, and Tanzania (30, 39–42). In fields such as pediatric surgery and obstetrics, short-term, specialized training courses have shown some success in knowledge retention (43, 44).

Standardized adult critical care programs have also been evaluated, both as educational instruments and as a means of transmitting knowledge (32). Training of Kenyan physicians using the Fundamental Critical Care Study (FCCS) course has been shown to increase the knowledge and confidence of new critical care skills (45). FCCS course participants in Zambia and Kenya felt that the material was site-appropriate and demonstrated an increase in clinical knowledge and confidence with procedures (46). There is less experience and evidence for pediatric standardized critical care curricula in RLS. However, a recent evaluation of Pediatric BASIC program in Northern Haiti showed post-course improvement in participants' ability to manage patients in all topics covered by the course. The topics which showed the greatest improvement were related to support for respiratory failure using noninvasive and invasive ventilator support as well as the interpretation of blood gases (Silverman AMP, Napolitano et al., unpublished data, 2017).

The issue of course evaluation begs the very important question of the appropriateness of these tools in RLS. Given the range of disease and variable shortages of materiel encountered in RLS, training programs developed and taught by physicians from higher resourced countries may lack relevance (47). Consider, for instance, the teaching of PALS in places without defibrillators, or only a fraction of the recommended medications. It is, therefore, essential that courses should be tailored to local needs and, to assure ongoing relevance, have feedback mechanisms allowing for new data to inform future course modifications (30, 48).

Cost-effectiveness analysis is another important consideration, since optimizing the effects of expenditures takes on greater significance in regions where such funds are scarce. This type of evaluation, however, is complicated by a general dearth of data as well as uncertainty over relevant outcomes. Although the BASIC course itself is free, accurately measuring the actual cost of the "inputs" (i.e., concrete and opportunity costs of volunteer staff, cost to the facilities, etc.) would be difficult. In fact, the significance of the burden borne by the host institution could be hard to contextualize. In any case, without funding for educational programs, organizing courses may be overly burdensome to partners in RLS, threatening the feasibility and sustainability of these initiatives.

Another challenge to teaching these courses is the task of simulating the core critical care concepts of teamwork and collaborative learning in settings where these are not commonly practiced (49). In some cases, these difficulties may be due to cultural and hierarchical attitudes, but, nevertheless, could hinder training in optimal resuscitation and ongoing care. Nurses and ancillary personnel have variable levels of education and training and little experience with programs that train and integrate personnel at different levels concurrently (50).

Language can present a further practical barrier, limiting the effectiveness of these courses (51). Recent data from Haiti suggest that even with variable levels of skill in English and the use of translators, language problems were seen to limit course effectiveness (Silverman AMP, Napolitano et al., unpublished data, 2017). PFCCS course materials have been translated into Japanese, Spanish, and Chinese. BASIC is currently only available in English, but plans are underway to translate the teaching material into French and Spanish, allowing greater applicability.

In the end, assumptions on the benefits of training may have to suffice pending further evidence. Achieving a sustainable teaching model, however, through a "train the trainer" approach could assure long-term educational gains (48). Over time, steadfast application and consistent reinforcement may show the greatest benefits (33, 52). Yet this strategy will only be possible in settings with strong local interest and support.

CONCLUSION

Training in the recognition and initial management of critical illness and injury may be an effective way to save the lives of countless children in RLS. Standardized courses in the fundamentals of critical care could be an effective component of this overall effort, helping to fill in gaps of trained personnel. Such courses should be adapted to local needs and resources. Also, while maintaining a consistent and readily reproducible, comprehensive curriculum, these courses should incorporate the feedback necessary to keep them locally relevant. In spite of the many challenges, standardized courses provide an opportunity to train large numbers of diverse personnel and achieve sustainability by instructing local trainers. Identifying relevant outcomes and gathering data will be an essential aspect of assuring future effectiveness and relevance.

AUTHOR CONTRIBUTIONS

AS and MC wrote the draft together and revised the contents. MC is primarily responsible for parts 1–3 and AS wrote the rest of the manuscript. Both authors revised the manuscript several times based on the feedback received from the coauthor.

REFERENCES

1. Shann F, Duke T. Twenty-three thousand unnecessary deaths every day: what are you doing about it? *Pediatr Crit Care Med* (2009) 10(5):608–9. doi:10.1097/PCC.0b013e3181ae4a95
2. Baker T. Pediatric emergency and critical care in low-income countries. *Paediatr Anaesth* (2009) 19(1):23–7. doi:10.1111/j.1460-9592.2008.02868.x
3. Duke T, Kelly J, Weber M, English M, Campbell H. Hospital care for children in developing countries: clinical guidelines and the need for evidence. *J Trop Pediatr* (2006) 52(1):1–2. doi:10.1093/tropej/fmk006
4. Molyneux E, Ahmad S, Robertson A. Improved triage and emergency care for children reduces inpatient mortality in a resource-constrained setting. *Bull World Health Organ* (2006) 84(4):314–9. doi:10.2471/BLT.04.019505
5. Nolan T, Angos P, Cunha AJ, Muhe L, Qazi S, Simoes EA, et al. Quality of hospital care for seriously ill children in less-developed countries. *Lancet* (2001) 357(9250):106–10. doi:10.1016/S0140-6736(00)03542-X
6. Manongi R, Mtei F, Mtove G, Nadjm B, Muro F, Alegana V, et al. Inpatient child mortality by travel time to hospital in a rural area of Tanzania. *Trop Med Int Health* (2014) 19(5):555–62. doi:10.1111/tmi.12294
7. Kadobera D, Sartorius B, Masanja H, Mathew A, Waiswa P. The effect of distance to formal health facility on childhood mortality in rural Tanzania, 2005–2007. *Glob Health Action* (2012) 5(1):19099. doi:10.3402/gha.v5i0.19099
8. Moisi JC, Nokes DJ, Gatakaa H, Williams TN, Bauni E, Levine OS, et al. Sensitivity of hospital-based surveillance for severe disease: a geographic information system analysis of access to care in Kilifi district, Kenya. *Bull World Health Organ* (2011) 89(2):102–11. doi:10.2471/BLT.10.080796
9. Jones G, Steketee RW, Black RE, Bhutta ZA, Morris SS, Bellagio Child Survival Study Group. How many child deaths can we prevent this year? *Lancet* (2003) 362(9377):65–71. doi:10.1016/S0140-6736(03)13811-1
10. Yeboah D, Mock C, Karikari P, Agyei-Baffour P, Donkor P, Ebel B. Minimizing preventable trauma deaths in a limited-resource setting: a test-case of a multidisciplinary panel review approach at the Komfo Anokye Teaching Hospital in Ghana. *World J Surg* (2014) 38(7):1707–12. doi:10.1007/s00268-014-2452-z
11. Paniker J, Graham SM, Harrison JW. Global trauma: the great divide. *SICOT J* (2015) 1:19. doi:10.1051/sicotj/2015019
12. Kissoon N. Out of Africa—a mother's journey. *Pediatr Crit Care Med* (2011) 12(1):73–9. doi:10.1097/PCC.0b013e3181ce74ef
13. Fowler RA, Adhikari NK, Bhagwanjee S. Clinical review: critical care in the global context—disparities in burden of illness, access, and economics. *Crit Care* (2008) 12(5):225. doi:10.1186/cc6984
14. Veirum JE, Biai S, Jakobsen M, Sandström A, Hedegaard K, Kofoed PE, et al. Persisting high hospital and community childhood mortality in an urban setting in Guinea-Bissau. *Acta Paediatr* (2007) 96(10):1526–30. doi:10.1111/j.1651-2227.2007.00467.x
15. Robison JA, Ahmad ZP, Nosek CA, Durand C, Namathanga A, Milazi R, et al. Decreased pediatric hospital mortality after an intervention to improve emergency care in Lilongwe, Malawi. *Pediatrics* (2012) 130(3):e676–82. doi:10.1542/peds.2012-0026
16. Mangia CM, Kissoon N, Branchini OA, Andrade MC, Kopelman BI, Carcillo J. Bacterial sepsis in Brazilian children: a trend analysis from 1992 to 2006. *PLoS One* (2011) 6(6):e14817. doi:10.1371/journal.pone.0014817
17. Rid A, Emanuel EJ. Why should high-income countries help combat Ebola? *JAMA* (2014) 312(13):1297–8. doi:10.1001/jama.2014.12869
18. Kissoon N, Argent A, Devictor D, Madden MA, Singhi S, van der Voort E, et al. World federation of pediatric intensive and critical care societies-its global agenda. *Pediatr Crit Care Med* (2009) 10(5):597–600. doi:10.1097/PCC.0b013e3181a704c6
19. Haque A, Bano S. Clinical profile and outcome in a paediatric intensive care unit in Pakistan. *J Coll Physicians Surg Pak* (2009) 19(8):534–5. doi:08.2009/JCPSP.534535
20. Campos-Mino S, Sasbón JS, Von Dessauer B. Pediatric intensive care in Latin America. *Med Intensiva* (2012) 36(1):3–10. doi:10.1016/j.medin.2011.07.004
21. Nakachi GSR, Cieza J. Assessment of survival in a pediatric intensive care unit in Lima, Peru. *Internet J Emerg Intensive Med* (2009) 12(1).
22. Pollack MM, Patel KM, Ruttimann E. Pediatric critical care training programs have a positive effect on pediatric intensive care mortality. *Crit Care Med* (1997) 25(10):1637–42. doi:10.1097/00003246-199710000-00011
23. Kaur G, Vinayak N, Mittal K, Kaushik JS, Aamir M. Clinical outcome and predictors of mortality in children with sepsis, severe sepsis, and septic shock from Rohtak, Haryana: a prospective observational study. *Indian J Crit Care Med* (2014) 18(7):437–41. doi:10.4103/0972-5229.136072
24. Riviello ED, Letchford S, Achieng L, Newton MW. Critical care in resource-poor settings: lessons learned and future directions. *Crit Care Med* (2011) 39(4):860–7. doi:10.1097/CCM.0b013e318206d6d5
25. Argent AC, et al. Pediatric intensive care in South Africa: an account of making optimum use of limited resources at the Red Cross War Memorial Children's Hospital. *Pediatr Crit Care Med* (2014) 15(1):7–14. doi:10.1097/PCC.0000000000000029
26. Biskup T, Phan P, Grunauer M. Lessons from the design and implementation of a pediatric critical care and emergency medicine training program in a low resource country. *J Pediatr Intensive Care* (2017) 6:60–5. doi:10.1055/s-0036-1584678
27. Baker T, Lugazia E, Eriksen J, Mwafongo V, Irestedt L, Konrad D. Emergency and critical care services in Tanzania: a survey of ten hospitals. *BMC Health Serv Res* (2013) 13:140. doi:10.1186/1472-6963-13-140
28. Duke T. Clinical care for seriously ill children in district hospitals: a global public-health issue. *Lancet* (2004) 363(9425):1922–3. doi:10.1016/S0140-6736(04)16438-6
29. Barasa EW. A multifaceted intervention to improve the quality of care of children in district hospitals in Kenya: a cost-effectiveness analysis. *PLoS Med* (2012) 9(6):e1001238. doi:10.1371/journal.pmed.1001238
30. Tchorz KM, Thomas N, Jesudassan S, Kumar R, Chinnadurai R, Thomas A, et al. Teaching trauma care in India: an educational pilot study from Bangalore. *J Surg Res* (2007) 142(2):373–7. doi:10.1016/j.jss.2006.07.010
31. Wright SW, Steenhoff AP, Elci O, Wolfe HA, Ralston M, Kgosiesele T, et al. Impact of contextualized pediatric resuscitation training on pediatric healthcare providers in Botswana. *Resuscitation* (2015) 88:57–62. doi:10.1016/j.resuscitation.2014.12.007
32. Joynt GM. A systematic review of short courses for nonspecialist education in intensive care. *J Crit Care* (2011) 26(5):533.e1–e10. doi:10.1016/j.jcrc.2011.01.007
33. Meaney PA, Sutton RM, Tsima B, Steenhoff AP, Shilkofski N, Boulet JR, et al. Training hospital providers in basic CPR skills in Botswana: acquisition, retention and impact of novel training techniques. *Resuscitation* (2012) 83(12):484–90. doi:10.1016/j.resuscitation.2012.04.014
34. Kissoon N, Uyeki TM. Sepsis and the global burden of disease in children. *JAMA Pediatr* (2016) 170(2):107–8. doi:10.1001/jamapediatrics.2015.3241

35. Waisman Y, Amir L, Mor M, Mimouni M. Pediatric advanced life support (PALS) courses in Israel: ten years of experience. *Isr Med Assoc J* (2005) 7(10):639–42.
36. Grant EC, Marczinski CA, Menon K. Using pediatric advanced life support in pediatric residency training: does the curriculum need resuscitation? *Pediatr Crit Care Med* (2007) 8(5):433–9. doi:10.1097/01.PCC.0000282044.78432.0B
37. Robertson MA, Molyneux EM. Description of cause of serious illness and outcome in patients identified using ETAT guidelines in urban Malawi. *Arch Dis Child* (2001) 85(3):214–7. doi:10.1136/adc.85.3.214
38. Tamburlini G, Di Mario S, Maggi RS, Vilarim JN, Gove S. Evaluation of guidelines for emergency triage assessment and treatment in developing countries. *Arch Dis Child* (1999) 81(6):478–82. doi:10.1136/adc.81.6.478
39. Bergman S, Deckelbaum D, Lett R, Haas B, Demyttenaere S, Munthali V, et al. Assessing the impact of the trauma team training program in Tanzania. *J Trauma* (2008) 65(4):879–83. doi:10.1097/TA.0b013e318184a9fe
40. Aboutanos MB, Rodas EB, Aboutanos SZ, Mora FE, Wolfe LG, Duane TM, et al. Trauma education and care in the jungle of Ecuador, where there is no advanced trauma life support. *J Trauma* (2007) 62(3):714–9. doi:10.1097/TA.0b013e318031b56d
41. Ali J, Adam R, Butler AK, Chang H, Howard M, Gonsalves D, et al. Trauma outcome improves following the advanced trauma life support program in a developing country. *J Trauma* (1993) 34(6):890–8. doi:10.1097/00005373-199306000-00022
42. Ali J, Adam RU, Gana TJ, Williams JI. Trauma patient outcome after the Prehospital Trauma Life Support program. *J Trauma* (1997) 42(6):1018–22. doi:10.1097/00005373-199706000-00005
43. Homaifar N, Mwesigye D, Tchwenko S, Worjoloh A, Joharifard S, Kyamanywa P, et al. Emergency obstetrics knowledge and practical skills retention among medical students in Rwanda following a short training course. *Int J Gynaecol Obstet* (2013) 120(2):195–9. doi:10.1016/j.ijgo.2012.07.031
44. Butler MW, Ozgediz D, Poenaru D, Ameh E, Andrawes S, Azzie G, et al. The Global Paediatric Surgery Network: a model of subspecialty collaboration within global surgery. *World J Surg* (2015) 39(2):335–42. doi:10.1007/s00268-014-2843-1
45. MacLeod JB, Gravelin S, Jones T, Gololov A, Thomas M, Omondi B, et al. Assessment of acute trauma care training in Kenya. *Am Surg* (2009) 75(11):1118–23.
46. Macleod JB, Jones T, Aphivantrakul P, Chupp M, Poenaru D. Evaluation of fundamental critical care course in Kenya: knowledge, attitude, and practice. *J Surg Res* (2011) 167(2):223–30. doi:10.1016/j.jss.2009.08.030
47. Ralston ME, Day LT, Slusher TM, Musa NL, Doss HS. Global paediatric advanced life support: improving child survival in limited-resource settings. *Lancet* (2013) 381(9862):256–65. doi:10.1016/S0140-6736(12)61191-X
48. Shah N, Bhagwanjee S, Diaz J, Gopalan PD, Appiah JA; ACART Group (Acute Care for Africa Research and Training). A roadmap for acute care training of frontline Healthcare workers in LMICs. *J Crit Care* (2017) 41:313–7. doi:10.1016/j.jcrc.2017.07.028
49. Shilkofski N, Hunt EA. Identification of barriers to pediatric care in limited-resource settings: a simulation study. *Pediatrics* (2015) 136(6):e1569–75. doi:10.1542/peds.2015-2677
50. Nicholas DD, Heiby JR, Hatzell TA. The Quality Assurance Project: introducing quality improvement to primary health care in less developed countries. *Qual Assur Health Care* (1991) 3(3):147–65. doi:10.1093/intqhc/3.3.147
51. Hategekimana C, Shoveller J, Tuyisenge L, Kenyon C, Cechetto DF, Lynd LD. Correlates of performance of healthcare workers in emergency, triage, assessment and treatment plus admission care (ETAT+) course in Rwanda: context matters. *PLoS One* (2016) 11(3):e0152882. doi:10.1371/journal.pone.0152882
52. Patocka C, Khan F, Dubrovsky AS, Brody D, Bank I, Bhanji F. Pediatric resuscitation training-instruction all at once or spaced over time? *Resuscitation* (2015) 88:6–11. doi:10.1016/j.resuscitation.2014.12.003

13

The Potential Harm of Cytomegalovirus Infection in Immunocompetent Critically Ill Children

Raidan Alyazidi[1,2], Srinivas Murthy[1], Jennifer A. Slyker[3] and Soren Gantt[1]*

[1] University of British Columbia and BC Children's Hospital, Vancouver, BC, Canada, [2] Department of Pediatrics, Faculty of Medicine, King Abdulaziz University, Jeddah, Saudi Arabia, [3] University of Washington, Seattle, WA, United States

Correspondence:
Raidan Alyazidi
raidan@dal.ca

Cytomegalovirus (CMV) is a ubiquitous infection that causes disease in congenitally infected children and immunocompromised patients. Although nearly all CMV infections remain latent and asymptomatic in immunologically normal individuals, numerous studies have found that systemic viral reactivation is common in immunocompetent critically ill adults, as measured by detection of CMV in the blood (viremia). Furthermore, CMV viremia is strongly correlated with adverse outcomes in the adult intensive care unit (ICU), including prolonged stay, duration of mechanical ventilation, and death. Increasing evidence, including from a randomized clinical trial of antiviral treatment, suggests that these effects of CMV may be causal. Therefore, interventions targeting CMV might improve outcomes in adult ICU patients. CMV may have an even greater impact on critically ill children, particularly in low and middle income countries (LMIC), where CMV is regularly acquired in early childhood, and where inpatient morbidity and mortality are inordinately high. However, to date, there are few data regarding the clinical relevance of CMV infection or viremia in immunocompetent critically ill children. We propose that CMV infection should be studied as a potential modifiable cause of disease in critically ill children, and that these studies be conducted in LMIC. Below, we briefly review the role of CMV in immunologically normal critically ill adults and children, outline age-dependent differences in CMV infection that may influence ICU outcomes, and describe an agenda for future research.

Keywords: cytomegalovirus, pediatric critical care, viremia, reactivation, immunocompetent, outcome, ganciclovir

INTRODUCTION

Cytomegalovirus (CMV) is a double-stranded DNA herpesvirus that infects most of the world's population (1, 2). Natural transmission is mostly through contact with viral shedding in breast milk, saliva, urine, or genital fluids (3–5). Similar to other herpesviruses, acute CMV infection is associated with high levels of lytic viral replication and dissemination throughout the body, followed by the establishment of viral latency in long-lived cell types that is responsible for lifelong persistence of infection (6).

Cytomegalovirus infection is typically diagnosed by serology (1, 7, 8). In addition to CMV IgG, use of CMV IgM and serial IgG avidity testing may help determine the timing of infection in selected situations (7, 9, 10). However, in infants, CMV serologic testing can be confounded presence of maternal IgG acquired passively *in utero* (3, 8). Therefore, diagnosis in infants requires either seroconversion (a change from negative to positive serologic testing) or, more often, by the detection of CMV in blood, saliva, or urine (3, 8). Isolation of CMV in culture or detection of CMV DNA or antigen in patient samples reflects lytic viral replication and is termed "active" infection (1, 2). Active CMV infection in a chronically infected person may be due to either reactivation of latent virus or reinfection with an exogenous strain of CMV (1, 2, 11, 12).

Acute CMV infection in healthy children or adults is nearly always asymptomatic or limited to mild non-specific illness. Periodic mucosal CMV reactivation and viral shedding is not uncommon during chronic infection, but systemic replication or viremia (detection of CMV in blood) is rare in immunologically normal individuals (4, 13, 14). By contrast, CMV viremia and end-organ disease is common in congenitally infected children and immunocompromised patients (15–18). More recent findings also suggest that CMV might have pervasive negative impact on health through indirect effects on the immune system (19–21). In particular, CMV has increasingly been recognized as a potential cause of disease in immunologically normal adults with critical illness (22–25). However, despite the fact that young children generally control CMV infection poorly compared to adults, little is known about the role of CMV in immunocompetent critically ill pediatric patients. Below, we review the evidence for CMV causing adverse clinical outcomes in immunocompetent critically ill adults, and provide a rationale for analogous studies to examine the impact of CMV on critical illness in immunocompetent children.

SYSTEMIC CMV REACTIVATION IN IMMUNOCOMPETENT CRITICALLY ILL ADULTS

Observational Studies Linking CMV Viremia With Adverse Adult Critical Care Outcomes

There have been more than 30 studies of immunologically normal, critically ill adult patients demonstrating an association between systemic CMV reactivation and worse outcomes in intensive care units (ICUs), as summarized in recent reviews (22–25). In these studies, CMV reactivation was defined as the detection of CMV in blood samples or, when feasible, in bronchoalveolar lavage (BAL) fluid, using CMV DNA PCR, antigen immunocytochemistry, or growth in shell vial culture. CMV viremia occurs in approximately 35% of seropositive adults following admission to the ICU. By contrast, fewer than 1% of adult blood donors with chronic CMV infection have detectable viremia (13, 14). CMV viremia and viral load are positively correlated with worse outcomes, including prolonged ICU stay, length of mechanical ventilation, secondary infections, and death. CMV viremia occurs over a wide spectrum of ICU admission diagnoses, such as infection, trauma, burns, and major surgery (26–35). In particular, patients with bacterial sepsis or pneumonia have been reported to have a higher likelihood of CMV viremia (28, 33, 36). The risk of CMV viremia is not clearly related to disease severity at the time of admission based on prognostic and organ dysfunction scores, and the onset of CMV viremia tends to precede or accompany clinical decline (37, 38), which support the possibility that CMV causes, rather than merely being a marker of, worse ICU outcomes in adults (23–25).

Mechanisms by Which Critical Illness May Cause CMV Viremia

Critical illness may impair immune control of CMV replication normally mediated by cytotoxic T cells and natural killer (NK) cells (39–41). Adults with sepsis show depletion of splenic T cells and reduced T cell responsiveness (42). Functional NK cell differences have also been reported between patients with septic shock or systemic inflammatory response syndrome and healthy controls (43). Furthermore, among patients with septic shock, those with CMV reactivation were found to have reduced NK cell function (44).

Exposure of latently infected cells to a pro-inflammatory environment contributes to CMV reactivation (6). Thus, inflammation, e.g., due to trauma or sepsis, may initiate CMV reactivation in critically ill patients, and CMV replication then might in turn drive more inflammation in a feed-forward manner (**Figure 1**). CMV replication is associated with production of pro-inflammatory cytokines, including interleukin (IL)-1, IL-6, IL-8, and TNF-α (45–47). In a cohort of young adults, IL-6 levels were significantly higher in the sera of CMV seropositive compared to seronegative subjects (48, 49). Interestingly, CMV-infected adults were more likely to have a pro-inflammatory profile at 3 months

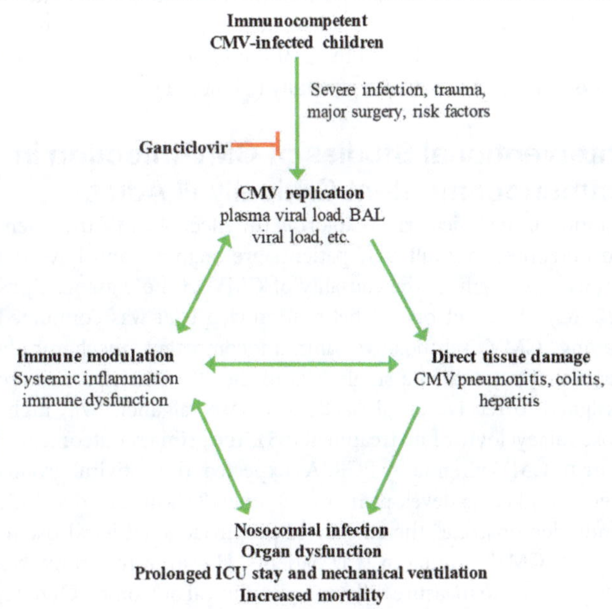

FIGURE 1 | Hypothesized model for cytomegalovirus (CMV) reactivation in critically ill children. Possible risk factors for systemic CMV replication include severity of illness, pneumonia, malnutrition, blood transfusion, corticosteroid treatment, and young age. BAL, bronchoalveolar lavage.

after discharge from ICU, even after adjusting for illness severity and underlying conditions (50).

Mechanisms by Which CMV Replication May Contribute to Clinical Decline

Adverse ICU outcomes often result from uncontrolled inflammation and/or impaired immunity (42). CMV infection may play a significant role in both of these processes through both direct and indirect mechanisms.

Cytomegalovirus replication in tissues of immunocompromised individuals is a well-recognized cause of end-organ damage, including pneumonitis, hepatitis, and colitis (11, 16–18). Although direct cytolytic effects of viral replication in tissues are central to the pathogenesis of CMV infection in the immunocompromised host, its role in immunocompetent critically ill individuals is relatively poorly defined. Some studies have reported frequent pulmonary CMV replication based on testing of BAL fluid and lung biopsies (26, 51). Histopathologic evidence of CMV colitis was also found in immunocompetent adult patients admitted to ICU for other causes (52). In addition, CMV has been reported to cause kidney and liver damage in immunocompetent adult ICU patients (53–55). Murine studies add further support to the hypothesis that CMV replication contributes to acute lung injury in adults with sepsis or severe trauma. Sepsis in immunocompetent mice causes murine CMV reactivation in the lungs, as well as pulmonary inflammation and fibrosis that is prevented by treatment with the antiviral drug ganciclovir (56, 57).

In transplant recipients, CMV is associated with the so-called "indirect" effects on the immune system, including increased risk of bacterial and fungal infections (52, 58, 59). Some studies suggest that CMV-induced immunomodulation may increase the risk of nosocomial infections in immunocompetent ICU patients (22, 53). These findings would seem to be consistent with our emerging understanding of the profound impact CMV infection has on the immune system generally (21, 60, 61).

Interventional Studies of CMV Infection in Immunocompetent Critically Ill Adults

Randomized clinical trials exploring the effect of CMV treatment on outcomes in adult ICU patients are ongoing, and have the ability to determine the causality of CMV in these associations (22, 62). A recent open-label randomized trial was conducted among CMV seropositive, immunocompetent mechanically ventilated patients in a single ICU in the UK. Participants were assigned to receive prophylactic low-dose valganciclovir, high-dose valacyclovir, or no treatment (63). The primary outcome was time to CMV viremia by PCR. As expected, the antiviral groups were less likely to develop viremia (8 versus 35% in controls). This study demonstrates the efficacy of prophylactic antiviral use to prevent CMV viremia in ICU patients. However, the study was not powered to measure differences in clinical outcomes. Of note, the valacyclovir arm was discontinued early due to higher mortality, though all deaths were judged to be expected and attributable to underlying disease rather than any adverse antiviral effects.

Subsequently, a phase 2, randomized controlled multicenter trial of prophylactic ganciclovir or valganciclovir versus placebo in immunocompetent CMV seropositive adult ICU patients with respiratory failure and severe sepsis or trauma was published (64). The study failed to detect a difference in the primary outcome, blood IL-6 level, which was chosen based on the reported association of elevated IL-6 with ICU mortality and ventilator-associated lung injury (65, 66). However, in addition to reduced viremia, subjects in the antiviral treatment arm had significantly more ventilation-free days, a predetermined secondary outcome. This effect was particularly marked in the subgroup admitted for sepsis. A composite end point of mortality and increased serum IL-6 by 50% or >7 days ventilation was significantly higher in placebo group, and there was a trend toward increased mortality in the placebo group. Notably, antiviral treatment was not associated with significant side effects. This study provides the strongest evidence to date for a causal association between CMV viremia and worse outcomes in and provides preliminary support for the possibility that antiviral treatment may be beneficial for selected immunocompetent adult ICU patients (62).

THE POTENTIAL ROLE OF CMV INFECTION IN IMMUNOCOMPETENT CRITICALLY ILL CHILDREN

Age-Dependent Differences in CMV Pathogenesis

There are qualitative and quantitative age-dependent differences in the immune responses of young children that impair the control of many viral infections, including CMV (67–69). Children with congenital CMV infection are most often asymptomatic, but commonly present with central nervous system disease, hepatitis, hematologic abnormalities, and pneumonitis. Sensorineural hearing loss and neurodevelopmental delay develop in approximately 20% of children with congenital CMV infection (15). Postnatal CMV infection rarely causes serious illness, though extremely premature infants can develop sepsis and severe end-organ disease (70–72). Even in the absence of CMV-related disease, compared with adults primary infection, children have substantially higher levels of viral replication as well as prolonged viremia and viral shedding in saliva or urine (4, 73). Though viral replication gradually declines over time, viral shedding during chronic infection remains substantially greater in children compared to adults (4, 73). Thus, as a result of more recent infection and differences in antiviral immunity, critically ill children might be expected to have worse control of CMV replication than adults.

CMV Infection in Critically Ill Children

There are very few data available about the frequency and effects of active CMV infection in critically ill, immunocompetent children. We performed a pilot study of CMV infection in children admitted to the ICU of BC Children's Hospital in Vancouver, Canada (unpublished data). Among the 27 children enrolled, the median age was 4 years (range 4 months–17 years). Only one child was CMV seropositive, and none were found to have viremia. This is consistent with the relatively low CMV seroprevalence among children in most high-income countries (74–77). By contrast, a study of children between 3 weeks and 2 years old hospitalized in Zambia found that 34% of HIV-uninfected children had CMV viremia (78). Of note, the prevalence of malnutrition was 36%, and being underweight was significantly associated with CMV viremia. In a retrospective study of Ugandan children 6 months–13 years old treated as outpatients for uncomplicated malaria, 11% had CMV viremia (79). Thus, even in the setting of moderate illness, systemic CMV replication is common in African children. In a prospective study that included 53 HIV-uninfected South African children ≤2 years old admitted to ICU with severe pneumonia, 12 (23%) were defined as having CMV pneumonitis based on DNA detection in BAL fluid and other clinical characteristics (80). Many of these children were treated with ganciclovir, but the published data are insufficient to determine whether disseminated CMV or antiviral treatment in HIV-uninfected children were associated with clinical outcomes (80).

DETERMINING THE IMPACT OF CMV INFECTION ON PEDIATRIC ICU OUTCOMES

General Considerations

Well-designed cohort studies are needed to understand the role of CMV in immunocompetent critically ill children, to estimate the potential benefits, and to inform the design of appropriate pediatric treatment trials. Given the differences between children and adults in the natural history and outcomes of CMV infection, extrapolation from adult studies is inappropriate. As an example, in the adult studies conducted to date, the clinical impact of CMV has been ascribed to reactivation and dissemination of chronic infection (23–25). However, CMV viremia in pediatric ICU patients might often represent systemic viral replication related to recent infection rather than reactivation. To distinguish between reactivation of chronic infection and exacerbation of recent infection would be challenging, but might provide insights into age-dependent differences should they exist. Thus, in pediatrics studies, it would be more appropriate to explicitly evaluate the role of disseminated CMV replication as opposed to reactivation of chronic infection.

Measuring CMV Replication in Pediatric ICU Patients

Quantitative CMV DNA PCR assays can reliably detect ≤50 international units/mL and have largely replaced older methods of detection (81, 82). Because high level CMV replication in saliva and urine is so prevalent in young children (73, 83), these measures are unlikely to be clinically meaningful for critically ill children except for confirming infection in infants with maternal antibody and concern for false-positive serology. As in adult studies, CMV replication in blood is likely to be the best measure of uncontrolled systemic viral infection in critically ill children. Although CMV in BAL fluid may simply represent shedding, high viral loads are predictive of CMV pneumonitis in transplant recipients and, perhaps, in critically ill children (80, 84, 85). Thus, pediatric ICU studies should incorporate CMV testing of BAL fluid, should it be collected for clinical purposes. In addition, detection of CMV in tissue biopsies (e.g., liver, colon), particularly by histopathology indicates invasive disease, and these specimens should be tested if available (**Table 1**).

The risk of CMV disease is correlated to the level of viremia in many clinical scenarios. For example, in HIV-infected individuals and transplant recipients, CMV viral load is proportionally associated with progression of disease (86, 87). However, the threshold of CMV replication that is clinically relevant or that might warrant intervention depends on the patient population. For example, antiviral treatment of newborns with symptomatic congenital CMV infection is indicated, regardless of viral load, to reduce the risk of hearing loss and neurocognitive delay (8, 88–90). Selected transplant patients are monitored using CMV blood PCR in order to trigger preemptive antiviral treatment before the onset of disease, but the viral load threshold used varies based on immunologic status and other clinical criteria (87, 91, 92). The antiviral studies performed so far in adults have randomized all CMV seropositive ICU patients with the intention of preventing, rather than treating, viremia (63, 64). The optimal approach to treating CMV infection in pediatric ICU patients would depend on the associations and dose–response that are found, but might conceivably utilize risk-stratification based on age, underlying illness, viral load, or other factors.

TABLE 1 | Suggested metrics for studies of cytomegalovirus (CMV) viremia in immunocompetent pediatric intensive care unit (ICU) patients.

CMV manifestations	Potential effects	CMV measures	Clinical outcome measures
Systemic inflammatory response syndrome	Multiorgan dysfunction	IgG, IgM, and urine PCR to diagnose infection	Mortality at 7, 14, and 28 days Ventilator-free days at 28 days
Pneumonitis Hepatitis	Prolonged ventilation Transaminitis, hyperbilirubinemia, impairment of synthetic liver function	Plasma/serum viral load If collected for clinical care: - BAL viral load - Histopathology (biopsies of lung, colon, liver, bone marrow)	Length of ICU/hospital stay Health-related quality of life at 28 days Organ dysfunction scores (PLEOD, SOFA, NPMOD, etc.)
Colitis	Enteric dysfunction, growth failure, nutritional deficiencies		Weight to height Z score Post-discharge mortality or readmission at 6 months
Myelosuppression, neutropenia, thrombocytopenia, anemia	Nosocomial infection Blood product transfusions		Inflammatory markers in blood, BAL, and stool Blood transfusions Nosocomial infections Antibiotic use

BAL, broncheoalveolar lavage; PLEOD, Pediatric Logistic Organ Dysfunction score; SOFA, Sequential Organ Failure Assessment score; NPMOD, New/Progressive Multiorgan Dysfunction.

Pediatric Populations of Greatest Interest

Studying the impact of CMV infection on critically ill immunocompetent children is anticipated to be both easier and more clinically relevant in low- and middle-income countries (LMIC), where CMV infection is holoendemic and mortality and morbidity rates from sepsis are often dismal. In LMIC, nearly all children acquire CMV infection within the first few years of life (74). By contrast, the national US survey found that while CMV prevalence increases linearly with age, it reaches only ~50% by 30 years of age (75, 76).

In addition to the relatively low rates of CMV infection in North American and European children, the excellent outcomes of pediatric ICU patients there hinder the ability to detect a clinically important impact of CMV infection on critically ill children (93–96). Furthermore, strategies to reduce mortality in critically ill children in LMIC are urgently needed. For example, in the Kenyatta National Hospital pediatric ICU in Nairobi, Kenya, overall mortality is 42% (unpublished data). Similarly, pediatric ICU mortality rates of 25–50% have been reported in other LMICs in Africa and Asia (97–100). Other outcomes of interest such as length of stay and need for invasive ventilation are also frequently higher in LMICs (99, 100). In Siriraj Hospital, one of the largest hospital in Thailand, median length of ICU stay and rate of mechanical ventilation are 4–5 days and 64%, respectively (Dr. K. Lapphra, personal communication), which are more than double those in the BC Children's Hospital ICU. Moreover, infections and sepsis account for most of pediatric ICU admission diagnoses in LMIC, which might again predispose to disseminated CMV infection and viremia (97, 98).

Outcome Measure Considerations

Importantly, appropriate studies in children require the incorporation of pediatric-specific illness severity scores and outcome measures (**Table 1**). Mortality and morbidity in pediatric patients are predicted by progressive or new organ dysfunction, using validated scores (101–103). Evaluation of mechanical ventilation outcomes should include invasive as well as non-invasive modalities, which are now commonly used in children (94). A longer follow-up duration that used in adults studies should also be considered, given the high rate of readmission and post-discharge mortality in children of African and Asian countries (104–106). Higher rates of CMV viremia as well as worse post-discharge outcomes have been observed in underweight children (78, 106). Therefore, including nutritional assessments in pediatric studies is also essential.

CONCLUSION

Strong evidence supports the association between CMV viremia and adverse outcomes in adult ICU patients (23–25), and early-phase interventional trial results suggest that antivirals in this population might be beneficial (62–64). Unfortunately, there are no studies yet in children that have adequately addressed this question. Not only is there an ethical obligation to include children in research according to the principle of justice (107–109), but we hypothesize that active systemic CMV infection might have an even greater negative impact on ICU outcomes in children than adults. Therefore, we propose that prospective observational studies should be conducted to characterize the association between CMV viremia and clinical outcomes in critically ill children, using metrics appropriate for pediatric populations. Furthermore, we suggest that such studies would best be performed in LMICs settings. Importantly, if CMV treatment were found to be beneficial for immunocompetent critically ill children, resource limitations would not preclude its implementation (110). If successful, studies in LMICs could result in reverse innovation to help targeting specific subpopulations of patients in high-income settings that might also benefit from CMV treatment. Studies in both adults and children should attempt to identify the mechanistic basis for the relationship between CMV and critical illness, and develop novel therapies to improve outcomes of critically ill patients.

ETHICS STATEMENT

The pilot study Reactivation of Cytomegalovirus in Pediatrics (ReCIPe) for the prevalence of CMV viremia among pediatric critical care patients in BC Children's Hospital was approved by BCCHR Ethics Board.

AUTHOR CONTRIBUTIONS

RA: literature review and writing; SG: reviewing, editing, writing, and knowledge check; JS: reviewing statistics and literature, editing, and writing; SM: checking literature and ICU data.

REFERENCES

1. Shenk TS, Mark F, et al. *Human Cytomegalovirus*. (Vol. 325). Springer.
2. Mocarski ES, Shenk T, Griffiths P, Pass RF. Cytomegaovirus. 6th ed. In: Knipe DM, Howley PM, editors. *Field's Virology*. Philadelphia: Lippincott Williams & Wilkins (2013).
3. Gantt S, Orem J, Krantz EM, Morrow RA, Selke S, Huang ML, et al. Prospective characterization of the risk factors for transmission and symptoms of primary human herpesvirus infections among Ugandan infants. *J Infect Dis* (2016) 214:36–44. doi:10.1093/infdis/jiw076
4. Cannon MJ, Hyde TB, Schmid DS. Review of cytomegalovirus shedding in bodily fluids and relevance to congenital cytomegalovirus infection. *Rev Med Virol* (2011) 21:240–55. doi:10.1002/rmv.695
5. Adler SP. Cytomegalovirus transmission among children in day care, their mothers and caretakers. *Pediatr Infect Dis J* (1988) 7:279–85. doi:10.1097/00006454-198804000-00009

6. Reeves M, Sinclair J. Aspects of human cytomegalovirus latency and reactivation. *Curr Top Microbiol Immunol* (2008) 325:297–313. doi:10.1007/978-3-540-77349-8
7. Ross SA, Novak Z, Pati S, Boppana SB. Diagnosis of cytomegalovirus Infections. *Infect Disord Drug Targets* (2011) 11:466–74. doi:10.2174/187152611797636703
8. American Academy of Pediatrics. Cytomegalovirus Infection. In: Kimberlin DW, Brady MT, Jackson MA, Long SS, editors. *Red Book® 2015: Report of the Committee on Infectious Diseases*. 30th ed. Elk Grove Village, IL: American Academy of Pediatrics (2015). p. 317–22.
9. Dollard SC, Keyserling H, Radford K, Amin MM, Stowell J, Winter J, et al. Cytomegalovirus viral and antibody correlates in young children. *BMC Res Notes* (2014) 7:776. doi:10.1186/1756-0500-7-776
10. Prince HE, Lape-Nixon M, Novak-Weekley SM. Performance of a cytomegalovirus IgG enzyme immunoassay kit modified to measure avidity. *Clin Vaccine Immunol* (2014) 21:808–12. doi:10.1128/CVI.00105-14
11. Ljungman P, Griffiths P, Paya C. Definitions of cytomegalovirus infection and disease in transplant recipients. *Clin Infect Dis* (2002) 34:1094–7. doi:10.1086/339329
12. Boucoiran I, Mayer BT, Krantz E, Marchant A, Pati S, Boppana S, et al. Nonprimary maternal CMV infection following viral shedding in infants. *Pediatr Infect Dis J* (2017). doi:10.1097/INF.0000000000001877
13. Roback JD, Drew WL, Laycock ME, Todd D, Hillyer CD, Busch MP. CMV DNA is rarely detected in healthy blood donors using validated PCR assays. *Transfusion* (2003) 43:314–21. doi:10.1046/j.1537-2995.2003.00312.x
14. Ziemann M, Thiele T. Transfusion-transmitted CMV infection – current knowledge and future perspectives. *Transfus Med* (2017) 27:238–48. doi:10.1111/tme.12437
15. Boppana SB, Ross SA, Fowler KB. Congenital cytomegalovirus infection: clinical outcome. *Clin Infect Dis* (2013) 57(Suppl 4):S178–81. doi:10.1093/cid/cit629
16. Ramanan P, Razonable RR. Cytomegalovirus infections in solid organ transplantation: a review. *Infect Chemother* (2013) 45:260–71. doi:10.3947/ic.2013.45.3.260
17. Bhat V, Joshi A, Sarode R, Chavan P. Cytomegalovirus infection in the bone marrow transplant patient. *World J Transplant* (2015) 5:287–91. doi:10.5500/wjt.v5.i4.287
18. Kovacs A, Schluchter M, Easley K, Demmler G, Shearer W, La Russa P, et al. Cytomegalovirus infection and HIV-1 disease progression in infants born to HIV-1-infected women. Pediatric pulmonary and cardiovascular complications of vertically transmitted HIV infection study group. *N Engl J Med* (1999) 341:77–84. doi:10.1056/NEJM199907083410203
19. Simanek AM, Dowd JB, Pawelec G, Melzer D, Dutta A, Aiello AE. Seropositivity to cytomegalovirus, inflammation, all-cause and cardiovascular disease-related mortality in the United States. *PLoS One* (2011) 6:e16103. doi:10.1371/journal.pone.0016103
20. Weltevrede M, Eilers R, de Melker HE, van Baarle D. Cytomegalovirus persistence and T-cell immunosenescence in people aged fifty and older: a systematic review. *Exp Gerontol* (2016) 77:87–95. doi:10.1016/j.exger.2016.02.005
21. Brodin P, Jojic V, Gao T, Bhattacharya S, Angel CJ, Furman D, et al. Variation in the human immune system is largely driven by non-heritable influences. *Cell* (2015) 160:37–47. doi:10.1016/j.cell.2014.12.020
22. Limaye AP, Boeckh M. CMV in critically ill patients: pathogen or bystander? *Rev Med Virol* (2010) 20:372–9. doi:10.1002/rmv.664
23. Papazian L, Hraiech S, Lehingue S, Roch A, Chiche L, Wiramus S, et al. Cytomegalovirus reactivation in ICU patients. *Intensive Care Med* (2016) 42:28–37. doi:10.1007/s00134-015-4066-9
24. Al-Omari A, Aljamaan F, Alhazzani W, Salih S, Arabi Y. Cytomegalovirus infection in immunocompetent critically ill adults: literature review. *Ann Intensive Care* (2016) 6:110. doi:10.1186/s13613-016-0207-8
25. Lachance P, Chen J, Featherstone R, Sligl WI. Association between cytomegalovirus reactivation and clinical outcomes in immunocompetent critically ill patients: a systematic review and meta-analysis. *Open Forum Infect Dis* (2017) 4:ofx029. doi:10.1093/ofid/ofx029
26. Chiche L, Forel JM, Roch A, Guervilly C, Pauly V, Allardet-Servent J, et al. Active cytomegalovirus infection is common in mechanically ventilated medical intensive care unit patients. *Crit Care Med* (2009) 37:1850–7. doi:10.1097/CCM.0b013e31819ffea6
27. Coisel Y, Bousbia S, Forel JM, Hraiech S, Lascola B, Roch A, et al. Cytomegalovirus and herpes simplex virus effect on the prognosis of mechanically ventilated patients suspected to have ventilator-associated pneumonia. *PLoS One* (2012) 7:e51340. doi:10.1371/journal.pone.0051340
28. Walton AH, Muenzer JT, Rasche D, Boomer JS, Sato B, Brownstein BH, et al. Reactivation of multiple viruses in patients with sepsis. *PLoS One* (2014) 9:e98819. doi:10.1371/journal.pone.0098819
29. Osawa R, Wagener M, Singh N. Cytomegalovirus infection in patients with sepsis due to bloodstream infections: lower risk and better outcomes in new versus already hospitalised intensive care unit admissions. *Anaesth Intensive Care* (2016) 44:571–80.
30. Heininger A, Jahn G, Engel C, Notheisen T, Unertl K, Hamprecht K. Human cytomegalovirus infections in nonimmunosuppressed critically ill patients. *Crit Care Med* (2001) 29:541–7. doi:10.1097/00003246-200103000-00012
31. Bordes J, Maslin J, Prunet B, d'Aranda E, Lacroix G, Goutorbe P, et al. Cytomegalovirus infection in severe burn patients monitoring by real-time polymerase chain reaction: a prospective study. *Burns* (2011) 37:434–9. doi:10.1016/j.burns.2010.11.006
32. Lopez Roa P, Hill JA, Kirby KA, Leisenring WM, Huang ML, Santo TK, et al. Coreactivation of human herpesvirus 6 and cytomegalovirus is associated with worse clinical outcome in critically ill adults. *Crit Care Med* (2015) 43:1415–22. doi:10.1097/CCM.0000000000000969
33. Cook CH, Martin LC, Yenchar JK, Lahm MC, McGuinness B, Davies EA, et al. Occult herpes family viral infections are endemic in critically ill surgical patients. *Crit Care Med* (2003) 31:1923–9. doi:10.1097/01.CCM.0000070222.11325.C4
34. Domart Y, Trouillet JL, Fagon JY, Chastre J, Brun-Vezinet F, Gibert C. Incidence and morbidity of cytomegaloviral infection in patients with mediastinitis following cardiac surgery. *Chest* (1990) 97:18–22. doi:10.1378/chest.97.1.18
35. Ishioka H, Sanui M, Tsutsumi Y, Yanase F, Shiotsuka J. Low prevalence of active cytomegalovirus infection in a cardiovascular intensive care unit. *J Intensive Care* (2014) 2:12. doi:10.1186/2052-0492-2-12
36. Heininger A, Haeberle H, Fischer I, Beck R, Riessen R, Rohde F, et al. Cytomegalovirus reactivation and associated outcome of critically ill patients with severe sepsis. *Crit Care* (2011) 15:R77. doi:10.1186/cc10069
37. Frantzeskaki FG, Karampi ES, Kottaridi C, Alepaki M, Routsi C, Tzanela M, et al. Cytomegalovirus reactivation in a general, nonimmunosuppressed intensive care unit population: incidence, risk factors, associations with organ dysfunction, and inflammatory biomarkers. *J Crit Care* (2015) 30:276–81. doi:10.1016/j.jcrc.2014.10.002
38. Kalil AC, Florescu DF. Prevalence and mortality associated with cytomegalovirus infection in nonimmunosuppressed patients in the intensive care unit. *Crit Care Med* (2009) 37:2350–8. doi:10.1097/CCM.0b013e3181a3aa43
39. Orr MT, Murphy WJ, Lanier LL. Unlicensed natural killer cells dominate the response to cytomegalovirus infection. *Nat Immunol* (2010) 11:321. doi:10.1038/ni.1849
40. La Rosa C, Diamond DJ. The immune response to human CMV. *Future Virol* (2012) 7:279–93. doi:10.2217/fvl.12.8
41. Klenerman P, Oxenius A. T cell responses to cytomegalovirus. *Nat Rev Immunol* (2016) 16:367. doi:10.1038/nri.2016.38
42. Boomer JS, To K, Chang KC, Takasu O, Osborne DF, Walton AH, et al. Immunosuppression in patients who die of sepsis and multiple organ failure. *JAMA* (2011) 306:2594–605. doi:10.1001/jama.2011.1829
43. Forel JM, Chiche L, Thomas G, Mancini J, Farnarier C, Cognet C, et al. Phenotype and functions of natural killer cells in critically-ill septic patients. *PLoS One* (2012) 7:e50446. doi:10.1371/journal.pone.0050446
44. von Muller L, Klemm A, Durmus N, Weiss M, Suger-Wiedeck H, Schneider M, et al. Cellular immunity and active human cytomegalovirus infection in patients with septic shock. *J Infect Dis* (2007) 196:1288–95. doi:10.1086/522429
45. Iwamoto GK, Konicek SA. Cytomegalovirus immediate early genes upregulate interleukin-6 gene expression. *J Investig Med* (1997) 45:175–82.
46. Craigen JL, Yong KL, Jordan NJ, MacCormac LP, Westwick J, Akbar AN, et al. Human cytomegalovirus infection up-regulates interleukin-8 gene expression and stimulates neutrophil transendothelial migration. *Immunology* (1997) 92:138–45. doi:10.1046/j.1365-2567.1997.00310.x
47. Humar A, St Louis P, Mazzulli T, McGeer A, Lipton J, Messner H, et al. Elevated serum cytokines are associated with cytomegalovirus infection and

disease in bone marrow transplant recipients. *J Infect Dis* (1999) 179:484–8. doi:10.1086/314602
48. Turner JE, Campbell JP, Edwards KM, Howarth LJ, Pawelec G, Aldred S, et al. Rudimentary signs of immunosenescence in cytomegalovirus-seropositive healthy young adults. *Age (Dordr)* (2014) 36:287–97. doi:10.1007/s11357-013-9557-4
49. Bengner M, Beziat V, Ernerudh J, Nilsson BO, Lofgren S, Wikby A, et al. Independent skewing of the T cell and NK cell compartments associated with cytomegalovirus infection suggests division of labor between innate and adaptive immunity. *Age (Dordr)* (2014) 36:571–82. doi:10.1007/s11357-013-9587-y
50. Griffith DM, Lewis S, Rossi AG, Rennie J, Salisbury L, Merriweather JL, et al. Systemic inflammation after critical illness: relationship with physical recovery and exploration of potential mechanisms. *Thorax* (2016) 71:820–9. doi:10.1136/thoraxjnl-2015-208114
51. Papazian L, Fraisse A, Garbe L, Zandotti C, Thomas P, Saux P, et al. Cytomegalovirus. An unexpected cause of ventilator-associated pneumonia. *Anesthesiology* (1996) 84:280–7. doi:10.1097/00000542-199602000-00005
52. Freeman RB Jr. The 'indirect' effects of cytomegalovirus infection. *Am J Transplant* (2009) 9:2453–8. doi:10.1111/j.1600-6143.2009.02824.x
53. Jaber S, Chanques G, Borry J, Souche B, Verdier R, Perrigault PF, et al. Cytomegalovirus infection in critically ill patients: associated factors and consequences. *Chest* (2005) 127:233–41. doi:10.1378/chest.127.1.233
54. Squizzato A, Ageno W, Cattaneo A, Brumana N. A case report and literature review of portal vein thrombosis associated with cytomegalovirus infection in immunocompetent patients. *Clin Infect Dis* (2007) 44:e13–6. doi:10.1086/509641
55. Siciliano RF, Castelli JB, Randi BA, Vieira RD, Strabelli TM. Cytomegalovirus colitis in immunocompetent critically ill patients. *Int J Infect Dis* (2014) 20:71–3. doi:10.1016/j.ijid.2013.11.008
56. Cook CH, Zhang Y, McGuinness BJ, Lahm MC, Sedmak DD, Ferguson RM. Intra-abdominal bacterial infection reactivates latent pulmonary cytomegalovirus in immunocompetent mice. *J Infect Dis* (2002) 185:1395–400. doi:10.1086/340508
57. Cook CH, Zhang Y, Sedmak DD, Martin LC, Jewell S, Ferguson RM. Pulmonary cytomegalovirus reactivation causes pathology in immunocompetent mice. *Crit Care Med* (2006) 34:842–9. doi:10.1097/01.CCM.0000201876.11059.05
58. Prentice HG, Gluckman E, Powles RL, Ljungman P, Milpied N, Fernandez Ranada JM, et al. Impact of long-term acyclovir on cytomegalovirus infection and survival after allogeneic bone marrow transplantation. European Acyclovir for CMV Prophylaxis Study Group. *Lancet* (1994) 343:749–53. doi:10.1016/S0140-6736(94)91835-X
59. Roman A, Manito N, Campistol JM, Cuervas-Mons V, Almenar L, Arias M, et al. The impact of the prevention strategies on the indirect effects of CMV infection in solid organ transplant recipients. *Transplant Rev (Orlando)* (2014) 28:84–91. doi:10.1016/j.trre.2014.01.001
60. Beziat V, Liu LL, Malmberg JA, Ivarsson MA, Sohlberg E, Bjorklund AT, et al. NK cell responses to cytomegalovirus infection lead to stable imprints in the human KIR repertoire and involve activating KIRs. *Blood* (2013) 121:2678–88. doi:10.1182/blood-2012-10-459545
61. Souquette A, Frere J, Smithey M, Sauce D, Thomas PG. A constant companion: immune recognition and response to cytomegalovirus with aging and implications for immune fitness. *GeroScience* (2017) 39:293–303. doi:10.1007/s11357-017-9982-x
62. Kumar D, Humar A. Time to consider cytomegalovirus prevention in critically ill patients? *JAMA* (2017) 318:709–10. doi:10.1001/jama.2017.10132
63. Cowley NJ, Owen A, Shiels SC, Millar J, Woolley R, Ives N, et al. Safety and efficacy of antiviral therapy for prevention of cytomegalovirus reactivation in immunocompetent critically ill patients: a randomized clinical trial. *JAMA Intern Med* (2017) 177:774–83. doi:10.1001/jamainternmed.2017.0895
64. Limaye AP, Stapleton RD, Peng L, Gunn SR, Kimball LE, Hyzy R, et al. Effect of ganciclovir on il-6 levels among cytomegalovirus-seropositive adults with critical illness: a randomized clinical trial. *JAMA* (2017) 318:731–40. doi:10.1001/jama.2017.10569
65. Parsons PE, Eisner MD, Thompson BT, Matthay MA, Ancukiewicz M, Bernard GR, et al. Lower tidal volume ventilation and plasma cytokine markers of inflammation in patients with acute lung injury. *Crit Care Med* (2005) 33:1–6; discussion 230–2. doi:10.1097/01.CCM.0000149854.61192.DC
66. Ranieri VM, Suter PM, Tortorella C, De Tullio R, Dayer JM, Brienza A, et al. Effect of mechanical ventilation on inflammatory mediators in patients with acute respiratory distress syndrome: a randomized controlled trial. *JAMA* (1999) 282:54–61. doi:10.1001/jama.282.1.54
67. Prendergast AJ, Klenerman P, Goulder PJ. The impact of differential antiviral immunity in children and adults. *Nat Rev Immunol* (2012) 12:636–48. doi:10.1038/nri3277
68. Schleiss MR. Cytomegalovirus in the neonate: immune correlates of infection and protection. *Clin Dev Immunol* (2013) 2013:501801. doi:10.1155/2013/501801
69. Muller WJ, Jones CA, Koelle DM. Immunobiology of herpes simplex virus and cytomegalovirus infections of the fetus and newborn. *Curr Immunol Rev* (2010) 6:38–55. doi:10.2174/157339510790231833
70. Lanzieri TM, Dollard SC, Josephson CD, Schmid DS, Bialek SR. Breast milk-acquired cytomegalovirus infection and disease in VLBW and premature infants. *Pediatrics* (2013) 131:e1937–45. doi:10.1542/peds.2013-0076
71. Capretti MG, Lanari M, Lazzarotto T, Gabrielli L, Pignatelli S, Corvaglia L, et al. Very low birth weight infants born to cytomegalovirus-seropositive mothers fed with their mother's milk: a prospective study. *J Pediatr* (2009) 154:842–8. doi:10.1016/j.jpeds.2008.12.046
72. Gunkel J, Wolfs TF, de Vries LS, Nijman J. Predictors of severity for postnatal cytomegalovirus infection in preterm infants and implications for treatment. *Expert Rev Anti Infect Ther* (2014) 12:1345–55. doi:10.1586/14787210.2014.966080
73. Matrajt L, Gantt S, Mayer BT, Krantz EM, Orem J, Wald A, et al. Virus and host-specific differences in oral human herpesvirus shedding kinetics among Ugandan women and children. *Sci Rep* (2017) 7:13105. doi:10.1038/s41598-017-12994-0
74. Cannon MJ, Schmid DS, Hyde TB. Review of cytomegalovirus seroprevalence and demographic characteristics associated with infection. *Rev Med Virol* (2010) 20:202–13. doi:10.1002/rmv.655
75. Staras SA, Dollard SC, Radford KW, Flanders WD, Pass RF, Cannon MJ. Seroprevalence of cytomegalovirus infection in the United States, 1988-1994. *Clin Infect Dis* (2006) 43:1143–51. doi:10.1086/508173
76. Bate SL, Dollard SC, Cannon MJ. Cytomegalovirus seroprevalence in the United States: the national health and nutrition examination surveys, 1988-2004. *Clin Infect Dis* (2010) 50:1439–47. doi:10.1086/652438
77. Hyde TB, Schmid DS, Cannon MJ. Cytomegalovirus seroconversion rates and risk factors: implications for congenital CMV. *Rev Med Virol* (2010) 20:311–26. doi:10.1002/rmv.659
78. Tembo J, Kabwe M, Chilukutu L, Chilufya M, Mwaanza N, Chabala C, et al. Prevalence and risk factors for betaherpesvirus DNAemia in children >3 weeks and <2 years of age admitted to a large referral hospital in sub-Saharan Africa. *Clin Infect Dis* (2015) 60:423–31. doi:10.1093/cid/ciu853
79. Gantt S, Huang ML, Magaret A, Bunts L, Selke S, Wald A, et al. An artesunate-containing antimalarial treatment regimen did not suppress cytomegalovirus viremia. *J Clin Virol* (2013) 58:276–8. doi:10.1016/j.jcv.2013.06.008
80. Govender K, Jeena P, Parboosing R. Clinical utility of bronchoalveolar lavage cytomegalovirus viral loads in the diagnosis of cytomegalovirus pneumonitis in infants. *J Med Virol* (2017) 89:1080–7. doi:10.1002/jmv.24730
81. Boeckh M, Huang M, Ferrenberg J, Stevens-Ayers T, Stensland L, Nichols WG, et al. Optimization of quantitative detection of cytomegalovirus DNA in plasma by real-time PCR. *J Clin Microbiol* (2004) 42:1142–8. doi:10.1128/JCM.42.3.1142-1148.2004
82. Kraft CS, Armstrong WS, Caliendo AM. Interpreting quantitative cytomegalovirus DNA testing: understanding the laboratory perspective. *Clin Infect Dis* (2012) 54:1793–7. doi:10.1093/cid/cis212
83. Stowell JD, Mask K, Amin M, Clark R, Levis D, Hendley W, et al. Cross-sectional study of cytomegalovirus shedding and immunological markers among seropositive children and their mothers. *BMC Infect Dis* (2014) 14:568. doi:10.1186/s12879-014-0568-2
84. Westall GP, Michaelides A, Williams TJ, Snell GI, Kotsimbos TC. Human cytomegalovirus load in plasma and bronchoalveolar lavage fluid: a longitudinal study of lung transplant recipients. *J Infect Dis* (2004) 190:1076–83. doi:10.1086/422327
85. Boeckh M, Stevens-Ayers T, Travi G, Huang ML, Cheng GS, Xie H, et al. Cytomegalovirus (CMV) DNA quantitation in bronchoalveolar lavage fluid from hematopoietic stem cell transplant recipients with CMV pneumonia. *J Infect Dis* (2017) 215:1514–22. doi:10.1093/infdis/jix048

86. Deayton JR, Sabin CA, Johnson MA, Emery VC, Wilson P, Griffiths PD. Importance of cytomegalovirus viraemia in risk of disease progression and death in HIV-infected patients receiving highly active antiretroviral therapy. *Lancet* (2004) 363:2116–21. doi:10.1016/S0140-6736(04)16500-8
87. Griffiths PD, Rothwell E, Raza M, Wilmore S, Doyle T, Harber M, et al. Randomized controlled trials to define viral load thresholds for cytomegalovirus pre-emptive therapy. *PLoS One* (2016) 11:e0163722. doi:10.1371/journal.pone.0163722
88. Kimberlin DW, Jester PM, Sanchez PJ, Ahmed A, Arav-Boger R, Michaels MG, et al. Valganciclovir for symptomatic congenital cytomegalovirus disease. *N Engl J Med* (2015) 372:933–43. doi:10.1056/NEJMoa1404599
89. Gantt S, Bitnun A, Renaud C, Kakkar F, Vaudry W. Diagnosis and management of infants with congenital cytomegalovirus infection. *Paediatr Child Health* (2017) 22:72–4. doi:10.1093/pch/pxx002
90. Rawlinson WD, Boppana SB, Fowler KB, Kimberlin DW, Lazzarotto T, Alain S, et al. Congenital cytomegalovirus infection in pregnancy and the neonate: consensus recommendations for prevention, diagnosis, and therapy. *Lancet Infect Dis* (2017) 17:e177–88. doi:10.1016/S1473-3099(17)30143-3
91. Solano C, Gimenez E, Pinana JL, Vinuesa V, Poujois S, Zaragoza S, et al. Preemptive antiviral therapy for CMV infection in allogeneic stem cell transplant recipients guided by the viral doubling time in the blood. *Bone Marrow Transplant* (2016) 51:718–21. doi:10.1038/bmt.2015.303
92. Razonable RR, Hayden RT. Clinical utility of viral load in management of cytomegalovirus infection after solid organ transplantation. *Clin Microbiol Rev* (2013) 26:703–27. doi:10.1128/CMR.00015-13
93. Jones S, Rantell K, Stevens K, Colwell B, Ratcliffe JR, Holland P, et al. Outcome at 6 months after admission for pediatric intensive care: a report of a national study of pediatric intensive care units in the United kingdom. *Pediatrics* (2006) 118:2101–8. doi:10.1542/peds.2006-1455
94. Namachivayam P, Shann F, Shekerdemian L, Taylor A, van Sloten I, Delzoppo C, et al. Three decades of pediatric intensive care: who was admitted, what happened in intensive care, and what happened afterward. *Pediatr Crit Care Med* (2010) 11:549–55. doi:10.1097/PCC.0b013e3181ce7427
95. Visser IH, Hazelzet JA, Albers MJ, Verlaat CW, Hogenbirk K, van Woensel JB, et al. Mortality prediction models for pediatric intensive care: comparison of overall and subgroup specific performance. *Intensive Care Med* (2013) 39:942–50. doi:10.1007/s00134-013-2857-4
96. Burns JP, Sellers DE, Meyer EC, Lewis-Newby M, Truog RD. Epidemiology of death in the PICU at five U.S. teaching hospitals*. *Crit Care Med* (2014) 42:2101–8. doi:10.1097/CCM.0000000000000498
97. Nyirasafari R, Corden MH, Karambizi AC, Kabayiza JC, Makuza JD, Wong R, et al. Predictors of mortality in a paediatric intensive care unit in Kigali, Rwanda. *Paediatr Int Child Health* (2017) 37:109–15. doi:10.1080/20469047.2016.1250031
98. Khanal A, Sharma A, Basnet S. Current state of pediatric intensive care and high dependency care in Nepal. *Pediatr Crit Care Med* (2016) 17:1032–40. doi:10.1097/PCC.0000000000000938
99. Abebe T, Girmay M, G/Michael G, Tesfaye M. The epidemiological profile of pediatric patients admitted to the general intensive care unit in an Ethiopian university hospital. *Int J Gen Med* (2015) 8:63–7. doi:10.2147/IJGM.S76378
100. Ballot DE, Davies VA, Cooper PA, Chirwa T, Argent A, Mer M. Retrospective cross-sectional review of survival rates in critically ill children admitted to a combined paediatric/neonatal intensive care unit in Johannesburg, South Africa, 2013–2015. *BMJ Open* (2016) 6:e010850. doi:10.1136/bmjopen-2015-010850
101. Proulx F, Fayon M, Farrell CA, Lacroix J, Gauthier M. Epidemiology of sepsis and multiple organ dysfunction syndrome in children. *Chest* (1996) 109:1033–7. doi:10.1378/chest.109.4.1033
102. Leteurtre S, Duhamel A, Grandbastien B, Lacroix J, Leclerc F. Paediatric logistic organ dysfunction (PELOD) score. *Lancet* (2006) 367:897. doi:10.1016/S0140-6736(06)68371-2
103. Matics TJ, Sanchez-Pinto LN. Adaptation and validation of a pediatric sequential organ failure assessment score and evaluation of the sepsis-3 definitions in critically ill children. *JAMA Pediatr* (2017) 171:e172352. doi:10.1001/jamapediatrics.2017.2352
104. Wiens MO, Pawluk S, Kissoon N, Kumbakumba E, Ansermino JM, Singer J, et al. Pediatric post-discharge mortality in resource poor countries: a systematic review. *PLoS One* (2013) 8:e66698. doi:10.1371/journal.pone.0066698
105. Nwankwor OC, Wiens MO, Kissoon N. Post-discharge morbidity and mortality in children with sepsis. In: Vincent JL, editor. *Annual Update in Intensive Care and Emergency Medicine 2017*. Cham: Springer (2017). p. 431–44.
106. Moisi JC, Gatakaa H, Berkley JA, Maitland K, Mturi N, Newton CR, et al. Excess child mortality after discharge from hospital in Kilifi, Kenya: a retrospective cohort analysis. *Bull World Health Organ* (2011) 89:725–32, 732A. doi:10.2471/BLT.11.089235
107. Taylor HA. Inclusion of women, minorities, and children in clinical trials: opinions of research ethics board administrators. *J Empir Res Hum Res Ethics* (2009) 4:65–73. doi:10.1525/jer.2009.4.2.65
108. Fernandez C. Ethical issues in health research in children. *Paediatr Child Health* (2008) 13:707–12. doi:10.1093/pch/13.8.707
109. Report B. *National Commission for the Protection of Human Subjects of Biomedical and Behavioral Research. Ethical Principles and Guidelines for the Protection of Human Subjects of Research*. Washington, DC: U.S. Government Printing Office (1978).
110. Farmer P, Walton D, Tarter L. Infections and inequalities. *Global Change Hum Health* (2000) 1:94–109. doi:10.1023/A:1010088804348

14

Clinical Presentation and Outcomes among Children with Sepsis Presenting to a Public Tertiary Hospital in Tanzania

Teresa Bleakly Kortz[1,2], Hendry R. Sawe[3], Brittany Murray[3,4], Wayne Enanoria[5], Michael Anthony Matthay[6] and Teri Reynolds[2,3,7]*

[1] Division of Critical Care, Department of Pediatrics, University of California, San Francisco, San Francisco, CA, United States, [2] Institute for Global Health Sciences, University of California, San Francisco, San Francisco, CA, United States, [3] Department of Emergency Medicine, Muhimbili University of Health and Allied Sciences, Dar es Salaam, Tanzania, [4] Division of Pediatric Emergency Medicine, Department of Pediatrics, Emory University School of Medicine, Atlanta, GA, United States, [5] Department of Epidemiology and Biostatistics, University of California, San Francisco, San Francisco, CA, United States, [6] Division of Pulmonary and Critical Care, Department of Medicine, University of California, San Francisco, San Francisco, CA, United States, [7] Department of Emergency Medicine, University of California, San Francisco, San Francisco, CA, United States

***Correspondence:**
Teresa Bleakly Kortz
teresa.bleakly@ucsf.edu

Background: Pediatric sepsis causes significant global morbidity and mortality and low- and middle-income countries (LMICs) bear the bulk of the burden. International sepsis guidelines may not be relevant in LMICs, especially in sub-Saharan Africa (SSA), due to resource constraints and population differences. There is a critical lack of pediatric sepsis data from SSA, without which accurate risk stratification tools and context-appropriate, evidence-based protocols cannot be developed. The study's objectives were to characterize pediatric sepsis presentations, interventions, and outcomes in a public Emergency Medicine Department (EMD) in Tanzania.

Methods: Prospective descriptive study of children (28 days to 14 years) with sepsis [suspected infection with ≥2 clinical systemic inflammatory response syndrome (SIRS) criteria] presenting to a tertiary EMD in Dar es Salaam, Tanzania (July 1 to September 30, 2016). Outcomes included: in-hospital mortality (primary), EMD mortality, and hospital length of stay. We report descriptive statistics using means and SDs, medians and interquartile ranges, and counts and percentages as appropriate. Predictive abilities of SIRS criteria, the Alert-Verbal-Painful-Unresponsive (AVPU) score and the Lambaréné Organ Dysfunction Score (LODS) for in-hospital, early and late mortality were tested.

Results: Of the 2,232 children screened, 433 (19.4%) met inclusion criteria, and 405 were enrolled. There were 247 (61%) subjects referred from an outside facility. Approximately half (54.1%) received antibiotics in the EMD, and some form of microbiologic culture was collected in 35.8% (*n* = 145) of subjects. In-hospital and EMD mortality were 14.2 and 1.5%, respectively, median time to death was 3 days (IQR 1–6), and median length of stay was 6 days (IQR 1–12). SIRS criteria, the AVPU score, and the LODS had low positive (17–27.1, 33.3–43.9, 18.3–55.6%, respectively) and high negative predictive values (88.6–89.8, 86.5–91.2, 86.8–90.5%, respectively) for in-hospital mortality.

Conclusion: This pediatric sepsis cohort had high and early in-hospital mortality. Current criteria and tested clinical scores were inadequate for risk-stratification and mortality prediction in this population and setting. Pediatric sepsis management must take into account the local patient population, etiologies of sepsis, healthcare system, and resource availability. Only through studies such as this that generate regional data in LMICs can accurate risk stratification tools and context-appropriate, evidence-based guidelines be developed.

Keywords: global health, resource-limited, low-resource setting, pediatric critical care, pediatric emergency medicine, pediatric sepsis

INTRODUCTION

Sepsis represents a spectrum of disease involving a systemic inflammatory response syndrome (SIRS) in the setting of infection, escalating in septic shock to cardiovascular and organ system dysfunction (1). It is the final common inflammatory pathway for most infectious disease-related deaths (2, 3) and incurs significant pediatric morbidity and mortality worldwide (1–9). Globally, there were 2.6 million deaths due to infectious diseases in children and adolescents in 2015, and 66% of these deaths occurred in sub-Saharan Africa (SSA) (10). A recent, global point prevalence study in children in pediatric intensive care units with severe sepsis from 128 sites in 26 countries, showed an aggregated in-hospital mortality rate of 25% (11). The identification and initial care of children with sepsis can significantly impact survival (12–14), and both delays in presentation (15) and delays in diagnosis have been shown to be risk factors for poor outcomes in low- and middle-income countries (LMICs) (14). The Surviving Sepsis Campaign's international guidelines set standards for early identification, resuscitation, and protocol-based management, which have been shown to substantially impact outcomes (16). Much of the recommended sepsis management, especially regarding goal-directed interventions, is dependent on frequent or invasive monitoring that is not reliably available in limited resource settings and healthcare providers in LMICs often face resource constraints that limit capacity to implement these guidelines (13).

Beyond resource gaps that may limit the usability of international management guidelines, there is recent evidence suggesting that the clinical effectiveness of some interventions may be context-dependent. In 2011, Maitland et al., published results from a large, multicenter, randomized controlled trial: Fluid Expansion as Supportive Therapy (FEAST) (8). In this trial, African children with severe febrile illness who received fluid bolus resuscitation had a significantly higher relative risk (RR) of mortality compared to children who received only maintenance fluids (RR for any bolus vs. control, 1.45; 95% CI, 1.13–1.86; $P = 0.003$) (8). Current international guidelines recommend fluid bolus resuscitation for severe sepsis and septic shock (1, 16–20), but the unexpected results from the FEAST trial call into question whether practice guidelines primarily developed in high-income countries (HICs) are appropriate for LMICs. This may be especially true in malaria endemic regions given the increased possibility of shock secondary to severe anemia as compared to septic shock due to bacteremia (21, 22).

There is a critical lack of region-specific and relevant pediatric sepsis data, and few pediatric sepsis cohorts exist in SSA (7). While we recognize pediatric sepsis to be a global burden, we lack a robust understanding of how best to identify and manage sepsis in settings where triage and goal-directed therapy are challenging given the scarcity of invasive monitoring, laboratory tests, and medical personnel and where HIV, malaria, malnutrition, and limited access to care frequently complicate management. Tanzania is one such setting with a paucity of data on the profile and outcomes of children with sepsis. Thus, the objective of this prospective study was to characterize the clinical presentation, emergency interventions received, and outcomes among children with sepsis presenting to Muhimbili National Hospital (MNH) in Tanzania. The generation of region-specific data is needed to accurately risk stratify patients, develop appropriate protocols for early recognition, and implement evidence-based treatment protocols.

MATERIALS AND METHODS

This prospective descriptive study included pediatric patients presenting with sepsis to an urban, tertiary Emergency Medicine Department (EMD) at the National Referral Hospital in Dar es Salaam, Tanzania (MNH) between July 1 and September 30, 2016. The EMD is the receiving department for all acutely ill and injured patients, and is the only 24-h, full capacity public EMD in Tanzania. It is also the training site for the only emergency medicine residency in the country and cares for an average of 60,000 patients annually, and children comprise approximately 25% of the patient population. Pediatric sepsis is common at MNH; the EMD cares for an estimated 150–200 children with sepsis monthly (23, 24).

The EMD is equipped to provide plain radiographs, bedside ultrasound, continuous cardiorespiratory monitoring, low-flow oxygen, bag mask ventilation, intubation, mechanical ventilation, blood product transfusions, vasoactive medications, and resuscitation medications. MNH has a large general pediatrics ward, a high-dependency unit (HDU), and no dedicated pediatric intensive care unit. In general, the MNH ward can administer intermittent medications, intravenous fluids, low-flow oxygen, and blood products and measure vital signs every shift. The HDU is similar to the ward with a more favorable nursing ratio. Vasoactive infusions, intubation and mechanical ventilation are not routinely available for children outside of the EMD.

Children were included if they were between 28 days and 14 years of age and met criteria for sepsis, defined as having two or more clinical SIRS criteria (**Box 1**) with a suspected infection. At MNH, patients younger than 28 days present directly to the maternity and neonatal ward, and those over 14 years are triaged to adult rooms and admitted to the adult ward. SIRS criteria is defined per international pediatric sepsis consensus definitions (1), adapted for resource-limited settings (12). All pediatric patients presenting to the EMD were screened. Patients in cardiac arrest on presentation or with acute trauma were excluded. Written consent was obtained prior to enrollment. The primary outcome was in-hospital mortality. Secondary outcomes included EMD mortality and hospital length of stay.

Patient data included: patient characteristics [age, sex, mid-upper arm circumference (MUAC), severity of illness]; patient comorbidities (HIV, malaria, TB, malnutrition); vital signs and SIRS criteria on admission; delay to care (onset of illness, facilities visited prior to MNH, duration of fever); socioeconomic status indicators (insurance status, parents' education levels, parental literacy, number of children in the household, number of children under 5 in the household); interventions and therapies received in the EMD; relevant laboratory results; and outcomes. All diagnostic and therapeutic decisions were made at the discretion of the treating physician. Severe malnutrition was defined as a MUAC of ≤11.5 cm and severe anemia was defined as a hemoglobin ≤5 g/dL. Level of consciousness was assessed with the AVPU score (alert, responds to verbal stimuli, responds to pain, unresponsive) and severity of illness was measured with the 4-point Lambaréné Organ Dysfunction Score (LODS) (**Box 2**) (25). The LODS is a simple clinical prediction score for mortality validated in African children ≤15 years, including malaria endemic regions (25, 26). Early and late mortality were defined as death within 48 and ≥48 h of presentation, respectively. Microbiological investigations including cultures are not routinely performed on all patients, but results were recorded when available.

Research personnel collected data from the electronic medical record, paper chart, care provider, and guardian. Study data were managed using REDCap electronic data capture tools (version 7.2.2) hosted at MNH (27). Data were deidentified prior to analysis. This study was carried out in accordance with the recommendations and approval of the Institutional Review Boards and Committees on Human Research at Muhimbili University of Health and Allied Sciences (Ref. No. 2016-03-30/AEC/Vol.X/201) and the University of California, San Francisco (IRB # 16-18977, Ref. No. 161295). We obtained written, informed consent from all guardians and assent from subjects when appropriate in accordance with the Declaration of Helsinki.

BOX 1 | Clinical SIRS Criteria for Resource-Limited Settings (12).

Presence of ≥2 of the following 4 criteria with a suspected or proven infection:

- Abnormal temperature (axillary >38 or <36.0°C) documented or by history.
- Abnormal heart rate for age: tachycardia OR bradycardia (<1 year).
- Respiratory insufficiency: tachypnea for age, hypoxia (S_pO_2 <92%), NIPPV, OR mechanical ventilation.
- Ill-appearing, in distress, OR not responsive.

BOX 2 | Lambaréné Organ Dysfunction Score (LODS) (2, 6, 25).

Validated in African children ≤15 years with and without malaria. The score assigns one point for each of the following:

- Prostration—defined as ≥1 of the following, depending on age: inability to breastfeed, sit, stand, or walk unsupported.
- Coma—Blantyre Coma Score ≤2.
- Deep breathing.

Statistical Analysis

All data analysis and descriptive statistics were performed using Stata/MP (14.2), including means and SDs, medians and interquartile ranges, and counts and percentages as appropriate for the data type and distribution. We evaluated the ability of number of SIRS criteria, the AVPU score and the LODS to predict in-hospital mortality in this population. Scoring system discrimination was evaluated by comparing positive and negative predictive values.

RESULTS

A total of 2,232 children presented to the EMD during the study period. There were 433 patients (19.4%) who had SIRS with a suspected infection, 28 children were excluded, and 405 subjects were successfully enrolled (**Figure 1**). Of those enrolled, 402 (99.3%) were followed to hospital discharge.

Baseline Patient Characteristics

The median age of children with sepsis at MNH was 25 months (IQR 11–63 months), and 73.1% were under 5 years of age (n = 296) (**Table 1**). Severe malnutrition was present in 12.6% (n = 51) of children, 6.9% (n = 28) tested positive for malaria by rapid diagnostic test (RDT) or microscopy, 1.7% (n = 7) had confirmed (by RDT or antibody testing) or a known history of HIV, and 12.8% (n = 52) of subjects were tested for HIV during hospitalization. The mean hemoglobin was 8.3 g/dL (n = 305), and 16.1% (n = 49) of children presented with severe anemia. The mean venous blood gas pH among those tested (n = 184) was 7.36 (SD 0.14), while the mean lactate (n = 177) was 3.2 mmol/L (SD 3.5). The majority of children (61.7%, n = 250) presented with fever: of these, 36.4% (n = 91) had fever only by history and 63.6% (n = 159) had a documented fever on arrival. Almost 66% of patients (205/311) reported a fever duration greater than 48 hours and the mean fever duration was 8.7 days (SD 27.5). Over half of the patients (61%, n = 247) were referred to MNH from an outside hospital or clinic. Among referred patients, 47.5% (116/244) had been administered antibiotics before arrival to MNH. Up-to-date immunization status was reported in 97.3% (n = 394) of patients.

Socioeconomic Status Indicators

Regarding insurance status, 42.5% (n = 172) of subjects were uninsured, though 76.2% (n = 131) of uninsured patients were categorically exempt from paying medical expenses by Tanzanian law based on age or disease status (**Table 1**). Paternal and maternal literacy rates were similar at 95.9 (n = 372) and 92.3% (n = 371), respectively, though more fathers completed secondary school or higher education than mothers (43.5 and 34.6%, n = 176 and 149, respectively). The median number of children younger than

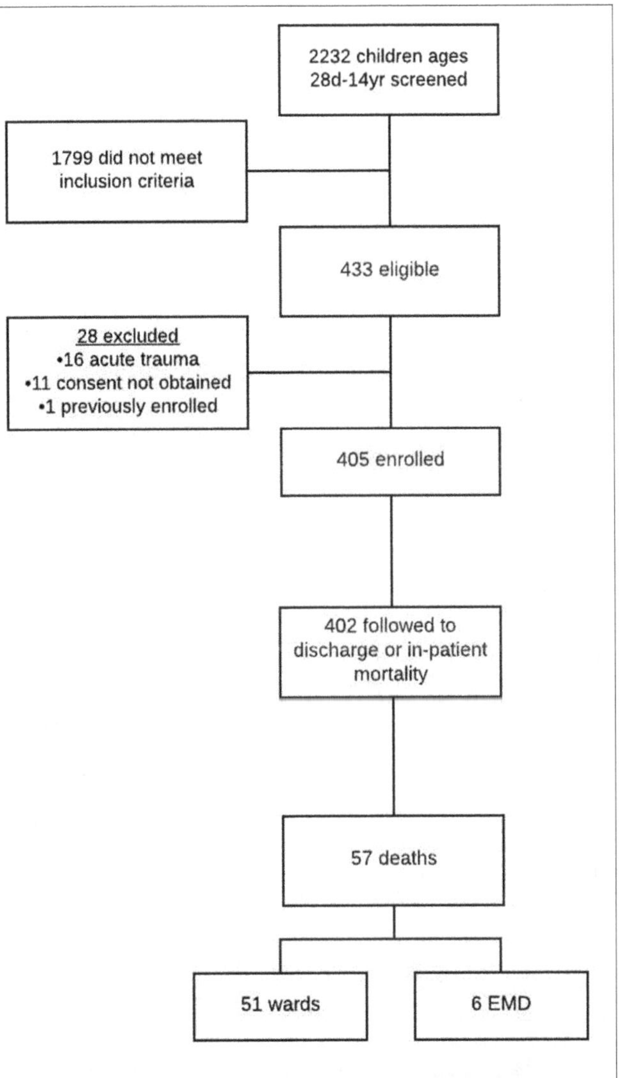

FIGURE 1 | Patient screening, enrollment, and outcomes flowchart.

18 years in the patient household was 2 (IQR 1–3). Ninety-five percent (n = 403) of families reported having regular access to an "improved" drinking water source, defined by the WHO/UNICEF Joint Monitoring Programme as a water source that is protected from sewage (28). Almost 71% (n = 283) of families had electricity, and 56.8% (n = 230) had toilets in the home.

Illness Severity

On arrival, 82% (n = 331) of children were "alert" by the AVPU score. Using the LODS as a measure of illness severity, 46.7% (n = 189) of subjects had the lowest severity score of zero, while 17.8% (n = 72) had a score of two or more. The median number of documented SIRS criteria was 3 (IQR 2–3), with 41.2 (n = 167), 41.0 (n = 166), and 17.8% (n = 72) of subjects meeting 2, 3, and 4 criteria, respectively. Respiratory insufficiency was the most common SIRS criteria, occurring in 86.4% (n = 350) of patients, followed by abnormal temperature, abnormal heart rate, and abnormal appearance occurring in 70.9 (n = 287), 60 (n = 243), and 53.3% (n = 216) of patients, respectively (**Table 2**).

TABLE 1 | Patient characteristics.

	Total (*N* = 405)
Demographics	
Age (months), median (IQR)	25 (11–63)
<2 years, *n* (%)	195 (48.2)
2–5 years, *n* (%)	101 (24.9)
>5 years, *n* (%)	109 (26.9)
Male sex, *n* (%)	236 (58.3)
MUAC, mean (SD)	14.7 (4.1)
≤11.5 cm, *n* (%)	51 (12.6)
Malaria positive, *n* (%)	28 (6.9)
HIV positive, *n* (%)	7 (1.7)
Fully immunized, *n* (%)	394 (97.3)
Illness severity and level of consciousness	
Lambaréné Organ Dysfunction Score	
LODS 0, *n* (%)	189 (46.7)
LODS 1, *n* (%)	144 (35.6)
LODS 2, *n* (%)	63 (15.6)
LODS 3, *n* (%)	9 (2.2)
AVPU score	
Alert, *n* (%)	331 (82.8)
Responds to verbal, *n* (%)	11 (2.8)
Responds to pain, *n* (%)	40 (10)
Unresponsive, *n* (%)	18 (4.5)
Missing	5 (1.3)
No. of SIRS criteria met, median (IQR)	3 (2–3)
2, *n* (%)	167 (41.2)
3, *n* (%)	166 (41)
4, *n* (%)	72 (17.8)
Laboratory values	
Hemoglobin (g/dL) (*n* = 305), mean (SD)	8.3 (3.0)
≤5 g/dL, *n* (%)	49/305 (16.1)
>10 g/dL, *n* (%)	85/305 (27.2)
WBC count ×10^3 (*n* = 305), mean (SD)	16.6 (22.4)
Platelet count ×10^3 (*N* = 304), mean (SD)	322 (201.6)
Venous blood gas pH (*n* = 184), mean (SD)	7.36 (0.14)
Bicarbonate (mEq/L) (*n* = 185), mean (SD)	21.3 (6.5)
Lactate (mmol/L) (*n* = 177), mean (SD)	3.2 (3.5)
Sodium (mEq/L) (*n* = 199), mean (SD)	132.5 (7.2)
Potassium (mEq/L) (*n* = 199), mean (SD)	4.1 (1.3)
Glucose (mmol/L) (*n* = 243), mean (SD)	6.6 (3.6)
Prehospital course	
Fever, *n* (%)	250 (61.7)
Documented, *n* (%)	159/250 (63.6)
By history, *n* (%)	91/250 (36.4)
Days of fever, mean (SD)	8.7 (27.5)
>2 days, *n* (%)	205/311 (65.9)
Hospital/clinic referral, *n* (%)	247 (61.0)
Antibiotics prearrival, *n* (%)	116/244 (47.5)
Socioeconomic status indicators	
Insured, *n* (%)	172 (42.5)
Exempt status, *n* (%)	131 (32.4)
Paternal literacy	372/388 (95.9)
Father's highest level of education	
No formal school	12 (3)
Primary school	190 (46.9)
Secondary school	95 (23.5)
University or advanced degree	81 (20)
Unknown	27 (6.7)
Maternal literacy	372/403 (92.3)
Mother's highest level of education	
No formal school	28 (6.9)
Primary school	228 (56.3)
Secondary school	78 (19.3)
University or advanced degree	62 (15.3)

(Continued)

TABLE 1 | Continued

	Total (*N* = 405)
Unknown	9 (2.2)
Number of children <18 in the household, median (IQR)	2 (1–3)
Number of children <5 in the household, median (IQR)	1 (1–2)
Electricity in the home	283/400 (70.8)
Improved water source, *n* (%)	403/423 (95.3)
Tap in the home, *n* (%)	96/403 (23.8)
Public tap, *n* (%)	214/403 (53.1)
Well, *n* (%)	93/403 (23.1)
Unimproved water source	20/423 (4.7)
Purchased water (bottled or truck)	9/20 (45.0)
Unprotected surface water	11/20 (55.0)
Toilet in the home	230 (56.8)

IQR, interquartile range; MUAC, mid-upper arm circumference; LODS, Lambaréné Organ Dysfunction Score; AVPU, alert-verbal-pain-unresponsive score; SIRS, systemic inflammatory response syndrome; WBC, white blood cell.

TABLE 2 | Frequency of SIRS criteria for patients enrolled in the study.

SIRS criterion	Total (*N* = 405)
Abnormal temperature, *n* (%)	287 (70.9)
Temperature, mean (SD)	37.7 (1.0)
Abnormal heart rate, *n* (%)	243 (60)
Tachycardia, *n* (%)	235 (58.0)
Bradycardia, *n* (%)	8 (2.0)
Respiratory insufficiency, *n* (%)	350 (86.4)
Tachypnea, *n* (%)	330 (81.5)
Hypoxia, *n* (%)	76 (18.8)
S_pO_2, mean (SD)	95.5 (10.3)
Abnormal appearance, *n* (%)	216 (53.3)
Ill-appearing, *n* (%)	203 (50.1)
Distress, *n* (%)	21 (5.2)
Prostrate, *n* (%)	7(1.7)

SIRS, systemic inflammatory response syndrome.

EMD Interventions

The most common EMD interventions included: antibiotic administration (54.1%, *n* = 219), fluid administration (38.8%, *n* = 157), oxygen therapy (24.5%, *n* = 99), chest radiograph (11.9%, *n* = 48), blood transfusion (11.2%, *n* = 45), and antimalarial medication administration (9.2%, *n* = 37) (**Table 3**). Three percent (*n* = 4) of pediatric sepsis patients had a blood culture drawn in the EMD, while 75.6% (*n* = 306) and 4.2% (*n* = 17) were tested with malaria and HIV RDTs, respectively. Few patients were intubated and received mechanical ventilation (1.2%, *n* = 5). While patients presenting in cardiac arrest were excluded, 1.2% (*n* = 5) of patients decompensated to require cardiopulmonary resuscitation (CPR) in the EMD.

Some form of microbiologic culture was collected during hospitalization in 35.8% (*n* = 145) of patients: blood, urine and cerebral spinal fluid (CSF) cultures were collected in 29.9, 14.8, and 4.0% of patients, respectively (**Table 4**). Of the cultures collected, 11.6, 10, and 0% of blood, urine and CSF were positive, respectively.

Outcomes

Of the 402 patients followed to discharge, 57 patients died in the hospital, yielding an in-hospital mortality of 14.2% (**Table 5**).

TABLE 3 | Interventions received in the EMD.

Intervention	*n* (%) (*N* = 405)
Fluid administration	157 (38.8)
Blood transfusion ordered	45 (11.1)
Blood initiated in EMD	25/45 (55.6)
Antibiotics received in the EMD	219 (54.1)
Antibiotics received prearrival, not in the EMD	40 (9.9)
Blood culture drawn in the EMD	4 (1.0)
HIV rapid diagnostic test	17 (4.2)
Malaria rapid diagnostic test	306 (75.6)
Vasoactive infusion	1 (0.2)
Hydrocortisone	1 (0.2)
Antimalarial medications	37 (9.1)
Oxygen	99 (24.4)
Chest radiograph	48 (11.9)
Ultrasound	12 (3.0)
Intubation and mechanical ventilation	5 (1.2)
CPR initiated	5 (1.2)
ROSC	1/5 (20)

EMD, Emergency Medicine Department; CPR, cardiopulmonary resuscitation; ROSC, return of spontaneous circulation.

TABLE 4 | Frequency of microbiologic tests performed and culture result positivity.

Microbiology	*n* (%)
Any microbiological culture performed	145/405 (35.8)
Blood culture	
Collected at any time during hospitalization	121/405 (29.9)
Culture positive	14/121 (11.6)
Urine culture	
Collected at any time during hospitalization	60/405 (14.8)
Culture positive	6/60 (10.0)
CSF culture	
Collected at any time during hospitalization	16/405 (4.0)
Culture positive	0/16 (0)

CSF, cerebral spinal fluid.

TABLE 5 | In-hospital outcomes for pediatric patients with sepsis.

Outcome	
EMD mortality, *n* (%)	6/402 (1.5)
In-hospital mortality, *n* (%)	57/402 (14.2)
Ward mortality, *n* (%)	51/57 (89.5)
EMD mortality	6/57 (10.5)
<48-h mortality, *n* (%)	20/57 (35.1)
≥48-h mortality, *n* (%)	37/57 (64.9)
Time to death (days), median (IQR)	3 (1–6)
Length of stay all subjects (days), median (IQR)	6 (1–12)

IQR, interquartile range.

Six subjects died in the EMD, representing 10.5% (6/57) of the patients who died, and the overall in-ED mortality was 1.5% (6/402). The median time to death was 3 days (IQR 1–6 days) and 35.1% (*n* = 20) of the patients who died did so within 48-h of presentation. The cumulative probability of mortality rose sharply until hospital day 7 (15.4%) and then rose gradually until hospital day 22 when it plateaued at 25.9% (**Figure 2**). The median length of stay for all patients was 6 days (IQR 1–12 days). SIRS criteria and LODS were available on all 402 subjects, while AVPU scores and in-hospital outcomes were available on 98.6% (397/402) of subjects. All five of the patients with missing AVPU scores survived to discharge. In this population, case-fatality rates increased with rising LODS and number of SIRS criteria, but less so with worsening AVPU score (**Figure 3**). We explored early mortality with respect to interventions received in the EMD: 80% (n = 16) received a fluid bolus, two of who were malnourished, and 85% (n = 17) received antibiotics in the EMD (**Table 6**). All three scores—AVPU, LODS, and SIRS—had low positive predictive values, and higher negative predictive values for in-hospital, early and late mortality (**Table 7**). This was also true in patient subgroups with malnutrition and severe anemia.

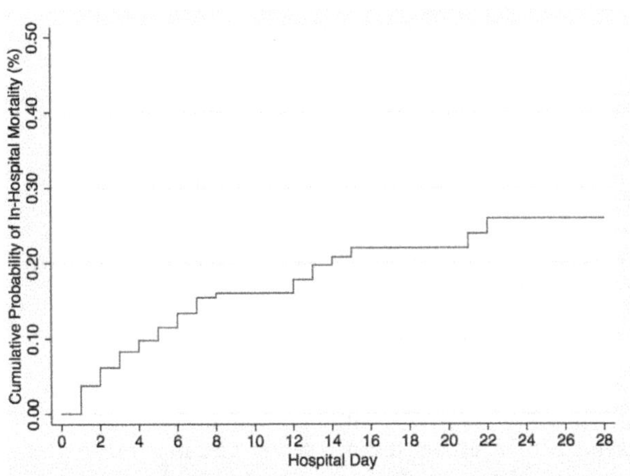

FIGURE 2 | Cumulative probability of in-hospital mortality by hospital day.

TABLE 6 | Early mortality due to sepsis and key EMD interventions.

	Early mortality (*N* = 20)
Fluid bolus in the EMD, *n* (%)	16 (80.0)
Malnourished, *n* (%)	2/11 (18.8)
Blood transfusion, *n* (%)	2 (10)
Severe anemia, *n* (%)	1/14 (7.1)
Antibiotics prearrival, *n* (%)	8/17 (34.5)
Antibiotics in the EMD, *n* (%)	17 (85.0)[a]
Antibiotics prearrival or EMD, *n* (%)	19 (95.0)
Antimalarial medication in the EMD, *n* (%)	4 (20.0)[b]
Malaria positive, *n* (%)	2 (10.0)

[a]*Six patients received antibiotics prearrival and in the EMD.*
[b]*Two patients tested negative and were treated.*
EMD, Emergency Medicine Department.

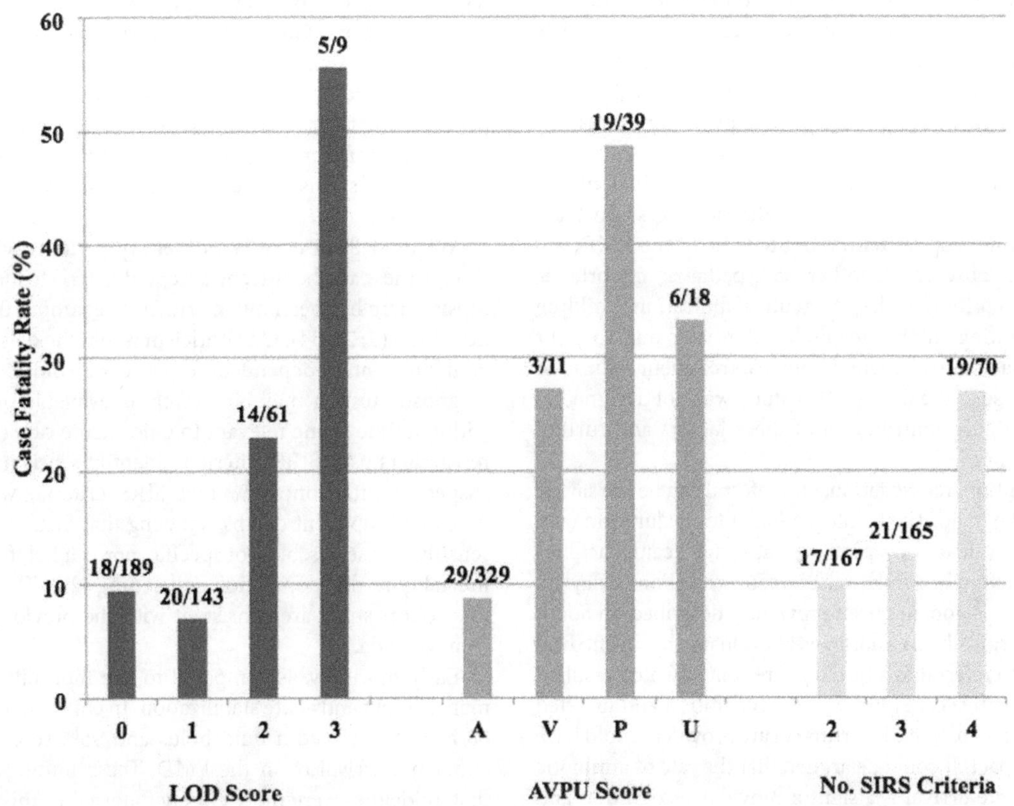

FIGURE 3 | Case fatality rates by Lambaréné Organ Dysfunction Score, best response by the Alert-Verbal-Painful-Unresponsive (AVPU) score, and number of SIRS criteria present on admission.

TABLE 7 | Positive and negative predictive values for clinical scores (LODS, AVPU, SIRS criteria) predicting in-hospital (subgroups malnutrition and severe anemia), early and late mortality.

Severity of illness measure	Positive predictive value					Negative predictive value				
	Total (%)	Malnutrition (%)	Severe anemia (%)	Early mortality (%)	Late mortality (%)	Total (%)	Malnutrition (%)	Severe anemia (%)	Early mortality (%)	Late mortality (%)
LODS										
≥1	18.3	21.7	21.4	40.0	10.6	90.5	87.5	90.0	77.8	92.6
≥2	27.1	37.5	12.5	47.4	13.9	88.6	87.0	82.5	71.8	91.9
3	55.6	19.4	50.0	60.0	22.2	86.8	[a]	84.8	67.9	91.2
AVPU score best response										
Verbal or worse	41.2	42.9	16.7	39.3	24.6	91.2	87.5	83.3	70.0	94.0
Pain or worse	43.9	40.0	20.0	40.0	25.9	90.6	84.6	83.7	69.7	93.6
Unresponsive	33.3	[a]	[a]	50.0	16.7	86.5	78.6	82.6	67.3	91.1
SIRS criteria										
≥3	17.0	20.0	19.4	37.5	10.5	89.8	81.2	88.2	72.2	92.8
4	27.1	25.0	25.0	42.1	15.3	88.6	81.5	87.5	69.2	92.2

[a]Too few subjects in a cell to calculate.
LODS, Lambaréné Organ Dysfunction Score; AVPU, alert-verbal-pain-unresponsive score; SIRS, systemic inflammatory response syndrome.

DISCUSSION

This pediatric sepsis cohort had a high overall in-hospital mortality of 14.2%, substantially greater than a recent sepsis cohort in Uganda (5.4%) (29) and 48-h mortality in the FEAST trial (approximately 10%) (8). Almost 85% of deaths occurred within the first seven days of hospitalization, and over half of all deaths were within 72 h. Using SIRS criteria as a screening tool and requirement for study inclusion, the addition of the LODS, AVPU, or additional SIRS criteria were not useful in predicting in-hospital, early or late mortality in any of the tested subgroups, illustrating the difficulty of risk-stratification and mortality prediction in this patient population and setting.

The overwhelming majority of children who died did so on the ward and not in the EMD. Pediatric sepsis mortality occurring early in hospitalization, but outside of the EMD, has previously been observed in other SSA pediatric cohorts (8, 29). This may signify that despite acute stabilization, children are decompensating in the hospital, potentially due to poor monitoring, a lack of treatment resources, treatment failure, or the natural course of the disease; this study was not designed to assess the individual contribution of these factors and further investigation is needed.

Early recognition, resuscitation, and referral can be life saving in sepsis; yet, the majority of children had a fever duration over 48 h and were evaluated by providers at other health facilities prior to presentation at MNH, raising concerns about delays to definitive care. This, too, has been previously described; in South Africa, 40% of critically ill children were evaluated by >1 medical provider prior to referral to a tertiary care center, which resulted in delays in definitive care (30). Earlier recognition and targeted referral of high-risk patients by primary care providers could have a significant impact. It could be argued that the rate of antibiotic administration pre-arrival is a sign of provider recognition and treatment of sepsis, though additional exploration of referral patterns and therapies received in primary and secondary health facilities are required to address these aspects of care.

There are several limitations to this study. This cohort presented to an urban, tertiary center and may not reflect the general population in Tanzania. Parents in this cohort had a higher literacy rate (>90%) than previously reported for the general Tanzanian population (80.4%) (31) and 95% of families reported using an "improved" water source, significantly more than the 2015 national average of 55.6% (28), though there are legitimate concerns regarding tap water quality and safety (32, 33) in Tanzania. Given the inclusion criteria, this cohort was likely to be a sicker cohort than the general pediatric population; therefore, results cannot be extrapolated and applied to a general pediatric population. However, since a primary objective was to inform therapy guidelines and recommendations for the treatment of sepsis at a tertiary center, this was an ideal cohort to study.

We used SIRS criteria to identify patients with sepsis, and though these are the current, accepted criteria to identify pediatric sepsis, there has been much criticism regarding this operational definition (7, 29, 34). One criticism is that the definition of sepsis is highly context-dependent, especially in LMIC settings where diagnostic testing may be entirely unavailable or not available within a time frame relevant to guide acute care (7). In Uganda, researchers used SIRS criteria to identify sepsis in children with suspected infection; 86% met SIRS criteria, which captured 94% of all inpatient deaths, showing that SIRS criteria is highly sensitive for sepsis, but not specific, nor is it helpful in predicting mortality in this population and setting (29). The findings from this cohort study are consistent with the previous study results from Uganda.

Early mortality, as compared to late mortality, reflects EMD management and acute stabilization. In children who died within 48-h, 80% received a fluid bolus and 95% received antibiotics either pre-arrival or in the EMD. These findings could signify that guidelines were more closely followed in this subgroup, but failed to alter disease progression. Another possibility is that the intervention (i.e., fluid bolus) may potentially be contributing to early mortality as was seen in the FEAST trial (8). Further analyses are required to determine guideline compliance and the association of fluid bolus with mortality.

We found that pathogen identification with conventional microbiological techniques were low-yield and not frequently used, making it difficult to determine the etiology of sepsis. A malaria RDT was far more likely to be performed than a blood culture in children with sepsis. This may be due to several factors. First, a significant percentage of children received antibiotics prior to arrival to the EMD Second, the majority of blood cultures were drawn in the ward and not in the EMD and cultures were not routinely drawn prior to initiation of antibiotics. Third, blood culture collection supplies, specifically the bottles, may not always be readily available. Finally, some clinicians expressed general distrust of the microbiologic results and did not think the results changed management.

We also found that 36% ($N = 146$) of children did not receive antibiotics in the EMD or prior to arrival despite antibiotic administration being an essential component of international guidelines (1, 16, 18). The low rate of antibiotic administration may have resulted from limited drug availability, failure to identify sepsis, the need for urgent treatment, incomplete documentation of drug administration, or some combination of these factors. Further work is necessary to elucidate the underlying cause of low antibiotic usage in this setting. Depending on the cause, early antibiotic administration in the EMD for children with sepsis is a potential future quality improvement project.

Some data were extracted from the chart and may not have captured all interventions performed; however, the presence of research assistants actively observing actions in the EMD likely minimized this effect. Simultaneously, having research assistants physically present in the EMD may have influenced providers' practices, producing an observer effect. The most likely results of such an effect would be increased provider awareness of sepsis and improved guideline compliance. We did not capture a metric for provider awareness, and guideline compliance in general was poor (not reported here), though antibiotic administration and blood culture collection are two indicators, which is consistent with prior pilot data from MNH.

In summary, pediatric sepsis management must take into account the local context; the unique patient population and its comorbidities, coinfections, and etiologies of sepsis; where and how the population accesses the healthcare system; and available resources including medical personnel and monitoring capabilities. Though there are many challenges to data collection in resource-limited settings—lack of research infrastructure, incomplete documentation, severe personnel shortages, inadequate funding, and technical difficulties performing follow-up—we have generated high-quality regional data that can be used to develop an accurate risk stratification tool and inform context-appropriate, evidence-based guidelines in this setting. This is the first, critical step towards improving pediatric sepsis outcomes in SSA.

ETHICS STATEMENT

Research personnel collected data from the electronic medical record, paper chart, care provider, and guardian and then entered it into REDCap (version 7.2.2). Data were deidentified prior to analysis. This study was carried out in accordance with the recommendations and approval of the Institutional Review Boards and Committees on Human Research at Muhimbili University of Health and Allied Sciences (Ref. No. 2016-03-30/AEC/Vol.X/201) and the University of California, San Francisco (IRB # 16-18977, Ref. No. 161295). We obtained written, informed consent from all guardians and assent from subjects when appropriate in accordance with the Declaration of Helsinki.

AUTHOR CONTRIBUTIONS

Author contributions are as follows: conception and design of the work (TK, HS, BM, WE, and TR); data acquisition (TK, HS, and BM); data analysis (TK); data interpretation (TK, HS, BM, MM, and TR); first draft of the manuscript (TK); and manuscript revision and editing, final approval of the version to be published, and agreement to be accountable for all aspects of the work (TK, HS, BM, WE, MM, and TR).

ACKNOWLEDGMENTS

We would like to acknowledge Victoria Mlele for her hard work and dedication to this project, as well as Jeff Fineman, Catherine Reuben, and the research assistants at Muhimbili National Hospital for their contributions. Some of the results in this manuscript were presented at the 2017 Pediatric Academic Society meeting (35) and the 2017 Consortium of Universities for Global Health conference (36) and published in an abstract that appeared in *Lancet Global Health* (37).

REFERENCES

1. Goldstein B, Giroir B, Randolph A. International pediatric sepsis consensus conference: definitions for sepsis and organ dysfunction in pediatrics. *Pediatr Crit Care Med* (2005) 6(1):2–8. doi:10.1097/01.PCC.0000149131.72248.E6
2. Kissoon N, Carcillo JA, Espinosa V, Argent A, Devictor D, Madden M, et al. World federation of pediatric intensive care and critical care societies: global sepsis initiative. *Pediatr Crit Care Med* (2011) 12(5):494–503. doi:10.1097/PCC.0b013e318207096c
3. Watson RS, Carcillo JA. Scope and epidemiology of pediatric sepsis. *Pediatr Crit Care Med* (2005) 6(3 Suppl):S3–5. doi:10.1097/01.PCC.0000161289.22464.C3
4. Jawad I, Luksic I, Rafnsson SB. Assessing available information on the burden of sepsis: global estimates of incidence, prevalence and mortality. *J Glob Health* (2012) 2(1):010404. doi:10.7189/jogh.02.010404
5. Liu L, Oza S, Hogan D, Perin J, Rudan I, Lawn JE, et al. Global, regional, and national causes of child mortality in 2000-13, with projections to inform post-2015 priorities: an updated systematic analysis. *Lancet* (2014) 388(10063):3027–35. doi:10.1016/S0140-6736(16)31593-8

6. Mangia CMF, Kissoon N, Carcillo JA. Sepsis and septic shock: a global overview. *J Pediatric Infect Dis* (2009) 4(2):71–6. doi:10.3233/JPI-2009-0157
7. Wiens MO, Kumbakumba E, Kissoon N, Ansermino JM, Ndamira A, Larson CP. Pediatric sepsis in the developing world: challenges in defining sepsis and issues in post-discharge mortality. *Clin Epidemiol* (2012) 4:319–25. doi:10.2147/CLEP.S35693
8. Maitland K, Kiguli S, Opoka RO, Engoru C, Olupot-Olupot P, Akech SO, et al. Mortality after fluid bolus in African children with severe infection. *N Engl J Med* (2011) 364(26):2483–95. doi:10.1056/NEJMoa1101549
9. Maitland K, George EC, Evans JA, Kiguli S, Olupot-Olupot P, Akech SO, et al. Exploring mechanisms of excess mortality with early fluid resuscitation: insights from the FEAST trial. *BMC Med* (2013) 11:68. doi:10.1186/1741-7015-11-68
10. Kassebaum N, Kyu HH, Zoeckler L, Olsen HE, Thomas K, Pinho C, et al. Child and adolescent health from 1990 to 2015: findings from the global burden of diseases, injuries, and risk factors 2015 study. *JAMA Pediatr* (2017) 171(6):573–92. doi:10.1001/jamapediatrics.2017.0250
11. Weiss SL, Fitzgerald JC, Pappachan J, Wheeler D, Jaramillo-Bustamante JC, Salloo A, et al. Global epidemiology of pediatric severe sepsis: the sepsis prevalence, outcomes, and therapies study. *Am J Respir Crit Care Med* (2015) 191(10):1147–57. doi:10.1164/rccm.201412-2323OC
12. Dunser MW, Festic E, Dondorp A, Kissoon N, Ganbat T, Kwizera A, et al. Recommendations for sepsis management in resource-limited settings. *Intensive Care Med* (2012) 38(4):557–74. doi:10.1007/s00134-012-2521-4
13. Baelani I, Jochberger S, Laimer T, Otieno D, Kabutu J, Wilson I, et al. Availability of critical care resources to treat patients with severe sepsis or septic shock in Africa: a self-reported, continent-wide survey of anaesthesia providers. *Crit Care* (2011) 15(1):R10. doi:10.1186/cc9410
14. Jacob ST, Moore CC, Banura P, Pinkerton R, Meya D, Opendi P, et al. Severe sepsis in two Ugandan hospitals: a prospective observational study of management and outcomes in a predominantly HIV-1 infected population. *PLoS One* (2009) 4(11):e7782. doi:10.1371/journal.pone.0007782
15. Wang Y, Sun B, Yue H, Lin X, Li B, Yang X, et al. An epidemiologic survey of pediatric sepsis in regional hospitals in China. *Pediatr Crit Care Med* (2014) 15(9):814–20. doi:10.1097/PCC.0000000000000247
16. Dellinger RP, Levy MM, Rhodes A, Annane D, Gerlach H, Opal SM, et al. Surviving sepsis campaign: international guidelines for management of severe sepsis and septic shock: 2012. *Crit Care Med* (2013) 41(2):580–637. doi:10.1097/CCM.0b013e31827e83af
17. de Oliveira CF. Early goal-directed therapy in treatment of pediatric septic shock. *Shock* (2010) 34(Suppl 1):44–7. doi:10.1097/SHK.0b013e3181e7e6d5
18. WHO. *Hospital Care for Children: Guidelines for the Management of Common Illnesses with Limited Resources*. Geneva: World Health Organization (2013).
19. Brierley J, Carcillo JA, Choong K, Cornell T, Decaen A, Deymann A, et al. Clinical practice parameters for hemodynamic support of pediatric and neonatal septic shock: 2007 update from the American College of Critical Care Medicine. *Crit Care Med* (2009) 37(2):666–88. doi:10.1097/CCM.0b013e31819323c6
20. de Oliveira CF, de Oliveira DSF, Gottschald AFC, Moura JDG, Costa GA, Ventura AC, et al. ACCM/PALS haemodynamic support guidelines for paediatric septic shock: an outcomes comparison with and without monitoring central venous oxygen saturation. *Intensive Care Med* (2008) 34(6):1065–75. doi:10.1007/s00134-008-1085-9
21. Barreiro P, Tiziano G, Fano H, Yohannes T, Gosa A, Reyes F, et al. Malaria and severe anemia over eight years at Gambo Rural Hospital, southern Ethiopia. *Pathog Glob Health* (2017) 111(4):195–9. doi:10.1080/20477724.2017.1322262
22. Calis JC, Phiri KS, Faragher EB, Brabin BJ, Bates I, Cuevas LE, et al. Severe anemia in Malawian children. *N Engl J Med* (2008) 358(9):888–99. doi:10.1056/NEJMoa072727
23. Reynolds TA, Mfinanga JA, Sawe HR, Runyon MS, Mwafongo V. Emergency care capacity in Africa: a clinical and educational initiative in Tanzania. *J Public Health Policy* (2012) 33(Suppl 1):S126–37. doi:10.1057/jphp.2012.41
24. UNAIDS. *HIV and AIDS Estimates 2014* (2014). Available from: http://www.unaids.org/en/regionscountries/countries/unitedrepublicoftanzania
25. Helbok R, Kendjo E, Issifou S, Lackner P, Newton CR, Kombila M, et al. The Lambarene Organ Dysfunction Score (LODS) is a simple clinical predictor of fatal malaria in African children. *J Infect Dis* (2009) 200(12):1834–41. doi:10.1086/648409
26. Conroy AL, Hawkes M, Hayford K, Namasopo S, Opoka RO, John CC, et al. Prospective validation of pediatric disease severity scores to predict mortality in Ugandan children presenting with malaria and non-malaria febrile illness. *Crit Care* (2015) 19:47. doi:10.1186/s13054-015-0773-4
27. Harris PA, Taylor R, Thielke R, Payne J, Gonzalez N, Conde JG. Research electronic data capture (REDCap) – a metadata-driven methodology and workflow process for providing translational research informatics support. *J Biomed Inform* (2009) 42(2):377–81. doi:10.1016/j.jbi.2008.08.010
28. UNICEF WHO. *WHO/UNICEF Joint Monitoring Programme (JMP) for Water Supply and Sanitation* (2015). Available from: https://www.wssinfo.org/
29. Wiens MO, Larson CP, Kumbakumba E, Kissoon N, Ansermino JM, Singer J, et al. Application of sepsis definitions to pediatric patients admitted with suspected infections in Uganda. *Pediatr Crit Care Med* (2016) 17(5):400–5. doi:10.1097/PCC.0000000000000708
30. Hodkinson P, Argent A, Wallis L, Reid S, Perera R, Harrison S, et al. Pathways to care for critically ill or injured children: a cohort study from first presentation to healthcare services through to admission to intensive care or death. *PLoS One* (2016) 11(1):e0145473. doi:10.1371/journal.pone.0145473
31. Bank W. *Adult Literacy Rate, Population 15+ Years, Both Sexes (%)*. The World Bank (2015). Available from: http://data.worldbank.org/indicator/SE.ADT.LITR.ZS?locations=TZ&view=chart
32. Kihupi CSM, Yohana L, Saria JA, Malebo HM. Fecal contamination of drinking-water in Tanzania's commercial capital, Dar Es Salaam: implication on health of the consumers. *SM J Public Health Epidemiol* (2016) 2(1):1025–9.
33. Mohamed H, Clasen T, Njee RM, Malebo HM, Mbuligwe S, Brown J. Microbiological effectiveness of household water treatment technologies under field use conditions in rural Tanzania. *Trop Med Int Health* (2016) 21(1):33–40. doi:10.1111/tmi.12628
34. Vincent JL, Opal SM, Marshall JC, Tracey KJ. Sepsis definitions: time for change. *Lancet* (2013) 381(9868):774–5. doi:10.1016/S0140-6736(12)61815-7
35. Kortz TB, Murray B, Matthay M, Reynolds T. *Pediatric Sepsis Risk Factors and Barriers to Care at a Referral Hospital in Tanzania: A Prospective Cohort Study*. San Francisco, CA: Pediatric Academic Society (2017).
36. Kortz TB, Murray B, Matthay M, Reynolds T. Surviving paediatric sepsis in Tanzania: a prospective cohort study to identify risk factors. *Consortium of Universities for Global Health*. Washington, DC (2017).
37. Kortz TB, Murray B, Matthay M, Reynolds T. Surviving paediatric sepsis in Tanzania: a prospective cohort study to identify risk factors. *Lancet Glob Health* (2017) 5(S14). doi:10.1016/S2214-109X(17)30121-3

15

Pediatric Critical Care in Resource-Limited Settings—Overview and Lessons Learned

Tina M. Slusher[1], Andrew W. Kiragu[1], Louise T. Day[2], Ashley R. Bjorklund[3†], Arianna Shirk[4], Colleen Johannsen[5] and Scott A. Hagen[6]*

[1] Department of Pediatrics, University of Minnesota and Hennepin County Medical Center, Minneapolis, MN, United States, [2] London School of Hygiene & Tropical Medicine, London, United Kingdom, [3] Walter Reed National Military Medical Center, Bethesda, MD, United States, [4] Department of Pediatrics AIC Kijabe Hospital, Kijabe, Kenya, [5] Cardiac Intensive Care Unit of Regions Medical Center, St. Paul, MN, United States, [6] Department of Pediatrics, University of Wisconsin, Madison, WI, United States

***Correspondence:**
Tina M. Slusher
tslusher@umn.edu

†The views expressed in this article are those of the authors and do not reflect the official policy of the Navy, Department of Defense, or US Government.

Pediatric critical care is an important component of reducing morbidity and mortality globally. Currently, pediatric critical care in low middle-income countries (LMICs) remains in its infancy in most hospitals. The majority of hospitals lack designated intensive care units, healthcare staff trained to care for critically ill children, adequate numbers of staff, and rapid access to necessary medications, supplies and equipment. In addition, most LMICs lack pediatric critical care training programs for healthcare providers or certification procedures to accredit healthcare providers working in their pediatric intensive care units (PICU) and high dependency areas. PICU can improve the quality of pediatric care in general and, if properly organized, can effectively treat the severe complications of high burden diseases, such as diarrhea, severe malaria, and respiratory distress using low-cost interventions. Setting up a PICU in a LMIC setting requires planning, specific resources, and most importantly investment in the nursing and permanent medical staff. A thoughtful approach to developing pediatric critical care services in LMICs starts with fundamental building blocks: training healthcare professionals in skills and knowledge, selecting resource appropriate effective equipment, and having supportive leadership to provide an enabling environment for appropriate care. If these fundamentals can be built on in a sustainable manner, an appropriate critical care service will be established with the potential to significantly decrease pediatric morbidity and mortality in the context of public health goals as we reach toward the sustainable development goals.

Keywords: pediatric critical care, low resource settings, low middle-income country, pediatric intensive care, partnership practice

Critical care is healthcare for the sickest patients. The concept of critical care developed during the poliomyelitis epidemic in the 1920–1950s when the number of critically ill patients led to the development of dedicated areas, "intensive care units," that provided continuous care and monitoring. Critical care services, with focused attention and expertise provided by medical and nursing staff for patients with multi-organ failure and life-threatening illness, quickly spread worldwide (1). Critical care services were extended to pediatric patients in high income countries (HICs) by the 1950s and early pioneers of critical care in low middle-income countries (LMICs) were only 15 years behind their HIC counterparts, opening the first African intensive care unit in 1969 (2).

Nearly 50 years later, however, a huge gap has emerged between the high quality pediatric critical care services available in most HIC settings and the inadequate pediatric critical care services available in most LMIC settings. Nearly 90% of the children who die globally each year below the age of 5 are living in 42 of the poorest countries. In these countries many illnesses and injuries are preventable and treatable diseases are widespread. In a call to action, Niranjan Kissoon described a journey of an African mother seeking care for her ill child filled with fear and frustration (3). The journey elegantly demonstrated how "accident of latitude" often determines whether one lives or dies (4).

HISTORY OF PEDIATRIC CRITICAL CARE IN HICs

The first pediatric intensive care units (PICU) were developed in 1955 in Sweden. This unit treated children with pneumonia and sepsis by extending knowledge gained from the adult ICUs (5). In HICs, PICUs developed rapidly over the subsequent decades with innovations in care and equipment as well as specialization of nursing and medical staff. In the 1990s, the American Academy of Pediatrics and the Pediatric Section of the Society for Critical Care Medicine published guidelines for establishment of pediatric critical care units (6) and for PICU admission criteria (7). The admission criteria were intentionally vague and broad, recommending admission for severe or life-threatening illness and/or illnesses requiring frequent monitoring or intensive intervention (8). The guidelines for establishing a PICU focused on staff training, nursing-to-patient ratio, equipment, and ancillary/support services needed to establish quality critical care. As the specialty advanced, critical care in HICs progressed from treating mostly curable acute, life-threatening illness to provide technologically advanced interventions and complicated coordination of care for patients with complex medical conditions. The interventions provided also evolved from relatively simple and inexpensive therapies, such as fluid resuscitation, oxygen, and medications to complex and expensive therapies, including organ transplantation, dialysis, and extracorporeal membrane oxygenation. The evolution of pediatric intensive care in HICs is a model for the development of the same care in LMICs; starting with inexpensive, simple, lifesaving care, and increasing capabilities as resources and training become available.

HISTORY OF PEDIATRIC CRITICAL CARE IN LMICs

The details of the first PICU and the development of specialized pediatric critical care services in LMICs are not as well documented as in HICs. A systematic review aimed at estimating ICU capacity in low resource settings reported a lack of critical care beds and pediatric intensive care services (9). Millennium Developmental Goal Four (MDG4) targeted a two-thirds reduction in childhood mortality in children less than 5 years of age by the year 2015. To achieve MDG4, UNICEF and WHO focused on the outpatient/ambulatory setting, aiming to improve hygiene, nutritional support, breastfeeding, and immunizations (10). The Integrated Management of Childhood Illness program was established to guide outpatient care. Based on these guidelines, an estimated 20% of children seen in the ambulatory setting met criteria for referral to a hospital for escalation of care (10). Hospital case mortality rates have decreased only slowly from the 1990s to early 2000s, highlighting the need for improved care of the sickest hospitalized children, including triage, emergency, and critical care services (8).

In response to the need for improved triage and emergency care, the WHO developed the Emergency Triage, Assessment, and Treatment (ETAT) guidelines (11). These guidelines emphasize the tenets of pediatric critical care with early recognition of children who needed immediate care and hospitalization. Implementation of these guidelines in a Malawi hospital decreased the mortality rate by half (10–18 to 6–8%) from 2001–2006 (12).

The WHO also published and updated *The Pocketbook of Hospital Care for Children for the Management of Common Illnesses with Limited Resources* (13), which provides many appropriate clinical guidelines for nurses and physicians caring for hospitalized children in these settings. The development of these guidelines and improvements in staff training clearly demonstrated that advances can be made in caring for critically ill children in LMICs by appropriate triage and rapid treatment using relatively inexpensive modalities, such as fluids, oxygen, and antibiotics.

CURRENT STATE OF PEDIATRIC CRITICAL CARE SERVICES IN LMICs SETTINGS

In LMIC settings, the burden of pediatric mortality remains high and a largely undocumented burden of critical illness exists (14). The "three delays" model, first developed to explain why maternal deaths occur may be applied to identify factors that are significant contributors to childhood mortality in LMICs (15). The three delays are (1) delay in deciding to seek care, (2) delay in reaching the appropriate facility, and (3) delay in receiving quality care at the facility. Examples of the third delay, with regards to pediatric critical care services in LMIC settings, are a lack of designated intensive care units with adequate numbers of healthcare staff trained to care for critically ill children, and rapid access to necessary medications, supplies, and equipments. Effective critical care in HICs relies on having a dedicated area, where close observation and frequent monitoring of pediatric patients leads to the provision of rapid, timely, appropriate interventions.

Despite the published guidelines for triage and fundamentals of care described above, the recognition and ability to provide rapid interventions still remains largely absent in many LMIC settings. Infections, such as sepsis, pneumonia, and malaria continue to have a high mortality and 90% of childhood trauma deaths occur in LMICs (16).

There are also significant disparities in pediatric critical care capabilities within regions of any given LMIC (8). In some African countries, university and private hospitals are capable of providing pediatric critical care comparable to PICUs in HICs

(8). In large cities throughout China, India, South Africa, South America, and the Middle East, emergency and intensive care services are often similar to HIC settings (8). The majority of hospitals in LMICs, however, do not have a designated PICU with pediatric trained nursing staff, adequate nurse to patient ratios to care for critical patients, appropriate equipment, monitoring capability, or ancillary support (9). Most pediatric critical care is performed in mixed adult-PICU and the majority of these units would be considered the lowest level ICU (pediatric level 2) (17). PICUs that are established in LMIC's are typically staffed by general pediatricians and lack specialized services.

Without a formal pediatric critical care training, curriculum, or certification process, there is a wide variation in understanding skills and care provided. Finally, rural hospitals and clinics in these same countries are not equipped with even the basic resources, such as oxygen, resuscitation equipment, and medication to provide pediatric emergency care, and appropriately trained staffs are rarely available (15).

THE ARGUMENTS AGAINST AND THE CASE FOR PICUs IN LMICs

Given the perceived high cost of developing and maintaining critical care services, questions naturally arise regarding the advisability or feasibility of establishing critical care units in LMICs. Indeed, financial instability was reported in 35% of established PICUs in the LMICs vs 2.6% of the HICs (13). One could argue that resources would be better employed in addressing the most common primary public health problems facing these communities. In addition, since many of the essential aspects of basic emergency care are not present in LMICs, provision of quality intensive care can be difficult (15). Critical care services in HICs involve a well-coordinated system including three components: triage, emergency medical care and intensive care. Such a comprehensive system is largely unattainable in many LMICs. Yet, despite the strain on resources and the difficulty in establishment of complex systems of care, there is a need to manage children with sudden, serious reversible disease in all settings (14).

An argument for developing critical care services is the potential for these services to translate to improvements in hospital care for all patients (18). Many of the conditions that contribute to the burden of disease in LMICs, such as dehydration and respiratory distress, can be mitigated through prompt, simple treatments (14). Pediatric emergency and critical care services do not need to be expensive, nor excessively dependent on complex technology (19). Critical care services can be utilized to improve outcomes if combined with a focus on community recognition of serious illness, early access to care, referral, and safe transport (15). A robust triage system, the first component of critical care, is still formally lacking in many hospitals in LMICs despite the WHO ETAT recommendations (19). The South African Triage Scale (SATS), for example, employs clinical signs and a triage early warning score to assist in the early identification of acute illness. Use of the SATS has led to better use of hospital resources and earlier discharge (8). Implementing simple tools and interventions such as these, can make a significant difference in the outcomes of critically ill children, supporting their use in LMICs.

Finally, a key argument for the provision of critical care services in resource-limited settings lies within an ideology that all human beings belong to a single community, based on a shared morality, and is based on three principles: the worth of individuals, equality, and the existence of obligations binding to all (8).

BASICS OF DEVELOPING A PICU IN A LMIC: LESSONS LEARNED

Preparing to set up a pediatric critical care unit in a LMIC setting requires planning, vision, specific resources, and most importantly investment by the nursing and permanent medical staff. While PICUs in LMIC settings may develop organically, led by national experts within a country, experts from HICs may be asked to provide focused training. It is essential that these visiting experts recognize the importance of collaboration with local medical staff. A needs assessment performed in collaboration with the local team provides important information to guide appropriate establishment of medical services and ensures that programs established are valued by the medical staff and community, making them more likely to be sustainable.

It is essential to recognize that preconceptions can be a barrier to developing pediatric critical care in resource-limited settings. An extreme example is one of "Medical Colonialism," a term first used by two medical students in 1987 to describe how they were allowed to perform procedures in a LMIC that they would not be allowed to perform in their home country (20). "Medical colonialism," as a concept, can be more subtle. Resentment and distrust may develop if medical personnel from HICs present themselves as knowing "what is best" for those in LMICs despite being visitors. To avoid this undesirable situation, it is critical to listen to, recognize and respect the expert guidance of the local medical staff, nurses, and healthcare workers and form a true partnership.

Borrowing from the work done by Dr. Paul Farmer and his model of four components required to solve epidemics, we have provided examples of lessons learned in developing pediatric critical care services in resource-limited settings (21, 22). The four S components of Dr. Farmer's model are: (1) staff: properly trained and compensated healthcare professionals; (2) stuff: appropriate medical equipments; (3) space: a clean environment to treat patients; and (4) systems: the infrastructure and logistical organization to provide the services. Although Dr. Farmer's model may not be fully applicable to development of sustainable systems of health care, it provides a contextual framework for discussion of the issues encountered and examples of pitfalls to avoid when developing pediatric critical care services.

Staff: Properly Trained and Compensated Healthcare Professionals

Critical care depends on a team of dedicated, well-trained, and compensated medical and nursing staff. The establishment of a standardized pediatric critical care curriculum and certification for healthcare professionals greatly improves provision of appropriate care. A specialized certification is not currently available in most low resource settings; however, standardized training should continue to be a focus of improving care. Trained nurses are essential to providing appropriate critical care services. Nurse roles in the intensive care unit include patient evaluation, medication administration, data collection and assessment, evaluation of the effectiveness of interventions, and communication with the health care team. There are often obstacles to establishing stable critical care nursing (see **Table 1**). It cannot be over-emphasized that recommended nurse to patient ratios should be at least 1 nurse to every 3–4 patients in the PICU setting, which may be a dramatic change from the 1:10–30 nurse to patient ratio (PC authors) in many LMIC hospital wards.

Focused team-based training is essential in establishing a PICU. Early in the partnership it is important to identify gaps in staff knowledge or skills. Performing a need assessment can provide a template to guide training and meet the objectives of the program. A necessary first step is to establish a solid foundation of basic critical care knowledge and skills. Early training should focus on basic life support skills, recognition of age-specific normal vital signs, input/output fluid balance calculation, and continuous monitoring of the cardiorespiratory system. Recognizing abnormalities in basic physiologic parameters is the first step in a chain of actions to improve outcomes in the PICU. Nurses who typically work in adult ICUs should receive pediatric-specific training focused on how to care for infants and children, knowledge of age-dependent vital signs, and the key differences in resuscitation of pediatrics patients. Simple resources, such as posters or binders with age appropriate vital signs, relevant assessments, and basic therapies are useful while establishing a new PICU. Once basic skills are mastered, it is natural to develop more advanced resuscitation skills. Training can progress to include goal-directed therapy and may include tracheal intubation, mechanical ventilation, use of vasopressors, and placement of central lines. Regular mock codes, critical cases review, and simulation not only reinforce training, but also provide team training and establish the importance of teamwork in the PICU.

A complementary set of skills and knowledge that can have great impact on sustaining a program are those associated with quality improvement (QI), teamwork and leadership. QI provides essential skills to monitor and make adjustments to the program over time as skills and knowledge change, equipment decisions are made, and to continually improve outcomes. As skills in caring for critically ill children are established, a parallel set of skills in teamwork and leadership also become essential in the development of pediatric critical care program. To complement formal teaching, physicians, nurses, and other ICU staffs will benefit from the guidance of mentors to model and help to develop effective teamwork and leadership skills. As critical care services are established in LMICs, mortality rates may remain high while quality care is developed. Therefore, providing emotional support for staff where issues, such as staff turnover, emotional fatigue, and burnout are at epidemic proportions is essential to the well-being of those working in the PICU. Support might include developing the capacity to provide services, such as event debriefing, when mortality or morbidity occurs in the PICU.

TABLE 1 | Obstacles to establishing critical care nursing.

- Lack of hospital and nursing administration understanding of nursing role in critical care
- Lack of funding for specialized training
- Inability to provide adequate staffing for ICU nurse to patient ratios
- The traditional role of nurses in the hospital including level of education, experience in critical care, cultural norms, and comfort surrounding communication with and respectfully challenging a physician's orders
- Inadequate compensation to encourage retention
- Allowing nurses who are fully trained and invested to be allowed to remain in the pediatric intensive care units without frequent rotation and reassignment
- The need for well-trained nurses to work as preceptors and mentors to new staff

Stuff: Appropriate Medical Equipment

In addition to staffing, medical equipment has an important role in pediatric critical care. When developing critical care services for children in LMICs, a step-wise approach to introducing equipment is an effective way to build a sustainable service without overwhelming the system. Use of low cost, simple technologies and techniques early in the development of critical care can be lifesaving, and improve quality of care in a sustainable long-term manner (19). Resuscitation kits containing an appropriate-sized neonatal and pediatric bag valve mask systems, adrenaline, cannulas, glucose containing fluids, and normal saline should be readily available in the PICU. Respiratory support is an essential aspect of pediatric care. Non-invasive positive pressure ventilation, including bubble CPAP, is likely a safer and more sustainable respiratory support option than ventilators. Non-invasive ventilation is preferred for many reasons, including conservation of oxygen, decreased need for sedation, decreased equipment/maintenance cost, use of battery power sources, and less monitoring needs. The use of "home" ventilators with internal compressors, instead of "hospital" ventilators that rely on high pressure air and oxygen sources to function, can conserve oxygen and resources. Since oxygen may be supplied in tanks, knowing how much oxygen is available is important. Some ventilators will deplete a large oxygen tank in less than an hour.

Using inexpensive, but appropriate, substitutes for costly medical equipment is a way to establish critical care services without the excessive cost found in some HIC. Examples of low cost medical equipment substitutes include adapting plastic water bottles as spacers for inhaler therapy and the use of sterile nasogastric tubes as umbilical vein catheters (19, 23, 24). When purchasing equipment, the availability in the LMIC or region should be considered, so that it may be maintained and repaired locally (19). Additionally, buying equipment locally supports the regional economy while providing a much-needed service to the hospital.

Space: A Clean Environment to Treat Patients

Providing critical care requires physical space in all settings. Caring for critically ill patients requires more space than caring for non-critically ill patients due to the space needed for equipment and higher number of medical personnel needed per patient.

Overestimating the number of patients that can be cared for in a given space is common. Crowded care areas can create an unorganized work environment that may promote infection, cause difficulty locating necessary equipment, and limit medical personnel and family access to patients. Due to the lack of infrastructure, such as pressurized gases and vacuum, more space may be required in LMICs for equipment that is not needed in HICs. Examples of extra equipment in LMICs may include oxygen tanks, oxygen concentrators, air compressors, and suction machines in addition to monitors, IV pumps, and ventilators that are needed to support the critically ill child in all environments.

Systems: The Infrastructure and Logistical Organization to Provide the Services

Having support to develop pediatric critical care services from the local leadership, both within the organization and from various levels of government, is essential to the success of the program. Support is necessary to develop and retain trained medical personnel.

Additionally, having a biomedical team that provides a reliable way to replace and repair equipment and the infrastructure to maintain the space and facility is invaluable. When supportive leadership is absent, trained personnel may end up leaving for other opportunities, equipment may fall into disrepair, and the facilities will become unusable. Since no pediatric critical care service works in isolation, relationships between the PICU services and the rest of the organization must also be clarified. Relationships are particularly essential between PICU and emergency medicine, anesthesiology, radiology, and surgery, but good working relationships with all the medical and surgical services that will interact with PICU are important.

Finally, in any medical environment that cares for critically ill children, difficult decisions over the use of limited resources will occur. The most difficult question is often the dilemma of "what can be done, what should be done and what will be done." Those making the decisions in a resource-limited setting need to be aware of anticipated outcomes for specific illnesses and should avoid the use of limited resources on patients that have a terminal illness (19). Additionally, long-term use of limited resources, such as pumps and ventilators needs to be considered part of resource stewardship. As these difficult situations are inevitable, admission and discharge guidelines should be established early, based on local experience and outcomes, and updated as outcomes change (20). When beds and supplies are limited, PICU admissions should be limited to illness and injury that are reversible or curable, such as shock secondary to dehydration, anemia, or malaria, and survivable trauma. Having admission criteria based on outcomes will prevent the use of limited critical care resources for children with terminal or untreatable conditions or for those unlikely to benefit from treatments (19). Some examples of situations that may deplete medical resources without benefit to the patient, include complex congenital heart disease in the absence of a cardiac surgery program, malignancies without effective therapy, and patients in persistent coma requiring mechanical ventilation. It is also important to ensure families don't utilize all of their resources, financial, or otherwise, since the health status of many LMIC individuals and families is closely tied to their ability to stay out of poverty (19). Therefore, ensuring financial support is available to a family should be part of the treatment plan for critically ill children in LMICs. Finally, local medical personnel are invaluable in understanding the limits of their system, knowing when to stop or limit resuscitation, or limit the use of supplies and medicines that might be considered unhelpful or wasteful. Listening to local medical providers is an important aspect of respecting their expertise and culture.

CONCLUSION

The principal goal of developing critical care services in LMICs is to progressively improve the outcomes of children presenting with a serious or life-threatening illness and to do it in a sustainable manner. This requires working together as partners with LMIC healthcare providers in a respectful and nurturing environment. A thoughtful approach to developing pediatric critical care services starts with fundamental skills and knowledge, inexpensive, but effective equipment, and supportive leadership. These fundamentals can be built on in a sustainable manner, having the potential to significantly decrease pediatric morbidity and mortality in LMICs through excellent, but appropriate critical care in the context of public health goals as we reach toward the 2030 SDGs.

AUTHOR CONTRIBUTIONS

TS substantial contributions to the conception or design of the work, or the acquisition of background articles and topics to be covered. Drafted work and revised it critically for important intellectual content. Provided approval for publication. Agreed to be accountable for all aspects of the work in ensuring that questions related to accuracy or integrity of any part of work are appropriately investigated and resolved. AK and CJ drafted work and added content critically for important intellectual content. Provided approval for publication of content. LD revised work and added content critically for important intellectual content. Provided approval for publication of content. AS drafted and revised the work and added content critically for important intellectual content. Provided approval for publication of the content. SH drafted work and revised it critically for important intellectual content. Provided approval for publication. Agreed to be accountable for all aspects of the work in ensuring that questions related to accuracy or integrity of any part of work are appropriately investigated and resolved. AB drafted work for the article and critically edited, reviewed and approved the final version.

REFERENCES

1. Marshall JC, Bosco L, Adhikari NK, Connolly B, Diaz JV, Dorman T, et al. What is an intensive care unit? A report of the task force of the World Federation of Societies of Intensive and Critical Care Medicine. *J Crit Care* (2017) 37:270–6. doi:10.1016/j.jcrc.2016.07.015
2. Meiring Pde V, Lumsden JD, Morrison AG, Furnham LA. An intensive care unit in a provincial general hospital. *S Afr Med J* (1969) 43(26):806–10.
3. Kissoon N. Out of Africa – a mother's journey. *Pediatr Crit Care Med* (2011) 12(1):73–9. doi:10.1097/PCC.0b013e3181ce74ef
4. Fowler RA, Adhikari NK, Bhagwanjee S. Clinical review: critical care in the global context – disparities in burden of illness, access, and economics. *Crit Care* (2008) 12(5):225. doi:10.1186/cc6984
5. Epstein D, Brill J. A history of pediatric critical care medicine. *Pediatr Res* (2005) 58(5):987–96. doi:10.1203/01.PDR.0000182822.16263.3D
6. Guidelines and Levels of Care for Pediatric Intensive Care Units. Committee on Hospital Care of the American Academy of Pediatrics and Pediatric Section of the Society of Critical Care Medicine. *Pediatrics* (1993) 92(1):166–75.
7. Guidelines for Developing Admission and Discharge Policies for the Pediatric Intensive Care Unit. Pediatric Section Task Force on Admission and Discharge Criteria, Society of Critical Care Medicine in conjunction with the American College of Critical Care Medicine and the Committee on Hospital Care of the American Academy of Pediatrics. *Crit Care Med* (1999) 27(4):843–5.
8. Turner EL, Nielsen KR, Jamal SM, von Saint Andre-von Arnim A, Musa NL. A review of pediatric critical care in resource-limited settings: a look at past, present, and future directions. *Front Pediatr* (2016) 4:5. doi:10.1080/09540121.2016.1139043
9. Murthy S, Leligdowicz A, Adhikari NK. Intensive care unit capacity in low-income countries: a systematic review. *PLoS One* (2015) 10(1):e0116949. doi:10.1371/journal.pone.0116949
10. Baker T. Pediatric emergency and critical care in low-income countries. *Paediatr Anaesth* (2009) 19(1):23–7. doi:10.1111/j.1460-9592.2008.02868.x
11. World Health Organization. *Emergency Triage Assessment and Treatment (ETAT) Manual for Participants*. Geneva, Switzerland: World Health Organization (2005).
12. Molyneux E, Ahmed S, Robertson A. Improved triage and emergency care for children reduces inpatient mortality in a resource-constrained setting. *Bull World Health Organ* (2006) 84(4):314–9. doi:10.2471/BLT.04019505
13. World Health Organization. *Pocketbook of Hospital Care for Children Guidelines for the Management of Common Illnesses with Limited Resources*. Geneva: World Health Organization (2013).
14. Tripathi S, Kaur H, Kashyap R, Dong Y, Gajic O, Murthy S. A survey on the resources and practices in pediatric critical care of resource-rich and resource-limited countries. *J Intensive Care* (2015) 3:40. doi:10.1186/s40560-015-0106-3
15. Thaddeus S, Maine D. Too far to walk: maternal mortality in context. *Soc Sci Med* (1994) 38(8):1091–110. doi:10.1016/0277-9536(94)90226-7
16. Baker T. Critical care in low-income countries. *Trop Med Int Health* (2009) 14(2):143–8. doi:10.1111/j.1365-3156.2008.02202.x
17. Rosenberg DI, Moss MM; American College of Critical Care Medicine of the Society of Critical Care M. Guidelines and levels of care for pediatric intensive care units. *Crit Care Med* (2004) 32(10):2117–27. doi:10.1097/01.CCM.0000142704.36378.E9
18. Amoateng-Adjepong Y. Caring for the critically ill in developing countries – our collective challenge. *Crit Care Med* (2006) 34(4):1288–9. doi:10.1097/01.CCM.0000208352.74208.75
19. Slusher T, Bjorklund A, Aanyu HT, Kiragu A, Christo P. The assessment, evaluation and management of the critically ill child in resource limited international settings. *J Pediatr Intensive Care* (2016) 06(01):066–076. doi:10.1055/s-0036-1584677
20. Holt TA, Adams TJ. Medical colonialism. *J Med Ethics* (1987) 13(2):102. doi:10.1136/jme.13.2.102
21. Farmer P. *The Ebola Suspect's Dilemma. Keynote Address for the MacLean Prize Lecture*. Chicago, IL (2017).
22. Farmer P. *Taking up the Challenges of Poverty: Why Accompaniment Matters*. Notre Dame: Lecture delivered at Kellogg Institute for International Studies (2016)
23. Simulation Use for Global Away Rotations (SUGAR). (2016). Available from: http://sugarprep.org/pearls/ (accessed January 27, 2018).
24. Bensman RS, Slusher TM, Butteris SM, Pitt MB, On Behalf of the Sugar Pearls Investigators, Becker A, et al. Creating online training for procedures in global health with PEARLS (Procedural Education for Adaptation to Resource-Limited Settings). *Am J Trop Med Hyg* (2017) 97(5):1285–8. doi:10.4269/ajtmh.16-0936

16

Decisions Parents Make When Faced With Potentially Life-Limiting Fetal Diagnoses and the Importance of Perinatal Palliative Care

*Krishelle L. Marc-Aurele**

Division of Neonatology, Department of Pediatrics, University of California, San Diego, San Diego, CA, United States

***Correspondence:**
Krishelle L. Marc-Aurele
kmaurele@health.ucsd.edu

When parents face a potentially life-limiting fetal diagnosis in pregnancy, they then have a series of decisions to make. These include confirmatory testing, termination, and additional choices if they choose to continue the pregnancy. A perinatal palliative team provides a safe, compassionate, and caring space for parents to process their emotions and discuss their values. In a shared decision-making model, the team explores how a family's faith, experiences, values, and perspectives shape the goals for care. For some families, terminating a pregnancy for any reason conflicts with their faith or values and pursuing life prolonging treatments in order to give their baby the best chances for survival is the most important. For others, having a postnatal confirmatory diagnosis of a life limiting or serious medical condition gives them the assurance they need to allow their child a natural death. Others want care to be comfort-focused in order to maximize the time they to be together as a family. Through this journey, a perinatal palliative team can provide the support and encouragement for families to express their goals and wishes, as well as find meaning and hope.

Keywords: perinatal palliative care (PPC), decision-making, pregnancy, life-limiting fetal diagnoses, decisions

INTRODUCTION

During pregnancy, ultrasounds and blood test results in the first two trimesters provide information about the fetus' health. When these results suggest a potentially life-limiting fetal diagnosis, parents are faced with a series of decisions. The first choices involve whether to obtain more diagnostic information via invasive or non-invasive tests during the pregnancy. Invasive testing includes chorionic villus sampling or amniocentesis in order to check for genetic mutations or aneuploidy. Parents need to weigh the risks of invasive testing against their desire for more information and greater certainty to help them with time-sensitive decisions. Although rates of pregnancy loss have been difficult to estimate, a recent meta-analysis suggests no significant risk of miscarriage with chorionic villus sampling and a miscarriage risk of 1:300 with amniocentesis (1). There are other risks associated with invasive testing, however, including bleeding, Rh sensitization, rupture of membranes, and infection (2). The recommended time frame to perform these invasive tests, between 10 and 20 weeks' gestation, is exactly when concerns about the fetus are raised and therefore a relatively narrow window of time in which to make decisions about testing (3). Diagnostic results may take up to 1–2 weeks to return. Although prenatal genetic testing has been expanded to include exome sequencing, it unfortunately cannot identify all possible abnormalities. Despite these limitations, the results may determine whether some families continue the pregnancy.

As an alternative, parents may first choose to decline invasive testing and opt for non-invasive testing which includes cell-free DNA screening and additional imaging. Cell-free DNA screening has a high sensitivity and specificity for Trisomy 21 and Trisomy 18, but lower performance for Trisomy 13, other chromosomal anomalies, and microdeletions (4). If non-invasive cell-free DNA screening is suggestive of a genetic abnormality, invasive testing is still needed to confirm the diagnosis before termination. Additional imaging includes fetal echocardiogram, three-dimensional fetal ultrasound, or fetal magnetic resonance imaging. For advice and opinion on the suspected diagnosis and outcomes, parents may also want to consult with pediatric subspecialists. What adds to the complexity of the situation is that maternal fetal medicine specialists have two patients: the mother and the fetus. Their duty is to separate information about the risks and benefits of various choices for both patients, recognizing that decisions made will have linked outcomes (5). As such, the maternal fetal medicine specialist will also review for the mother potential pregnancy complications associated with fetal anomalies: preeclampsia, preterm labor, polyhydramnios, and mirror syndrome (6–10).

After gathering as much data as possible, parents will consider whether or not to terminate the pregnancy. This decision often must be made within days or a couple of weeks after learning about a fetal abnormality. While many technologies offer to improve diagnostic certainty or prognostication, parents need to know about limitations in predicting survival and outcome variability. Each test, imaging modality, and consultation is an option for parents to pursue or decline. For some families, terminating a pregnancy is not consistent with their faith or values so undergoing invasive or non-invasive testing to inform a decision to terminate does not make sense. It is possible that a life-limiting fetal diagnosis may not be discovered until after termination is no longer an option, but families may still want information to prepare themselves for possible outcomes. Other families may feel the degree of uncertainty associated with some information acquired during pregnancy is not worth the additional stress. And some families want more time to process the news before obtaining more data.

PERINATAL PALLIATIVE CONSULTATION

"Perinatal palliative care refers to a coordinated care strategy that comprises options for obstetric and newborn care that include a focus on maximizing quality of life and comfort for newborns with a variety of conditions considered to be life-limiting in early infancy. With a dual focus on ameliorating suffering and honoring patient values, perinatal palliative care can be provided concurrently with life-prolonging treatment" (11). There is a misconception that palliative care applies only to cases where the goals are to allow a natural death. In fact, perinatal palliative teams advocate primarily for respect of parental wishes, supporting a spectrum of goals from comfort-focused to life-prolonging care. A perinatal palliative team is typically multidisciplinary including a physician, nurse, social worker, and spiritual counselor (12). Some palliative teams are imbedded within fetal diagnostic centers, enabling simultaneous palliative consultation (13). For centers without integrated palliative teams, however, there are barriers to early referral and palliative consultation might not occur for weeks (14). Because decisions to terminate often need to occur relatively quickly, families who chose termination are likely to miss the opportunity for perinatal palliative consultation. In practice, consultation with a perinatal palliative team most frequently occurs after parents have declined termination with plans instead to continue the pregnancy (15). No matter which decision parents make (i.e., to terminate or continue the pregnancy), however, all parents experience losses, find themselves planning for a future they did not hope for or expect, and can benefit from the additional support for decision-making that perinatal palliative teams can provide (16).

Providing support to parents as they make decisions is central to the perinatal palliative consultation. Amidst the variable and sometimes overwhelming emotions that parents can experience, the perinatal palliative team allows parents to explore their goals in order to promote shared decision-making with regard to obstetric management as well as postnatal care for the baby. Mixed, changing, and sometimes conflicting feelings of shock, concern, disbelief, denial, anger, love, shame, hope, and guilt are normal for parents to experience when hearing serious news about their baby (17). The perinatal palliative team fosters a safe, compassionate, and supportive environment for parents to process their emotions and discuss their values (18). Without the ability to address their feelings or spiritual distress, parents may not be ready to explore their hopes for their baby's care, let alone make changes to the plan of care. For example, a spiritual counselor on the perinatal palliative team is especially important if a parent is worried about the "right" thing to do with respect to her faith. Addressing the meaning of the situation in the context of her faith is necessary before approaching decision-making about treatment options for the baby. By validating and reflecting what parents express and in turn building trust, the perinatal palliative team can support a parent's voice in decision-making and facilitate communication between parents and other medical teams (19).

BIRTH PLANS

One way in which the perinatal palliative team supports a parent's voice and decisions is to collaborate on a birth plan. A birth plan is similar to an advanced directive for the pregnancy, delivery, and neonatal care. By sharing their birth plan with the medical team, families create additional opportunities for informed and shared decision-making. A birth plan documents parental hopes, wishes, and goals of care, serving as a communication tool for the entire medical team. Personalized birth plans vary in content but generally address the following components: pain control for the mother, preference for fetal monitoring, mode of delivery, who to be present in the delivery room, resuscitation measures desired at birth, medical management for the baby, as well as wishes for memory making, and ceremonies (20). **Table 1** presents suggested topics for a birth plan. Writing a birth plan allows parents to identify and articulate goals ahead of time before a potentially overwhelming emotional moment. Parents have reported that creating and using a birth plan gave

TABLE 1 | Suggested topics for a birth plan.

Plan of care for mother
Maternal information including medical record number and date of birth
Preference for fetal monitoring and mode of delivery
Requested persons to be present in the delivery room
Music choices for labor and delivery
Requests for any limitations in medical personnel
Pain control preferences
Request for information regarding maintenance and suppression of lactation
Plan of care for baby
Planned name
Designated person to cut the umbilical cord
Resuscitation measures desired at birth
Goals for medical management for the baby
Code status
Anticipated location for care
Expectations for respiratory and nutrition support
Desired diagnostic testing, imaging, consultations
Symptom management
Any limitations for routine newborn care (i.e. screening and prophylaxis)
Selected persons to be present with the baby
Memory making including caregiving activities, photography, and creation of mementos
Desired spiritual care or ceremonies
End-of-Life Plan
Plans for home hospice care
Organ donation
Autopsy
Preference regarding use of a cooling bassinet
Final Arrangements
Requests for bereavement counseling resources

them a sense of control, was therapeutic, and helped them feel prepared (21).

The most challenging sections of the birth plan to complete usually address fetal monitoring, mode of delivery, and goals of care for baby's management. The 2019 ACOG Committee Opinion on Perinatal Palliative Care states that, "Decisions regarding the appropriateness of intrapartum fetal monitoring in cases like this should be individualized" (11). Some families are willing to accept the possibility of their baby's death during unmonitored labor in order to avoid the operative risks of cesarean section. Other families would rather have fetal monitoring during labor and if necessary, cesarean delivery for fetal distress, to increase the chances for their baby to be born alive. For example, some may want the opportunity for the entire family to meet the baby or to perform a ceremony at birth. For some families, having a postnatal confirmatory diagnosis of a life-limiting or serious medical condition gives them the assurance they need to allow their child to have a natural death. And other families may want to pursue life-prolonging treatments in order to give their baby the best chances for survival.

The uncertainty of whether the baby will survive the pregnancy and birth can make planning for the neonatal period challenging. Some families are ready to consider in detail the choices for baby's care after birth while other families want to defer those decisions until after the baby is born. The perinatal palliative team can help to explain how care for the newborn can be adapted to align with the goals of care. For example, families may want a time-limited trial of respiratory and nutrition support in order to see if the baby can breathe or eat on her or his own. If the baby is unable to breathe independently or feed by mouth safely, then families will need to consider whether providing long-term ventilation or artificial nutrition aligns with their goals for care. As it was during pregnancy, each test, imaging modality, and consultation for the baby is an option for parents to pursue or decline.

The birth plan will vary based on a family's faith, values, and experiences. For example, some families will want specific spiritual care or ceremonies after birth to honor their faith. But there are also some universal themes (22). Janvier et al. found that among families with children who lived with Trisomy 13 or 18, there were "common hopes to bring their child home, give their child a good life, and be together/a family" (23). Parents often have an intrinsic need to feel that they have "done the best that they could" for their child and want to avoid having regrets in the future (24). Maintaining hope is an important source of strength for parents when facing difficult situations (25). A parent's hope can change with time and new information, from hoping for a normal pregnancy, to hoping the baby will be healthier than predicted, to hoping that the baby will be alive at birth to meet the family. During goals of care planning, the perinatal palliative team can encourage and help families to maintain hope as circumstances change. Nearing the day of delivery, parents may worry about future regrets in choosing comfort-focused care, and want time-limited trials of therapy until the baby's diagnosis is confirmed. It is important to validate that concerns about regret can inform the goals of care and to acknowledge that allowing time to pass might reduce parental decision regret (26). There is also the possibility that at birth, the baby's presentation may not match the prenatal diagnosis thereby suggesting a different prognosis. Health care providers need to be flexible and remember that the birth plan serves as a guide for both mother and baby care providers, but it can be modified at any point before and after delivery. Ultimately, what is most important is that parents are supported, ideally by perinatal palliative teams alongside other medical teams, to discuss and express the rationale behind their decisions.

MEMORY MAKING

Whether the goals of care are focused on life-prolongation or comfort, most families whose baby may have a short life want to plan for memory making. The perinatal palliative team offers expertise and experience to support parents in the many ways they want to make memories. Memory making includes "any intervention or experience that encourages contact or interaction between the parents and newborn and any intervention that results in the creation or collection of mementos" (27). Mementos include molds of the baby's hands and feet, foot and handprints, blankets, hats, and clothing that the baby touched, as well as crib cards, hospital bands, and other personal items that were associated with the baby in the hospital. Now I Lay Me Down to Sleep is a non-profit international organization which offers free professional retouched photography to families who have a baby with a life-limiting condition (28). Families may want to take their own photographs or hire a photographer instead. Although parents may not want to see photos of their child right away, the portrait sessions give them the opportunity to have documentation of their child's life available for when they are ready. After the death of an infant, interviewed families emphasize the importance of having as many parenting experiences as possible to reflect upon in bereavement (29). Opportunities for caregiving can include bathing, dressing, and holding their baby as well as talking, singing, and playing music with their baby (30). Families recall that they needed encouragement and guidance to overcome their hesitation in order to spend time with their newborn (31). Some families introduce their baby to siblings and relatives to officially welcome him or her into the family. Making memories can not only validate the importance of the newborn's life and death but also create a sense of identity for individuals as parents, siblings, and grandparents.

COMFORT FOCUSED-CARE

If families choose comfort-focused care for their baby, there may be an opportunity to continue the caregiving at home with hospice support. A hospice physician and team provide expertise in end-of-life care at home and ongoing bereavement counseling for the immediate family. A designated pediatrician is customarily not needed unless the goals of care change to include life-prolonging interventions. If the baby is unlikely to survive the trip home, some parents may want to room-in with the baby in the hospital while some families may not have the financial or logistical capacity to room-in. The perinatal palliative team can provide inpatient support to the primary neonatal team who will attend to the baby's pain and symptom management as well as support the family through the dying process. Many parents have little to no experience with death and will want to know what their baby will look like and feel in the last hours of living (32). Generally, babies in the dying process will become less active, sleeping more as time goes on. Any ability to swallow saliva will become impaired. With less intake, decreased urine and stool output is expected. Cool hands and feet along with mottling of the skin is normal. Less commonly, newborns may need treatment for seizures in the dying process. Eventually, when the baby is no longer conscious, periods of apnea, or Cheyne-Stokes pattern respirations will occur. Ordinary techniques to soothe babies, such as holding, rocking, and swaddling, are usually successful to minimize discomfort. Occasionally, morphine or lorazepam may be needed for symptom management of pain or agitation, respectively. Normalizing the signs of dying for families may reduce their anxiety and distress when the time comes. It is not possible to predict when death will occur, but it is possible to prepare families for the unpredictability of death. Using words such as "weeks not months," "days not weeks," or "hours not days," can be helpful (33).

If medically possible, families can choose organ or tissue donation to create a hopeful and positive legacy. Organ procurement teams have specialized training and are the preferred communicators to maintain ethical and clinical standards while initiating organ donation discussions. Referrals to organ procurement organizations should be made in a timely manner when death is anticipated and may occur before birth (34). In addition, some families may agree to a full or limited autopsy to inform subsequent pregnancies or to improve medical knowledge for future families. Others may decline autopsy because they do not need more information, or their faith and values are not congruent with allowing an autopsy. Families may choose final arrangements based on family or faith traditions as well as their budget. Generally, cremation is less expensive than burial but the cost can vary by mortuary and location (35). Some parents will want to designate a relative or friend to do research and get quotes on available services and some families will prefer to do this work on their own.

After a baby dies, some families will want extended time with the baby and may want to use a cooling bassinet to decrease the rate that the body deteriorates (36). Others will say goodbye a few hours after the baby dies. There are physical and emotional aspects of lactation that need to be addressed. Some mothers will want to suppress breast milk production but need education on how to avoid painful engorgement and mastitis. Others will want to continue expressing and donate breast milk as a way to help other families and find meaning in the context of their loss and grief (37). It is important to recommend grief resources and counseling for families whether they go home with hospice or stay in the hospital setting. Some families may prefer to visit online bereavement resources first and others will want to start mental health therapy immediately (38, 39). The perinatal palliative team continues to support families as they make choices to honor their baby that may include a funeral, celebration of life, and donations to charities or research. Additionally, the team often maintains contact with families in bereavement. It is important to share with families that there are no right or wrong ways to grieve or feel when a baby dies.

CONCLUSION

Through the journey with a potentially life-limiting fetal diagnosis in pregnancy, a perinatal palliative team can provide the encouragement families need to make decisions based on their faith, values, and experiences. The team has the expertise to create a safe, compassionate, and caring environment for parents to process a number of intense emotions and discuss their values. Although parents must confront uncertainty and complex decision-making for both the mother and baby, perinatal palliative teams support parents to express their goals as well as find meaning and hope.

AUTHOR CONTRIBUTIONS

KM-A agrees to be accountable for and conceived, drafted, revised, and approved all aspects of the work.

REFERENCES

1. Salomon LJ, Sotiriadis A, Wulff CB, Odibo A, Akolekar R. Risk of miscarriage following amniocentesis or chorionic villus sampling: systematic review of literature and updated meta-analysis. *Ultrasound Obstet Gynecol.* (2019) 54:442–51. doi: 10.1002/uog.20353
2. Alfirevic Z, Mujezinovic F, Sundberg K. Amniocentesis and chorionic villus sampling for prenatal diagnosis. *Cochrane Database Syst Rev.* (2003) 2003:CD003252. doi: 10.1002/14651858.CD003252
3. American College of Obstetricians and Gynecologists' Committee on Practice Bulletins—Obstetrics, Committee on Genetics, Society for Maternal–Fetal Medicine. Practice bulletin No. 162: prenatal diagnostic testing for genetic disorders. *Obstet Gynecol.* (2016) 127:e108–22. doi: 10.1097/AOG.0000000000001405
4. Palomaki GE, Deciu C, Kloza EM, Lambert-Messerlian GM, Haddow JE, Neveux LM, et al. DNA sequencing of maternal plasma reliably identifies trisomy 18 and trisomy 13 as well as down syndrome: an international collaborative study. *Genet Med.* (2012) 14:296–305. doi: 10.1038/gim.2011.73
5. Marty CM, Carter BS. Ethics and palliative care in the perinatal world. *Semin Fetal Neonatal Med.* (2018) 23:35–8. doi: 10.1016/j.siny.2017.09.001
6. Burwick RM, Pilliod RA, Dukhovny SE, Caughey AB. Fetal hydrops and the risk of severe preeclampsia. *J Matern Fetal Neonatal Med.* (2019) 32:961–5. doi: 10.1080/14767058.2017.1396312
7. Nelson DB, Chalak LF, McIntire DD, Leveno KJ. Is preeclampsia associated with fetal malformation? A review and report of original research. *J Matern Fetal Neonatal Med.* (2015) 28:2135–40. doi: 10.3109/14767058.2014.980808
8. Kornacki J, Adamczyk M, Wirstlein P, Osiński M, Wender-Ozegowska E. Polyhydramnios — frequency of congenital anomalies in relation to the value of the amniotic fluid index. *Ginekol Polska.* (2017) 88:442–5. doi: 10.5603/GP.a2017.0081
9. Norton ME, Chauhan SP, Dashe JS. Society for maternal-fetal medicine (SMFM) clinical guideline #7: nonimmune hydrops fetalis. *Am J Obstetrics Gynecol.* (2015) 212:127–39. doi: 10.1016/j.ajog.2014.12.018
10. Quaresima P, Homfray T, Greco E. Obstetric complications in pregnancies with life-limiting malformations. *Curr Opin Obstetrics Gynecol.* (2019) 31:375–87. doi: 10.1097/GCO.0000000000000583
11. Perinatal palliative care: ACOG COMMITTEE OPINION, Number 786. *Obstet Gynecol.* (2019) 134:e84–9. doi: 10.1097/AOG.0000000000003425
12. Balaguer A, Martín-Ancel A, Ortigoza-Escobar D, Escribano J, Argemi J. The model of palliative care in the perinatal setting: a review of the literature. *BMC Pediatr.* (2012) 12:25. doi: 10.1186/1471-2431-12-25
13. Kukora S, Gollehon N, Laventhal N. Antenatal palliative care consultation: implications for decision-making and perinatal outcomes in a single-centre experience. *Arch Dis Child Fetal Neonatal Ed.* (2017) 102:F12–6. doi: 10.1136/archdischild-2016-311027
14. Marc-Aurele KL, Nelesen R. A five-year review of referrals for perinatal palliative care. *J Palliat Med.* (2013) 16:1232–6. doi: 10.1089/jpm.2013.0098
15. Marc-Aurele KL, Hull AD, Jones MC, Pretorius DH. A fetal diagnostic center's referral rate for perinatal palliative care. *Ann Palliat Med.* (2017) 7:177–85. doi: 10.21037/apm.2017.03.12
16. Lou S, Jensen LG, Petersen OB, Vogel I, Hvidman L, Møller A, et al. Parental response to severe or lethal prenatal diagnosis: a systematic review of qualitative studies. *Prenat Diagn.* (2017) 37:731–43. doi: 10.1002/pd.5093
17. Luz R, George A, Spitz E, Vieux R. Breaking bad news in prenatal medicine: a literature review. *J Reprod Infant Psychol.* (2017) 35:14–31. doi: 10.1080/02646838.2016.1253052
18. O'Connell O, Meaney S, O'Donoghue K. Anencephaly; the maternal experience of continuing with the pregnancy. incompatible with life but not with love. *Midwifery.* (2019) 71:12–8. doi: 10.1016/j.midw.2018.12.016
19. Moro TT, Kavanaugh K, Savage TA, Reyes MR, Kimura RE, Bhat R. Parent decision making for life support decisions for extremely premature infants: from the prenatal through end-of-life period. *J Perinat Neonatal Nurs.* (2011) 25:52–60. doi: 10.1097/JPN.0b013e31820377e5
20. Limbo DR, Wool C, Carter B, (editors). *Handbook of Perinatal and Neonatal Palliative Care: A Guide for Nurses, Physicians, and Other Health Professionals.* 1 ed. New York, NY: Springer Publishing Company (2019). doi: 10.1891/9780826138422
21. Cortezzo DE, Bowers K, Cameron Meyer M. Birth planning in uncertain or life-limiting fetal diagnoses: perspectives of physicians and parents. *J Palliat Med.* (2019) 22:1337–45. doi: 10.1089/jpm.2018.0596
22. Blakeley C, Smith DM, Johnstone ED, Wittkowski A. Parental decision-making following a prenatal diagnosis that is lethal, life-limiting, or has long term implications for the future child and family: a meta-synthesis of qualitative literature. *BMC Med Ethics.* (2019) 20:56. doi: 10.1186/s12910-019-0393-7
23. Janvier A, Farlow B, Barrington KJ. Parental hopes, interventions, and survival of neonates with trisomy 13 and trisomy 18. *Am J Med Genet Part C Semin Med Genet.* (2016) 172:279–87. doi: 10.1002/ajmg.c.31526
24. Côté-Arsenault D, Denney-Koelsch E. "Have no regrets:" parents' experiences and developmental tasks in pregnancy with a lethal fetal diagnosis. *Soc Sci Med.* (2016) 154:100–9. doi: 10.1016/j.socscimed.2016.02.033
25. Janvier A, Barrington K, Farlow B. Communication with parents concerning withholding or withdrawing of life-sustaining interventions in neonatology. *Semin Perinatol.* (2014) 38:38–46. doi: 10.1053/j.semperi.2013.07.007
26. Wool C, Limbo R, Denny-Koelsch EM. "I would do it all over again" : cherishing time and the absence of regret in continuing a pregnancy after a life-limiting diagnosis. *J Clin Ethics.* (2018) 29:227–36.
27. Thornton R, Nicholson P, Harms L. Scoping review of memory making in bereavement care for parents after the death of a newborn. *J Obstet Gynecol Neonatal Nurs.* (2019) 48:351–60. doi: 10.1016/j.jogn.2019.02.001
28. *Now I Lay Me Down to Sleep | Now I Lay Me Down To Sleep.* (2019). Available online at: https://www.nowilaymedowntosleep.org/ (accessed August 29, 2019).
29. Tan JS, Docherty SL, Barfield R, Brandon DH. Addressing parental bereavement support needs at the end of life for infants with complex chronic conditions. *J Palliat Med.* (2012) 15:579–84. doi: 10.1089/jpm.2011.0357
30. Wool C, Catlin A. Perinatal bereavement and palliative care offered throughout the healthcare system. *Ann Palliat Med.* (2018) 8(Suppl. 1):S22–9. doi: 10.21037/apm.2018.11.03
31. Abraham A, Hendriks MJ. "You can only give warmth to your baby when it's too late" : parents' bonding with their extremely preterm and dying child. *Qual Health Res.* (2017) 27:2100–15. doi: 10.1177/1049732317721476
32. Catlin A, Carter B. Creation of a neonatal end-of-life palliative care protocol. *J Perinatol.* (2002) 22:184–95. doi: 10.1038/sj.jp.7210687
33. Bodtke S, Ligon K. *Hospice and Palliative Medicine Handbook: A Clinical Guide.* 1st ed. Lexington: CreateSpace Independent Publishing Platform (2016).
34. Medicare Medicaid programs; hospital conditions of participation; identification of potential organ, tissue, eye donors transplant hospitals' provision of transplant-related data–HCFA. Final rule. *Fed Regist.* (1998) 63:33856–75.
35. *How Much Does it Cost to Cremate? The Living Urn.* Available online at: https://www.thelivingurn.com/blogs/news/how-much-does-it-cost-to-cremate
36. Smith P, Vasileiou K, Jordan A. Healthcare professionals' perceptions and experiences of using a cold cot following the loss of a baby: a qualitative study in maternity and neonatal units in the UK. *BMC Pregnancy Childbirth.* (2020) 20:175. doi: 10.1186/s12884-020-02865-4
37. Cole JCM, Schwarz J, Farmer M-C, Coursey AL, Duren S, Rowlson M, et al. Facilitating milk donation in the context of perinatal palliative care. *J Obstet Gynecol Neonatal Nurs.* (2018) 47:564–70. doi: 10.1016/j.jogn.2017.11.002
38. *Still Standing Magazine.* Available online at: https://stillstandingmag.com/
39. *Glow in the Woods.* Available online at: http://www.glowinthewoods.com/

17

Pediatric Critical Care Medicine Training in India: Past, Present and Future

Utpal Bhalala[1] and Praveen Khilnani[2]*

[1] Baylor College of Medicine at the Children's Hospital of San Antonio, San Antonio, TX, United States, [2] Rainbow Children's Hospital, New Delhi, India

Correspondence:
Utpal Bhalala
utpal.bhalala@bcm.edu

Pediatric critical care services in India have grown with leaps and bounds. There has been a growing need of physicians specially trained in pediatric critical care medicine (PCCM) in India. Physicians returning to India after their formal training in PCCM abroad have partly supported this growing need. Development of formal PCCM training programs in India has been a huge step toward supporting the growing clinical needs. This article focuses on advances in pediatric critical care training in India and its future directions.

Keywords: pediatric critical care, training, fellowship, simulation, India, resource-limited settings

INTRODUCTION

Until 2002, formal fellowship training in pediatric critical care medicine (PCCM), accredited by a national governing body did not exist in India. Therefore, pediatricians interested in such training, explored options outside of India for formal PCCM fellowship. Over the subsequent 15 years, the scenario of PCCM changed dramatically in India. Quite a few physicians after completing a formal PCCM fellowship and gaining some experience working as senior house officers or faculty abroad returned to India to lead the PCCM programs in major metropolitan areas of India. Also, a very good number of hospitals established formal fellowship training in PCCM. This article focuses on formal, curriculum-based PCCM training as well as recent advances in simulation-based PCCM training in India.

GROWTH OF PEDIATRIC CRITICAL CARE SPECIALTY IN INDIA (FIGURE 1)

In 1997, Vidyasagar and co-authors summarized the evolution of neonatal and pediatric critical care in India (1) (**Figure 1**). The initiative to upgrade neonatal and pediatric critical care came primarily from major teaching hospitals, especially government sponsored institutions (1). Around the turn of the century, India witnessed a boom in the field of healthcare (2, 3). There was a significant growth in number of corporate hospitals capable of providing state-of-the-art services to patients in metropolitan areas of India (3). These corporate hospitals took the lead in establishing units based on Western standards of equipment and personnel, thereby moving the PCCM specialty in a favorable direction in India (1, 4). The establishment of these hospitals created newer opportunities and attracted well-trained and experienced physicians and surgeons to either return to India or move from government hospitals to corporate hospitals to establish specialty and subspecialty divisions. In 2010, Lodha and co-authors reported a few centers in government and private hospitals in India with separate pediatric intensive care units (PICUs) (5). Now there are multiple, small-to-medium size PICUs all over India, which are run by pediatric intensivists formally trained either abroad or within India. In fact, Dr. Khilnani under auspices of Indian Academy of Pediatrics (IAPs) published consensus guidelines for design and operation of PICUs in India (6). Needless to say, large proportions

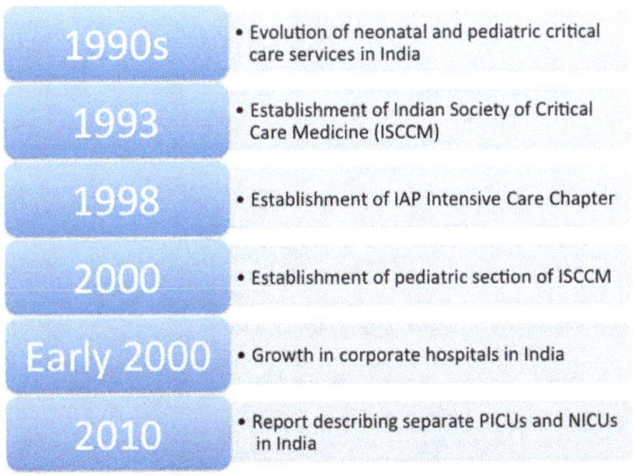

FIGURE 1 | A flow diagram of growth of pediatric critical care medicine in India.

of children in rural and remote parts of India are still deprived of timely critical care services and succumb to the illness.

CONTRIBUTIONS OF NATIONAL SOCIETIES IN SUPPORTING THE PEDIATRIC CRITICAL CARE TRAINING IN INDIA

Indian Society of Critical Care Medicine (ISCCM) was established in Mumbai, India in 1993. It is the largest non-profit association of Indian physicians, nurses, physiotherapists, and other allied health care professionals involved in the care of the critically ill. ISCCM, which started with a small group of intensivists, from Mumbai, has grown to membership of 7,440, comprising of 67 city branches all across the India with headquarter in Mumbai (7). The pediatric section of ISCCM was established in 2000. It has more than 200 members. Indian College of Critical Care Medicine was established by ISCCM to implement and carry out all the educational activities, including Indian fellowship in critical care medicine and Indian diploma in critical care medicine (7). The intensive care chapter of IAPs was established in 1998 (8). Since then, IAP Intensive Care Chapter has been successful in promoting the field of pediatric critical care. It has more than 500 members. The chapter has established guidelines for PICUs and education programs (8). ISCCM in coordination with the IAP intensive care chapter has developed PCCM fellowship with an established curriculum and training at the approved PICUs all over the country (9). The pediatric section of ISCCM and IAP has been active in beginning Diplomat in National Board certification in PCCM (7, 10). The national bodies have been active in organizing critical care conferences, workshops, and courses such as basic pediatric intensive care in India (8). This has not only improved networking opportunities connecting the potential PCCM fellows to the appropriate fellowship programs but also reinforced their clinical and academic training.

PCCM TRAINING IN INDIA

There are now 22 official PCCM fellowship programs listed on the college of pediatric critical care website and the number is growing every year (8) (**Figure 2**). There are different curriculum-based PCCM fellowships—a 1-year fellowship and a 2-year fellowship, each heavily clinically focused. There are only a handful of institutions in India, which have started a 3-year PCCM fellowship with curriculum similar to that of PCCM training in the West. The 3-year fellowship provides sufficient time for accomplishing a meaningful research project. The 3-year fellowship programs, which offer Doctor of Medicine degree upon successful completion of the fellowship, have been restricted to large, esteemed, government-run teaching institutions (10).

During fellowship, the fellows work closely with pediatric critical care consultants, pediatric cardiologists, surgeons, and other specialists. In India, traditional bedside teaching is still far more prevalent than classroom teaching. Apart from fundamental critical care training, the fellows also get exposed to counseling families, delivering difficult news, quality, and safety in PICU and end of life care. The fellows also get trained in designing a PICU, understanding a need for PICU in rural setting, creating, managing and maintaining a new PICU, and working on a budget for building a new PICU, implementing PICU protocols and a teaching program. Critical care ultrasound has been increasingly utilized in India (10–12). A significant number of PICUs in India have started using bedside ultrasound for assessment of critically ill children and monitoring of the therapies (13, 14). But the training of the PCCM fellows in India occurs largely based on the traditional "see one, do one and teach one" model. A handful of PCCM fellows attend critical care ultrasound workshop or course (15) but there is no formal curriculum or credentialing process for critical care ultrasound (16).

For PCCM fellows in India, majority of clinical learning, including procedural skills occur on the job. In the USA, a large number of PCCM fellowship training programs have adopted a formal fellow orientation process, which often includes hands-on airway skills in the operating room under supervision of a pediatric anesthesiologist and simulation-based training before they actually begin to work in the PICU. Similar to the West, majority of PCCM fellowship programs in India offer hands-on airway skills training in the operating room in the first year of fellowship. Recently, there is an increase in awareness and use of simulation-based teaching and training methodologies in pediatric emergency and critical care medicine.

SIMULATION-BASED PCCM TRAINING IN INDIA

Over last 5 years, there is a significant growth in simulation-based PCCM training. Pediatric Simulation Training and Research Society (pediSTARS) has played vital role in introducing and spreading the simulation-based pediatric training in India (17). Back in 2011, the society introduced the first simulation workshop focused on pediatric emergencies as a pre-congress workshop prior to National Conference of Pediatric Critical

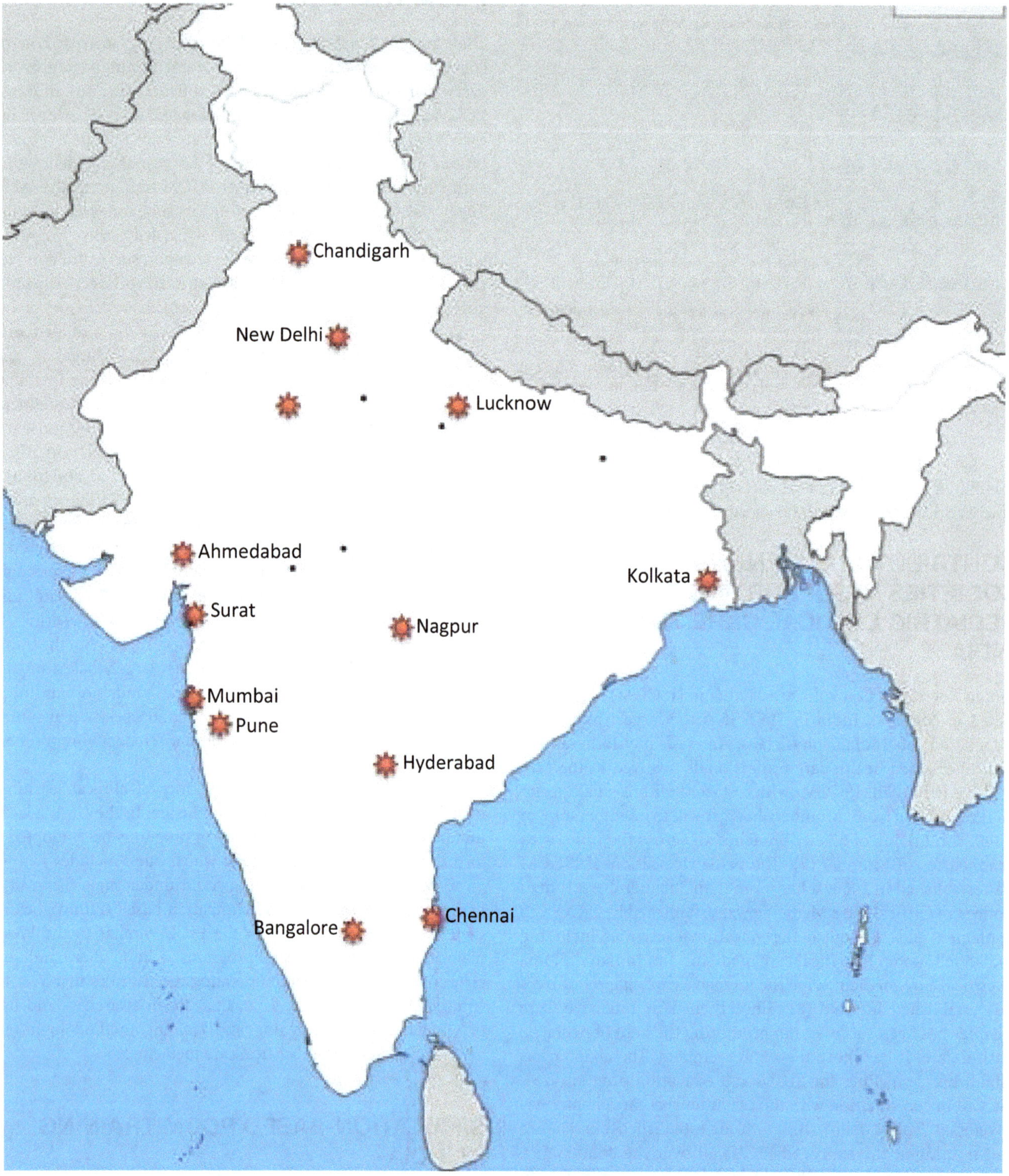

FIGURE 2 | Map of major cities of India with pediatric critical care medicine fellowship training centers.

Care (NCPCC) (17). But the simulation-based training in PCCM remained largely dormant in India for a couple of years beyond the initial attempt at introducing the concept of simulation. Our first regional pediatric critical care simulation workshop organized and conducted by us in Mumbai in 2013 (18) drew a significant interest and enthusiasm in simulation-based PCCM training in rest of the India. Ever since then, the IAP intensive care chapter adopted it as a standing pre-congress workshop for the NCPCC. Also, following this, pediSTARS launched the first national conference in pediatric simulation, SIMULUS along with the first pediatric simulation training of trainers' workshop in 2014 in India (17). PediSTARS India has played a prominent role in organizing SUCCESS—Simulation Course for Critical care Emergencies for pediatric intensive care trainees (17). Moving forward, simulation-based PCCM training must focus on basic and advanced PCCM training in keeping with the challenges of critical care delivery unique to the developing world, such as limitation of resources (19), fulminant infections unique to the developing world (20) and transportation of critically ill children (21).

Simulation training of PICU fellows should also focus on training them on multidisciplinary care, prevention, and management of team conflicts, dealing with difficult situation, delivering bad news, dealing with hostile and uncooperative family.

FUTURE OF PCCM TRAINING IN INDIA

A rapid growth of PCCM training programs in India has paralleled and complemented the rapid growth of healthcare sector in India. Two national societies—ISCCM and IAPs have played pivotal role in growing and supporting PCCM fellowship programs all over India and in future they will continue to advance the field. In future, it is likely that a larger number of teaching institutions in India will adopt a 3-year fellowship curriculum with balanced clinical and academic PCCM training. Critical care ultrasound training, simulation-based training, training in advanced therapies, such as renal replacement and extracorporeal life support, training in quality and safety, and research methodologies are likely to become integral part of the PCCM fellowship in India in future. Western influence is likely to bring less hierarchy in healthcare. Therefore, a formal, 360° evaluation system within PCCM fellowship is likely to be introduced in India in future. Similar to what western countries witnessed in the last decade, PCCM subspecialty services in India, such as pediatric cardiac critical care and pediatric neurocritical care, are likely to grow and branch out from the general pediatric critical care. Separate pediatric cardiac intensive care units already exist in a good number of private and government hospitals since last few years. It is likely that special critical care training programs focused on pediatric cardiac critical care and pediatric neurocritical care will begin in India in the near future. In short, since the beginning of the new century, the PCCM training in India has grown with leaps and bounds and it is still growing. The contributions of national societies and quality of standards of PCCM fellowship programs maintained by national societies and governing bodies, such as ISCCM, IAP intensive care chapter, Medical Council of India, and National Board of Examinations, will define the future of pediatric critical care training in India.

AUTHOR CONTRIBUTIONS

Each author contributed equally to this manuscript.

REFERENCES

1. Vidyasagar D, Singh M, Bhakoo ON, Paul VK, Narang A, Bhutani V, et al. Evolution of neonatal and pediatric critical care in India. *Crit Care Clin* (1997) 13(2):331–46. doi:10.1016/S0749-0704(05)70313-4
2. Sengupta A, Nundy S. The private health sector in India is burgeoning, but at the cost of public health care. *BMJ* (2005) 331(7526):1157–8. doi:10.1136/bmj.331.7526.1157
3. Data from: India Brand Equity Foundation. *Healthcare*. Source: Deloitte by TechSci Research Inc. (2017). Available from: https://www.ibef.org/download/Healthcare-January-2017.pdf
4. Khilnani P. Pediatric critical care in the 21st century. *Indian J Pediatr* (1998) 65:707–8. doi:10.1007/BF02731046
5. Lodha R, Kabra SK. Protocol based treatment in pediatric intensive care units. *Indian J Pediatr* (2010) 77:1277–8. doi:10.1007/s12098-010-0269-9
6. Khilnani P. Consensus guidelines for pediatric intensive care units in India. *Indian Pediatr* (2002) 39(1):43–50.
7. Data from: Education and College, Indian Society of Critical Care Medicine (2017). Available from: http://www.isccm.org/education_and_college.aspx
8. Data from: Training, Pediatric Intensive Care Chapter (2017). Available from: http://www.piccindia.com/default.shtml
9. Data from: Guidelines for Competency Based Training Programme in FNB-Pediatric Intensive Care (2017). Available from: https://nbe.edu.in/mainpdf/curriculum/Pediatric-Intensive-Care.pdf
10. Data from: DM courses, Post Graduate Institute of Medical Education and Research (2017). Available from: http://pgimer.edu.in/PGIMER_PORTAL/PGIMERPORTAL/GlobalPages/JSP/Page_Data.jsp?dep_id=43
11. Agarwal A, Singh DK, Singh AP. Ultrasonography: a novel approach to central venous cannulation. *Indian J Crit Care Med* (2009) 13(4):213–6. doi:10.4103/0972-5229.60174
12. Chacko J, Brar G. Bedside ultrasonography: applications in critical care: part I. *Indian J Crit Care Med* (2014) 18(5):301–9. doi:10.4103/0972-5229.132492
13. Khilnani P. Bedside ultrasound and echocardiography by the pediatric intensivist: an evolving tool and a feasible option in a pediatric ICU. *Indian J Crit Care Med* (2013) 17(4):201–2. doi:10.4103/0972-5229.118405
14. Khilnani P. The pediatric BUS has arrived: is bedside ultrasound in the pediatric intensive care unit a feasible option? *Pediatr Crit Care Med* (2011) 12(6):681–3. doi:10.1097/PCC.0b013e31822f1140
15. Data from: Courses, The International Council for Critical Emergency Sonography (2017). Available from: http://aiimsultrasound.com/courses/
16. Khilnani P. Is it time for training and accreditation of an intensivist sonographer? *Pediatr Crit Care Med* (2014) 15(7):678–9. doi:10.1097/PCC.0000000000000183
17. Data from: Training Programs, Pediatric Simulation Training and Research Society (2017). Available from: http://www.pedistarsindia.com/
18. Bhalala US, Sadawarte J, Sadawarte S, Baldua V, Garekar S, Pandit R, et al. Development and implementation of pediatric critical care focused simulation workshop and program in India. *J Pediatr Crit Care* (2014) 1(4):240–4. doi:10.21304/2014.0104.00039
19. Turner EL, Nielsen KR, Jamal SM, von Saint André-von Arnim A, Musa NL. A review of pediatric critical care in resource-limited settings: a look at past, present, and future directions. *Front Pediatr* (2016) 4:5. doi:10.3389/fped.2016.00005
20. Khilnani P, Singhi S, Lodha R, Santhanam I, Sachdev A, Chugh K, et al. Pediatric sepsis guidelines: summary for resource-limited countries. *Indian J Crit Care Med* (2010) 14(1):41–52. doi:10.4103/0972-5229.63029
21. Khilnani P, Chhabra R. Transport of critically ill children: how to utilize resources in the developing world. *Indian J Pediatr* (2008) 75(6):591–8. doi:10.1007/s12098-008-0115-5

18

A Review of the Integrated Model of Care: An Opportunity to Respond to Extensive Palliative Care Needs in Pediatric Intensive Care Units in Under-Resourced Settings

Michelle Grunauer[1,2] and Caley Mikesell[1]*

[1] *Escuela de Medicina, Colegio de Ciencias de la Salud, Universidad San Francisco de Quito, Quito, Ecuador,*
[2] *Pediatric Intensive Care Unit, Hospital de los Valles, Quito, Ecuador*

Correspondence:
Michelle Grunauer
mgrunauer@usfq.edu.ec

It is estimated that 6.3 million children who die annually need pediatric palliative care (PPC) and that only about 10% of them receive the attention they need because about 98% of them live in under-resourced settings where PPC is not accessible. The consultative model and the integrated model of care (IMOC) are the most common strategies used to make PPC available to critically ill children. In the consultative model, the pediatric intensive care unit (PICU) team, the patient, or their family must request a palliative care (PC) consultation with the external PC team for a PICU patient to be evaluated for special care needs. While the consultation model has historically been more popular, issues related to specialist availability, referral timing, staff's personal biases, misconceptions about PC, and other factors may impede excellent candidates from receiving the attention they need in a timely manner. Contrastingly, in the IMOC, family-centered care, PC tasks, and/or PC are a standard part of the treatment automatically available to all patients. In the IMOC, the PICU team is trained to complete critical and PC tasks as a part of normal daily operations. This review investigates the claim that the IMOC is the best model to meet extensive PPC needs in PICUs, especially in low-resource settings; based on an extensive review of the literature, we have identified five reasons why this model may be superior. The IMOC appears to: (1) improve the delivery of PPC and pediatric critical care, (2) allow clinicians to better respond to the care needs of patients and the epidemiological realities of their settings in ways that are consistent with evidence-based recommendations, (3) facilitate the universal delivery of care to all patients with special care needs, (4) maximize available resources, and (5) build local capacity; each of these areas should be further researched to develop a model of care that enables clinicians to provide pediatric patients with the highest attainable standard of health care. The IMOC lays out a pathway to provide the world's sickest, most vulnerable children with access to PPC, a human right to which they are entitled by international legal conventions.

Keywords: pediatric palliative care, integrated model of care, pediatric critical care, pediatric intensive care, Pediatric Palliative Screening Scale, low-resource settings, consultative model

---

Abbreviations: ICU, intensive care unit; PICU, pediatric intensive care unit; PC, palliative care; PPC, pediatric palliative care; IMOC, integrated model of care; DNR, do not resuscitate; WHO, World Health Organization; LMICs, low-middle income countries; HDLV, Hospital de los Valles; PCCEM, Pediatric Critical Care and Emergency Medicine; PaPaS, Pediatric Palliative Screening Scale.

PALLIATIVE CARE (PC) IN THE INTENSIVE CARE UNIT (ICU)

The silo thinking that underpins much of western medicine cannot universally facilitate the enforcement of the human right to the highest possible standard of health care and, in many cases, may be antagonistic to the pursuit of that goal; ICUs in under-resourced settings characterized by great health-care-related inequalities, poor infrastructure, and limited personnel are one such context in which silo thinking cannot structure care to appropriately meet the multifaceted needs of patients (1). The tendency to isolate medical specialties under this framework has led to a division between intensive and PC—two branches of medicine that are essential to the treatment of critically ill patients in ICUs. This common practice has contributed to the perception that adding PC tasks to intensivists' daily responsibilities will burden them, unnecessarily absorb valuable time and resources, and take away from their "real care goals." On the contrary, a breadth of evidence shows that adopting a holistic care strategy can conserve valuable resources in the ICU (2–4) and improve patients', their families', and caretakers' well-being (5).

Silo thinking is the foundation of the most popular strategy used to make PC available in the ICU: the consultative model (5). In purely consultative models, the hospital uses its resources to hire additional specialists and perhaps even create a stand-alone PC department. This external team is brought into the ICU to care for patients who are identified as having PC needs. The patient, their family, or their health-care providers must first identify the need for PC and then request a consultation with the external PC team for such attention to be provided.

According to the consultative model, ICU staff are positioned as gatekeepers to PC access; if they lack training, have negative attitudes or false beliefs about PC, do not understand its applications and potential benefits, or cannot recognize the "triggers" that signal a patient's PC needs, external PC resources may not be used when indicated and, consequently, PC may not be normalized in a given ICU (6, 7). Lynn explains, "The course of care is much more strongly associated with the service supply and habit patterns of the local care system than with the particular preferences or prognoses of the individual patient" (8). If consultative models do not involve the intentional training of ICU staff in holistic care, the personnel's attitudes, knowledge, and practices may impede the treatment of patients' PC needs (6, 7).

Contrastingly, in the integrated model of care (IMOC), family-centered care, PC tasks, and/or PC are a standard part of the treatment automatically available to all patients. In the IMOC, the ICU team is trained in holistic critical care and PC tasks are embedded in the unit's protocols. As a part of normal daily operations, team members simultaneously initiate PC and critical care, screen for PC needs regularly, and design plans to meet those needs as they arise. Although the consultative model is overall more common (5), the IMOC appears to offer distinct benefits to patients with pediatric palliative care (PPC) needs and, in pediatric ICUs, "is rapidly becoming the standard for high quality care of critically ill children" (4). While both models can make PC available in ICUs and pediatric intensive care units (PICUs), the IMOC may be more beneficial to patients/their families and may be better suited to under-resourced settings where hiring outside specialists may be impossible.

To date, there is little research that directly compares the effectiveness of the IMOC and the consultative model. However, one compelling 2011 study comparing models of PC in the United States found family members' opinions of their loved ones' last month of life correlated with the model according to which they were treated. The family of patients who had received integrated PC services were the most likely to report that the deceased had an "excellent" quality of life during their last month, followed by those who had received consultative PC services, and then by those who had only received usual care (no PC) (9). The group that received integrated PC services also appeared to receive more holistic attention; they were more likely to have accessed chaplain services and prepared do not resuscitate orders before death; their families also received more bereavement contact following their passing (9). This study presents direct evidence that the IMOC may be superior to the consultative model across various dimensions of care (9), even in industrialized countries where more PC specialists, superior infrastructure, greater education, and more medical resources are available (10).

This review investigates the claim that the IMOC is the best model to meet extensive PPC needs in PICUs, especially in low-resource settings; based on an extensive review of the literature, we have identified five reasons why this model may be superior. The IMOC appears to: (1) improve the delivery of PPC and critical care, (2) allow clinicians to better respond to the care needs of patients and the epidemiological realities of their settings in ways that are consistent with evidence-based recommendations, (3) facilitate the universal delivery of care to all patients with special care needs, (4) maximize available resources, and (5) build local capacity in a way that responds to the current shortage of PC specialty education; each of these areas requires further investigation to improve PPC delivery.

This review integrates evidence from countries around the world, but especially focuses on under-resourced settings like Ecuador, the authors' country of residence. The need for improved PPC and pediatric critical care (PCC) delivery is particularly urgent in contexts like ours because the high burden of PPC needs overwhelms our underdeveloped health-care infrastructure. Unfortunately, as this review will highlight, the majority of PC-related studies have been completed in industrialized countries and, as such, do not always accurately reflect the realities of PC and health-care professionals in our context. The skewed perspective of the academic discipline of PC was evidenced by a 2016 review of the last 20 years of publications in the field of PC, which revealed that over 90% of all documents published on the topic originated in industrialized nations classified as Group 4 countries by the World Palliative Care Alliance, meaning that they have already achieved integration of hospice-PC into their health-care systems (10, 11). When industrialized countries' practices, beliefs, and customs are assumed to be the neutral standard for medical care and subsequently applied to different cultural contexts, health professionals may disregard the unique assets, traditions, and needs of under-resourced communities in which they work. Such dynamics have the potential to further oppress already disadvantaged groups, waste resources, and create additional barriers between PC and the patients who need it. For this reason, we integrate as much pertinent data from our context as possible, but significantly supplement it with findings from industrialized nations.

RESISTANCE TO PC IN THE ICU

The direct integration of PC into the PICU/ICU through the IMOC is commonly met with resistance because of prevalent myths, discipline-based bias, and a lack of knowledge of evidence-based recommendations (12, 13). Although the specific barriers to implementing PC in the ICU vary from culture to culture and unit to unit, some of the particularly problematic misconceptions that keep this specialty out of the ICU are the ideas that PC is (1) ineffective and unimportant for most ICU patients, (2) synonymous with hospice and hopelessness on the part of the family, patients, and/or clinician, (3) equivalent to the "soft skills" that health-care professionals already innately have, and (4) wasteful in that it absorbs valuable time and resources from intensivists. Although prevalent, none of these ideas are consistent with decades of research about PC. **Table 1** provides a summary of key articles highlighting the importance of the PC in the ICU.

Contrary to the first myth, evidence shows that PC has major implications for the well-being of patients, their families, and practitioners (4, 5, 9, 18–25). PC is an interdisciplinary field that seeks to prevent and relieve the multifaceted suffering that critically ill patients and their families experience as a result of acute, chronic, life-limiting, and life-threatening conditions. PC addresses physical, psychosocial, ethical, spiritual, cultural, familial, and communication-related distress, as well as death and bereavement issues (21, 26–28). The timely initiation of PC is associated with (1) improved symptom management (18–20), (2) positive outcomes in patients (4, 18, 20), (3) improved quality of life for patients, families, and caregivers (18, 20), (4) better communication between professionals, patients, and their families (1, 4, 29, 30), and (5) longer life survival times among patients (4, 29).

Furthermore, PC belongs in the PICU/ICU because virtually all critically ill patients exhibit some level of PC need throughout their hospitalization (4, 5, 14, 31); to meet patients' extensive PPC needs, PICUs may benefit from making PPC universally accessible through an IMOC. PC is indicated in a wide range of patients, not only those confronting the terminal stages of illness (4). Because PC is inaccurately equated with hospice, it is commonly and erroneously thought to signal imminent death and therefore may provoke anxiety among patients, families, and practitioners. Combined with the lack of knowledge about PC recommendations, this reputation fodders the incorrect idea that PC—care supposedly directed only at the dying—is not applicable to most patients in the ICU. However, the World Health Organization (WHO) (22), United Nations (32), and together for Short Lives' PC charity (28) recommend that PPC should be extended to children with life-limiting conditions and not solely to those who are terminally ill. Cook and Rocker explain, "The coexistence of palliative care and critical care may seem paradoxical in the

TABLE 1 | Summary of key articles.

Reference	Summary
Nelson et al. (14)	Rapid response teams (RRTs) or emergency medical teams are common in intensive care unit (ICU) settings and seek to prevent morbidity and mortality among already hospitalized patients who may be deteriorating. While there are conflicting data about the effectiveness of RRTs in accomplishing these goals, RRTs are well positioned to meet the palliative care (PC) needs of patients in the ICU. RRTs can, and in many cases, already perform a range of PC tasks related to communication, emotional/psychological support, symptom control, and pain management. RRTs should also be given the tools necessary to facilitate family conferences in emergencies, provide family-centered care, support distressed caregivers, foster shared decision-making, and help colleagues to administer measures of self-care. Considering their already extensive skillsets and proximity to patients, their families, and professional caretakers, RTTs should be trained to provide PC to patients admitted to ICUs and emergency departments
Boss et al. (4)	This article reviews the benefits that patients, their families, and pediatric intensive care unit (PICU) staff experience "when PC is intentionally incorporated into the PICU." (4) PC is indicated in a large share of children admitted to PICUs; as epidemiological shifts occur across the world, an increasingly large number of children become eligible for PC to address the needs that arise from their complex, chronic diseases. PC is interdisciplinary and addresses a range of needs of patients, families, and their professional caregivers, including pain management, symptom control, family and patient-centered communication and decision-making, psychological care, and other types of support key to the well-being of patients, their families, and PICU personnel. This review also highlights some of the gaps in care in PICUs, including accurate pain assessment, poor communication between families and PICU staff, inadequate psychosocial treatment, high levels of unaddressed psychological morbidity among family members, and other issues; intentionally integrating PC into PICUs is an excellent opportunity to meet such needs
O'Brien et al. (15)	This article examines the potential impact and methodology for a future intervention in 26 PICUs from Canada, Australia, and New Zealand to change the role of parents in neonatal care. Based on data from previous similar interventions, O'Brien et al. hypothesized that integrating parents into the NICU team as providers of all, but the most advanced medical interventions would result in faster weight gain, greater rates of breastfeeding, and improved clinical outcomes for infants as well as reduced levels of stress and anxiety for parents. The FICare intervention program requires primary care givers to undergo extensive training to learn how to properly care for their neonates, commit to 6 h daily to caring for their babies, record their interactions with their babies in a special journal, and interact with "veteran parents," who give personal support to parents whose babies are in the NICU. Previous data evidence the great positive potential for this intervention

(Continued)

TABLE 1 | Continued

Reference	Summary
Curtis (16)	ICU personnel should be trained to provide PC in their units because it plays an important role in the care of critically ill patients, not merely those at risk for dying. PC is important because it allows us to better facilitate intentional discussions about treatment plans, other types of communication, patient-focused/family-centered decision-making, symptom management, multidisciplinary collaborations in patient treatment, end-of-life decisions, logistical planning, and other aspects of care. Implementing PC in the ICU could help to address diverse unmet symptoms or patients and their families, improper communication techniques employed by ICU personnel, conflicts/lack of communication within the ICU, and many other difficulties. To improve PC in ICUs, Curtis suggests educating ICU personnel in PC and how to overcome PC implementation barriers, establishing institutional policies to promote PC, and providing ICU staff with feedback from families of their patients. PC should be implemented in the ICU to improve the experiences and well-being of patients, their families, and the ICU staff itself
Aslakson et al. (17)	PC is used to address the complex care needs of critically ill individuals, regardless of their prognoses or diagnoses; as such, this type of care should be initiated for various critically ill individuals upon ICU admission to better address psychosocial, spiritual, and physical symptom management; coordinate, plan and communicate about multidisciplinary treatment that reflects the patient's and their family's preferences; provide family-centered care and extensive care planning; and facilitate the family caregivers' and ICU personnel's own self-care. Aslakson et al. identified clinician's subpar communication skills, unrealistic expectations related to patients and treatment, clinicians' time constraints, decision-making difficulties, and other areas as opportunities for care improvement within the ICU which PC could address. The authors suggest that further research needs to be completed to determine the best methods for providing patients and their families with PC in situations of critical illness both inside and outside of the ICU

technological ICU. However, contemporary critical care should be as concerned with palliation as with the prevention, diagnosis, monitoring, and treatment of life-threatening conditions" (33). PC not only improves the quality of patients' deaths but also of their lives.

Palliative care can be beneficial to a wide range of patients regardless their prognoses and diagnoses (16, 17, 22, 28). Boss et al. explain that PC should begin at the time of diagnosis of a potentially life-limiting condition and continue throughout the disease trajectory, regardless of the expected outcome (4). Although this type of care is particularly important to the terminally ill, it also plays a complementary role in the care of critically ill patients who may be able to make a complete recovery (22, 32). Together for Short Lives, a leading charity in the United Kingdom for children with life-limiting and life-threatening conditions, developed a categorization of pediatric conditions for which PC is indicated; these include potentially curable diseases (in which life is at risk and treatment may or may not succeed), progressive conditions, irreversible conditions causing severe disability, and morbidities that inevitably cause premature death (28). PC is applicable in all stages of such diseases and conditions (10, 34–39) and represents the evolution of hope, rather than the extinguishment of it—in some illness. Through impeccable assessment, treatment, and communication carried out by multidisciplinary teams, PC enhances the quality of life for a diverse range of patients and their loved ones, independent of what the future may hold for them (4, 5, 21, 22). Through PC, we can focus our hope on a better quality of life, death, and other realistic goals rather than wish for impossible outcomes.

In addition, considering that PC involves a range of multidisciplinary tasks to address various needs common among most PICU patients (4, 5, 31), health-care professionals should not be expected to be innately prepared to address all PC needs. Special training is required to address any one of the many areas that PC seeks to address in a way that is consistent with evidence-based recommendations. Unsurprisingly, several studies have shown that ICU staff's beliefs about PC, knowledge of the field, and their actual practices in the ICU are deeply interconnected. One study of ICU nurses' attitudes about PC found that participants had "moderately negative to neutral attitudes toward PC," especially with regards to patient preferences and withholding/withdrawing treatment (7). Unsurprisingly, Razban et al. found that nurses' beliefs were significantly correlated with their own "...personal study about palliative care, level of education, and experience of caring for a dying family member" (7). These findings suggest that education is key to creating an environment receptive to PC. Another study of nurses, intensivists, and advanced practice providers at three large academic hospitals found the "triggers" for initiating PC consultation to be an important barrier: the staff most frequently relied on triggers that resulted in late-stage PC application (6), which is inconsistent with best-practice recommendations that PC should be applied early and concurrently with disease-directed treatment (2, 22, 28). Again, education is key to implementing evidence-based practices; if ICU staff are expected to bridge the gaps in PC in their units, they must be properly trained to do so.

Finally, contrary to the popular myth that it is wasteful and unnecessarily burdensome for intensivists, PC is actually a resource-saving strategy in the ICU (2, 3). In under-resourced contexts like ours, distributive justice in medical care is perhaps the most prominent ethical principle that we encounter on a day-to-day basis. PC saves valuable resources because it prevents morbidities like depression and anxiety (3) and prevents futile treatments (2), thereby conserving resources to treat other patients. Well-managed PC patients are able to enjoy an improved quality of life, may have better outcomes, and are empowered to make long-term care plans if necessary; this, in turn, helps PC to maximize local resources on the population level because it prevents unnecessary emergency room visits and keeps precious ICU beds open (3). In countries with limited medication access, health-care personnel, and ICU capacity, PC stands to have a dramatic impact on the well-being of individuals and communities alike.

PPC ACROSS THE GLOBAL SOUTH

In light of their effectiveness, the international community has declared PC and PPC basic human rights, maintaining that they are fundamental to the appropriate treatment of adults and children with special care needs in any stage of disease (20, 21, 23, 32, 35, 36, 39–42). Furthermore, "Palliative care is a recognized component of the right to the highest attainable standard of health, which is protected in article 12 of the International Covenant on Economic, Social and Cultural Rights, and in article 24 of the Convention on the Rights of the Child" (32). The WHO's inclusive definition of PPC echoes this sentiment (22):

- PC for children is the active total care of the child's body, mind, and spirit, and also involves giving support to the family.
- It begins when illness is diagnosed and continues regardless of whether or not a child receives treatment directed at the disease.
- Health providers must evaluate and alleviate a child's physical, psychological, and social distress.
- Effective PC requires a broad multidisciplinary approach that includes the family and makes use of available community resources; it can be successfully implemented even if resources are limited.
- It can be provided in tertiary care facilities, in community health centers and even in children's homes.

As described by the United Nations (43) and the WHO (22), the holistic focus of PPC makes it indispensable to achieving the highest attainable standard of care in many critical pediatric cases.

Despite the overwhelming evidence of its effectiveness, the vast majority of children who require PPC never receive it (10, 44); in part, this is because nearly 98% of pediatric patients who have PC needs come from low-middle income countries (LMICs) where it is simply not available (10). While many of these patients receive treatment directed at the disease, few receive concomitant PC (24, 25). Overall, around 6.3 million children requiring PPC die annually, but only about 10% of them receive the attention they need (10). The lack of PPC availability across the world results in the unnecessary suffering of the world's most vulnerable children.

PPC NEED IN ECUADOR

To better elucidate the urgent need for improved, more accessible PPC in contexts like Ecuador, it is vital to identify aspects of our context which may result in more extensive PC needs (10) and which may be unexpected for readers from industrialized contexts. The combination of issues unique to LMICs may contribute to an overall higher need for PPC which might not be seen in industrialized countries, where PICUs may commonly receive many children who need an intermediate level of care or postoperative stabilization (4). The level of development and fragmentation of the Ecuadorian health-care system leads to the deterioration of patients before they arrive to the hospital and therefore contribute to a greater need for PC. These challenges can be grouped into three categories, including: (1) insufficient Infrastructure, (2) lack of trained specialists, and (3) socioeconomic factors (20, 44).

With respect to infrastructure issues, the number of PICU beds and emergency transport vehicles are major hurdles for providing appropriate, timely care. Ecuador only has 36 PICU beds available throughout the entire country (45); therefore, the patients who take priority for these few precious spots are often in extremely critical states. Because of the severity of these cases, the average national PICU mortality rate in 2012 was around 15% (as compared with a 5% mortality rate in European PICUs) (45). Similarly, Ecuador has a fragmented emergency transport system which contributes to the severity of cases that arrive to the PICU. Aside from a menagerie of ambulances of varying quality from the private sector, Ecuador only has 714 medical emergency transport vehicles from the public sector, which are insufficient to meet the population's needs (46).

Similarly, a lack of trained pediatric intensivists and PC specialists in Ecuador makes it more difficult for children to receive the care they need. In Ecuador, there are approximately 33 pediatric intensivists (45) who are responsible for a pediatric population of nearly 5,000,000 (47). Unsurprisingly, the majority of these specialists are located in cities, further exacerbating regional inequalities in care.

Finally, socioeconomic factors reduce the quality of care available to pediatric patients. The lack of development of quality health care in rural areas, historical discrimination, poverty, and a lack of general health education especially among vulnerable groups are barriers (44). In addition, Ecuadorian children are also at great risk for comorbidities that can aggravate their conditions including parasitic infestations (48), malnutrition (49), and anemia (49). Similarly, the main causes of death common among Ecuadorian children include acute respiratory infections, traffic accidents, congenital malformations, leukemia, and other external causes, each of which can entail PPC needs before death (50, 51).

THE IMOC: A PATHWAY TO MEET INTERNATIONAL PPC NEEDS

Considering the extensive PPC needs of PICU patients (especially in LMIC countries like Ecuador), the IMOC may be the best strategy to make PC available to all of those patients who may require it because the IMOC appears to (1) improve the delivery of PPC and PCC, (2) allow clinicians to better respond to the care needs of patients and the epidemiological realities of their settings in ways that are consistent with evidence-based recommendations, (3) facilitate the universal delivery of care to all patients with special care needs, (4) maximize available resources, and (5) build local capacity. The IMOC lays out a pathway to provide the world's sickest, most vulnerable children with access to PPC, a human right to which they are entitled by international legal conventions (20, 22, 32, 34–39, 41).

The IMOC may improve the delivery of PPC in under-resourced environments because it bypasses those barriers which often impede the timely application of PPC. The advantage of the IMOC as compared with other models is that it already has PC embedded in its protocols. While the consultation model can make PPC available to patients, issues such as the timing of referral, physicians' personal perspectives, ethical dilemmas, decision-making difficulties, lack of screening tools and trained personnel, communication issues, and misconceptions about PC can impede excellent candidates from receiving the attention they need in a timely manner (4, 52).

The IMOC also improves the delivery of PPC in settings like ours because it does not assume that patients, families, or even health-care workers innately know what PPC is and when to request a consultation for such care. In many countries, most families do not know of the existence of PPC or understand what it involves; thus, they may never ask for the care or even accept it when it is offered (53). Worse yet, some families and many medical professionals may believe damaging myths about PC, such as the erroneous idea that PC hastens death (12); a plethora of evidence, including the low mortality rate in our own center which uses the IMOC (4.8%) (54), discredits this notion. In an IMOC, the aforementioned obstacles are non-existent because all patients, regardless of their disease state, prognosis, and diagnosis, are regularly screened for PPC needs.

Moreover, we speculate that the IMOC is the best model to meet patients' needs in the PICU because it better responds to epidemiological trends around the world and to patients' needs in ways that are consistent with evidence-based recommendations. As epidemiological transitions occur across the world, an increasingly large share of patients with complex, chronic diseases are being seen more frequently and repeatedly in ICUs/PICUs; Lynn argues that current health systems that bifurcate curative treatment and PC do not adequately respond to patients', families, and communities' care needs in an appropriate or sustainable way (8). Rather, models of care ought to focus on early intervention, continuity, family-centeredness, and patients' psychosocial suffering to create care pathways that help patients to avoid unnecessary suffering and that allow communities to conserve their precious medical resources (8, 15).

In addition, embedding PPC directly into PICU care models sidesteps the resistance against PC initiatives common in low-resource settings and maximizes local resources. Because the IMOC necessitates that PICU teams themselves are trained to carry out PC tasks, this model does not require additional staff or a new department as the consultation model does. PC consultation models are commonly met with resistance because cost-related hurdles can impede the establishment of new departments, pain and suffering are often normalized in low-resource settings (20), and PC may be viewed as a "luxury" for industrialized countries (20). By hybridizing PCC and PPC, it is possible to avoid such hurdles that can prevent the establishment of important PC programs.

Furthermore, the consultative PC model is ineffective in many settings because it relies on communities' current capacity; the IMOC is more effective in meeting PC needs because it involves and trains all ICU personnel and therefore necessitates capacity-building in every unit in which it is implemented. Evidence indicates that the consultative model is limited in its capacity to meet communities' PC needs even in resource-rich industrialized countries. For example, in a 2017 study, Wysham et al. reported that up to 35% of ICU patients in the United States needed PC; however, even in such a resource-rich setting, this level of need still overwhelmed the available 5,500 PC specialists' capacity (6). In other words, even in the United States, there are not enough PC specialists to make the consultative model effective in addressing national PC need. Wysham et al. explain, "In this context, it is estimated that <5% of ICU patients receive specialist palliative care" (6).

The apparent dominance of the consultative PC model in ICUs seems even less appropriate when examined through the lens of pediatric intensive care in under-resourced settings like ours. Ecuador is categorized as a 3A country in the provision of PC (meaning that it has isolated provision in level of PC development) (10) and a high burden of conditions, diseases, and accidents that require PC (47, 49, 50). The burden of PC need combined with a lack of specialists renders the consultative model ineffective in addressing national and international PC needs.

While it is easy to point to a need for more training programs as a solution to the gross mismatch between PPC needs and specialist availability across the world, this idealistic thought process follows the paradigm that heralds the consultative model as king. It is true that there is great global need for more PPC training programs; however, international conventions entitle the world's sickest children to pathways of care that provide more immediate access to the highest available standard of health care (which must include access to PC services) (22, 43). The IMOC proposes a paradigm shift that would make it possible to begin meeting children's PC needs more rapidly and effectively than the consultative model.

Although trained PPC specialists may have greater expertise than health-care professionals who do not have the same level of formal training, many PICU personnel already unknowingly engage in some dimensions PC and can learn tasks to improve the level of care that they already provide (14). Shifting from the consultative model to the IMOC requires us to honestly appraise and develop the PC skills of all PICU/ICU staff, not only those of highly trained specialists. While a breadth of evidence demonstrates that beliefs and practices incongruent with the goals of PC abound in ICUs (6, 7, 34, 53), this does not indicate that intensive care staff lack the valuable foundations necessary to learn how better perform PC tasks. In Ecuador (45), the United States (6), and probably in most other settings, pediatric intensivists, nurses, and other support personnel present in PICUs greatly outnumber the trained PPC specialists. Whereas the consultative model frames this reality as damning, the IMOC frames it as a latent possibility for PC expansion. Ecuador has 33 pediatric intensivists (45) and countless other health-care professionals that work in PICUs—according to the IMOC, these health-care professionals ought to be considered potential PPC providers.

THE IMOC IN ECUADOR

While it may seem foolishly idealistic to paint non-specialist PICU/ICU personnel as potential PPC providers, in recent years our team has pioneered a number of training programs that hybridize PCC and PPC. In 4 years, these programs have disseminated the IMOC and increased the national Pediatric Critical Care and Emergency Medicine (PCCEM) and PPC capacity by 560% (54). Without making formal policy changes, gaining new specialists, or adding new subspecialist training in our country, we were able to exact systematic change by training non-specialist personnel to work together to identify and complete PC tasks in the PICU. Our programs have been massively successful in improving the quality and accessibility of PCC and PPC care to pediatric patients throughout Ecuador and further support the hypothesis IMOC is the best model to meet extensive PPC needs.

The extensive PC need in our context (20, 46, 49, 51, 55) and new data supporting the effectiveness of the IMOC (9) lead the principal investigator (Michelle Grunauer) to implement the IMOC in the PICU of the Hospital de los Valles (HDLV) when it was established in Quito, Ecuador in 2013. HDLV's PICU was the first PICU in Ecuador to use a family-centered IMOC. She integrated the IMOC into the PICU because there is no known evidence that the external consultation strategy provides better patient care and because the IMOC is particularly well suited to under-resourced settings like ours, where there are no resources available to create an external PC service.

Michelle Grunauer incorporated the IMOC into this unit primarily through a certificate training program she launched in conjunction with physicians from the United States trained in PCCEM to elevate local medical professionals' expertise in critical care and PC (54). "The Laude in PCCEM employs a family-centered approach by integrating pediatric critical care (PCC), mental health, and palliative medicine. It is innovative in that any critically ill (not merely dying) child benefits from family involvement [in an IMOC] so that family might understand the disease process and take part in treatment decisions" (54). In essence, participants learned how to provide care to critically ill patients according to the framework of the IMOC.

Various methods are effective in integrating health-care professionals into the IMOC. In the first program launched in HDLV, instructors used a combination of pre-readings, classroom instruction, bedside didactics, and simulation drills to teach professionals about the IMOC (54). These activities integrated PC and family-centered care techniques into PCCEM by focusing on case-based learning, interdisciplinary/interprofessional teamwork, individual confidence, and skill competency (54). The activities themselves emphasized techniques and tasks key to the IMOC, including communication, symptom management, planning, ethical dilemmas, and other topics. Integrating these themes into the standardly available Advanced Pediatric Life Support curriculum is also an effective introduction to the IMOC (54).

A number of indicators pointed to the IMOC's success in HDLV's PICU. Improved holistic care provided through the IMOC seems to have impacted the satisfaction of patients and families that are admitted; this PICU has not had a single medical lawsuit during its 5 years of existence. Staff appear to provide better care and patients seem to have better symptom management, greater familial involvement, and improved overall outcomes since the implementation of the IMOC (54). In addition, the unit's mortality rate decreased from 10 to 4.8% after the staff were fully trained in the IMOC [Ecuador's average PICU mortality rate is 15% (45)]. These unit-wide improvements suggest that the IMOC may better meet the extensive special care needs of HDLV's PICU patients. Further studies are needed to determine the effectiveness of the IMOC in other settings, but this may be a better care model for other settings as well.

CONCLUSION

This article has identified reasons why the IMOC is well designed to meet the extensive PPC needs in PICUs across different contexts, especially in under-resourced settings like Ecuador. Currently, the direct integration of PC into the PICU is met with resistance because of prevalent myths and misconceptions about PC, discipline-related bias, and ignorance of evidence-based recommendations related to the application of PC. However, evidence (4, 5, 31) indicates that virtually all patients admitted to the PICU have some level of PC need; thus, PICU models must make PC highly accessible to all patients who may develop special care needs throughout their stay in the unit. Training difficulties, lack of specialists, consultation barriers, and a number of other factors appear to impede the consultative model from meeting this goal both in industrialized contexts (6) and in the global south. Considering the propriety of the IMOC to meet extensive PPC needs across different settings, the authors recommend further research related to the establishment of the IMOC in other centers, the effects of this model on quality of care, and comparisons of the IMOC with the consultative model. Employing the IMOC in PICUs around the world could represent an important paradigm shift within pediatric intensive medicine which could elevate care to a superior level, especially in under-resourced contexts.

AUTHOR CONTRIBUTIONS

MG contributed to the following in the elaboration of this investigation:

- Substantial contributions to the conception or design of the work and the acquisition, analysis, or interpretation of data for the work.
- Critical revision for important intellectual content.
- Final approval of the version to be published.
- Agreement to be accountable for all aspects of the work in ensuring that questions related to the accuracy or integrity of any part of the work are appropriately investigated and resolved.

CM contributed to the following in the elaboration of this investigation:

- Substantial contributions to the conception or design of the work and the acquisition, analysis, or interpretation of data for the work.
- Drafting the work and revising it critically for important intellectual content.
- Final approval of the version to be published.
- Agreement to be accountable for all aspects of the work in ensuring that questions related to the accuracy or integrity of any part of the work are appropriately investigated and resolved.

ACKNOWLEDGMENTS

The authors extend their deepest gratitude to all of the health-care professionals who selflessly dedicate their lives to caring for critically ill children in the Hospital de los Valles' PICU.

REFERENCES

1. Curtis K, Foster K, Mitchell R, Van C. Models of care delivery for families of critically ill children: an integrative review of international literature. *J Pediatr Nurs* (2016) 31(3):330–41. doi:10.1016/j.pedn.2015.11.009
2. Gaertner J, Maier BO, Radbruch L. Resource allocation issues concerning early palliative care. *Ann Palliat Med* (2015) 4(3):156–61. doi:10.3978/j.issn.2224-5820.2015.07.02
3. Meier DE. Increased access to palliative care and hospice services: opportunities to improve value in health care. *Milbank Q* (2011) 89(3):343–80. doi:10.1111/j.1468-0009.2011.00632.x
4. Boss R, Nelson J, Weissman D, Campbell M, Curtis R, Frontera J, et al. Integrating palliative care into the PICU: a report from the improving palliative care in the ICU advisory board. *Pediatr Crit Care Med* (2014) 15(8):762–7. doi:10.1097/PCC.0000000000000209
5. Nelson JE, Bassett R, Boss RD, Brasel KJ, Campbell ML, Cortez TB, et al. Models for structuring a clinical initiative to enhance palliative care in the intensive care unit: a report from the IPAL-ICU project (improving palliative care in the ICU). *Crit Care Med* (2010) 38(9):1765–72. doi:10.1097/CCM.0b013e3181e8ad23
6. Wysham NG, Hua M, Hough CL, Gundel S, Docherty SL, Jones DM, et al. Improving ICU-based palliative care delivery: a multicenter, multidisciplinary survey of critical care clinician attitudes and beliefs. *Crit Care Med* (2017) 45(4):e372–8. doi:10.1097/CCM.0000000000002099
7. Razban F, Iranmanesh S, Rafiei H. Nurses' attitudes toward palliative care in south-east Iran. *Int J Palliat Nurs* (2013) 19(8):403–10. doi:10.12968/ijpn.2013.19.8.403
8. Lynn J. Living long in fragile health: the new demographics shape end of life care. *Hastings Cent Rep* (2005) Spec No:S14–8. doi:10.1353/hcr.2005.0096
9. Casarett D, Johnson M, Smith D, Richardson D. The optimal delivery of palliative care: a national comparison of the outcomes of consultation teams vs inpatient units. *Arch Intern Med* (2011) 171(7):649–55. doi:10.1001/archinternmed.2011.87
10. World Palliative Care Alliance, World Health Organization. *Global Atlas of Palliative Care at the End of Life*. London: Worldwide Palliative Care Alliance (2014).
11. Chang HT, Lin MH, Chen CK, Hwang SJ, Hwang IH, Chen YC. Hospice palliative care article publications: an analysis of the Web of Science database from 1993 to 2013. *J Chin Med Assoc* (2016) 79(1):29–33. doi:10.1016/j.jcma.2015.05.012
12. Meier DE, Brawley OW. Palliative care and the quality of life. *J Clin Oncol* (2011) 29(20):2750–2. doi:10.1200/JCO.2011.35.9729
13. Perrin KO, Kazanowski M. Overcoming barriers to palliative care consultation. *Crit Care Nurse* (2015) 35(5):44–52. doi:10.4037/ccn2015357
14. Nelson JE, Mathews KS, Weissman DE, Brasel KJ, Campbell M, Curtis JR, et al. Integration of palliative care in the context of rapid response: a report from the improving palliative care in the ICU advisory board. *Chest* (2015) 147(2):560–9. doi:10.1378/chest.14-0993
15. O'Brien K, Bracht M, Robson K, Ye XY, Mirea L, Cruz M, et al. Evaluation of the Family Integrated Care model of neonatal intensive care: a cluster randomized controlled trial in Canada and Australia. *BMC Pediatr* (2015) 15:210. doi:10.1186/s12887-015-0527-0
16. Curtis JR. Caring for patients with critical illness and their families: the value of the integrated clinical team. *Respir Care* (2008) 53(4):480–7.
17. Aslakson RA, Curtis JR, Nelson JE. The changing role of palliative care in the ICU. *Crit Care Med* (2014) 42(11):2418–28. doi:10.1097/CCM.0000000000000573
18. Somerville M. Human rights and human ethics: health and health care. *Death Talk: The Case against Euthanasia and Physician-Assisted Suicide*. Montreal: McGill-Queen's University Press (2014). p. 327–44.
19. Gans D, Kominski GF, Roby DH, Diamant AL, Chen X, Lin W, et al. Better outcomes, lower costs: palliative care program reduces stress, costs of care for children with life-threatening conditions. *Policy Brief UCLA Cent Health Policy Res* (2012) (PB2012-3):1–8.
20. Human Rights Watch. *"Please, Do Not Make Us Suffer any More..." Access to Pain Treatment As a Human Right*. Washington, DC: Human Rights Watch (2009).
21. American Academy of Pediatrics, American College of Emergency Physicians, O'Malley P, Mace SE, Brown K. Patient- and family-centered care and the role of the emergency physician providing care to a child in the emergency department. *Ann Emerg Med* (2006) 48(5):643–5. doi:10.1016/j.annemergmed.2006.09.011
22. World Health Organization. *WHO Definition of Palliative Care*. (2016). Available from: http://www.who.int/cancer/palliative/definition/en/
23. Zernikow B, Hasan C, Hechler T, Huebner B, Gordon D, Michel E. Stop the pain! A nation-wide quality improvement programme in paediatric oncology pain control. *Eur J Pain* (2008) 12(7):819–33. doi:10.1016/j.ejpain.2007.12.002
24. Feudtner C, Kang TI, Hexem KR, Friedrichsdorf SJ, Osenga K, Siden H, et al. Pediatric palliative care patients: a prospective multicenter cohort study. *Pediatrics* (2011) 127(6):1094–101. doi:10.1542/peds.2010-3225
25. De Lima L. Palliative care and pain treatment in the global health agenda. *Pain* (2015) 156(Suppl 1):S115–8. doi:10.1097/01.j.pain.0000460349.23083.0b
26. Loscalzo MJ. Palliative care: an historical perspective. *Hematology Am Soc Hematol Educ Program* (2008) 2008:465. doi:10.1182/asheducation-2008.1.465
27. Rushton CH. A framework for integrated pediatric palliative care: being with dying. *J Pediatr Nurs* (2005) 20(5):311–25. doi:10.1016/j.pedn.2005.03.003
28. Together for Short Lives, AfCsPCTfS. *A Framework for the Development of an Integrated Care Pathway for Children and Young People with Life Threatening or Life-Limiting Conditions and Their Families*. (2013). Available from: http://www.togetherforshortlives.org.uk/assets/0000/4121TfSL_A_Core_Care_Pathway__ONLINE_pdf
29. Stewart MA. Effective physician-patient communication and health outcomes: a review. *CMAJ* (1995) 152(9):1423–33.
30. Davidson JE, Powers K, Hedayat KM, Tieszen M, Kon AA, Shepard E, et al. Clinical practice guidelines for support of the family in the patient-centered intensive care unit: American College of Critical Care Medicine Task Force 2004–2005. *Crit Care Med* (2007) 35(2):605–22. doi:10.1097/01.CCM.0000254067.14607.EB
31. Campbell ML, Weissman DE, Nelson JE. Palliative care consultation in the ICU #253. *J Palliat Med* (2012) 15(6):715–6. doi:10.1089/jpm.2012.9582
32. Schmidlin E, Oliver D. Palliative care as a human right: what has the Prague Charter achieved? *EJPC* (2015) 22(3):141–3.
33. Cook D, Rocker G. Dying with dignity in the intensive care unit. *N Engl J Med* (2014) 370(26):2506–14. doi:10.1056/NEJMra1208795
34. Adams V; Worldwide Palliative Care Alliance. Access to pain relief: an essential human right. A report for World Hospice and Palliative Care Day 2007. Help the hospices for the Worldwide Palliative Care Alliance. *J Pain Palliat Care Pharmacother* (2008) 22(2):101–29. doi:10.1080/15360280801992025
35. Breitbart W. Palliative care as a human right: update. *Palliat Support Care* (2011) 9(4):345–9. doi:10.1017/S1478951511000356
36. Brennan F. Palliative care as an international human right. *J Pain Symptom Manage* (2007) 33(5):494–9. doi:10.1016/j.jpainsymman.2007.02.022
37. Gwyther L, Brennan F, Harding R. Advancing palliative care as a human right. *J Pain Symptom Manage* (2009) 38(5):767–74. doi:10.1016/j.jpainsymman.2009.03.003
38. Larkin P. Far, far away land: palliative care as a human right. *Int J Palliat Nurs* (2013) 19(6):263. doi:10.12968/ijpn.2013.19.6.263
39. Radbruch L, Payne S, de Lima L, Lohmann D. The Lisbon challenge: acknowledging palliative care as a human right. *J Palliat Med* (2013) 16(3):301–4. doi:10.1089/jpm.2012.0394
40. Hannon B, Zimmermann C, Knaul FM, Powell RA, Mwangi-Powell FN, Rodin G. Provision of palliative care in low- and middle-income countries: overcoming obstacles for effective treatment delivery. *J Clin Oncol* (2016) 34(1):62–8. doi:10.1200/JCO.2015.62.1615
41. Shrivastava SR, Shrivastava PS, Ramasamy J. Palliative care: an integral component of human right to health. *Int J Prev Med* (2016) 7:15. doi:10.4103/2008-7802.173916
42. Donnelly JP, Huff SM, Lindsey ML, McMahon KA, Schumacher JD. The needs of children with life-limiting conditions: a healthcare-provider-based model. *Am J Hosp Palliat Care* (2005) 22(4):259–67. doi:10.1177/104990910502200406
43. UN Commisioner on Human Rights, Office of the High Commisioner, United Nations, editors. *International Covenant on Economic, Social and Cultural Rights*. New York: United Nations (1966). 2200A (XXI) p.
44. Baker T. Critical care in low-income countries. *Trop Med Int Health* (2009) 14(2):143–8. doi:10.1111/j.1365-3156.2008.02202.x
45. Campos-Miño S, Sasbon JS, von Dessauer B. [Pediatric intensive care in Latin America]. *Med Intensiva* (2012) 36(1):3–10. doi:10.1016/j.medin.2011.07.004
46. Ministerio de Salud Pública del Ecuador. *Dirección Nacional de Unidades Móviles y Atención Pre-Hospitalaria del MSP*. Quito, Ecuador: Ministerio de Salud Públic del Ecuador (2017).

47. The World Bank. *World Development Indicators.* (2016). Available from: http://databank.worldbank.org/data/reports.aspx?source=world-development-indicators
48. Cartelle Gestal M, Holban AM, Escalante S, Cevallos M. Epidemiology of tropical neglected diseases in Ecuador in the last 20 years. *PLoS One* (2015) 10(9):e0138311. doi:10.1371/journal.pone.0138311
49. The World Bank. *Ecuador – Nutrition at a Glance.* Washington, DC: The World Bank (2011).
50. Ministerio de la Salud Pública, Presidencia de la República del Ecuador, Instituto Nacional de Estadística y Censos, Organización Panamericana de la Salud. *Indicadores Básicos de Salud.* Quito, Ecuador: Ministerio de Salud Pública (2010).
51. Pan American Health Organization. *Ecuador.* Quito, Ecuador: Pan American Health Organization (2012).
52. Mohanti BK. Ethics in palliative care. *Indian J Palliat Care* (2009) 15(2):89–92. doi:10.4103/0973-1075.58450
53. Connor S, Sisimayi C, Downing J, King E, Lim Ah Ken P, Yates R, et al. Assessment of the need for palliative care for children in South Africa. *Int J Palliat Nurs* (2014) 20(3):130–4. doi:10.12968/ijpn.2014.20.3.130
54. Biskup T, Phan P, Grunauer M. Lessons from the design and implementation of a pediatric critical care and emergency medicine training program in a low resource country—the South American experience. *J Pediatr Intensive Care* (2017) 6(1):60–5. doi:10.1055/s-0036-1584678
55. Ministerio de Salud Pública del Ecuador. *Modelo de Gestión, Organización y Funcionamiento del Servicio de Atención de Salud Móvil.* Quito, Ecuador: Dirección Nacional de Atención Prehospitalaria y Unidades Móviles (EC) (2016). 59 p.

19

Successful Deployment of High Flow Nasal Cannula in a Peruvian Pediatric Intensive Care Unit Using Implementation Science—Lessons Learned

Katie R. Nielsen[1,2], Rosario Becerra[3], Gabriela Mallma[3] and José Tantaleán da Fieno[3,4]*

[1] *Department of Pediatrics, Critical Care Medicine, University of Washington, Seattle, WA, United States,* [2] *Department of Global Health, University of Washington, Seattle, WA, United States,* [3] *Departamento de Cuidados Intensivos Pediátricos, Instituto Nacional de Salud del Niño, Lima, Peru,* [4] *Universidad Nacional Federico Villarreal, Lima, Peru*

***Correspondence:**
Katie R. Nielsen
ktruth@uw.edu

Acute lower respiratory infections are the leading cause of death outside the neonatal period for children less than 5 years of age. Widespread availability of invasive and non-invasive mechanical ventilation in resource-rich settings has reduced mortality rates; however, these technologies are not always available in many low- and middle-income countries due to the high cost and trained personnel required to implement and sustain their use. High flow nasal cannula (HFNC) is a form of non-invasive respiratory support with growing evidence for use in pediatric respiratory failure. Its simple interface makes utilization in resource-limited settings appealing, although widespread implementation in these settings lags behind resource-rich settings. Implementation science is an emerging field dedicated to closing the know-do gap by incorporating evidence-based interventions into routine care, and its principles have guided the scaling up of many global health interventions. In 2016, we introduced HFNC use for respiratory failure in a pediatric intensive care unit in Lima, Peru using implementation science methodology. Here, we review our experience in the context of the principles of implementation science to serve as a guide for others considering HFNC implementation in resource-limited settings.

Keywords: high flow nasal cannula, implementation science, resource-limited setting, peru, pediatrics, acute respiratory failure

INTRODUCTION

Acute lower respiratory infections remain the leading cause of death outside the neonatal period for children less than 5 years of age, and the majority of these deaths occur in low- and middle-income countries (1). These large discrepancies in mortality are due, at least in part, to a lack of availability of basic supplies like oxygen and antibiotics and more advanced technology such as invasive and non-invasive mechanical ventilation (2–4). Despite efficacy of many types of advanced pediatric respiratory support (5, 6), widespread implementation of these technologies in resource-limited settings has lagged behind (7). Implementation science is a rapidly growing field dedicated to improving quality of health care delivery by incorporating evidence-based practices into routine care. Implementation science principles have guided the scale-up of interventions such as prevention of maternal-to-child transmission of HIV in resource-limited settings and could be applied to respiratory technologies to help ensure their success (8, 9).

High flow nasal cannula (HFNC) is an alternative form of non-invasive respiratory support with increasing use for respiratory failure in neonates, children, and adults (6, 10). Due to the non-occlusive nature of the nasal cannula, HFNC is easier to manage by bedside providers than CPAP or BiPAP because there is no need to readjust the interface to maintain a seal. In fact, HFNC has been used for pediatric patients outside the ICU setting with great success (11–13). In resource-limited settings where high patient:provider ratios limit clinicians' ability to be at the bedside, the simple HFNC interface has the potential to be successful in supporting children with respiratory failure. This, as well as evidence that HFNC may be more comfortable for pediatric patients (14, 15), led us to pursue implementation of HFNC in the Pediatric Intensive Care Unit (PICU) at Instituto Nacional de Salud del Niño (INSN) in Lima, Peru. A prior study in Ghana demonstrated substantial challenges in sustaining CPAP in that resource-limited setting (16), so we decided to use implementation science principles to guide our deployment strategy. In this article, we describe our implementation science approach to guide others planning to introduce pediatric advanced respiratory care in resource-limited settings, so that they may avoid common pitfalls.

SETTING

Instituto Nacional de Salud del Niño is the largest freestanding children's hospital in Peru with approximately 400 inpatient beds and 15 PICU beds. It is a major tertiary care referral center for children covered by the government insurance program, Seguro Integral de Salud. The PICU has approximately 400 admissions annually, of which, 50% are surgical and 50% medical, and a mortality rate of 18%. Children up to 18 years of age with any medical or surgical pathology may be admitted, although oncology and burn patients are typically admitted to other facilities, and postoperative cardiac surgery patients are admitted to the cardiac intensive care unit. Pediatric critical care physicians are in-house 24 h a day, 7 days a week. The nurse:patient ratio is 1:2, and there is one respiratory therapist available during day shift. HFNC was implemented as part of a larger research study to determine whether post-extubation use of HFNC would decrease the duration of invasive mechanical ventilation. According to the research protocol, all children less than 5 years of age who required invasive mechanical ventilation during the first 24 h of PICU admission were eligible for the study unless they had craniofacial malformations that would preclude HFNC use. Informed consent was obtained while children were still intubated. If they developed respiratory distress after extubation, the treating physician could decide to support them with HFNC according to our study protocol (**Figure 1**). This study was approved by the Seattle Children's Hospital IRB and the Ethics Committee at Instituto Nacional de Salud del Niño.

PREPARATION

Identify Champions

Anyone who has attempted to enact change in an organization acknowledges the necessity of identifying local champions to oversee the intervention. Borrowing from the engineering industry, many health care organizations have adopted systems analysis and improvement approaches to improve the quality of health care delivery (9, 17). These principles focus on involving frontline health care workers in both identifying problems in the current system as well as suggesting possible solutions to streamline the process. Prior studies in resource-limited settings have shown that participation of local providers in the quality improvement process leads to more effective and sustainable solutions (18). Although we had access to a HFNC protocol from a resource-rich setting, we knew that direct implementation of that protocol would not be effective. Instead, we formed a core group of PICU providers at INSN to lead the HFNC project and used the protocol as a starting point to talk with locals to understand the process of caring for pediatric patients with respiratory failure at INSN.

Map the Process

Process mapping is the systematic creation of flow maps to understand how patients move through the health care system and is used to identify bottlenecks and prioritize interventions. To be most effective, all stakeholders involved in the system should be represented in the final process map. We did not use formal process mapping during the preparation phase. Instead, a core group of INSN physicians and respiratory therapists with nearly 20 years experience in direct patient care in the PICU at INSN helped our team understand how HFNC could fit into their process of providing advanced respiratory care. This local perspective allowed us to design a HFNC protocol appropriate for their environment, increasing the chance of a successful intervention. Because implementation occurred in the context of a physician-led research study, nurses were not included in the early preparation phase. In retrospect, the addition of nurses to the core group from the beginning would have been extremely helpful in identifying potential issues for bedside providers prior to HFNC introduction.

Determine Resource Needs

Prior to implementing any new technology for advanced respiratory care, it is essential to determine the availability of resources in the particular environment. As others have suggested, use of advanced respiratory care is only appropriate in settings that have the capability to closely monitor vital signs including oxygenation, have adequately trained staff, and have all equipment necessary to provide the specific type of respiratory support (19). Given that INSN has enough nurses to maintain a nurse:patient ratio of 1:2 and is able to provide invasive and non-invasive mechanical ventilation at each bed within the PICU, we focused on procurement of HFNC equipment and staff training. Detailed discussion about the selection of HFNC system is beyond the scope of this article, but gathering information about upfront and ongoing supply costs in addition to established processes for equipment purchasing and maintenance should inform discussions with local leadership. Ultimately, the choice of HFNC system should be left to local experts.

Training

Local staff training is paramount to successful implementation, and the specific training module should be tailored to the needs of

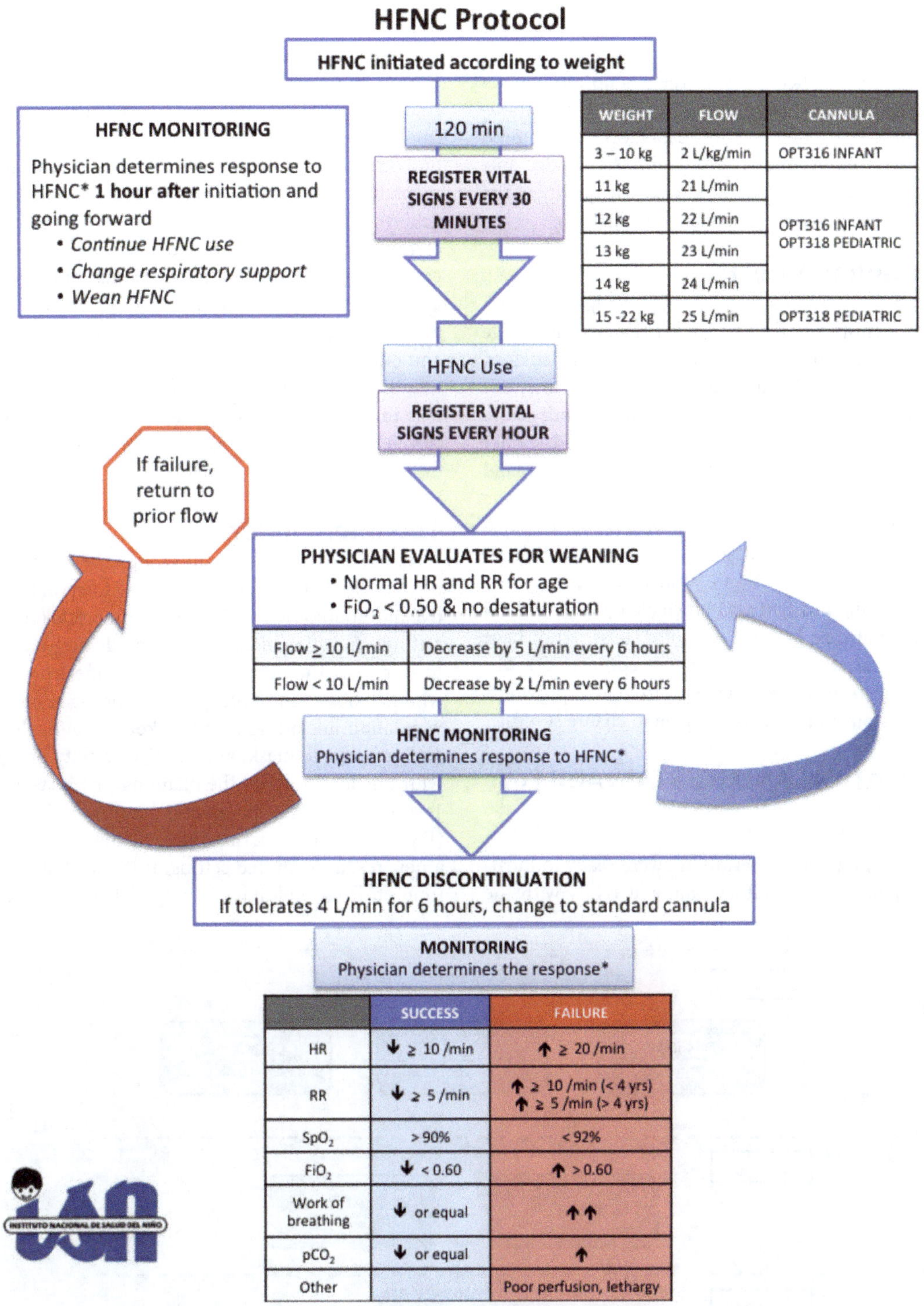

FIGURE 1 | High flow nasal cannula protocol at Instituto Nacional de Salud del Niño.

the specific environment. Adapting to the local context is part of the pre-implementation action cycle described by the Knowledge to Action Framework (20), which has guided implementation studies from Canada to the Democratic Republic of Congo (21). Because the educational needs of physicians and nurses are different, we chose to develop separate training modules for each group. The physician module provided more details regarding scientific evidence for HFNC mechanisms of action and efficacy in different patient populations, whereas the nursing module provided a summary of the evidence with more practical aspects of HFNC setup and management. We trained physicians first because they would be the ones to make the decision to use HFNC, and we knew their buy-in would be required in order to start using the technology. We then trained nurses over the course of 1 week, with morning and afternoon training sessions daily so that they could attend during scheduled shifts, as there is no mechanism in place to compensate them for additional hours spent on training. Although somewhat onerous, this adaptation was required in order to reach as many nurses as possible. All participants completed pre- and post-tests to both evaluate the quality of the training sessions as well as assess knowledge acquisition.

Identify Potential Barriers

The next pre-implementation step in the Knowledge to Action Framework is to identify and address any barriers to knowledge use (20). We used qualitative methods to explore these barriers, conducting focus groups with nurses and one-on-one semistructured interviews with physicians after the training and before the introduction of HFNC. Qualitative research methods gather information in more depth, allowing participants to expand upon ideas, which are then organized into themes using thematic analysis (22). Some of the most prevalent themes were innate to the local health care system. For instance, the frequency of physician handoffs and a siloed health care system with insufficient interdisciplinary communication make it challenging to create a uniform, longitudinal care plan for patients. These issues have been reported in a variety of other health care contexts (23, 24), but having these up-front discussions with front-line providers helped us strategize our implementation plan to ensure success.

IMPLEMENTATION AND SUSTAINABILITY

Interrogate the Process

After the 18-month preparation period, we were ready to introduce HFNC for pediatric respiratory failure at INSN with the goal of shortening the duration of invasive mechanical ventilation. It is important to recognize that many interventions that are effective in research studies fail to translate into improved patient outcomes. To address that discrepancy, implementation research emphasizes the need to evaluate the effectiveness of the implementation process in addition to monitoring the primary outcome of the intervention. In real life scenarios, the implementation process has a direct effect on whether an intervention achieves its desired outcome. Determinant frameworks, such as the Consolidated Framework for Implementation Research, can be used to understand factors that influence the success of an intervention. This framework describes five important components: the intervention, the individuals involved, the inner and outer settings, and the implementation process (25). Given that these components will influence the success of deployment, it is important to develop ways to assess each of these factors throughout the implementation process. Each component is discussed in more detail below.

The Intervention

As we learned from the focus groups, the intervention itself must be seen as beneficial for locals. Not all interventions that are effective in resource-rich settings are appropriate for resource-limited settings, and all implementation should be guided by local needs. In our case, the desire for HFNC came from INSN providers who had observed challenges with management of non-invasive ventilation, including skin breakdown, difficulty maintaining a seal around the mask, and relative scarcity of equipment. Even with this local buy-in, the planning phase lasted approximately 1 year to ensure the intervention would meet local needs (**Figure 2**). If considering implementation of an intervention in a new resource-limited setting, it is essential to spend adequate time up-front building a strong collaboration to maximize the

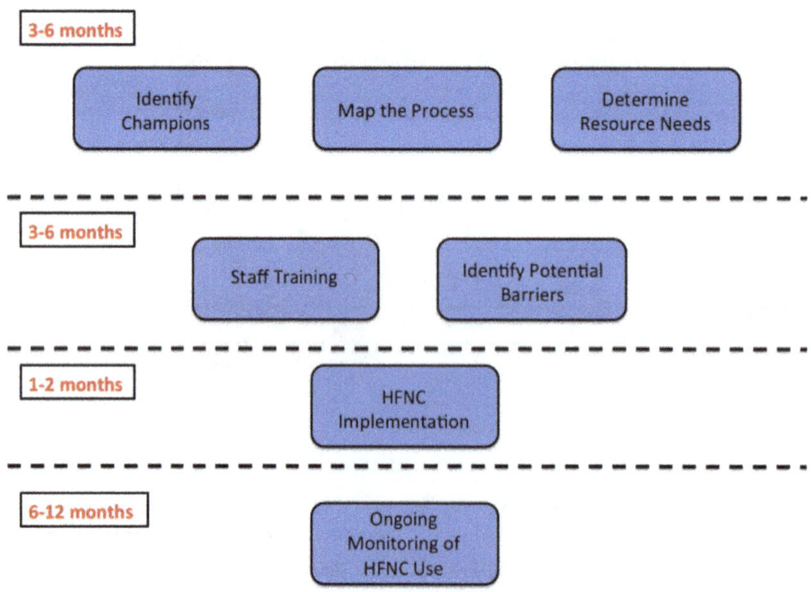

FIGURE 2 | High flow nasal cannula implementation timeline.

chances of success. In addition, checking in with the local team periodically can identify any unanticipated challenges that need to be addressed. During our follow-up focus group discussions, we learned that it was difficult for staff to remember the details of the HFNC protocol. To address this, we hung large flow charts of the protocol throughout the PICU to serve as a resource for clinicians.

The Individuals

The individuals involved in the intervention play a key role in the outcome of the intervention. Above, we emphasized the importance of local champions in the planning process, but these individuals need to demonstrate strong leadership throughout the intervention. Our core group of PICU providers filled many different rolls throughout the intervention. They responded to questions about HFNC, organized ongoing training sessions, encouraged local "hold-outs" to try using HFNC, and addressed any new issues that arose. In addition, the individuals using the intervention are also key players in its outcome. Adopting new practices is challenging for people in any setting, but in resource-limited settings, it can sometimes seem impossible. This can lead to resistance to change, which is why it is so important to have local leaders who can lead by example. Finally, a lack of familiarity with a new technology can contribute to hesitancy to use it. By organizing regular training sessions, nurses and physicians had the opportunity to ask questions related to their experience and go over specific case studies to highlight important aspects of HFNC management. After the training sessions, many nurses reported a desire for more frequent opportunities to review competencies, even beyond HFNC use. This emphasizes the importance of incorporating periodic review sessions to any implementation project to ensure individuals continue to feel comfortable with the new technology and/or protocol.

The Inner and Outer Settings

The inner and outer settings also influence the effectiveness of a new technology. Although the differences can be subtle, the inner setting generally consists of the structural, political, and cultural context in which the implementation will take place. The outer setting encompasses the greater economic, political, and cultural context surrounding the organization responsible for implementation (26). In Peru, this meant determining whether or not the Ministry of Health would be involved in our project since INSN is under their control. The Ministry of Health had minimal influence over our study; however, in other settings, government oversight may play more of a role and these representatives need to be included in regular organizational meetings. The leadership structure and culture of the PICU at INSN includes both physician and nursing leaders who we engaged prior to implementation. One unanticipated challenge we faced was an unexpected PICU medical director leadership transition, and the position was filled with interim individuals for several months. Fortunately, these individuals were also supportive of our study; however, this transition could just as easily have been detrimental to the success of our project. This highlights the necessity of extra efforts during times of transition to ensure the inner and outer settings remain supportive.

The Implementation Process

Finally, the implementation process itself greatly impacts the outcome of the intervention. This is where the work of the core group of providers at INSN paid off. With their recommendations, we implemented HFNC during respiratory season to increase the chance of finding eligible patients. Initially, the uptake of the intervention was slow, with some physicians hesitant to change their practice and adopt new technology. However, with on-site support of colleagues involved in the implementation process, HFNC use increased over time. Similar to other interventions, as providers witnessed successes with HFNC and its ease of use, they were more willing to try it for other patients. The type of support the implementation team provides must fit within the cultural context of the clinical setting. In some settings, direct hands-on guidance may be welcomed whereas in other settings, this may be perceived as interfering with clinical care. At INSN, the local team provided "behind-the-scenes" support, meaning they provided subtle suggestions about trying HFNC for some patients while emphasizing that the ultimate decision was up to the treating physician. Again, this emphasizes the importance of guidance by a team of local champions to determine what is appropriate for their setting.

Sustainability

After implementation, it is important to maintain ongoing support for HFNC use. This includes many of the concepts described above: having a group of local experts to address clinical concerns, organizing ongoing staff training, and maintaining a consistent supply chain. At INSN, HFNC was implemented in the context of a research project with a specific research protocol. Over the 17-month study period, 29 patients received HFNC support for post-extubation respiratory failure. Study enrollment closed November 30, 2017, so our team of local experts is currently working on developing a protocol for HFNC use for general clinical care. This process will also be more successful if implementation science principles are utilized.

CONCLUSION

Overall, our implementation experience at INSN has shown that HFNC can be successfully introduced in resource-limited settings. Utilizing tools of implementation science to engage key stakeholders during the planning process, understand the local process and identify its unique challenges, recruit local champions to facilitate training and support throughout the implementation process, and check-in with providers periodically after implementation greatly increases the chance of successful implementation. It is important to recognize that the timeline will likely be slower than anticipated, so maintaining momentum throughout the process is essential to keep local stakeholders engaged. As with all new interventions, sustainability is challenging and requires substantial ongoing effort to maintain. Our experience has taught us that with a core group of dedicated individuals, changing practice to improve the care of critically ill children is possible.

AUTHOR CONTRIBUTIONS

All authors contributed to the design of the work as well as the drafting and/or revising of this work and have approved this final version for publication.

ACKNOWLEDGMENTS

The authors would like to thank Dr. Laura E. Ellington, MD for her contributions to the design and implementation of the HFNC training program and in conducting focus groups and one-on-one interviews with INSN nurses and physicians.

REFERENCES

1. GBD 2016 Causes of Death Collaborators. Global, regional, and national age-sex specific mortality for 264 causes of death, 1980–2016: a systematic analysis for the Global Burden of Disease Study 2016. *Lancet* (2017) 390(10100):1151–210. doi:10.1016/S0140-6736(17)32152-9
2. Duke T, Wandi F, Jonathan M, Matai S, Kaupa M, Saavu M, et al. Improved oxygen systems for childhood pneumonia: a multihospital effectiveness study in Papua New Guinea. *Lancet* (2008) 372:1328–33. doi:10.1016/S0140-6736(08)61164-2
3. Towey RM, Ojara S. Intensive care in the developing world. *Anaesthesia* (2007) 62(Suppl 1):32–7. doi:10.1111/j.1365-2044.2007.05295.x
4. Murthy S, Adhikari NK. Global health care of the critically ill in low-resource settings. *Ann Am Thorac Soc* (2013) 10(5):509–13. doi:10.1513/AnnalsATS.201307-246OT
5. Hull J. The value of non-invasive ventilation. *Arch Dis Child* (2014) 99(11):1050–4. doi:10.1136/archdischild-2013-305322
6. Lee JH, Rehder KJ, Williford L, Cheifetz IM, Turner DA. Use of high flow nasal cannula in critically ill infants, children, and adults: a critical review of the literature. *Intensive Care Med* (2013) 39(2):247–57. doi:10.1007/s00134-012-2743-5
7. Jensen EA, Chaudhary A, Bhutta ZA, Kirpalani H. Non-invasive respiratory support for infants in low- and middle-income countries. *Semin Fetal Neonatal Med* (2016) 21(3):181–8. doi:10.1016/j.siny.2016.02.003
8. Mate KS, Ngubane G, Barker PM. A quality improvement model for the rapid scale-up of a program to prevent mother-to-child HIV transmission in South Africa. *Int J Qual Health Care* (2013) 25(4):373–80. doi:10.1093/intqhc/mzt039
9. Rustagi AS, Gimbel S, Nduati R, Cuembelo MF, Wasserheit JN, Farquhar C, et al. Impact of systems engineering intervention on PMTCT service delivery in Cote d'Ivoire, Kenya, Mozambique: a cluster randomized trial. *J Acquir Immune Defic Syndr* (2016) 72(3):e68–76. doi:10.1097/QAI.0000000000001023
10. DeMauro SB, Millar D, Kirpalani H. Noninvasive respiratory support for neonates. *Curr Opin Pediatr* (2014) 26(2):157–62. doi:10.1097/MOP.0000000000000066
11. Bressan S, Balzani M, Krauss B, Pettenazzo A, Zanconato S, Baraldi E. High-flow nasal cannula oxygen for bronchiolitis in a pediatric ward: a pilot study. *Eur J Pediatr* (2013) 172(12):1649–56. doi:10.1007/s00431-013-2094-4
12. Mayfield S, Bogossian F, O'Malley L, Schibler A. High-flow nasal cannula oxygen therapy for infants with bronchiolitis: pilot study. *J Paediatr Child Health* (2014) 50(5):373–8. doi:10.1111/jpc.12509
13. Wing R, James C, Maranda LS, Armsby CC. Use of high-flow nasal cannula support in the emergency department reduces the need for intubation in pediatric acute respiratory insufficiency. *Pediatr Emerg Care* (2012) 28(11):1117–23. doi:10.1097/PEC.0b013e31827122a9
14. Collins CL, Barfield C, Horne RS, Davis PG. A comparison of nasal trauma in preterm infants extubated to either heated humidified high-flow nasal cannulae or nasal continuous positive airway pressure. *Eur J Pediatr* (2014) 173(2):181–6. doi:10.1007/s00431-013-2139-8
15. Klingenberg C, Pettersen M, Hansen EA, Gustavsen LJ, Dahl IA, Leknessund A, et al. Patient comfort during treatment with heated humidified high flow nasal cannulae versus nasal continuous positive airway pressure: a randomised cross-over trial. *Arch Dis Child Fetal Neonatal Ed* (2014) 99(2):F134–7. doi:10.1136/archdischild-2013-304525
16. Wilson PT, Brooks JC, Otupiri E, Moresky RT, Morris MC. Aftermath of a clinical trial: evaluating the sustainability of a medical device intervention in Ghana. *J Trop Pediatr* (2014) 60(1):33–9. doi:10.1093/tropej/fmt074
17. Sherr K, Gimbel S, Rustagi A, Nduati R, Cuembelo F, Farquhar C, et al. Systems analysis and improvement to optimize pMTCT (SAIA): a cluster randomized trial. *Implement Sci* (2014) 9:55. doi:10.1186/1748-5908-9-55
18. Weinberg M, Fuentes JM, Ruiz AI, Lozano FW, Angel E, Gaitan H, et al. Reducing infections among women undergoing cesarean section in Colombia by means of continuous quality improvement methods. *Arch Intern Med* (2001) 161(19):2357–65. doi:10.1001/archinte.161.19.2357
19. Duke T. CPAP: a guide for clinicians in developing countries. *Paediatr Int Child Health* (2014) 34(1):3–11. doi:10.1179/2046905513Y.0000000102
20. Graham ID, Logan J, Harrison MB, Straus SE, Tetroe J, Caswell W, et al. Lost in knowledge translation: time for a map? *J Contin Educ Health Prof* (2006) 26(1):13–24. doi:10.1002/chp.47
21. Field B, Booth A, Ilott I, Gerrish K. Using the knowledge to action framework in practice: a citation analysis and systematic review. *Implement Sci* (2014) 9(172):1–14. doi:10.1186/s13012-014-0172-2
22. Chapman AL, Hadfield M, Chapman CJ. Qualitative research in healthcare: an introduction to grounded theory using thematic analysis. *J R Coll Physicians Edinb* (2015) 45:201–5. doi:10.4997/JRCPE.2015.305
23. Rosenthal JL, Doiron R, Haynes SC, Daniels B, Li ST. The effectiveness of standardized handoff tool interventions during inter- and intra-facility care transitions on patient-related outcomes: a systematic review. *Am J Med Qual* (2018) 33(2):193–206. doi:10.1177/1062860617708244
24. Khowaga-Punjwani S, Smardo C, Hendricks MR, Lantos JD. Physician-nurse interactions in critical care. *Pediatrics* (2017) 140(3):e20170670. doi:10.1542/peds.2017-0670
25. Damschroder LJ, Aron DC, Keith RE, Kirsh SR, Alexander JA, Lowery JC. Fostering implementation of health services research findings into practice: a consolidated framework for advancing implementation science. *Implement Sci* (2009) 4(50):1–15. doi:10.1186/1748-5908-4-50
26. Pettigrew AM, Woodman RW, Cameron KS. Studying organizational change and development: challenges for future research. *Acad Manage J* (2001) 44(4):697–713. doi:10.2307/3069411

20

Pediatric Trauma Care in Low Resource Settings: Challenges, Opportunities and Solutions

Andrew W. Kiragu[1*], *Stephen J. Dunlop*[2,3], *Njoki Mwarumba*[4], *Sanusi Gidado*[5], *Adesope Adesina*[6], *Michael Mwachiro*[7], *Daniel A. Gbadero*[8] *and Tina M. Slusher*[1,9]

[1] *Department of Pediatrics, Hennepin Healthcare, Minneapolis, MN, United States,* [2] *Department of Emergency Medicine, Hennepin Healthcare, Minneapolis, MN, United States,* [3] *Division of Global Medicine, University of Minnesota, Minneapolis, MN, United States,* [4] *Department of Political Science, Oklahoma State University, Stillwater, OK, United States,* [5] *Department of Surgery, Bingham University Teaching Hospital, Jos, Nigeria,* [6] *Department of Surgery, Bowen University Teaching Hospital, Ogbomosho, Nigeria,* [7] *Department of Surgery, Tenwek Hospital, Bomet, Kenya,* [8] *Department of Pediatrics, Bowen University Teaching Hospital, Ogbomosho, Nigeria,* [9] *Division of Global Pediatrics, University of Minnesota, Minneapolis, MN, United States*

***Correspondence:**
Andrew W. Kiragu
andrew.kiragu@hcmed.org

Trauma constitutes a significant cause of death and disability globally. The vast majority -about 95%, of the 5.8 million deaths each year, occur in low-and-middle-income countries (LMICs) 3–6. This includes almost 1 million children. The resource-adapted introduction of trauma care protocols, regionalized care and the growth specialized centers for trauma care within each LMIC are key to improved outcomes and the lowering of trauma-related morbidity and mortality globally. Resource limitations in LMICs make it necessary to develop injury prevention strategies and optimize the use of locally available resources when injury prevention measures fail. This will lead to the achievement of the best possible outcomes for critically ill and injured children. A commitment by the governments in LMICs working alone or in collaboration with international non-governmental organizations (NGOs) to provide adequate healthcare to their citizens is also crucial to improved survival after major trauma. The increase in global conflicts also has significantly deleterious effects on children, and governments and international organizations like the United Nations have a significant role to play in reducing these. This review details the evaluation and management of traumatic injuries in pediatric patients and gives some recommendations for improvements to trauma care in LMICs.

Keywords: low- and middle-income countries, trauma, pediatrics, injury prevention, emergency management, surgical management, child abuse, disasters

INTRODUCTION

The global emphasis on reductions in childhood mortality and meeting the Sustainable Developmental Goals (SDGs), has resulted in significant gains in reducing childhood deaths around the world (1). However, an epidemiologic shift has been noted, with relative increases in deaths from injuries and declines in deaths from poor nutrition and infections such as pneumonia and diarrheal diseases (2).

Trauma constitutes a significant cause of death and disability globally. About 95%, of the 5.8 million deaths each year occur in low-and-middle-income countries (LMICs) (3–6). Almost 1 million of these deaths are children. The World Health Organization (WHO) reports that the top five etiologies for unintentional injuries are road traffic accidents (RTAs), falls, burns, drowning and poisoning (3–6) (**Figure 1**). An alarming number of children are also injured or killed in war-zones, in disasters, and from child abuse (3, 7). Resource limitations in LMICs necessitate trauma prevention and thoughtful resource allocation and utilization in the care of injured children. This review details the evaluation and management of pediatric trauma in LMICs.

EMERGENCY RESPONSE TO TRAUMA

Pre-hospital Systems and Triage

In high-income countries (HICs), caring for injured patients involves well-coordinated systems of triage, emergency medical care, and critical care. While such systems are currently unfeasible in many LMICs, it is essential that capabilities for managing acute onset, severe but reversible disease and injuries are available in any country around the world (8).

Wholesale, poorly planned imitations of HIC-type pre-hospital systems in LMICs often result in expensive, ineffective systems (9). There are, alternatively, low-cost interventions, for example, first responder training programs in Uganda and Mexico. These have resulted in excellent outcomes for relatively low costs (9). In LMICs, successful systems of pre-hospital trauma care take into careful consideration local financial resources and capitalize on them and also are broadly acceptable in the local societal context (9). Initiatives to improve or implement pre-hospital or trauma systems in LMICs must recognize domestic resource constraints to minimize financial strain and improve efficiencies in the distribution of these resources (10). Emergency care depends on recognition of severe injury or illness and timely intervention. It involves the ability to quickly obtain care, rapid and appropriate referrals and the safe transportation of patients (11). The absence of a formal triage system in many hospitals in LMICs often leads to potentially life-threatening delays in obtaining needed care for patients who are severely injured or critically ill (12). The WHO, to bridge this gap in pre-hospital care that is present in many LMICs, recommends the establishment of first-responder programs to train laypeople as the first step toward building pre-hospital systems in LMICs (13). There are examples of such programs that have successfully used local resources to educate laypersons with little formal education (14). Effective triage and emergency care have also been described in some LMICs. The South African Triage Scale (SATS) for children is one such tool. It is used to prioritize children requiring emergency treatment. By employing a triage early warning score in combination with clinical signs and symptoms, the SATS helps to identify acute illness earlier, improves emergency department patient flow and allows better stewardship of hospital resources (15).

Emergency Department Management

Inadequate staffing levels coupled with huge patient loads lead to delays in assessment and treatment in many hospitals in LMIC's (16). While most hospitals have a dedicated emergency or casualty department, few have emergency medicine-trained

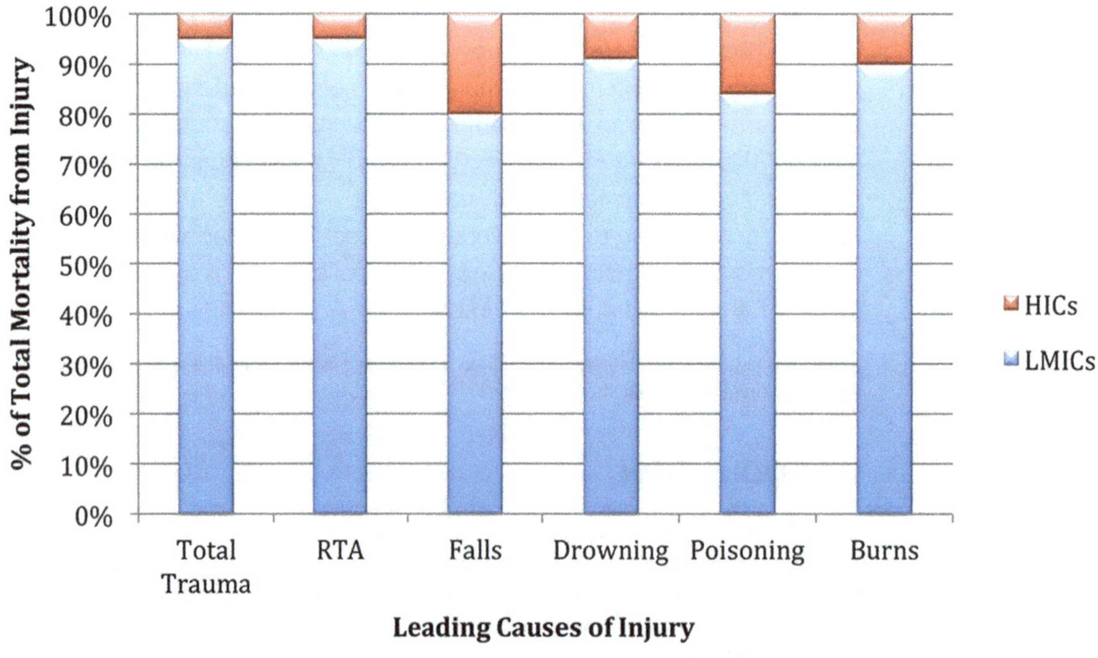

FIGURE 1 | Illustration of the burden of trauma-related mortality borne by LMICs in comparison to HICs.

specialists. Even more rare are dedicated trauma centers. This means that healthcare providers with no specialized training in the management of pediatric trauma provide the majority of pediatric trauma care. This has a significantly negative impact on outcomes, which are dependent more on the speed and appropriateness of the medical care received than how severe of an injury was sustained (17). There are significant differences even within the same LMICs with regards to available resources for emergency room care between public and private hospitals (**Figure 2**). Public hospitals, which usually have fewer resources, are often overwhelmed. A recent study of 7 EDs in Pakistan noted that on average, only about 17% of patients were appropriately triaged, and fewer than 25% had any vital signs documented (18). To improve patient flow in overcrowded EDs, a recent study employed LEAN methodologies in a teaching hospital in Ghana (19).

Like the previously noted SATS, the Emergency Triage, Assessment, and Treatment plus (ETAT+) training in LMICs has resulted in better prioritization of pediatric trauma cases in the ED (20). Improved outcomes have also been achieved in some institutions in LMICs that have developed protocols for trauma management (21–25). Comprehensive Advanced Life Support (CALS®) and Advanced Trauma Life Support (ATLS)® are two examples of guidelines for the management of trauma. Organizations such as the African Federation of Emergency Medicine (AFEM) and the WHO have also provided guidelines on the appropriate resources needed for the care of pediatric trauma patients which are adjustable based on local resources (13, 22–25). Given the expense associated with maintenance of CALS and ATLS training, locally developed standardized trauma protocols have been found to be effective in achieving increased use of timely appropriate interventions for trauma patients and associated with decreased mortality rates particularly in patients with severe traumatic brain injuries (26).

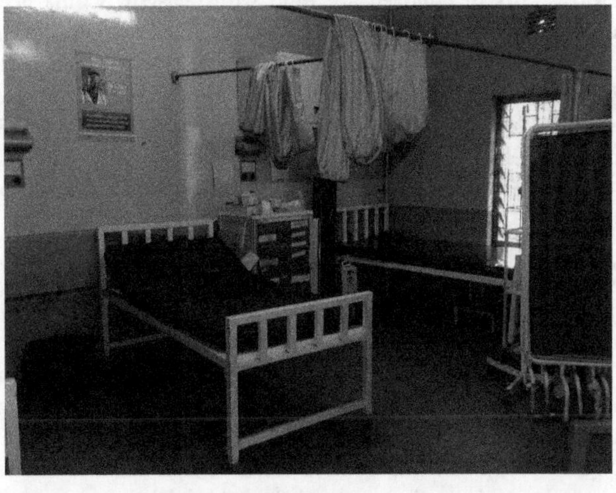

FIGURE 2 | Example of an Emergency Room in a public hospital in a LMIC. Courtesy Benjamin Wachira, MD Aga Khan University Hospital, Nairobi Kenya.

Surgical Management

Surgical management is the cornerstone of trauma care. In HICs the ready availability of multispecialty surgical teams as key members of the trauma management team facilitates timely surgical intervention when needed and the improved outcomes that this translates to. Given the lack of even basic surgical services in many LMICs, the surgeon-led trauma team and related resources remain a dream in most low-resource areas of the world. Globally, an estimated 2 billion people lack access to even the most basic surgical care (5). A recent study by Higashi et al. found that 1 million deaths and the loss of 52.3 million DALYs could have been averted in all LMICs if a basic menu of surgical services were made universally available (27). These services included basic resuscitation, advanced life support including the provision of surgical airways, peripheral venous access, laceration, and wound management, needle decompression and chest tube placement, fracture reduction, escharotomy and fasciotomy, skin grafting and trauma-related laparotomies (27). Governments in LMICs in conjunction with international partners have a significant role to play. Many essential physical resources, including equipment and supplies, are low cost and can be better supplied through improved planning and logistics (5). Enhanced durability, lower purchasing and operating costs as well as increased capabilities for local manufacture, maintenance and repair could enhance the availability of more expensive equipment like x-ray machines and ventilators (5). The poorest LMICs will require international assistance for the initial purchase of basic essential equipment and supplies (5). In the interim, surgical services in some LMICs, particularly during crisis situations, have been provided by non-governmental organizations (NGOs) (5). This assistance has varied from short-term mission trips by groups like Operation Smile to mobile, self-contained surgical platforms provided by Médecins Sans Frontières that remain in-country for months to years (5). There are also examples of more permanent specialty surgical hospitals established by NGOs in-country (5).

Trauma teams adapted to local conditions and resources in each LMIC should be developed. This will also require financial commitments to facilitate training and equipment purchases (28). Tele-simulation is another option for teaching and developing pediatric trauma resuscitation skills to healthcare providers in LMICs (25). An excellent resource for online learning and simulation is OPEN Pediatrics, an online community of clinicians that share best practices from all around the world (29). Incorporation of trauma management training into the undergraduate medical school curriculum will help ensure on-going widespread dissemination of the skills required to manage pediatric trauma.

ADDRESSING SPECIFIC CAUSES OF PEDIATRIC INJURY

Road Traffic Injuries

Each year there are over 1 million deaths associated with RTAs and an estimated 20–50 million non-fatal road traffic injuries

(RTIs) around the world (30). These RTAs result in the deaths of 186,300 children (ages 0–17 years) (31). Boys are twice as likely to be killed in RTAs as girls. LMICs account for approximately 95% of all children killed by RTAs, with the brunt of this burden borne by countries in Sub-Saharan Africa. Over 35% of global child deaths from RTAs are in Sub-Saharan Africa (31). To address this significant problem, several steps should be taken. These include building road safety management capacity, improved infrastructure, and enhanced vehicle safety. Also, improved road user behaviors with enforcement of speed limits, seat belt and laws prohibiting driving under the influence of alcohol could also make an impact (30, 31). Improved pre-hospital, hospital and rehabilitation systems would help reduce the mortality and morbidity associated with RTIs (31).

Falls

Over 400,000 fatal falls occur each year globally. This makes them the second-leading cause of unintentional injury-related deaths after RTAs. More than 80% of fall-related fatalities occur LMICs (32). While not all fall injuries are fatal, every year more than 37 million fall-related injuries are severe enough to require medical attention. They account for over 17 million DALYs (32). Children living in countries with poor infrastructure and unsafe housing conditions are especially at risk for injuries from falls (3). Other fall risk factors include male sex and age. In LMICs infants have significantly higher rates of fall-related injuries than older children (5). Efforts to prevent falls include developing and promoting local manufacture of inexpensive measures to prevent falls such as window guards, building regulations and enforcement that prevent unsafe housing, access to safe playgrounds, and better supervision of children (5).

Drowning

According to the WHO, worldwide there are 370,000 deaths from drowning making it the 3rd leading cause of unintentional injury-related mortality. Ninety-one percent of these deaths occur in LMICs (33). Children at the greatest risk of drowning are unsupervised boys in rural areas with little formal swimming instruction. Strategies to prevent drowning include placing barriers around bodies of water, covering wells, increased supervision, providing formal swimming lessons, and increasing community awareness about the risks of drowning (33, 34).

Comprehensive boating regulations and enforcement, improved signage including designation of dangerous water bodies, enhanced water rescue and resuscitation, water safety requirements including the use of personal flotation devices and improved supervision of swimming areas used for recreation are also important (34).

Poisoning

Poisoning is a leading cause of morbidity and mortality globally. There are multiple causes of poisoning ranging from pesticides and industrial chemicals to lead and mercury poisoning. LMICs bear the larger part of the burden with regards to poisoning. According to WHO data, in 2012, over 190,000 people died worldwide from unintentional poisoning. Of these deaths, 84% occurred in LMICs (35). Unintentional poisoning also resulted in the loss of over 10.7 million years of DALYs (35).

Poverty, lack of education, poor quality controls and absent legislation regarding certain products are some of the challenges that exacerbate this problem. Suicide from intentional poisoning point to the significant challenge of mental illness in LMICs and the inadequate resources available to combat this problem (35, 36). Nearly a million people die each year as a result of suicide, and chemicals account for a significant number of these deaths. Deliberate ingestion of pesticides causes approximately 370,000 deaths each year' and self-poisoning is the most common method of suicide attempt in youth in LMICs (35, 36).

EVALUATION AND MANAGEMENT OF SPECIFIC SYSTEM-BASED INJURIES

Traumatic Brain Injuries

Traumatic brain injuries (TBIs) constitute a significant public health problem and a leading cause of death and disability worldwide (37, 38). They affect over 3 million children annually, impacting every population and demographic group (38). RTAs are the leading cause of TBIs worldwide followed by falls (38). The vast majority of TBIs occur in LMICs where inadequate pre-hospital and hospital-based care and poor rehabilitation facilities result in unsatisfactory outcomes (37, 39). The mortality rate for TBI patients in LMICs is twice that in HICs (40) with most of these deaths being of patients with severe TBI (40).

There are recently published guidelines for the management of severe traumatic brain injury in infants and children (41). However, the dearth of resources in LMICs means that the application of these guidelines is variable (37). Given the limited neurosurgical and neurocritical care capacity in most LMICs, consideration should be given to regionalization to optimize neurosurgical resources. Resource-adapted courses similar to the Advanced Life Support in Brain Injury (ALSBI) course may lead to broader dissemination of the knowledge needed to improve outcomes from pre-hospital to rehabilitation (42).

Most TBIs in children are mild with Glasgow Coma Scale scores of $\geq$13. These children usually have no significant findings on radiographic evaluation (38). In situations where the injuries are more severe, the most common findings are skull fractures, brain parenchymal hemorrhages, and contusions (38). Unfortunately, these patients have poorer outcomes particularly in LMICs where neurosurgical intervention is often unavailable (38).

Management of TBI

The goal of TBI management is to treat the primary injury, when indicated, including the evacuation of subdural and extradural hematomas and repairing significant skull fractures. Treatment is aimed at preventing any secondary insults to the brain through improvements in cerebral perfusion and provision of adequate oxygen (41, 43). To achieve this, placement of an advanced airway and mechanical ventilation may be required. The capacity to do this is absent in many LMIC settings where even provision of supplemental oxygen might be difficult. To maintain cerebral perfusion, patients often need intravenous fluids and sometimes might require initiation of vasopressor agents. In patients with a severe TBI defined as a GCS ≤8, the optimal evaluation would ideally include a head computed tomography (CT) to visualize any skull fractures and intracranial pathology (44, 45). In many LMICs, CT scanners are often not available or are out of the financial reach of most of the general population. In such situations, there may be some utility to skull x-rays which can at least identify fractures but do not reveal intracranial injuries (45, 46). In situations where clinical examination or, when available, intracranial pressure monitoring, reveals increased intracranial pressure and evidence for cerebral edema, hyperosmolar therapy is initiated (41, 43). The hyperosmolar therapy used in LMICs is most often mannitol although in some countries hypertonic saline is also used (41, 43). Ventriculostomy catheters to monitor ICP are usually indicated when the GCS ≤8. In many resource-limited areas, the capability to do this is frequently absent. Ultrasonographic optic nerve sheath diameter measurement can be used to detect elevated ICP, although in most low-resource settings the equipment and expertise to perform this evaluation are lacking (47). Nonetheless, ultrasound is available in many hospitals thus making this training possible and potentially very valuable. The BESTTRIP study offers an example of how to manage patients when a ventriculostomy is not available (48). This study revealed no substantial difference in outcome between patients with invasive monitoring of ICP and those evaluated with clinical exams and repeat CT scans (48). Unfortunately, this would be difficult to replicate in most LMICs. In HICs the ready availability of neurosurgical expertise means that any required surgical interventions such as evacuation of subdural and extradural hematomas and decompressive craniectomy for ICP elevation unresponsive to medical therapy are easily accomplished. In LMICs this is significantly more difficult to achieve. Other aspects of care that could be accomplished even in low resource settings include elevation of head-of-bed, maintenance of euthermia, provision of adequate pain control and sedation, provision of adequate nutrition and seizure prophylaxis and control (40, 41, 43).

Abdominal Injuries

Abdominal injuries (AI) are associated with a significantly increased risk of death and disability especially when other injuries and in particular TBI are present (49). The majority of AI result from motor vehicle-related crashes and falls (49, 50). Clinical signs and symptoms concerning for AI include abdominal tenderness and distention, absent bowel sounds and peritoneal signs. The presence of the latter may indicate a need for surgical exploration (49, 51). In children who present with the classic abdominal wall bruising consistent with a seat-belt injury, a high index of suspicion for bowel, kidney, and vertebral injuries is required (50). Splenic and hepatic injuries are the most frequently noted AI's. A system of classification established by the American Association for the Surgery of Trauma (AAST) for these visceral injuries helps guide prognosis and management (52). Bowel injuries are found in approximately 1–5% of blunt abdominal injuries (49). Most commonly injured is the jejunum, which accounts for about 30% of all hollow-viscous injuries. The second most commonly injured part of the bowel is the duodenum (49).

Management of Abdominal Injuries

Initial management of an AI involves ensuring a patent airway, adequate oxygenation, and IV fluid resuscitation if indicated (49). Ongoing evaluations including of vital signs, neurologic and abdominal exams and urine output are important (49). In HICs, initial imaging after an AI involves a Focused Assessment with Sonography for Trauma (FAST) evaluation (49). This helps to identify intraperitoneal blood or fluid from a visceral injury (49). However, FAST exams potentially miss about a third of visceral injuries in children (50). A potential impediment in LMICs is that ultrasound machines are not always available and expertise in their use is variable. CT scans are standard in the evaluation of abdominal trauma in HIC's but less likely to be available in LMICs (51). Ultrasonography is, however, despite the limitations noted, more readily available and additional training in ultrasound use is invaluable to clinicians in these settings. In HIC's, over 90% of blunt AIs are managed non-operatively (49). However, non-operative management has been made possible by advanced imaging techniques that are limited in LMIC's which itself has led to higher rates of surgical exploration (50). Otherwise, clinicians must rely on their physical diagnostic skills in combination with peritoneal taps. If urgent surgical intervention is needed in these patients, then transfer to centers offering a higher level of surgical and critical care should be done expeditiously as possible once resuscitation has begun.

Thoracic Injuries

Thoracic injuries (TIs) constitute an ongoing challenge to the trauma or general surgeon practicing in LMICs and have associated high morbidity and mortality (53). The majority of these are blunt thoracic injuries and most often results from RTAs. Penetrating trauma is mainly related to gunshot wounds and other projectiles (54). Young children have more compliant, cartilaginous chest walls and therefore even significant force injuries are less likely to result in fractures. However, there is a greater transmission of these forces to the child's internal organs and these patients will still have associated pulmonary and cardiac contusions, pneumothoraces, hemothoraces and mediastinal injuries (54, 55). Given the disproportionately smaller size of the thorax in comparison to the cranium and abdomen, it is imperative to assess the entire patient when thoracic trauma is present to rule out TBIs and abdominal injuries (56–59).

Management of Thoracic Injuries

Evaluation of thoracic injuries begins with primary and secondary surveys. In addition to the FAST exam, a basic x-ray of the chest is required. CT scan imaging and other advanced imaging techniques can be useful adjuncts but are frequently not readily available in many LMICs. Again, where available the value and use of ultrasound should be capitalized on, and the FAST exam taught. They are also a strain on resources for both patients and healthcare facilities and increase radiation exposure to children (57, 60). Initial resuscitation should follow the usual trauma protocol attention to airway, breathing, and circulation (ABCs) while ensuring C-spine immobilization for polytrauma patients. Clinical presentation of thoracic injuries is dependent on the type of injury. An underlying pulmonary contusion is usually more prognostic than the chest wall injury itself (56). (**Figure 3**) Rib fractures are usually very painful because of the inability to immobilize them. The extent of the multisystem injury is directly proportional to the number of rib fractures. Scapular, clavicular and rib 1-3 fractures are linked to cardiovascular injury and indicate a high-energy mechanism (61). A high index of suspicion for traumatic asphyxia for patients who present with tachypnea and facial petechiae is important (56). Children are more likely to develop hypoxia than adults due to their lower functional residual capacity and relatively higher tissue oxygen consumption (54). Additionally, their more mobile mediastinum allows for the faster conversion of a simple pneumothorax to a tension pneumothorax (54). Proper airway management takes priority in patients with tracheobronchial injuries. Other more rare injuries include esophageal injuries, traumatic diaphragmatic rupture, and cardiac injuries. A plain chest x-ray can diagnose diaphragmatic injury with herniated viscera, and esophageal tears commonly with left sided pleural effusions (54). Algorithms have been developed for these that can be adapted to the LMIC setting (55). Blunt cardiac injury (BCI) is often under-diagnosed due to a lack of diagnostic tools including troponin laboratory screening, electrocardiography, and echocardiography, as well as a low index of suspicion (62, 63). Persistent tachycardia or other arrhythmia in the face of thoracic trauma should prompt an evaluation for BCI. In HIC, emergency thoracotomy has been described and has been shown to be lifesaving for children with penetrating cardiac injuries (64, 65). Indications for ER thoracotomy are well defined and include massive hemothorax, initial chest tube output >20 mls/kg, and pericardial effusion on ultrasound in the setting of shock (66). In many LMIC settings, the absence of equipment and trained staff means that ER thoracotomy is not currently feasible. However, temporizing measures such as pericardiocentesis or pericardial catheter placement may be possible. Whenever possible, early referral to a better-equipped trauma unit should be made after initial stabilization.

Orthopedic Injuries

Orthopedic injuries have a significant impact on DALYs in LMICs since those most commonly injured are typically younger, potentially more productive persons (2, 3, 67). The causes of these injuries include falls, RTAs, workplace accidents, child abuse, and injuries sustained in conflicts or other disasters (1–3). Fractures in pediatric patients are distinct from those in adult patients. Young children have a growth plate, and physeal fractures represent ~18% of fractures (68). Four distinct types of fractures seen in children include plastic deformity, torus fractures, greenstick fractures, and physeal fractures (68). Thoughtful evaluation with attention to the child's neurovascular status is key. Radiologic evaluation of the fracture when radiographic

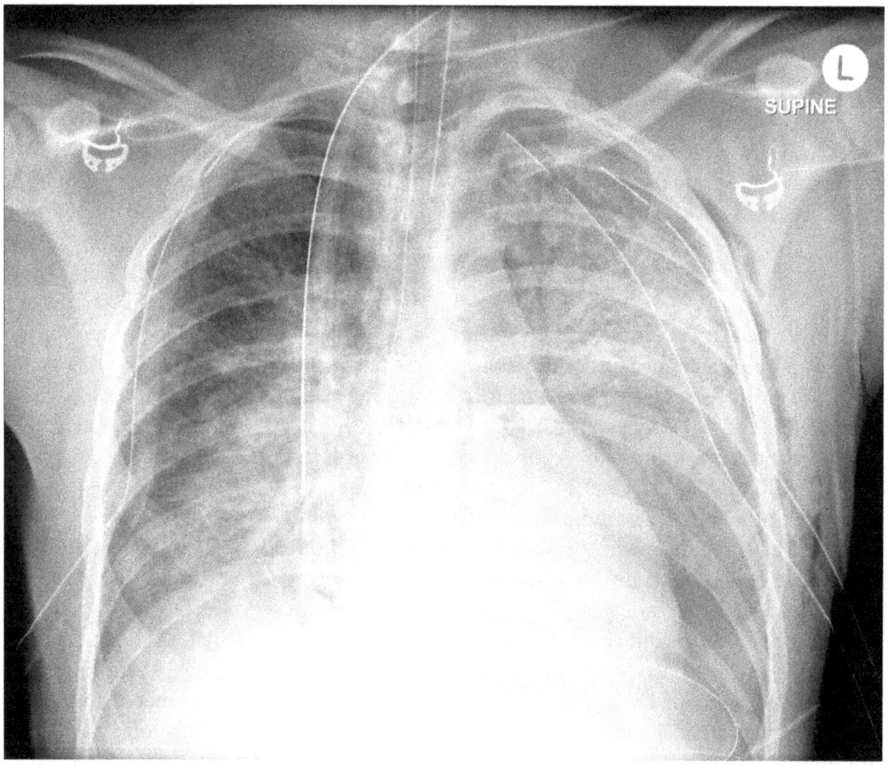

FIGURE 3 | Chest x-ray showing bilateral pulmonary contusions and pneumothoraxes requiring chest tube placement.

equipment is available requires at least two planes, including the joint above and below, if necessary (68) (**Figure 4**).

Management of Orthopedic Injuries in LMICs

Management of these fractures begins with stabilization of the fractured extremity. Consideration may be given to pelvic binding, if indicated for hemodynamic stability, and should be performed as part of the circulation assessment in the primary survey. Any open wounds should be irrigated with large amounts of sterilized water, and antibiotic therapy started if indicated, in addition to tetanus prophylaxis (69, 70). Adequate analgesia is important in children. This can vary from acetaminophen and other non-steroidal anti-inflammatory drugs for mild pain to opioids for more severe pain.

Management is conservative in closed uncomplicated fractures. External fixation and wound care for open fractures, and open reduction and internal fixation in selected cases may be required. In HICs, interdisciplinary management decisions are made by orthopedic surgeons in collaboration with plastic, vascular, trauma, and general surgeons as well as physiotherapists and occupational therapists (71). However, in many LMICs, it is difficult for most patients to access this interdisciplinary care.

A large burden of care in these countries is borne by general surgeons as there is not a large pool of orthopedic surgeons and even fewer vascular or plastic surgeons. The surgeon is faced with patients whose initial care is not by trained first responders (72). Sometimes the surgeon may care for patients who elected to initially be managed by "traditional bone healers." There is also delay in obtaining consent from families for any procedures other than initial stabilization and wound care (73). There is, therefore, a higher rate of limb amputations from orthopedic injuries. This increases costs and length of stay due to additional care needs and rehabilitation (73). The surgical care of orthopedic injuries is increasingly being recognized as a more cost-effective modality of treatment than more conservative methods in many LMICs. Previously, surgeons improvised with old-fashioned implants and equipment donated to their hospitals from HICs with varying results. More recently, there are centers in LMICs that have access to appropriate implants and training through programs like SIGN Fracture Care International. This has resulted in fracture treatments and outcomes that are comparable to those in HICs (74). One impediment to appropriate orthopedic care is the fact that most orthopedic surgeons are located in urban areas with practices that are out of the reach of most of the general population. Governmental policies and financial investments are needed to facilitate the training of more surgeons in all specialties, and making these surgeons available and accessible at most public access hospitals. General surgeons in LMICs should also receive more training in the management of orthopedic injuries. Consideration should also be given to providing additional training in basic orthopedic stabilization, to nurses and medical officers who typically are the initial healthcare providers for injured children in most public access facilities in LMICs.

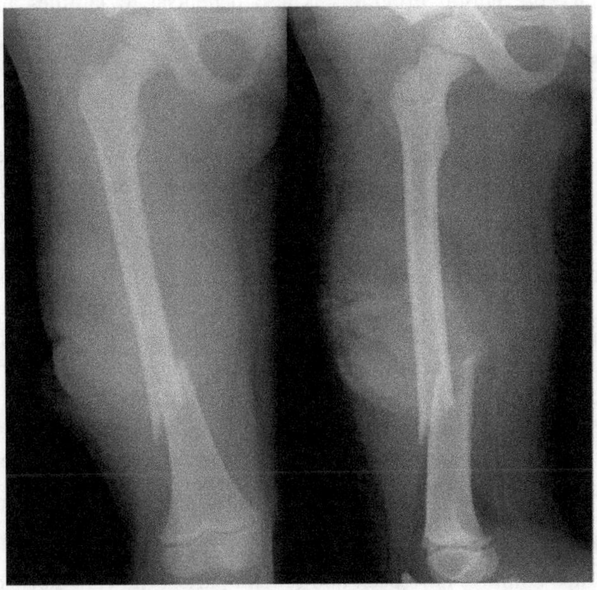

FIGURE 4 | X-ray showing right femur fracture.

Burn Injuries

Burns, especially those that leave a child permanently disfigured or disabled, represent the most catastrophic events to happen to a child (75). Globally, over 11 million people are estimated to suffer burn injuries leading to over 265,000 deaths annually (75, 76). As with other traumatic injuries, the vast majority of burn injuries and deaths occur in LMICs (76, 77). Children <5 years of age are usually at the greatest risk for burn injuries, with an estimated 100,000 admissions annually. This number is likely a significant underestimation (78). In HICs, improvements in burn management have led to decreases in morbidity and mortality with most burn centers in HICs reporting an LA50 (lethal total body burn surface area [TBSA] for 50% of patients) >90% TBSA (79). These improvements have not universally been seen in LMICs where there is large variability in outcomes, with most centers reporting an aggregate LA50 <40% and many reporting 100% mortality with burns >40% TBSA (80). If LMIC center outcomes matched those in the best performing HIC centers, over 34,000 additional lives could be saved worldwide (81). These poor outcomes are multifactorial but are most often related to delayed presentation, lack of trained personnel and a paucity of burn centers (80). One regional referral center in Tanzania found that almost half of burns arrived >72 h after injury (82).

Management of Burns in LMICs

Management of burn injuries includes the early recognition of major burns (>10–20% partial thickness and full thickness burns), evaluation and management of airway involvement, provision of oxygen and recognition of carbon monoxide and cyanide poisoning, and fluid resuscitation for management of burn shock.

A survey of burn resuscitation in the African continent revealed that parenteral fluid resuscitation protocols using lactated Ringers solution based upon the Parkland formula are the most commonly utilized (83). There was also an increased utilization of enteral hydration in the form of oral rehydration solution (ORS), along with a focus on clinical endpoints such as urine output, rather than invasive monitoring in comparison with higher resourced counterparts. ORS is a viable option for burn resuscitation for burns <20% TBSA (84). Patients with significant burns have better outcomes when treated at centers with expertise in burn care, and therefore, after stabilization immediate transfer whenever possible is encouraged. These centers, employ typical burn therapies such as protocolized resuscitation, topical antibiotics, skin grafting and have a mean daily cost per 1% total burn surface per patient as low as $2.65 (85, 86). Airway management and management of inhalation injuries can be challenging in many LMICs where access to intensive care resources like mechanical ventilation and bronchoscopy is limited. Carbon monoxide and cyanide poisoning can be managed with administration of supplemental oxygen (84). Burn wound care is particularly challenging in low resource areas where adequate access to clean water is often problematic. Daily cleaning with Dakin's solution helps to ensure sterility of the water and is bactericidal against most bacteria in the wound (84). The burn wounds are then dressed with antibiotic incorporated dressings (84). The antimicrobial agents used include silver sulfadiazine, mafenide acetate, silver nitrate, and even medical grade honey (84). The need for adequate analgesia cannot be overstated. Opioid analgesia for pain control and ketamine to facilitate wound care are key adjuncts (84). Fevers are common in burn patients but there is no evidence that supports the routine use of prophylactic parenteral antibiotics in the absence of clear evidence of infection (87). In addition, burn centers are more likely to employ contracture avoidance techniques like splinting and physiotherapy to prevent further morbidity.

However, the importance of early recognition, resuscitation initiation, maintenance of euthermia, and basic wound dressings can and should be initiated at the first point of contact. Early referral to tertiary burn centers in LMICs whenever possible is key. Burn prevention and education continue to lead the way in reducing the morbidity and mortality. The majority of childhood burns occur in the home, and therefore public health interventions that target changing the type of fuel used for cooking/lighting, location of these fires, and storage of the fuel have preliminarily resulted in a reduction of burns (88).

Disasters: Pediatric Implications

While disasters are often unpredictable, they are neither a fixed singular event nor are they all sudden onset events (89–91). What differentiates them is the scale and magnitude of the impact on families and communities (90, 92). Disasters are increasing in frequency intensity including climate change and environmental degradation related disasters (93). How well families, communities, and government systems prepare for and respond to disasters, determines response and recovery (94). Allocation of technical, financial, and personnel resources during a disaster life cycle (mitigation, preparedness, response, and recovery) is critically important to minimizing mortality and morbidity in extreme events. LMICs are often resource-strapped from poor governance or narrow resource options, and this results in minimal support for disaster cycle provision. Socially vulnerable populations are the most affected by the failure to support disaster cycle planning and implementation (95–97). Children below age 18 and in particular those with disabilities are an especially vulnerable population during and after disasters (95–100).

While the Convention on the Rights of the Child supported by majority countries commit to the right of protecting children from unsafe environments, injury, and violence, the reality in LMIC's and disasters is quite different than envisaged (98, 101). During and after disasters children's needs and protections are more an afterthought, despite the reality that children experience disasters uniquely (102). Children are more susceptible to disaster trauma because of their dependence on adults for information, decision-making, transportation, protection from abuse, and provision of mental support. The assumption that adults promptly inform and make decisions for children in disasters overlooks the reality that children spend substantial amounts of time alone or with their peers or are homeless children living without adults (103). The number of children affected by disasters is projected to triple in coming decades due to factors such as climate change, which UNICEF refers to as a "threat multiplier that exacerbates inequality of children" (93).

In disaster situations, adults, family members, and caregivers are the first responders to children. This is especially true in LMIC's where lag time between disaster impact and response by official responders is substantial or non-existent. Additionally, in complex emergencies population displacement, collapse of health systems and inaccessibility may result in an even larger response lag. Consequently, child-focused training and exercise drills are imperative for mitigating disaster-related injuries or aggravating existing injuries.

Disaster Preparation

Integrating pediatric disaster planning into regular child injury prevention programs is also beneficial to families and communities. Disaster planning learned at school, and other institutions by children benefit families and communities, e.g., who do not speak the dominant disaster planning language (99, 103).

In complex emergencies, mortality rates for unaccompanied minors at refugee camps or shelters increase. Immediate triage and trauma care during intake remain critically important for saving impacted children's lives. Post evacuation to shelters, reunification protocols to protect children from the high risk of abuse, victimization, and trafficking minimizes additional trauma (104). Expeditious reunification (102) to legal guardians is critically important for the commencement of the child's recovery process. Place attachment is a critical component in the recovery processes of children. If evacuation is necessary, or stays in locations other than their places of attachment, creating new place ties bolsters recovery and resilience (95, 98, 105).

War and Its Effects on Children

Armed conflicts have been and remain part of the very fabric of human history. All around the world wars between nations, civil war, acts of terrorism and other forms of armed conflict persist.

The United Nations Children's Fund (UNICEF) estimates that 10% of the world's children (almost 250 million) live in regions affected by war and other armed conflicts (106). The majority of these conflicts are in LMICs (106). Of major concern is the fact that modern warfare is increasingly having a significant impact on the lives of children worldwide (106, 107). The violence is often indiscriminate. There is frequently no defined battlefield, and in most modern conflicts, civilians are directly targeted leading to a marked increase in pediatric injuries and deaths (107). Millions of children have been disabled or killed by this indiscriminate use of force (107). Notably, from 2005 to 2015 the average number of 0–19 disability-adjusted life years (DALYs) due to war and legal intervention increased by 582% (3). The conflicts in Iraq and Afghanistan and in particular the ongoing conflict in Syria, paint a stark portrait of the effects of war on children (**Figure 5**) (7, 108). Also quite troubling in a number of conflicts, has been the use of children as child soldiers and suicide bombers (106, 107). In addition to physical injuries, psychological wounds including post-traumatic stress disorder and other emotional and behavioral problems result from children's exposure to war (108). Children are also impacted by the disruption to the access to care caused by the conflict and the disruption that additionally results when they become refugees (106). According to the United Nations High Commission for Refugees (UNHCR), by 2015 there were over 65 million people displaced from their homes as they attempted to escape armed conflicts in their countries. About 50% of these are children under the age of 18 (106). It is imperative that children and other civilian non-combatants are protected and that governments and their international partner organizations make every effort to prevent armed conflicts and help end existing conflicts quickly. It is also important that the rights of children are recognized and that those who target children or use them deliberately in armed conflict are brought to justice.

Child Abuse

Child maltreatment occurs in all human communities and across all financial, ethnic, and religious boundaries (109). A recent systematic review of the literature by Hillis et al. found that the actual prevalence of violence against children is higher in LMICs than HICs (59% vs. 44%) (110). This same article reports a minimum of 64, 50, and 34% of children (2–17 yo) in Asia, Africa, and Latin America experienced past-year violence respectively (110). Globally, in 2014 at least 1 billion children were exposed to violence (110). The WHO Global Status report stated that in selected African countries one in three girls are victims of childhood sexual abuse and up to 76% of childhood physical abuse in both boys and girls (111).

A group of children at particularly high risk of abuse in LMICs, are those with disabilities. These children are often socially excluded and prevented from attending schools and are often unable to communicate the violence against them (112).

According to the WHO report, the knowledge of the true extent of the problem is hindered by gaps in knowledge with much of the data coming from high and middle-income countries (111). According to the WHO, a meta-analysis of global data finds self-reported child sexual abuse 30 times higher and physical abuse 75 times higher than official reports would suggest (109).

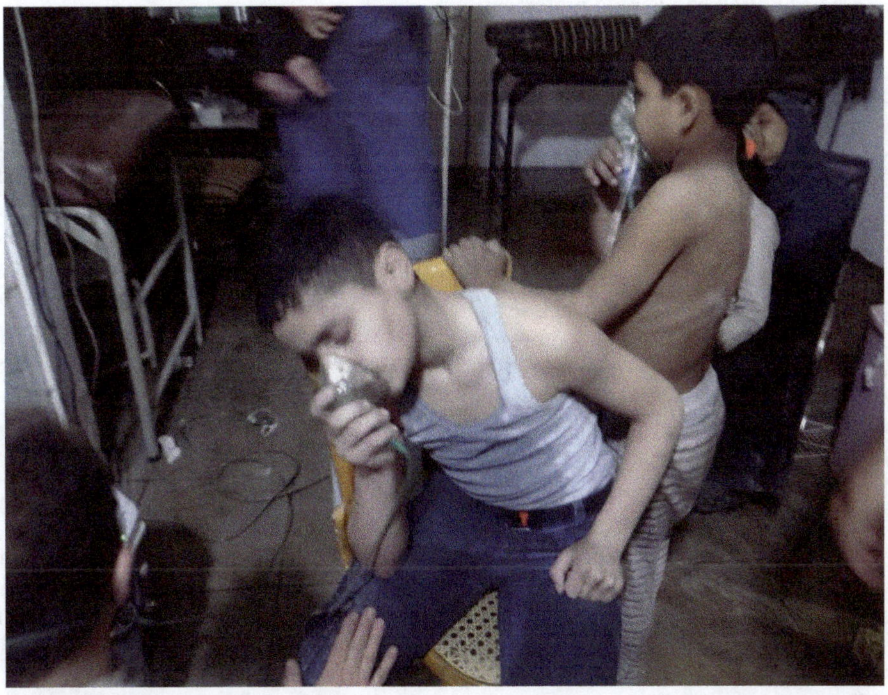

FIGURE 5 | Children being treated after suspected chemical weapon attack in Syria. Image courtesy of Muhammad Ghbeis, Boston Children's Hospital.

Recognizing Child Abuse

Although the prevalence and type of abuse may vary by location, the signs and symptoms are similar. We must consider abuse in all children presenting to us with symptoms consistent with abuse such as the triad of retinal hemorrhages, subdural hemorrhage, and encephalopathy or evidence of diffuse axonal injury (113). It is important to note that abusive head trauma can sometimes present with much more subtle findings such as vomiting (113). Additionally, child abuse must be considered in children presenting with features not consistent with the history provided, such as rib fractures from wrestling with another child, or bruises on the ears, under the toes, or in the form of a handprint (111). A helpful mnemonic for assessing which bruises are more concerning is the "TEN 4" rule (Torso, Ear, Neck and 4 (<4 yo or any bruising <4 mo) (113). Worrisome fractures include posterior or lateral rib fractures, "bucket handle" fractures and fractures such as sternal, spine, and scapula (113) unless the child has been in a major motor vehicle or similar accident. (**Figure 6**) In children, with elevated liver function tests, pancreatic enzymes or otherwise unexplained hematuria abuse with abdominal trauma should be considered (113). Other signs and symptoms that should trigger a careful exam include unusual scars in the form of hand and belt prints, cigarette burns, burns in an unusual distribution, or swelling that is unexplainable such as swollen painful thigh in a young infant (114). (**Figure 7**) Each of the seven strategies in the INSPIRE strategies, elucidated below are important in prevention as well as specific treatment for the injuries sustained (109, 113). It is also important to differentiate abuse from traditional treatment and practices such as tattooing, cupping and coining prevalent in many cultures (115).

While viewed by many as abusive, female circumcision continues to occur (116). In cultures where this is considered the normal practice, widespread education and laws to protect girls against this practice are needed (116). Another challenging area of child maltreatment is the use of child labor. UNICEF estimates that as many as 246 million children are engaged in child labor with 70% working in hazardous conditions[1]. Child labor may expose children to physical and traumatic maltreatment whether they are involved in hawking wares on the streets, hired as domestic workers or working in factory production lines.

Sexual abuse is common in all cultures but as noted above can be a common form of abuse in LMICs especially in girls. Numerous studies highlight significant rates of unwanted sexual encounters in children. An article by Summer et al. notes rates from 11.3–21.5% depending on age range and country (117). It is important to remember that lack of physical evidence of sexual abuse does not equate to lack of sexual abuse. These children need appropriate counseling and treatment (114, 117).

Child soldiering is a terrible form of maltreatment of children and youth[2]. Children are exploited to achieve the nefarious ends of the abusers as they expose them to violence and rape. These children suffer from post-traumatic stress disorder (PTSD) made worse by the lack of supportive mental health services in many LMICs (118).

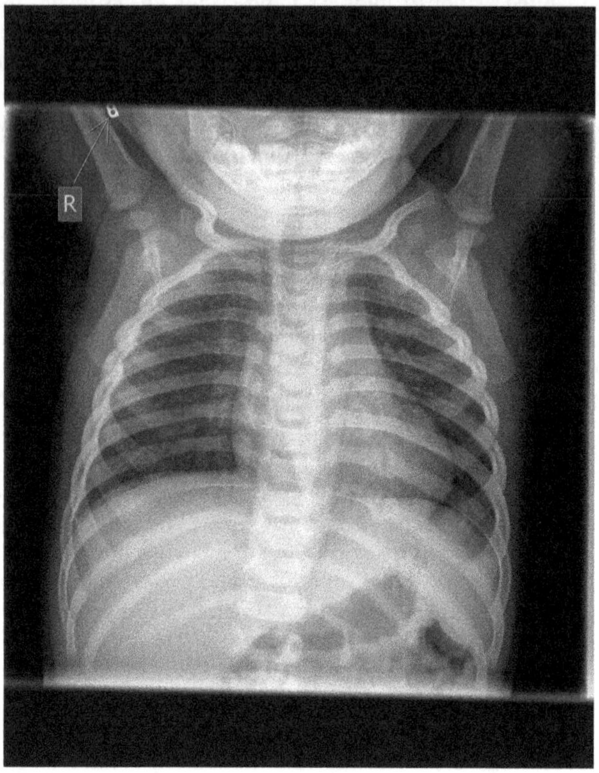

FIGURE 6 | Chest x-ray showing multiple rib fractures from child abuse. Fractures of ribs 3, 4, and 10 on the right and ribs 8, 9, and 10 on the left. Image courtesy of Nancy Harper, MD Masonic Children's Hospital, Minneapolis, MN and Sonja Eddleman, RN, Driscoll Children's Hospital, Corpus Christi, TX.

Cultures differ in their views about what is appropriate discipline. In some cultures, women and children may be viewed as the property of the husband and therefore virtually nothing constitutes abuse. Male abusers in these cultures are viewed as unquestionable authority figures. Changing norms and values as suggested by the INSPIRE strategies, is likely the most important measure to decrease this abuse. However, laws and their enforcement will also be imperative (109).

Education surrounding inappropriate corporal punishment is needed, as is guidance on the use of other appropriate methods of discipline both at home and in school. Guidelines about age-appropriate discipline are also needed (119).

Prevention

Given the dearth of available resources, the role of injury prevention in LMICs is vitality important. There are significant human and financial implications for reducing the number of people injured and killed around the world. If injury prevention efforts and improvements in trauma care in LMICs led to injury mortality rates similar to those in HICs, 2 million fewer children would die worldwide (120). The WHO in its *World Report on Child Injury Prevention* (6) set recommendations for prevention of injuries around the world:

[1]https://www.unicef.org/protection/files/child_labour.pf
[2]https://www.unicef.org/sowc96/2csoldrs.htm

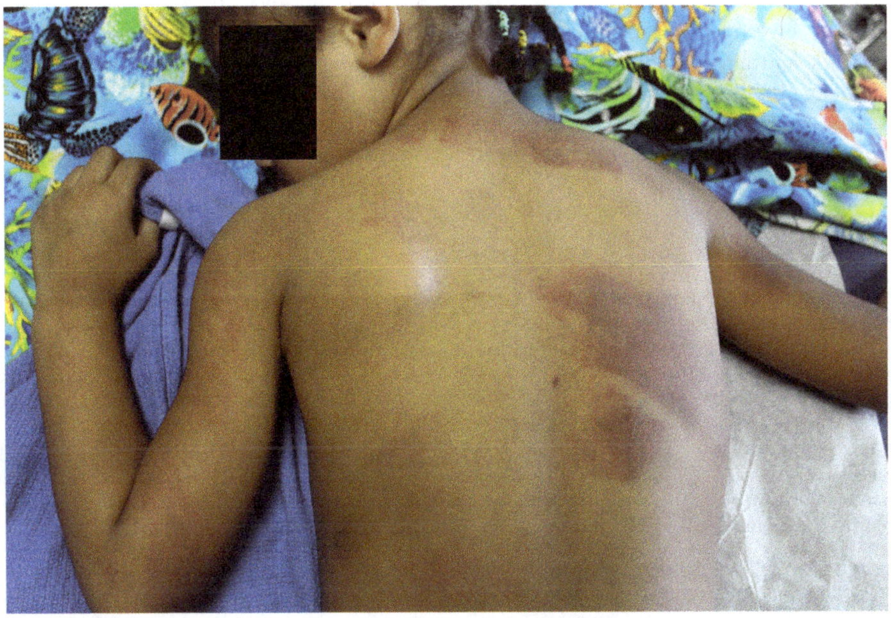

FIGURE 7 | Child with multiple bruises from a belt. Image courtesy of Nancy Harper, MD Masonic Children's Hospital, Minneapolis, MN and Sonja Eddleman, RN, Driscoll Children's Hospital, Corpus Christi, TX.

(a) Integrating childhood injury into an all-inclusive approach to child health and development
(b) Developing and implementing child-injury prevention policies and plans of action
(c) Implementing specific actions to prevent and control child injuries
(d) Strengthening of health systems to address childhood injuries
(e) Enhancement of the quality and quantity of data for child-injury prevention
(f) Defining research priorities
(g) Increasing awareness of and target investments toward child-injury prevention

The recommendations are a foundation for injury prevention efforts. Injury prevention in children is best achieved by blending education, legislation, law enforcement, environmental modifications and the use of safer products and safety devices (117). Governments in LMICs are increasingly aware of the importance of injury prevention. In Vietnam, where motorbikes are the principal mode of transportation, legislation mandating helmet use by all riders and passengers on motorcycles has the potential to decrease morbidity and mortality in motorcycle-involved RTIs (121). There have also been significant impacts on reduction of injuries from RTIs made by the Road Safety in 10 Countries project (2). The SwimSafe Project which is being implemented in Thailand, Bangladesh, and Vietnam, has taught over 525,000 children how to swim (122). In Bangladesh, one of the largest drowning prevention projects undertaken in an LMIC, the Saving of Lives from Drowning (SoLiD) Project, aims to reduce childhood drowning (123). In addition, given the increasing numbers of children who are injured and killed in armed conflicts, it is imperative that governments and international organizations such as the United Nations, make every effort to end these armed conflicts and minimize their impact on children.

CONCLUSIONS

Trauma is a leading cause of morbidity and mortality globally. Children in LMICs bear the greatest burden of unintentional and intentional injury. LMICs often lack adequate resources for managing trauma. Following trauma care protocols and adapting treatment based on local resources is important. Emphasizing injury prevention, regionalizing care and developing centers of excellence through multispecialty collaboration within each country is vital to improving outcomes and lowering trauma-related morbidity and mortality globally. War is increasingly having a devastating effect on children. A commitment by governments in LMICs in collaboration with international health organizations as well as partners in HICs to provide adequate healthcare services to their populations will be a safeguard against the devastation of infectious diseases and will also lead to improved outcomes for injured children.

AUTHOR CONTRIBUTIONS

AK: Substantial contributions to the conception or design of the work and the acquisition of background articles and topics to be covered; drafted work and revised it critically for important intellectual content; provided approval for publication; agreed to be accountable for all aspects of the work in ensuring that questions related to accuracy or integrity of any part of work are appropriately investigated and resolved. SD, NM, and AA: Drafted work and added content critically for important intellectual content; provided approval for publication of content. SG, MM and DG: Drafted and revised the work and added content critically for important intellectual content; provided approval for publication of the content. TS: Drafted work and revised it critically for important intellectual content; provided approval for publication; agreed to be accountable for all aspects of the work in ensuring that questions related to accuracy or integrity of any part of work are appropriately investigated and resolved.

REFERENCES

1. Kassebaum NJ, Kyu HH, Zoeckler L, Olsen HE, Thomas K, Pinho C, et al. Child and adolescent health from 1990 to 2015 findings from the global burden of diseases, injuries, and risk factors 2015 study. *JAMA Pediatr.* (2017) **171**:573–92. doi: 10.1001/jamapediatrics.2017.0250
2. Rivara FP. Prevention of death and disability from injuries to children and adolescents. *Int J Inj Contr Saf Promot* (2012) **19**:226–30. doi: 10.1080/17457300.2012.686919
3. He S, Lunnen JC, Puvanachandra P, Amar-Singh, Zia N, Hyder AA. Global childhood unintentional injury study: multisite surveillance data. *Am J Public Health* (2014) **104**:e79–84. doi: 10.2105/AJPH.2013.301607
4. Chandran A, Hyder AA, Peek-Asa C. The global burden of unintentional injuries and an agenda for progress. *Epidemiol Rev.* (2010) **32**:110–20. doi: 10.1093/epirev/mxq009
5. Debas HT, Donkor P, Gawande A, Jamison DT, Kruk ME, Mock CN, editors. *Essential Surgery. Disease Control Priorities.* 3rd ed. Washington, DC: World Bank (2015). doi: 10.1596/978-1-4648-0346-8
6. PedenM, Oyegbite K, Ozanne-Smith J, Hyder AA, Branche C, Rahman AKMF, et al. *World Report on Child Injury Prevention.* Geneva: World Health Organization (2008).
7. Carlson LC, Lafta R, Al-Shatari S, Stewart BT, Burnham G, Kushner AL. Pediatric injury during conflict and prolonged insecurity in Iraq from 2003–2014. *Surgery* (2016) **160**:493–500. doi: 10.1016/j.surg.2016.03.022
8. Baker T. Critical care in low-income countries. *Trop. Med. Int. Health.* (2009) **14**:143–8. doi: 10.1111/j.1365-3156.2008.02202.x
9. Debenham S, Fuller M, Stewart M, Price RR. Where there is no EMS: lay providers in Emergency Medical Services care - EMS as a public health priority. *Prehosp Disaster Med.* (2017) **32**:1–3. doi: 10.1017/S1049023X17006811
10. Callese TE, Richards CT, Shaw P, Schuetz SJ, Paladino L, Issa N, et al. Trauma system development in low- and middle-income countries: a review. *J Surg Res.* (2015) **193**:300–7. doi: 10.1016/j.jss.2014.09.040
11. Duke T, Cheema B. Paediatric emergency and acute care in resource poor settings. *J Paediatr Child Health* (2016) **52**:221–6. doi: 10.1111/jpc.13105
12. Osifo OD, Iribhogbe PE, Ugiagbe EE. Epidemiology and pattern of paediatric and adolescent trauma deaths in a level 1 trauma centre in Benin city, Nigeria. *Injury* (2012) **43**:1861–4. doi: 10.1016/j.injury.2011.07.016
13. Molyneux E, Ahmad S, Robertson A. Improved triage and emergency care for children reduces inpatient mortality in a resource constrained setting. *Bull World Health Organ.* (2006) **84**:314–9. doi: 10.2471/BLT.04.019505
14. Kotwal RS, Howard JT, Orman JA, Tarpey BW, Bailey JA, Champion HR, et al. The effect of a golden hour policy on the morbidity and mortality of combat casualties. *JAMA Surg* (2016) **151**:15–24. doi: 10.1001/jamasurg.2015.3104
15. Turner EL, Nielsen KR, Jamal SM, von Saint André-von Arnim A, Musa NL. A review of pediatric critical care in resource-limited settings: a look at past, present, and future directions. *Front. Pediatr.* (2016) **4**:5. doi: 10.3389/fped.2016.00005
16. Mock C, Lormand JD, Goosen J, Joshipura M, Peden M, editors. *Guidelines for Essential Trauma Care.* Geneva: World Health Organization (2004).
17. Callese TE, Richards CT, Shaw P, Schuetz SJ, Issa N, Paladino L, et al. Layperson trauma training in low- and middle-income countries: a review. *J Surg Res* (2014) **190**:104–10. doi: 10.1016/j.jss.2014.03.029
18. Hyder AA, He S, Zafar W, Mir MU, Razzak JA. One hundred injured patients a day: multicenter emergency room surveillance of trauma in Pakistan. *Public Health* (2017) **148**:88–95. doi: 10.1016/j.puhe.2017.03.006
19. Aaronson E, Mort E, Soghoian S. Mapping the process of emergency care at a teaching hospital in Ghana. *Healthcare* (2016) **5**:214–20. doi: 10.1016/j.hjdsi.2016.12.001
20. *Emergency Triage Assessment and Treatment (ETAT): Manual for Participants.* Geneva: World Health Organization; 2005. Available online at: http://www.who.int/maternal_child_adolescent/documents/9241546875/en/
21. Otieno T, Woodfield JC, Bird P, Hill AG. Trauma in rural Kenya. *Injury* (2004) **35**:1228–33. doi: 10.1016/j.injury.2004.03.013
22. Mock CN, Quansah R, Addae-Mensah L, Donkor P. The development of continuing education for trauma care in an African nation. *Injury* (2005) **36**:725–32. doi: 10.1016/j.injury.2004.12.044
23. Ali J, Adam R, Butler AK, Chang H, Howard M, Gonsalves D, et al. Trauma outcome improves following the advanced trauma life support program in a developing country. *J Trauma* (1993) **34**:890–8. discussion: 898–9.
24. Mikrogianakis A, Kam A, Silver S, Bakanisi B, Henao O, Okrainec A, et al. Telesimulation: an innovative and effective tool for teaching novel intraosseous insertion techniques in developing countries. *Acad Emerg Med.* (2011) **18**:420–7. doi: 10.1111/j.1553-2712.2011.01038.x
25. Reynolds TA, Calvello EJB, Broccoli MC, Sawe HR, Mould-Millman NK, Teklu S, et al. AFEM consensus conference 2013 summary: emergency care in Africa – where are we now? *Afr J Emerg Med.* (2014) **4**:158–63. doi: 10.1016/j.afjem.2014.07.004
26. Kesinger MR, Nagy LR, Sequeira DJ, Charry JD, Puyana JC, Rubiano AM. et al. A standardized trauma care protocol decreased in-hospital mortality of patients with severe traumatic brain injury at a teaching hospital in a middle-income country. *Injury, Int. J. Care Injured* (2014) **45**:1350–4. doi: 10.1016/j.injury.2014.04.037
27. Higashi H, Barendregt JJ, Kassebaum NJ, Weiser TG, Bickler SW, Vos T. Burden of injuries avertable by a basic surgical package in low and middle-income regions: a systematic analysis from the global burden of disease 2010 study. *World J Surg.* (2015) **39**:1–9. doi: 10.1007/s00268-014-2685-x
28. Sethi D, Aljunid S, Sulong SB, Zwi AB. Injury care in low- and middle-income countries: identifying potential for change. *Inj Control Saf Promot.* (2000) **7**: 153–64. doi: 10.1076/1566-0974(200009)7:3;1-N;FT153
29. OPENPediatrics. Homepage. Available online at: http://www.openpediatrics.org (Accessed November 2, 2017).
30. Banstola A, Mytton J. Cost-effectiveness of interventions to prevent road traffic injuries in low- and middle-income countries: a literature review. *Traffic Injury Prevent.* (2017) **18**:357–62. doi: 10.1080/15389588.2016.1212165
31. Li Q, Alonge O, Hyder AA. Children and road traffic injuries: can't the world do better? *Arch Dis Child.* (2016) **101**:1063–70. doi: 10.1136/archdischild-2015-309586
32. Gupta S, Gupta SK, Devkota S, Ranjit A, Swaroop M, Kushner AL, et al. Fall injuries in nepal: a countrywide population-based survey. *Ann. Global Health* (2015) **81**:487–94. doi: 10.1016/j.aogh.2015.07.004
33. Tyler MD, Richards DB, Reske-Nielsen C, Saghafi O, Morse EA, Carey R, et al. The epidemiology of drowning in low- and middle-income countries: a systematic review. *BMC Public Health* (2017) **17**:413. doi: 10.1186/s12889-017-4239-2
34. Hossain M, Mani KKC, Sidik SM, Hayati KS, Rahman AK. Randomized controlled trial on drowning prevention for parents with children aged below five years in Bangladesh: a study protocol. *BMC Public Health* (2015) **15**:484. doi: 10.1186/s12889-015-1823-1
35. WHO. *Poisoning Prevention and Management Program.* Available online at: http://www.who.int/ipcs/poisons/en/ (Accessed November 30, 2017).
36. Aggarwal S, Patton G, Reavley N, Sreenivasan SA, Berk M. Youth self-harm in low- and middle-income countries: systematic review of the risk and protective factors. *Int J Soc Psychiatry* (2017) **63**:359–75. doi: 10.1177/0020764017700175
37. Rubiano AM, Puyana JC, Mock CN, Bullock MR, Adelson PD. Strengthening neurotrauma care systems in low and middle-income countries. *Brain Inj.* (2013) **27**:262–72. doi: 10.3109/02699052.2012.750742

38. Dewan MC, Mummareddy, N, Wellons JC, Bonfield CM. Epidemiology of global pediatric traumatic brain injury: qualitative review. *World Neurosurg.* (2016) **91**:497–509. doi: 10.1016/j.wneu.2016.03.045
39. De Silva MJ, Roberts I, Perel P, Edwards P, Kenward MG, Fernandes J, et al. CRASH Trial Collaborators. Patient outcome after traumatic brain injury in high-, middle- and low-income countries: analysis of data on 8927 patients in 46 countries. *Int J Epidemiol.* (2009) **38**:452–8. doi: 10.1093/ije/dyn189
40. Staton CA, Msilanga D, Kiwango G, Vissoci JR, de Andrade L, Lester R, et al. A prospective registry evaluating the epidemiology and clinical care of traumatic brain injury patients presenting to a regional referral hospital in Moshi, Tanzania: challenges and the way forward. *Int J Inj Control Safety Promot.* (2017) **24**:69–77. doi: 10.1080/17457300.2015.1061562
41. Kochanek PM, Carney N, Adelson PD, Ashwal S, Bell MJ, Bratton S, et al.. Guidelines for the acute medical management of severe traumatic brain injury in infants, children, and adolescents—second edition. *Pediatr Crit Care Med* (2012) **13**(1 Suppl 1):S1–82.
42. Basso A, Previgliano I, Duarte JM, Ferrari N. Advances in management of neurosurgical trauma in different continents. *World J Surg.* (2001) **25**:1174–8. doi: 10.1007/s00268-001-0079-3
43. Brain Trauma Foundation. Guidelines for the management of severe traumatic brain injury. *J Neurotrauma* (2007) **24**(1 Suppl): S1–106.
44. Orliaguet GA, Meyer PG, Baugnon T. Management of critically ill children with traumatic brain injury. *Paediatr Anaesth* (2008) **18**:455–61. doi: 10.1111/j.1460-9592.2008.02507.x
45. Atabaki SM. Updates in the general approach to pediatric head trauma and concussion. *Pediatr Clin North Am* (2013) **60**:1107–22. doi: 10.1016/j.pcl.2013.06.001
46. Morrison J, Mâsse B, Ouellet P, Décarie JC, Gravel J. Four-film X-ray series is more sensitive than 2-film for diagnosis of skull fractures in children. *Pediatr Emerg Care* (2013) **29**:1189–93. doi: 10.1097/PEC.0b013e3182a9f7c1
47. Sahoo SS, Agrawal D. Correlation of optic nerve sheath diameter with intracranial pressure monitoring in patients with severe traumatic brain injury. *Indian J Neurotrauma* (2013) **10**:9–12. doi: 10.1016/j.ijnt.2013.05.010
48. Chesnut RM, Temkin N, Carney N, Dikmen S, Rondina C, Videtta W, et al. Global Neurotrauma Research Group. A trial of intracranial-pressure monitoring in traumatic brain injury. *N Engl J Med.* (2012) **367**:2471–81. doi: 10.1056/NEJMoa1207363
49. Gutierrez IM, Ben-Ishay O, Mooney DP. Pediatric thoracic and abdominal trauma. *Minerva Chir.* (2013) **68**:263–74.
50. Chirdan LB, Uba AF, Yiltok SJ, Ramyil VM. Paediatric blunt abdominal trauma: challenges of management in a developing country. *Eur J Pediatr Surg* (2007) **17**:90–5. doi: 10.1055/s-2007-965008
51. Adelgais KM, Kuppermann N, Kooistra J, Garcia M, Monroe DJ, Mahajan P, et al. Intra-Abdominal Injury Study Group of the Pediatric Emergency Care Applied Research Network (PECARN). Accuracy of the abdominal examination for identifying children with blunt intra-abdominal injuries. *J Pediatr.* (2014) **165**:1230–5.e5. doi: 10.1016/j.jpeds.2014.08.014
52. Moore EE, Cogbill TH, Jurkovich GJ, Shackford SR, Malangoni MA, Champion HR. Organ injury scaling: spleen and liver (1994 revision). *J Trauma* (1995) **38**:323–4. doi: 10.1097/00005373-199503000-00001
53. Nwafor IA, Eze JC, Ezemba N, Onyekwulu OC, Brown A, Anyanwu CH. The profile of chest injuries in a southeastern Nigeria teaching hospital, a 10-year experience. *Niger J Med.* (2014) **23**:162–9.
54. Pearson EG, Fitzgerald CA, Santore MT, Pediatric thoracic trauma: current trends. *Semin Pediatr Surg.* (2017) **26**:36–42. doi: 10.1053/j.sempedsurg.2017.01.007
55. Ameh EA, Bickler SW, Lakhoo K, Nwomeh, B, Poenaru D, editors. *Paediatric Surgery: A Comprehensive Text for Africa.* Seattle, WA: Global HELP Organization (2011).
56. Holcomb GW, Murphy JP, Ostlie DJ, editors. *Ashcraft's Pediatric Surgery.* 5th ed. Philadelphia, PA: Elsevier (2010).
57. Skinner DL, den Hollander D, Laing GL, Rodseth RN, Muckart DJ. Severe blunt thoracic trauma: differences between adults and children in a level I trauma centre. *S Afr Med J.* (2015) **105**:47–51. doi: 10.7196/SAMJ.8499
58. Coran AG, Caldamone A, Adzick NS, Krummel TM, Laberge JM, Shamberger R, et al. editors. *Pediatric Surgery.* 7th ed. Philadelphia, PA: Elsevier (2012)
59. Peclet MH, Newman KD, Eichelberger MR, Gotschall CS, Garcia VF, Bowman LM. Thoracic trauma in children: an indicator of increased mortality. *J Pediatr Surg.* (1990) **25**:961–5. discussion: 965–6.
60. Holscher CM, Faulk LW, Moore EE, Cothren Burlew C, Moore HB, Stewart CL, et al. Chest computed tomography imaging for blunt pediatric trauma: not worth the radiation risk. *J Surg Res.* (2013) **184**:352–7. doi: 10.1016/j.jss.2013.04.044
61. Moore MA, Wallace EC, Westra SJ. Chest trauma in children: current imaging guidelines and techniques. *Radiol Clin North Am.* (2011) **49**:949–68. doi: 10.1016/j.rcl.2011.06.002
62. Clancy K, Velopulos C, Bilaniuk JW, Collier B, Crowley W, Kurek S, et al. Eastern Association for the Surgery of Trauma. Screening for blunt cardiac injury: an Eastern Association for the Surgery of Trauma practice management guideline. *J Trauma Acute Care Surg.* (2012) **73**(5 Suppl 4):S301–6. doi: 10.1097/TA.0b013e318270193a
63. Dowd MD, Krug S. Pediatric blunt cardiac injury: epidemiology, clinical features, and diagnosis. Pediatric Emergency Medicine Collaborative Research Committee: Working Group on Blunt Cardiac Injury. *J Trauma* (1996) **40**:61–7. doi: 10.1097/00005373-199601000-00012
64. Rielly JP, Brandt ML, Mattox KL, Pokorny WJ. Thoracic trauma in children. *J Trauma* (1993) **34**:329–31. doi: 10.1097/00005373-199303000-00003
65. Hanafi M, Al-Sarraf N, Sharaf H, Abdelaziz A. Pattern and presentation of blunt chest trauma among different age groups. *Asian Cardiovasc Thorac Ann* (2011) **19**:48–51. doi: 10.1177/0218492310395954
66. Burack JH1, Kandil E, Sawas A, O'Neill PA, Sclafani SJ, Lowery RC, et al. Triage and outcome of patients with mediastinal penetrating trauma. *Ann Thorac Surg.* (2007) **83**:377–82. doi: 10.1016/j.athoracsur.2006.05.107
67. *Global Status Report on Road Safety: Time for Action.* Geneva: World Health Organization (2009). Available online at: www.who.int/violence_injury_prevention/road_safety_status/2009
68. Thornton MD, Della-Giustina K, Aronson PL. Emergency department evaluation and treatment of pediatric orthopedic injuries. *Emerg Med Clin North Am.* (2015) **33**:423–49. doi: 10.1016/j.emc.2014.12.012
69. Komlatsè AN, Azanledji BM, Abossisso SK, Anani MA, Komla G, Hubert T. Elastic stable intramedullary nailing of femoral shaft fractures in children: particularities and results at Sylvanus Olympio Teaching Hospital of Lomé, Togo. *Afr J Paediatr Surg.* (2014) **11**:8–11. doi: 10.4103/0189-6725.129202
70. Akinyoola AL, Orekha OO, Taiwo FO, Odunsi AO. Outcome of non-operative management of femoral shaft fractures in children. *Afr J Paediatr Surg.* (2011) **8**:34–9. doi: 10.4103/0189-6725.78666
71. Conway DJ, Coughlin R, Caldwell A and Shearer D. The institute for global orthopedics and traumatology: a model for academic collaboration in orthopedic surgery. *Front. Public Health.* (2017) **5**:146. doi: 10.3389/fpubh.2017.00146
72. Young S. Orthopaedic trauma surgery in low-income countries: follow-up, infections, and HIV. *Acta Ortho.* (2014) **85**:1–35. doi: 10.3109/17453674.2014.937924
73. Omololu AB, Ogunlade SO, Gopaldasani VK. The practice of traditional bone setting: Training algorithm. *Clin Orthop Relat Res.* (2008) **466**:2392–8. doi: 10.1007/s11999-008-0371-8
74. Phillips J, Zirkle LG, Gosselin RA. Achieving locked intramedullary fixation of long bone fractures: Technology for the developing world. Int Orthop. (2012) **36**:2007–13. doi: 10.1007/s00264-012-1625-3
75. Gali BM, Madziga AG, Naaya HU. Epidemiology of childhood burns in Maiduguri north-eastern Nigeria. *Niger J Med.* (2004) **13**:144–7.
76. Argenta A, Demos J. Burn management in the developing world international volunteerism. *Clin Plastic Surg.* (2017) **44**:875–83. doi: 10.1016/j.cps.2017.05.019
77. *World Health Organization.* Available online at: http://www.who.int/violence_injury_prevention/other_injury/burns/en/ (Accessed November 2, 2017).
78. Atiyeh BS, Costagliola M, Hayek SN. Burn prevention mechanisms and outcomes: pitfalls, failures, and successes. *Burns* (2009) **35**:181–93. doi: 10.1016/j.burns.2008.06.002
79. Kasten KR, Makley AT, Kagan RJ. Update on the critical care management of severe burns. *J Intensive Care Med* (2011) **26**:223–36. doi: 10.1177/0885066610390869
80. Tyson AF, Boschini LP, Kiser MM, Samuel JC, Mjuweni SN, Cairns BA, et al. Survival after burn in a sub-saharan burn unit: challenges and opportunities. *Burns* (2013) **39**:1619–25. doi: 10.1016/j.burns.2013.04.013
81. Sengoelge M, El-Khatib Z, Laflamme L. The global burden of child burn injuries in light of country-level economic development

and income inequality. *Prevent Med Rep.* (2017) **6**:115–20. doi: 10.1016/j.pmedr.2017.02.024
82. Ringo Y, Chilonga K. Burns at KCMC: epidemiology, presentation, management, and treatment outcome. *Burns* (2014) **40**:1024–9. doi: 10.1016/j.burns.2013.10.019
83. Rode H, Rogers AD, Cox SG, Allorto NL, Stefani F, Bosco A, et al. Burn resuscitation on the African continent. *Burns* (2014) **40**:1283–91. doi: 10.1016/j.burns.2014.01.004
84. Jeng J, Gibran N, Peck M. Burn care in disaster and other austere settings. *Surg Clin North Am.* (2014) **94**:893–907. doi: 10.1016/j.suc.2014.05.011
85. Atiyeh B, Masellis A, Conte C. Optimizing burn treatment in developing low- and middle-income countries with limited health care resources (part 2). *Ann Burns Fire Disasters* (2009) **22**:189–95.
86. Gallaher JR, Mjuweni S, Cairns BA, Charles AG. Burn care delivery in a sub-Saharan African unit: a cost analysis study. *Int J Surg.* (2015) **19**:116e120. doi: 10.1016/j.ijsu.2015.05.015
87. Stewart BT, Gyedu A, Agbenorku P, Amankwa R, Kushner AL, Gibran N. Routine systemic antibiotic prophylaxis for burn injuries in developing countries: a best evidence topic (BET). *Int J Surg.* (2015) **21**:168e172. doi: 10.1016/j.ijsu.2015.08.002
88. World Health Organization. *Burn Prevention: Success Stories Lessons Learned.* Available online at: http://apps.who.int/iris/bitstream/10665/97938/1/9789241501187_eng.pdf (Accessed November 2, 2017)
89. Barton A. *Community in Disaster.* Garden City, NY: Anchor (1970).
90. Quarantelli EL. *Disaster Planning, Emergency Management, and Civil Protection: The Historical Development and Current Characteristics of Organized Efforts to Prevent and to Respond to Disasters.* University of Delaware Disaster Research Center (1998) p. 227.
91. Miletti DS. *Disasters by Design: A Reassessment of Natural Hazards in the United States.* Washington, DC: Joseph Henry Press (1999).
92. Quarantelli EL. *The Disasters of the 21st Century: A Mixture of New, Old, and Mixed Types.* University of Delaware Research Center. (2006) p. 353.
93. United Nations Children's Fund (UNICEF). *Learning to Live in a Changing Climate: The Impact of Climate Change on Children in Bangladesh.* Dhaka (2016).
94. Waugh WL, Terrorism homeland security, and the national emergency management network. *Public Organ Rev. Glob J.* (2003) **3**:373–85. doi: 10.1023/B:PORJ.0000004815.29497.e5
95. Wisner B, Blaikie P, Cannon T, Davis I. *At Risk: Natural Hazards, People's Vulnerability and Disasters.* 2nd ed. Routledge:Taylor & Francis Group (2004).
96. Dash N, Gladwin H. Evacuation decision making and behavioral responses: individual and household. *Nat Hazards Rev.* (2007) **8**:3. doi: 10.1061/(ASCE)1527-6988(2007)8:3(69)
97. Peek L, Stough M. Children with disabilities in the context of disaster: a Social Vulnerability perspective. *Child Dev.* (2010) **81**:1260–70. doi: 10.1111/j.1467-8624.2010.01466.x
98. Penrose A, Takaki M. Children's rights in emergencies and disasters. *Lancet* (2006) **33367**:698–99. doi: 10.1016/S0140-6736(06)68272-X
99. Ronan KR, Alisic E, Towers B, Johnson VA, Johnston MD. Disaster preparedness for children and families: a critical review. *Curr Psychiatry Rep.* (2015) **17**:58. doi: 10.1007/s11920-015-0589-6
100. Cartwright C, Hall M, Lee ACK. The changing health priorities of earthquake response and implications for preparedness: a scoping review. *Public Health* (2017) **150**:60–70. doi: 10.1016/j.puhe.2017.04.024
101. State *of the Worlds Children.* Geneva: UNICEF (2008).
102. National Commission on Children and Disasters. *2010 Report to the President and the Congress. AHRQ Publication No. 10-M*Rockville, MD: Agency for Healthcare Research and Quality (2010).
103. Phillips BD, Morrow BH. Social science research needs: focus on vulnerable populations, forecasting, and warnings. *Nat Hazards Rev.* (2007) **8**:61–8. doi: 10.1061/(ASCE)1527-6988(2007)8:3(61)
104. Enarson E. Fothergill A. Peek L. Gender and disaster: foundations and directions. In: Rodriguez H, Quarantelli, EL, Dynes RR, editors. *Handbook of Disaster Research* (2007). P. 130–46.
105. Scannell L, Cox RS, Fletcher S., Heykoop C. "That was the last time I saw my house": the importance of place attachment among children and youth in disaster contexts. *Am J Commun Psychol.* (2016) **58**:158–73. doi: 10.1002/ajcp.12069
106. Brown FL, de Graaf AM, Annan J, Betancourt TS. Annual research review: breaking cycles of violence –a systematic review and common practice elements analysis of psychosocial interventions for children and youth affected by armed conflict. *J Child Psychol Psychiatry* (2017) **58**:507–24. doi: 10.1111/jcpp.12671
107. Slone M and Mann S. Effects of war, terrorism and armed conflict on young children: a systematic review. *Child Psychiatry Hum Dev.* (2016) **47**:950–65. doi: 10.1007/s10578-016-0626-7
108. Celikel A, Karbayez K, Karsalan B, Arslan MM, Zeren C. Childhood casualties during civil war: syrian experience. *J Foren Legal Med* (2015) **34**:1–4. doi: 10.1016/j.jflm.2015.04.021
109. *WHO. INSPIRE: Seven Strategies for Ending Violence Against Children.* Available online at: www.who.int/violence_injury_prevention/violence/inspire/en/; (*WHO Global Status Report on Violence Prevention 2014.* Available online at: www.who.int/violence_injury_prevention/violence/status_report/2014/en/
110. Hillis S, Mercy J, Amobi A, Kress H. Global prevalence of past-year violence against children: a systematic review and minimum estimates. *Pediatrics* (2016) **137**:e20154079. doi: 10.1542/peds.2015-4079
111. *WHO Global Status Report on Violence Prevention 2.* Available online at: www.who.int/violence_injury_prevention/violence/status_report/2014/en/)
112. Banks LM, Kelly SA, Kyegombe N, Kuper H, Devries K. "If he could speak, he would be able to point out who does those things to him": experiences of violence and access to child protection among children with disabilities in Uganda and Malawi. *PLoS ONE* (2017) **12**:e0183736. doi: 10.1371/journal.pone.0183736
113. Gonzalez D, McCall JD. *Child Abuse and Neglect. StatPearls [Internet].* Treasure Island, FL: StatPearls Publishing (2017).
114. What is child abuse and neglect. *Recognizing the Signs and Symptoms.* Available online at: https://www.childwelfare.gov/pubPDFs/whatiscan.pdf
115. Lilley E, Kundu RV. Dermatoses secondary to Asian cultural practices. *Int J Dermatol.* (2012) **51**:372–9. doi: 10.1111/j.1365-4632.2011.05170.x
116. Gordon JS. Reconciling female genital circumcision with universal human rights. *Dev World Bioeth.* (2017). doi: 10.1111/dewb.12173. [Epub ahead of print].
117. Summer SA, Marcelin LH, Cela T, Mercy JA, Lee V, Kress H,et al. Sentinel events predicting later unwanted sex among girls: a national survey in Haiti, 2*Child Abuse Negl.* (2015) **50**:49–55.
118. Ovuga E, Oyok TO, Moro EB. Post-traumatic stress disorder among former child soldiers attending a rehabilitative service and primary school education in northern Uganda. *Afric Health Sci.* (2008) **8**:136–41.
119. Salami B, Ali Hirani SA, Meherali A, Amodu O, Chamber T. Parenting practices of african immigrants in destination countries: a qualitative research synthesis. *J Pediatric Nurs.* (2017) **36**:20–30. doi: 10.1016/j.pedn.2017.04.016
120. Kotagal M, Agarwal-Harding KJ, Mock C, Quansah R, Arreola-Risa C, et al. Health and economic benefits of improved injury prevention and trauma care worldwide. *PLoS ONE* (2014) **9**:e91862. doi: 10.1371/journal.pone.0091862
121. Boufous S, Ali M, Nguyen HT, et al. Child injury prevention in Vietnam: achievements and challenges. *Int J Inj Contr Saf Promot.* (2012) **19**:123–9. doi: 10.1080/17457300.2011.603426
122. *Preventing Drowning: An Implementation Guide.* Geneva: WHO (2017).
123. Hyder AA, Alonge O, He S, Wadhwaniya S, Rahman F, El Arifeen S. A framework for addressing implementation gap in global drowning prevention interventions: experiences from Bangladesh. *J Health Popul Nutr.* (2014) **32**:564–76.

21

Neonatal End-of-Life Symptom Management

DonnaMaria E. Cortezzo [1,2,3,4] and Mark Meyer[2,3,4,5]*

[1] Division of Neonatal and Pulmonary Biology, Cincinnati Children's Hospital Medical Center, Cincinnati, OH, United States, [2] Division of Pain and Palliative Medicine, Cincinnati Children's Hospital Medical Center, Cincinnati, OH, United States, [3] Department of Pediatrics, University of Cincinnati College of Medicine, Cincinnati, OH, United States, [4] Department of Anesthesiology, University of Cincinnati College of Medicine, Cincinnati, OH, United States, [5] Division of Anesthesia, Cincinnati Children's Hospital Medical Center, Cincinnati, OH, United States

Correspondence:
DonnaMaria E. Cortezzo
donnamaria.cortezzo@cchmc.org

Purpose of review: Despite advances in technology and treatment options, over 15,000 neonates die each year in the United States. The majority of the deaths, with some estimates as high as 80%, are the result of a planned redirection of care or comfort measures only approach to care. When curative or life-prolonging interventions are not available or have been exhausted, parents focus on preserving quality of life and eliminating needless suffering. Parents hope their child will have a peaceful death and will not feel pain. A significant component of end-of-life care is high quality symptom evaluation and management. It is important that neonatal providers are knowledgeable in symptom management to address common sources of suffering and distress for babies and their families at the end-of-life (EOL).

Recent findings: Medically complex neonates with life-threatening conditions are a unique patient population and there is little research on end-of-life symptom assessment and management. While there are tools available to assess symptoms for adolescents and adults, there is not a recognized set of tools for the neonatal population. Nonetheless, it is widely accepted that neonates experience significant symptoms at end-of-life. Most commonly acknowledged manifestations are pain, dyspnea, agitation, and secretions. In the absence of data and established guidelines, there is variability in their clinical management. This contributes to provider discomfort and inadequate symptom control.

Summary: End-of-life symptom assessment and management is an important component of neonatal end-of-life care. While there remains a paucity of studies and data, it is prudent that providers adequately manage symptoms. Likewise, it is important that providers are educated so that they can effectively guide families through the dying process by discussing disease progression, physical changes, and providing empathetic support. In this review, the authors make recommendations for non-pharmacological and pharmacological management of end-of-life symptoms in neonates.

Keywords: Perinatal palliative care, neonatal, end-of-life, symptom management, pharmacological management

INTRODUCTION

Neonatal end-of-life care is pivotal for the patient, parents, and providers. Whether the need for end-of-life care is the result of a comfort measures only approach with a known life-limiting diagnosis, the result of redirection of care after a trial of therapy, or the end result despite maximal invasive medical interventions, it is an incredibly difficult time filled with emotions and uncertainty. At a time typically filled with joy and hopes for the future they will have with their child, parents of neonates at EOL are grieving the loss of their baby even before death occurs (1). Parents note that when goals have transitioned to end-of-life care, they worry that their child will experience pain and physical suffering. They hope for a peaceful death with minimal discomfort for their child (2–8). One of the focuses of palliative care is the prevention and alleviation of symptoms including physical, emotional, and perceived suffering of the patient (9). In addition to providing support, it is paramount that providers focus on pain and symptom management (10, 11). At the same time, there can be many unknowns. For clinicians as well as families this is a time of uncertainty. It is often difficult to predict the timing of death, whether it be hours, minutes, days, or more (8). Effective management requires anticipation of the disease manifestations as well as the severity of symptoms for each patient. This can vary greatly and is often related in part to the underlying diagnoses and conditions leading to death. For any patient population, anticipating the symptom burden can be challenging even with a strong understanding of the pathophysiology. There is an added layer of complexity when caring for neonates as they cannot communicate their symptoms or express how they are feeling. For older children, adolescents, and adults, the gold standard of symptom assessment is self-report. However, there is no such standard that exists for preverbal patients. In neonates, there are few reliable tools to accurately assess symptoms and observational measures can be blunted depending on the gestational age and underlying disease process. This makes it difficult for providers to know if a neonate is experiencing symptoms at the EOL and if interventions are alleviating the symptoms to a satisfactory and acceptable level. In spite of all of these challenges, it is pertinent that providers are able to assess and treat symptoms a neonate may have at EOL so that the baby, the parents, and family have a peaceful experience.

SCOPE OF NEONATAL END-OF-LIFE CARE AND SYMPTOM MANAGEMENT

In the United States, there are over 15,000 neonatal deaths each year (12). The majority of these deaths are the result of congenital malformations or chromosomal anomalies, with up to 3% of pregnancies being complicated by a fetal life-limiting diagnosis (13–15). While some families opt for a comfort measures approach to care at home, the majority of neonatal deaths occur in the neonatal intensive care unit (NICU). Regardless of the location of care, most deaths, with some estimates as high as 80%, are the result of a comfort measures only approach to care or a redirection of care after a trial of therapy (16). As a result, there is a unique opportunity to thoughtfully and methodically plan to treat symptoms based on the anticipated needs unique to the pathophysiology effecting each neonate (8, 17–20).

Likely in part due to the paucity of data, there is significant variability in neonatal EOL comfort practices. A recent survey of members of the American Academy of Pediatrics Section on Neonatal-Perinatal Medicine inquired about neonatal end-of-life practices across America (21). Of the respondents, nearly half did not have institutional guidelines for comfort care. Of those that did, 80.9% addressed pain management and over 75% discussed non-pharmacological management. Other symptoms, such as secretions and anxiety, were addressed less than half the time.

END-OF LIFE SYMPTOMS

Symptoms experienced during EOL care that can be applicable to the neonatal population include agitation, dyspnea, neuroirritability, pain, and increased secretions (20, 22). Agitation and neuroirritability, generally speaking, are unpleasant states of arousal. They can be the result of the underlying disease process or from interventions and medications. Common manifestations include autonomic signs, increased motor activity, restlessness, and disturbed or disrupted sleep. Dyspnea is discomfort with breathing and is largely a subjective experience or sensation. Though subjective, a majority of verbal patients report dyspnea at the end-of-life and family members frequently perceive the patient is having dyspnea (23–26). As a result, it is reasonable to associate physical signs of increased work of breathing and tachypnea with the subjective experience of dyspnea at EOL. Pain, defined as an unpleasant sensation that results in discomfort and distress, is commonly experienced by pediatric patients in the last days of life (19, 22, 23, 26). The etiology and degree of pain experienced can vary greatly. It is important to know that there are different types of pain. Nociceptive pain is the result of tissue damage or inflammation and can be somatic, localized to a specific region, or visceral, affecting the internal organs. Neuropathic pain is the result of damage or irritation to the nerves. Identifying the type of pain that is occurring and understanding the etiology and underlying mechanism can help direct more effective approaches to therapy. Much of the early work of Anand was focused on understanding the neuroanatomy, neurophysiology, and neurochemistry of pain in fetuses and neonates (27). At 20–22 weeks gestation fetuses have developed their peripheral pain sensors and the neuronal migration of the ascending pathway to connect with the thalamus and sensory cortex has occurred. The peripheral nervous system and spinal cord are well-developed by 30 weeks gestation. The descending pathways develops later. This would indicate that neonates as young as 22 weeks gestation have the same number of pain receptors as an adult on a much smaller surface area and without the complete development of the inhibitory pathways. In addition, substance

---

Abbreviations: NICU, Neonatal Intensive Care Unit; EOL, end-of-life; PPS, Proportionate Palliative Sedation; PST, Sedation Therapy; PSU, Palliative Sedation to Unconsciousness.

P and other neurotransmitters can also cause excitation of uninvolved neurons leading to lower pain thresholds and more robust, increased and longer pain responses in even the youngest neonates. These findings were accompanied by recognition in the clinical setting of pain responses and led to the acceptance the neonates are capable of experiencing pain and a change in practice around assessing and treating pain in neonates. With the understanding and acceptance that neonates experience pain, it is appropriate to assume that neonates should be properly monitored for signs of pain and treated accordingly (27–30). Excessive secretions are not as commonly seen but can be experienced if the neonate is unable to effectively swallow. This can be the result of the underlying disease process or from overall decreased tone, alertness, and activity during the dying process.

ASSESSMENT OF SYMPTOMS

While there are approved and validated methods to evaluate EOL symptoms for adults and older children, there are limited data and methods for neonates (20, 22, 31). Considering the clinical circumstances surrounding death, neonates may not be able to mount the normal physiologic response to pain that is seen in older populations. Similarly, neonates may not display other symptoms in the same manner other individuals do, making it difficult for providers to assess and effectively manage them. As a result, the methods and tools utilized in adolescents and adults cannot be translated to this population. The evaluation is largely reliant on clinician and family perception of symptoms. A recent qualitative exploratory study interviewed NICU nurses about the EOL care their patients received (32). While small, this study displayed themes of uncertainty, discomfort, and chaos. Nurses were not always certain, based on the physical signs they were seeing and on the clinical situation, if their patient was experiencing pain or any other symptoms. Lack of education, resources, and consistency in the approach to EOL care contributed to overall provider discomfort. In addition, providers may be focused on other tasks such as supporting the family which lend to subtle physical signs going unnoticed (8).

These challenges, along with historically limited documentation, makes it difficult to draw conclusions or to come to a consensus about standardized approaches to symptom assessment in neonates. One study of 20 neonates with planned redirections of care described the documentation of symptoms exhibited and the treatment of those symptoms during the dying process (8). The authors noted that all patient documentation had missing data related to EOL care and that there was a varying amount of detail with regard to the infant's symptoms and use of medications. Specifically, no pain scores were documented after invasive medical interventions were withdrawn or care was redirected. With gaps in documentation, providers may not be able to accurately assess the baby. Furthermore, this leads to significant limitations in research. Without detailed documentation regarding symptoms and interventions, there are challenges in drawing conclusions about current assessment and management of neonatal EOL care, as well as challenges in developing innovative or consistent guidelines and approaches to that care.

Pain, one of the most common symptoms discussed at EOL in older populations, has been historically challenging to assess in neonates. Additionally, there is concern that pain has been underappreciated and undertreated at baseline in this population. Research shows that fetuses and neonates have well-developed peripheral nervous systems and pain-related neurotransmitters are present as early as 22 weeks gestation; it has been accepted that neonates, even when born premature, can experience pain (27, 33, 34). In recent years, there have been improvements in assessment and management of neonatal pain, especially post-operatively (28, 29, 34–37). While not specific to EOL care, it is pertinent that providers utilize a neonatal specific pain assessment tool (9, 20). Carter describes at length the various pain assessment tools available for neonates and concludes that the evidence does not allow for recommendation of one specific tool but that using a validated tool is pertinent (20). It is pertinent that providers have been trained to use the tool and are experienced with it to increase the reliability of the reported results. An ideal tool is one that is validated in both premature and term neonates for subacute and chronic pain. Given the challenges of assessing pain in neonates, strong tools combine both behavioral and physiological data in the assessment. Common pain assessment tools suitable for this population are COMFORTneo, CRIES (Cry, Requirement for more oxygen, Increased vital signs, Expressions, Sleeplessness), N-PASS (Neonatal Pain, Agitation, and Sedation Scale), NIPS (Neonatal Infant Pain Scale), and PIPP (Premature Infant Pain Profile) (20, 38). While there is a paucity of data regarding pain and comfort in neonates at the end-of-life, one study showed that significantly fewer neonates had their pain evaluated with a pain assessment scale routinely used in other pediatrics patients receiving end-of-life care (20, 39, 40).

Other symptoms, such as agitation, dyspnea, and secretions are evaluated based on the clinical circumstance and physical assessment. Agitation or neuroirritability are suspected when there is self-reported or perceived increased motor activity, restlessness, and disturbed sleep. Similarly, assessment of dyspnea is reliant on a subjective report either by the patient or a visual assessment by another individual based on markers such as respiratory rate, the presence of hypoxia, and work of breathing.

To date, there remains little research on symptom assessment, symptom management, and the evaluation of interventions used in EOL care of neonates (41). Although there is a lack of standardized assessment tools or standards for interventions for neonatal EOL care, some providers advocate for treating common distressing conditions at the EOL in neonates whether or not they appear to be in distress. In these conditions, older, verbal populations commonly experience a high symptom burden from the same sources of suffering and their self-report and observations scores correspond to the severity of their burden. Providers suggest that neonates experience the same symptom burden and ought to be treat similarly (17, 42). For example, in verbal pediatric patients there is a high likelihood of dyspnea occurring after ventilator withdrawal, and there is also a high likelihood of dyspnea causing additional secondary symptoms that can be alleviated with pain medications (43). The same can be assumed with neonatal populations experiencing similar distressing symptoms after going through similar clinical experiences.

Parent Perception

Parental perception of suffering is extremely important as parents know their baby better than anyone and are sensitive to signs of pain or distress others may not be aware of. Parents may perceive their baby is distressed by physical changes they observe during the dying process. They often equate these changes with pain or discomfort (32, 44, 45). As symptom assessment has a component of subjectivity, there can be differing opinions from those interacting with the baby. In fact, one small study of EOL experiences for neonates revealed that 85% of providers felt symptoms were well-managed while only 57% of parents felt their baby was comfortable (44). Another study asked the bereaved parents of 40 neonates about their observations of symptoms during the last week of life (46). Mothers and fathers were given a list of 22 symptoms and on average the mothers reported 6.63 symptoms in their baby's last week of life while the fathers reported and average of 5.67 symptoms. Mothers most often noted respiratory distress, agitation, and pain while fathers most often noted respiratory distress, agitation, and lethargy. Both reported respiratory distress as the worst symptom in severity and the most difficult symptom to watch as they perceived it as the most uncomfortable symptom. On average parents reported their baby experienced a moderate amount of suffering. Only 6 of the symptoms inquired about where routinely documented in the medical record and of those there was no significant difference between parenteral or provider report. While parents and providers may not agree on the extent of suffering, provider initiated discussion around EOL care with parents allows for improved care of the neonate and reduction in anxiety of parents and possible tension between parents and the care team.

MANAGEMENT OF END-OF-LIFE SYMPTOMS

While there is a body of evidence and guidance for the treatment of EOL symptoms in adults and adolescents, there is limited data for neonates (20). As a result, there is a great deal of variability in pharmacological and non-pharmacological end-of-life symptom management for neonates (32, 47, 48). While there is variability, it is important that symptoms including pain are addressed by both pharmacological and non-pharmacological means (49). Other symptoms seen that may need to be addressed include dyspnea, agitation, neuroirritability, and secretions (20, 22).

Non-pharmacological Management

Preparing the family for what to expect during the dying process helps to alleviate parental anxiety. As a result, effective communication with families that supports the parental role and conveys empathy is required. Providers must prepare families for the dying process with clear and honest conversations, realizing that families will want varying degrees of information about the physiologic changes (9, 49). By understanding the changes that may occur, some families are less distressed by symptoms such as gasping and color changes (50, 51). They are able to appreciate that the physical changes occurring do not necessarily mean their child is experiencing dyspnea. They feel more prepared for the death, have less grief, and are more satisfied with the care their child received (2, 52–54). One study of 131 bereaved caregivers of children who died of cancer revealed that they did not feel prepared for the medical needs of their child as they approached death (55). Parent who felt unprepared for the changes at the time of death perceived their child suffered more. They expressed that they desire clear, honest communication about the medical issues around the time of death. Without an understanding of these changes, they may feel powerless or unsure of what their child is experiencing. By fostering open communication, providers can set expectations, address misconceptions, and encourage the family to convey when they are concerned that their baby is having symptoms so that they are addressed in a timely fashion. This is important not only for the comfort of the baby and the parent's experience with their child, but also for how the parents process the death of their baby. Parent perception of suffering has a lasting impact that can prolong and complicate their grief. Parents who are uncertain about what to expect at the EOL have more severe grief afterwards (56, 57).

Care should be taken to reduce uncomfortable procedures or invasive touching/stimulation (58). When symptoms occur, interventions such as decreasing stimulation, massage, skin care, mouth care, elevating the head or repositioning for dyspnea, fluid restriction, and gentle suctioning may be beneficial (9, 42, 49). Gentle suction and repositioning, for example, are more effective than pharmacological therapy the majority of the time for secretion management and noisy breathing. Swaddling, skin-to-skin contact, and non-nutritive sucking can be beneficial for agitation and pain. These measures help to meet the basic needs of neonates and promote positive bonding experiences (59). Families appreciate the opportunity to bond with and parent their baby (60). Eighteen nurses in Scandinavia were interviewed about their practices around skin-to-skin contact for parents and neonates during EOL care (61). Skin-to-skin interaction is known to decrease pain, improve labored breathing, and have positive psychosocial effects. Providers believe facilitating this care promotes comfort and bonding for both the mother and baby. This, in conjunction with promoting emotional and physical intimacy for families, can be very effective in alleviating dyspnea and agitation as hypoxia and hypercapnia that can occur during this time also have natural sedative effects (39). While there is expressed knowledge of the benefit of non-pharmacological interventions, documentation of their use in the medical chart remains limited (8). This makes it difficult to know the true extent to which these techniques are utilized and are effective.

Pharmacological Management

Non-pharmacological interventions will often alleviate some but not all symptoms neonates experience at the EOL. If anticipated and discussed ahead of time, parental apprehension and resistance to using medications to treat symptoms can be alleviated. Historically, providers have been hesitant to administer medications, specifically opioids and benzodiazepines, out of concern that they will hasten death. This concern of providing medications that have respiratory depression as a side effect in a medically fragile neonate has led to inadequate treatment of symptoms (39). However, there is a commonly accepted ethical notion known as the principle of double-effect which states that an action is justifiable if the nature of the act is good, the good effects are the intended effects as opposed to the bad effects, and that the good effects outweigh the bad given the circumstances (20, 47). Along these lines, it is considered good medical practice and standard of care to alleviate symptoms and pain during the dying process. In addition, multiple studies have shown that administering opioids and sedatives in appropriate doses to treat EOL symptoms does not hasten death, carries little risk of respiratory depression, and increases perceived comfort during the dying process (20, 62, 63).

While there remains variability in practice around administering medications for EOL symptoms in neonates, many providers give some type of medication. Typical classes of medications utilized are opioids, benzodiazepines, antipyretics, anticholinergics, diuretics, hypnotics, and anticonvulsants (9, 42, 64). The majority of studies in neonates are limited to intravenous administration in a hospital setting. A study of 20 neonates with planned redirections of care noted that most babies received pharmacological therapy. Eighty-five percent received opioids or benzodiazepines prior to withdrawal of invasive medical interventions and 60% received them afterwards. The majority received intravenous medications with one receiving oral medications, and five receiving aerosolized forms (8). One of the earliest studies looking at practices around neonatal EOL care reviewed deaths over a 3 year period in the NICU secondary to withdrawal of or withholding invasive medical interventions (18). Eight-four percent of neonates were given opioid analgesia. When care was redirected in the setting of perceived suffering or with major surgical or congenital anomalies, infants were more likely to receive opioids, most commonly morphine or fentanyl. If deaths outside of the delivery room were excluded, birth weight had no impact on the likelihood of receiving analgesia. Doses of opioids given were consistent with typical the pharmacological range when taking in to account previous opioid exposure. There was no significant difference in the time from withdrawal of invasive medical interventions to death for those who received no opioids or <0.2 mg/kg of morphine compared to those who received >0.2 mg/kg of morphine. In the institution at that time, the nurses would routinely ask physicians for opioid analgesia if they felt the neonate was in pain based on their assessment. The use of benzodiazepines was not typical and as a result there was no use of them documented in the study.

Other studies similarly found that there was no difference in birth weight or gestational age in whether or not infants received medications for symptoms as part of EOL care and that the vast majority of patients who died in the delivery room did not receive opioids (39). A study of 171 neonates at a level III NICU showed that 27.5% did not receive opioids or benzodiazepines for EOL care (17). Those in the group weighing <800 g were less likely to receive these medications. However, those weighing >1,500 g did not receive pain medications as often as those weighing 800–1,500 g. It was thought that potentially those in the 800–1,500 g group more often had diagnoses associated with pain. The fact that any died without comfort medications, though, was concerning to the authors.

One study retrospectively reviewed practices around medication administration for neonates at four NICUs in the United States, Canada, and the Netherlands (47). Of note, similar to previous studies, none of the babies who died in the delivery room received medications. Outside of the delivery room setting, most neonates received some type of medication for comfort, an opioid and/or benzodiazepine, in the 48 hours prior to redirection of care and after the redirection of care. Benzodiazepines were utilized more frequently in the NICUs in the United States than in the other countries. However, only the NICUs outside of the United States increased the dose of comfort medications prior to redirection of care. If a neuromuscular blockade was already being used, it was discontinued at two of the centers but continued at the other two. Only the NICU in the Netherlands administered a neuromuscular blockade after redirection of care and that was only to relieve suffering at the request of family.

While it is well-known that there is significant variability in the assessment and approach to treatment of pain in neonates in other countries, there is little evidence with regards to variations in practices around EOL care for neonates. The largest difference in the literature around EOL practices in other countries is related to euthanasia. While a rare occurrence, there are instances where the Dutch and Belgium consider euthanasia of neonates to be acceptable. The prognosis must be certain, there must be evidence of undue suffering, and parents must give consent. While this topic is sensitive, complex, and wrought with ethical debate, it is an acceptable practice for the Dutch and Belgium under rare circumstances that are tightly regulated (65–67).

Classes of Commonly Used Medications

Alpha 2 adrenergic agonists, clonidine, and dexmedetomidine, have analgesic and sedative properties. They been used in the neonatal population, particular after cardiac surgery, for some time (36). These options are appealing as they are usually well-tolerated and have minimal effect on respiratory drive.

Anticholinergics block acetylcholine either centrally or peripherally. As a result, they can cause fever, tachycardia, and other physiologic symptoms. In proper doses these side effects can be minimized and the effect of anhidrosis can be beneficial. Specific to EOL care this can reduce the amount of secretions. It is important to note, though, that there is little evidence that pharmacological therapy is effective for secretion management or the death rattle during the dying process (20).

Anticonvulsants have properties that lend themselves to EOL care in certain circumstances. Seizures themselves are unlikely during the dying process unless there is a preexisting condition. However, some of these medications can be effective at treating agitation or neuroirritability. Gabapentin, which works on the voltage dependent calcium channel, can be beneficial for neonates with difficult to control agitation or neuroirritability (68–71).

Benzodiazepines work by activating the gamma aminobutyric acid A receptors. They are commonly used in neonates for sedative purposes and have no analgesic properties. Side effects can be myoclonic jerks, hypotension, and, at higher doses, respiratory depression, or excessive sedation. In end-of-life care, they can be used to treat agitation and dyspnea.

Cyclooxygenase-2 enzyme inhibitors, acetaminophen and non-steroidal anti-inflammatory drugs, have been well-studied in the neonatal population and as a result have been used to treat fevers and mild pain, or as an adjuvant for pain treatment plans. They could have similar roles in end-of-life symptom management. Non-steroidal anti-inflammatory medications convert arachidonic acid to prostaglandin and are known to have anti-inflammatory, analgesic, and antipyretic properties. They can inhibit platelet function and lead to renal impairment. If already part of an analgesic treatment plan, they would likely be beneficial to continue for EOL care.

Dissociative anesthetics such as ketamine, have amnetic, analgesic, and sedative properties. Ketamineis is not known to cause hypotension or respiratory depression in neonates. However, there have been concerns at higher doses in animal models of apoptosis which has led to limited use until recently in the neonatal population (72, 73). In human models and in the presence of painful stimuli, it has been shown to have a possible protective effect (74). Given the limited data, its use had been limited to invasive procedures. In opioid exposed patients, it could be beneficial to treat pain, dyspnea, and agitation at the EOL.

Opioids are a class of medications that act on the opioid receptors in the body. Depending on the specific medication, they work on the mu, kappa, and delta portion of the receptors with varying degrees of affinity. They have effective analgesic and sedative properties and are readily used in neonates (29, 36). They are most commonly used for and most effective in treating pain, dyspnea, and agitation during the dying process.

Routes of Administration

Historically, in the hospital setting, IV access has been maintained though EOL care as a stable way to provide comfort medications either as continuous or intermittent infusions (64). Both methods can lead to adequate symptom control but some providers feel intermittent infusions, if possible, may make it easier for families to hold their babies and may be more conducive to memory-making. As for subcutaneous drug administration in neonates, there is very little data (75). Recently, there has been a focus on alternative and less invasive routes to provide medications for EOL care. The reasoning is largely to remove invasive equipment such an intravenous needles, aid in memory-making, allow EOL care to occur outside to the NICU, and to allow the option for EOL care in the home setting while still effectively managing symptoms. The route of administration with the most data and experience in these circumstance is oral administration. There are well-established dosage guidelines of oral medications in neonates. Alternately, while oral transmucosal (buccal or sublingual) administration provides several benefits, there are very few medications concentrated or designed for this route of administration making its utility limited (76). One center utilized the limited data available to develop a protocol for neonates receiving EOL care (76). Medications used included morphine, midazolam, lorazepam, scopolamine, and glycopyrrolate with doses equivalent to intravenous dosing. There were clear criteria on when to administer the medications and which dosages to use. While compliance with utilizing the pain assessment tool was low, by report, all survey respondents felt symptoms were controlled with oral transmucosal administration and no adverse side effects were noted. The vast majority said they would recommend this protocol. Similarly, a small retrospective study looking for non-invasive methods of controlling symptoms examined intranasal fentanyl in neonates (77). This medication and mode was evaluated because of the rapid onset of action, ease of administration, and because opioids are utilized to treat two of the most common symptoms-pain and dyspnea. There is more data available on the intranasal route of administration in children as opposed to the sublingual or buccal route. Doses were similar to intravenous doses while accounting for incomplete bioavailability. In the 11 neonates who received intranasal fentanyl for treatment of EOL pain or dyspnea, they received an average of 4.5 doses and had symptom control without the need for intravenous medications. There were no noted side effects and some were able to be cared for in settings outside of the NICU. Another route that is at times utilized in the neonatal population is transdermal. While there are transdermal forms of opioids and alpha 2 agonists available, there are is limited data of their use in neonates to make clear recommendations. The dosages in which these medications are available may be one limitation to the use in the neonatal population.

PALLIATIVE SEDATION

While it is accepted and expected that symptoms should be appropriately managed during EOL care, there is a clear distinction between appropriately managing symptoms and providing the medication with the intent of ending life or hastening death (78–80). This is particularly true when there is a high symptom burden refractory to typical medications and doses. One article looking at Dutch practices found that the intent is not always obvious by reviewing the type and dose of medications used (78). In this nationwide study, the authors utilized retrospective chart review and physician interviews to describe the type, dose, and reason for medication administration surrounding EOL care in the Dutch NICUs. Comparable to other studies, roughly 14% did not receive medications. They found that doses of opioids and sedatives were generally increased following EOL discussions and that documentation of the reasons for this were present <50% of the time despite the physicians explaining the reasoning in interviews. Per interviews, medications were usually titrated to mitigate or prevent symptoms such as pain, agitation, and gasping. In 10% of cases the intent was to hasten the dying process. Opioids were administered above what they considered normal dosages in 5% of patients before EOL decisions were made and in 17% afterwards. Benzodiazepines dosages were above the considered normal dosage in 12% of patients after EOL decisions were made. Roughly 16% of neonates received neuromuscular blockades as part of the EOL care. In interviews reasons included to prevent gasping, per parental request, and to limit suffering. While there has been debate over the years around the use of neuromuscular blockade at the EOL, it is generally accepted that they should not be utilized after redirection of care as the principle of double effect typically cannot be justified and it would bring the patient to his death (9, 81). In cases where a paralytic has recently been given, if time is not allowed for the paralytic to wear off, there should be discussions with the family, the intent should be to relieve suffering, and it should be clear that the burden of waiting an extended period of time for the effects of the paralytic to completely wear off would significantly outweigh the benefits (9, 20, 47). Another study from Europe examining the use of medications with the intent of hastening death in neonates concluded that the medications used are highly effective, the infants were moribund at the time they received the medications, and there was a discrepancy in documentation of the reported intent and effect (79). Furthermore, they felt that it is not easy to distinguish between intent to end life and provide adequate symptom control during the dying process.

When sedation is utilized at the EOL as a means to decrease and control symptom burden, it has been referred to as terminal sedation, palliative sedation therapy, controlled sedation for intractable patients, EOL sedation, and continuous sedation for the dying (82, 83). Palliative sedation can occur across a continuum from anxiolysis to deep sedation with loss of consciousness. As pediatric palliative care has evolved, the field is able to articulate the terminology, objectives and methods to provide effective and ethical management of severe symptoms at the EOL. Providing an effective level of symptom control to match the symptom burden without hastening death through respiratory depression is the objective. The provision of palliative sedation has been supported by numerous professional organizations including the American Medical Association, National Hospice and Palliative Care Organization, American Academy of Hospice and Palliative Medicine, and American Academy of Pediatrics.

Many pediatric palliative care providers apply criteria for patients under consideration for palliative sedation prior to initiation of sedation including limited prognosis of hours to weeks, confirmation that the target symptom is refractory, parental consent, and a goal of comfort care and foregoing resuscitative efforts. Accurately determining prognosis can be challenging for providers and discussion with specialists and colleagues can produce an accurate perspective. While not often utilized in the NICU, palliative sedation may have a role for patients who have refractory symptoms and/or a lengthy history of exposure to pharmacological therapies typically used

TABLE 1 | Neonatal end-of-life symptom management: suggested pharmacologic medications.

Medication	Class	Symptom	Starting dose (per kg) with route and frequency	Comments
Acetaminophen	COX2 inhibitor	Fever Mild pain	15 mg PO/PR q6 6–8 mg IV q8	As an adjuvant for pain
Atropine	Anticholinergic	Secretions	0.01–0.02 mg PO q2	No strong evidence
Dexmedetomidine	Selective alpha 2 agonist	Agitation Pain	0.5–1 mcg IV/IN q2 0.5–1 mcg/kg/hr IV continuous	
Fentanyl	Opioid	Pain Dyspnea	0.5–2 mcg IN/IV q2 1–4 mcg/kg/hr IV continuous	Quicker onset of action
Gabapentin	anticonvulsant	Agitation Neuroirritability	5–15 mg PO q8	
Glycopyrrolate	Anticholinergic	Secretions	0.01–0.02 mg IV q4 0.04–0.1 mg PO q4	No strong evidence
Ketamine	Dissociative anesthetic	Agitation Pain	0.5–1 mg PO/IV q2-4	
Lorazepam	Benzodiazepine	Agitation Dyspnea	0.05–0.1 mg PO/IV q4-6	
Methadone	Opioid	Pain	0.05–0.2 mg IV/PO q12-24 (initially q4 for 3 doses)	
Midazolam	Benzodiazepine	Agitation Dyspnea	0.05–0.1 mg IV q2-4 0.2–0.3 mg Sublingual q2-4 0.25 mg IN q2-3 0.05 mg/kg/hr IV continuous	Short acting
Morphine	Opioid	Pain Dyspnea Agitation	0.05–0.2 mg IV/IM q2-4 0.15–0.5 mg PO/Sublingual q2-4 0.01–0.05 mg/kg/hr IV continuous	

COX-2 inhibitor, Cyclooxygenase-2 enzyme inhibitor; IN, intranasal; IM, intramuscular; IV, intravenous; PO, per oral; PR, per rectum; q2, every 2 h; q2-4, every 2–4 h; q4-6, every 4–6 h; q6, every 6 h; q8, every q hours; q12-24, every 12–24 h.

It may not be appropriate to continue feedings. They can be difficult to digest and cause fluid overload.

to treat EOL symptoms. The latter often results in tolerance and resistance to conventional symptom management. Beyond light sedation, palliative sedation can be classified as proportionate palliative sedation and palliative sedation to unconsciousness.

Proportionate Palliative Sedation

Proportionate Palliative Sedation (PPS) is symptom management that directly targets a specific symptom with a medication's identified mechanism of action while accepting that the side effects of the medication will cause sedation. Pain treated with analgesia is a common scenario in which the symptom is managed with a class of medications that directly targets the symptom. Opioids, for example, provide analgesia and can induce sedation at higher doses. Opioid analgesics directly reduce the suffering caused by pain while the use of hypnotics, such as midazolam, would mask the manifestations of the pain. Alternatively, seizure management, a less common threat to comfort at the EOL, can be complicated by antiepileptic therapy that can induce sedation at levels needed to optimally treat refractory seizures. In PPS the antiepileptic therapy that targets the source of suffering is appropriate and the end-point is relief of suffering while causing the minimum amount of sedation necessary.

The Level of Sedation and Titration

Sedation may vary from intermittent to continuous as the patient may waken spontaneously or may not waken once sedation is initiated. The depth of sedation can vary from light in which the patient readily wakens to voice and light touch to deep. In the latter, the patient is unable to be awake at all. In deep sedation, respiratory depression may be marked by decreased respiratory rate, tidal volumes, and obstructive breathing. In all scenarios, the objective is to provide relief of symptoms. The process for achieving adequate dosing is based upon medication titration proportional to the severity of the symptoms. When a symptom breaks through a previously achieved level of control, dosing increases can be based on the severity. Many providers use the following guide to make medication increases that are proportional to the severity: mild breakthrough −10 to 20% increase, moderate breakthrough −20 to 30% increase, and severe −30 to 50% increase. Any increase in dosing, whether intermittent dosing or continuous infusion, is followed by a period of reassessment to ensure the symptom has been addressed. The term Palliative Sedation Therapy (PST) has been advocated for to describe the active management that is required to adequately treat evolving symptoms in that frequent assessment of symptoms coupled with titration of medications to achieve the balance is needed. This active management process involves parents and family by including them in the symptom assessment.

Palliative Sedation to Unconsciousness (PSU)

There are clinical circumstances in which proportional palliative sedation is inadequate and suffering persists despite adequate titration and dosing. If the symptom is refractory, obtaining comfort can be achieved by using agents that alter the level

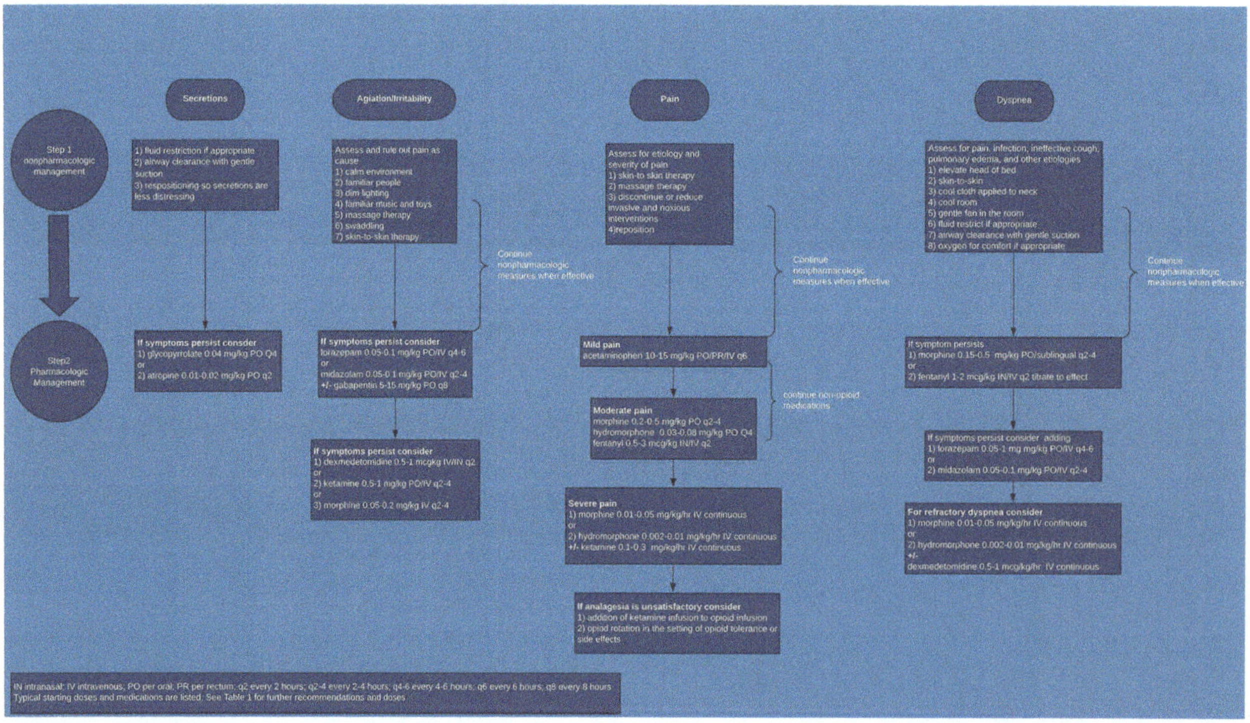

FIGURE 1 | Neonatal end-of-life symptom management.

of consciousness but do not directly reduce the symptom itself. PSU is provided using classes of sedative and hypnotic medications in conjunction with the medication targeted to treat the specific symptom. Distinct from PPS, the intent is to induce loss of consciousness to eliminate suffering. Agents commonly used included propofol, phenobarbital, ketamine, and dexmedetomidine. The addition of a hypnotic is often done only after all measures to treat symptoms have been exhausted and is administered in an addition to the current regimen.

DISCUSSION

Appropriate EOL symptom management, while challenging at times, is important for neonates. Every individual deserves to have their symptoms addressed so they can have as peaceful of a dying process as possible. Not only does it improve comfort for the neonate, it also improves the EOL experience for the family. This allows them to focus on spending time with their baby and make meaningful memories which can help lead to less complicated grief and a positive experience for the limited time they have with their baby. While there are challenges associated with identifying and quantifying some of the symptoms that neonates experience during the dying process, many providers and families report common symptoms including respiratory distress, pain, and agitation. These are the same EOL symptoms that are often experienced in adolescents and adults.

It is important, especially when there is time such as with a planned redirection of care, that the healthcare team clearly communicates with the family about the dying process. Clear communication can lead to an open dialogue to address some of the concerns and fears of the family. By understanding the changes they will see in their baby, they can better prepare themselves and begin to understand the difference between physiologic changes and signs of distress or discomfort. When they perceive less suffering surrounding the death of their child, they have less guilt and less complicated grief.

It is pertinent that symptoms be regularly assessed during the dying process. If EOL care takes place in the NICU, routine assessment by staff should occur. If EOL care occurs outside of the NICU, family and staff should be educated as to the common signs of agitation, dyspnea, neuroirritability, pain, and increased secretions. For agitation and neuroirritability, signs of restlessness, abnormal movements, and disturbed sleep should be monitored closely. With dyspnea, common associations in a non-verbal patient are tachypnea and increased work of breathing. For secretions, increased saliva coming out of the mouth, gagging, and the "death-rattle" are common signs. Pain is the symptom that has the most validated assessment tools in the neonatal population. While not specific to EOL, institutions should have an agreed upon tool routinely used for preterm and term neonates that evaluates chronic and subacute pain. If EOL care is occurring outside of the hospital, family should be educated about ways in which their baby manifests signs of pain or discomfort. Despite the challenges associated with adequately assessing symptoms in neonates, when symptoms appear they should be adequately treated in a multidisciplinary approach. Many of the therapies that are beneficial for treating these symptoms in adults have been utilized in neonates with perceived benefit. Environmental and non-pharmacological factors are incredibly important. Promoting bonding, holding, and skin-to-skin contact is therapeutic for both the neonate and family. Implementing interventions such as decreasing painful procedures, decreasing stimulation, ensuring normothermia, and repositioning can be quite effective. Often times, though, non-pharmacological interventions are not adequate. This is particularly true outside of the delivery room or in situations where a neonate is being compassionately extubated. Identifying if there is a treatable cause of the symptom is important in developing an effective treatment plan. For example, dyspnea that is secondary to a pneumonia may be treated differently than dyspnea secondary to congestive heart failure. Based on current literature, institutional expertise, and clinical experience of the authors, suggestions for common medications are included (see **Table 1**). **Figure 1** is an algorithm for a practical application of and approach to EOL symptom management in the NICU population. Medication choices and doses used may need to be adjusted based on prior exposures. For example, if the neonate is already on an opioid drip the dose may need to be increased. At times, higher doses are needed to achieve adequate symptom management or alternative medications need to be utilized. In rare circumstances, where there is a high symptom burden and traditional treatment options have not achieved appropriate symptom control, palliative sedation may be appropriate. In either of these situations, if the provider is not comfortable or familiar with alternatives such as ketamine, dexmedetomidine, or gabapentin, or if the provider is not experienced with providing palliative sedation, expert input should be sought ahead of time.

Despite the recent focus on neonatal palliative care, there remains a scarcity of data in the literature about EOL symptom assessment and management in neonates. Some providers are still concerned about the possibility of medications causing respiratory depression and hastening the dying process. Studies have not shown this to be the case and it is accepted that it is ethically appropriate and medically necessary to treat EOL symptoms. While this is true, there are disagreements about the classes of or doses of medications to use and providers are left with little guidance on pharmacological management. This contributes largely to the wide variations in practices. Future research is needed to develop standardized tools to assess EOL symptoms in neonates. This would help providers and families have an objective way to evaluate symptoms. Beyond that, further research on the pharmacokinetics and pharmacodynamics and efficacy of the medications used is needed to better guide dosing recommendations and treatment options for these patients. A better understanding could lead to better symptom control and alternative medications, as well as alternative routes for administration. This could potentially lead to more choices for the location of EOL care for certain neonates.

With further research, institutions could develop more comprehensive guidelines for the assessment and management of EOL symptoms in neonates. In order to accomplish this, clinicians must take care in documenting their assessment of symptoms surrounding EOL as well as the interventions used. This includes noting the indication for the intervention and how effective it was at alleviating the symptom. This will lead to overall better control of symptoms, more consistency in the care provided, and less discomfort among staff and parents. One approach would be to develop an EOL symptom flowsheet in the electronic medical record where the various symptoms are listed along with the established mode of assessment. In this flowsheet, staff can easily document if symptoms are present, their severity, interventions used and a reassessment of the symptoms after interventions. This will provide valuable insight for patient care and for research. Even now in the absence of clear data for assessment and management of EOL symptoms in neonates, institutions should have guidelines in place. As part of that process, there should be education for staff around the dying process, EOL symptoms, and symptom management. With a better understanding, provider distress can be decreased. It also serves as an avenue to increase comfort and empower providers to have discussions with families around EOL care. While these discussions can be difficult, they promote a unified understanding of what to expect as well as shared decision-making that can ultimately translate to a better EOL experience for the neonate and the family.

AUTHOR CONTRIBUTIONS

DC conceptualized and designed the report, drafted the initial manuscript, and approved the final manuscript as submitted. MM aided in designing the manuscript, contributed to the content, and approved the final manuscript as submitted. All authors contributed to the article and approved the submitted version.

REFERENCES

1. Cortezzo DE, Bowers K, Cameron Meyer M. Birth planning in uncertain or life-limiting fetal diagnoses: perspectives of physicians and parents. *J Palliat Med.* (2019) 22:1337–45. doi: 10.1089/jpm.2018.0596
2. Midson R, Carter B. Addressing end of life care issues in a tertiary treatment centre: lessons learned from surveying parents' experiences. *J Child Health Care.* (2010) 14:52–66. doi: 10.1177/1367493509347060
3. Meyer EC, Ritholz MD, Burns JP, Truog RD. Improving the quality of end-of-life care in the pediatric intensive care unit: parents' priorities and recommendations. *Pediatrics.* (2006) 117:649–57. doi: 10.1542/peds.2005-0144
4. Brosig CL, Pierucci RL, Kupst MJ, Leuthner SR. Infant end-of-life care: the parents' perspective. *J Perinatol.* (2007) 27:510–6. doi: 10.1038/sj.jp.7211755
5. Seecharan GA, Andresen EM, Norris K, Toce SS. Parents' assessment of quality of care and grief following a child's death. *Arch Pediatr Adolesc Med.* (2004) 158:515–20. doi: 10.1001/archpedi.158.6.515
6. Widger K, Picot C. Parents' perceptions of the quality of pediatric and perinatal end-of-life care. *Pediatr Nurs.* (2008) 34:53–8.
7. Davies B, Connaughty S. Pediatric end-of-life care: lessons learned from parents. *J Nurs Adm.* (2002) 32:5–6. doi: 10.1097/00005110-200201000-00001
8. Fortney CA, Steward DK. Medical record documentation and symptom management at the end of life in the NICU. *Adv Neonatal Care.* (2015) 15:48–55. doi: 10.1097/ANC.0000000000000132
9. Catlin A, Carter B. Creation of a neonatal end-of-life palliative care protocol. *J Perinatol.* (2002) 22:184–95. doi: 10.1038/sj.jp.7210687
10. Davis MP, Gutgsell T, Gamier P. What is the difference between palliative care and hospice care? *Cleve Clin J Med.* (2015) 82:569–71. doi: 10.3949/ccjm.82a.14145
11. WHO. *WHO Definition of Palliative Care.* (2015). Available online at: http://www.who.int/cancer/palliative/definition/en/ (accessed August 3, 2020).
12. MacDorman MF, Gregory EC. Fetal and perinatal mortality: United States, 2013. *Natl Vital Stat Rep.* (2015) 64:1–24.
13. Osterman MJ, Martin JA, Curtin SC, Matthews TJ, Wilson EC, Kirmeyer S. Newly released data from the revised U.S. birth certificate 2011. *Natl Vital Stat Rep.* (2013) 62:1–22.
14. Lorenz JM, Ananth CV, Polin RA, D'Alton ME. Infant mortality in the United States. *J Perinatol.* (2016) 36:797–801. doi: 10.1038/jp.2016.63
15. Heron M. Deaths: leading causes for 2016. *Natl Vital Stat Rep.* (2018) 67:1–77.
16. Cook LA, Watchko JF. Decision making for the critically ill neonate near the end of life. *J Perinatol.* (1996) 16:133–6.
17. Matthews AL, O'Conner-Von S. Administration of comfort medication at end of life in neonates: effects of weight. *Neonatal Netw.* (2008) 27:223–7. doi: 10.1891/0730-0832.27.4.223
18. Partridge JC, Wall SN. Analgesia for dying infants whose life support is withdrawn or withheld. *Pediatrics.* (1997) 99:76–9. doi: 10.1542/peds.99.1.76
19. Carter BS, Howenstein M, Gilmer MJ, Throop P, France D, Whitlock JA. Circumstances surrounding the deaths of hospitalized children: opportunities for pediatric palliative care. *Pediatrics.* (2004) 114:e361–6. doi: 10.1542/peds.2003-0654-F
20. Carter BS, Jones PM. Evidence-based comfort care for neonates towards the end of life. *Semin Fetal Neonatal Med.* (2013) 18:88–92. doi: 10.1016/j.siny.2012.10.012
21. Haug S, Farooqi S, Wilson CG, Hopper A, Oei G, Carter B. Survey on neonatal end-of-life comfort care guidelines across America. *J Pain Symptom Manage.* (2018) 55:979–84.e2. doi: 10.1016/j.jpainsymman.2017.10.023
22. Komatz K, Carter B. Pain and symptom management in pediatric palliative care. *Pediatr Rev.* (2015) 36:527–34. doi: 10.1542/pir.36-12-527
23. Wolfe J, Grier HE, Klar N, Levin SB, Ellenbogen JM, Salem-Schatz S, et al. Symptoms and suffering at the end of life in children with cancer. *N Engl J Med.* (2000) 342:326–33. doi: 10.1056/NEJM200002033420506
24. Ullrich CK, Mayer OH. Assessment and management of fatigue and dyspnea in pediatric palliative care. *Pediatr Clin North Am.* (2007) 54:735–56. doi: 10.1016/j.pcl.2007.07.006
25. Blume ED, Balkin EM, Aiyagari R, Ziniel S, Beke DM, Thiagarajan R, et al. Parental perspectives on suffering and quality of life at end-of-life in children with advanced heart disease: an exploratory study*. *Pediatr Crit Care Med.* (2014) 15:336–42. doi: 10.1097/PCC.0000000000000072
26. Eche IJ, Eche IM, Aronowitz T. An integrative review of factors associated with symptom burden at the end of life in children with cancer. *J Pediatr Oncol Nurs.* 2020:1043454220909805. doi: 10.1177/1043454220909805
27. Anand KJ, Carr DB. The neuroanatomy, neurophysiology, and neurochemistry of pain, stress, and analgesia in newborns and children. *Pediatr Clin North Am.* (1989) 36:795–822. doi: 10.1016/S0031-3955(16)36722-0
28. Witt N, Coynor S, Edwards C, Bradshaw H. A guide to pain assessment and management in the neonate. *Curr Emerg Hosp Med Rep.* (2016) 4:1–10. doi: 10.1007/s40138-016-0089-y
29. Bhalla T, Shepherd E, Tobias JD. Neonatal pain management. *Saudi J Anaesth.* (2014) 8(Suppl. 1):S89–97. doi: 10.4103/1658-354X.144085
30. Craig KD, Whitfield MF, Grunau RV, Linton J, Hadjistavropoulos HD. Pain in the preterm neonate: behavioural and physiological indices. *Pain.* (1993) 52:287–99. doi: 10.1016/0304-3959(93)90162-I
31. Kuhn P, Strub C, Astruc D. [Problems for assessing the newborns' pain in palliative care]. *Arch Pediatr.* (2010) 17(Suppl. 3):S59–66. doi: 10.1016/S0929-693X(10)70903-9
32. Fortney CA, Steward DK. A qualitative study of nurse observations of symptoms in infants at end-of-life in the neonatal intensive care unit. *Intensive Crit Care Nurs.* (2017) 40:57–63. doi: 10.1016/j.iccn.2016.10.004

33. Anand KJ. Clinical importance of pain and stress in preterm neonates. *Biol Neonate.* (1998) 73:1–9. doi: 10.1159/000013953
34. Anand KJ, Pain IE-BGfN. Consensus statement for the prevention and management of pain in the newborn. *Arch Pediatr Adolesc Med.* (2001) 155:173–80. doi: 10.1001/archpedi.155.2.173
35. Deindl P, Unterasinger L, Kappler G, Werther T, Czaba C, Giordano V, et al. Successful implementation of a neonatal pain and sedation protocol at 2 NICUs. *Pediatrics.* (2013) 132:e211–8. doi: 10.1542/peds.2012-2346
36. Hall RW, Anand KJ. Pain management in newborns. *Clin Perinatol.* (2014) 41:895–924. doi: 10.1016/j.clp.2014.08.010
37. American Academy of Pediatrics Committee on Fetus and Newborn. Prevention and management of pain in the neonate. an update. *Adv Neonatal Care.* (2007) 7:151–60. doi: 10.1097/01.ANC.0000278214.49133.7d
38. Committee On Fetus And Newborn And Section On Anesthesiology And Pain Medicine. Prevention and management of procedural pain in the neonate: an update. *Pediatrics.* (2016) 137:e20154271. doi: 10.1542/peds.2015-4271
39. Garten L, Daehmlow S, Reindl T, Wendt A, Münch A, Bührer C. End-of-life opioid administration on neonatal and pediatric intensive care units: nurses' attitudes and practice. *Eur J Pain.* (2011) 15:958–65. doi: 10.1016/j.ejpain.2011.03.009
40. Pierucci RL, Kirby RS, Leuthner SR. End-of-life care for neonates and infants: the experience and effects of a palliative care consultation service. *Pediatrics.* (2001) 108:653–60. doi: 10.1542/peds.108.3.653
41. Carter BS. Pediatric palliative care in infants and neonates. *Children.* (2018) 5:21. doi: 10.3390/children5020021
42. Uthaya S, Mancini A, Beardsley C, Wood D, Ranmal R, Modi N. Managing palliation in the neonatal unit. *Arch Dis Child Fetal Neonatal Ed.* (2014) 99:F349–52. doi: 10.1136/archdischild-2013-305845
43. Abe N, Catlin A, Mihara D. End of life in the NICU. a study of ventilator withdrawal. *MCN Am J Matern Child Nurs.* (2001) 26:141–6. doi: 10.1097/00005721-200105000-00010
44. Cortezzo DE, Sanders MR, Brownell EA, Moss K. End-of-life care in the neonatal intensive care unit: experiences of staff and parents. *Am J Perinatol.* (2015) 32:713–24. doi: 10.1055/s-0034-1395475
45. McHaffie HE, Lyon AJ, Hume R. Deciding on treatment limitation for neonates: the parents' perspective. *Eur J Pediatr.* (2001) 160:339–44. doi: 10.1007/PL00008444
46. Shultz EL, Switala M, Winning AM, Keim MC, Baughcum AE, Gerhardt CA, et al. Multiple perspectives of symptoms and suffering at end of life in the NICU. *Adv Neonatal Care.* (2017) 17:175–83. doi: 10.1097/ANC.0000000000000385
47. Janvier A, Meadow W, Leuthner SR, Andrews B, Lagatta J, Bos A, et al. Whom are we comforting? an analysis of comfort medications delivered to dying neonates. *J Pediatr.* (2011) 159:206–10. doi: 10.1016/j.jpeds.2011.01.022
48. Stringer M, Shaw VD, Savani RC. Comfort care of neonates at the end of life. *Neonatal Netw.* (2004) 23:41–6. doi: 10.1891/0730-0832.23.5.41
49. Cortezzo DE, Carter B. *Palliative Care. Avery's Disease of the Newborn.* Philadelphia, PA: Elsevier. (2018) p. 446–52.
50. Kompanje EJ, van der Hoven B, Bakker J. Anticipation of distress after discontinuation of mechanical ventilation in the ICU at the end of life. *Intensive Care Med.* (2008) 34:1593–9. doi: 10.1007/s00134-008-1172-y
51. Williams C, Munson D, Zupancic J, Kirpalani H. Supporting bereaved parents: practical steps in providing compassionate perinatal and neonatal end-of-life care. a North American perspective. *Semin Fetal Neonatal Med.* (2008) 13:335–40. doi: 10.1016/j.siny.2008.03.005
52. Thompson AL, Young-Saleme TK. Anticipatory guidance and psychoeducation as a standard of care in pediatric oncology. *Pediatr Blood Cancer.* (2015) 62(Suppl. 5):S684–93. doi: 10.1002/pbc.25721
53. Brooten D, Youngblut JM, Seagrave L, Caicedo C, Hawthorne D, Hidalgo I, et al. Parent's perceptions of health care providers actions around child ICU death: what helped, what did not. *Am J Hosp Palliat Care.* (2013) 30:40–9. doi: 10.1177/1049909112444301
54. Mack JW, Wolfe J, Grier HE, Cleary PD, Weeks JC. Communication about prognosis between parents and physicians of children with cancer: parent preferences and the impact of prognostic information. *J Clin Oncol.* (2006) 24:5265–70. doi: 10.1200/JCO.2006.06.5326
55. Wiener L, Tager J, Mack J, Battles H, Bedoya SZ, Gerhardt CA. Helping parents prepare for their child's end of life: a retrospective survey of cancer-bereaved parents. *Pediatr Blood Cancer.* (2020) 67:e27993. doi: 10.1002/pbc.27993
56. Aschenbrenner AP, Winters JM, Belknap RA. Integrative review: parent perspectives on care of their child at the end of life. *J Pediatr Nurs.* (2012) 27:514–22. doi: 10.1016/j.pedn.2011.07.008
57. Mack JW, Joffe S. Communicating about prognosis: ethical responsibilities of pediatricians and parents. *Pediatrics.* (2014). 133(Suppl. 1):S24–30. doi: 10.1542/peds.2013-3608E
58. National Association of Neonatal Nurse Practitioners. Palliative care of newborns and infants. position statement #3051. *Adv Neonatal Care.* (2010) 10:287–93. doi: 10.1097/ANC.0b013e3181fc24ab
59. Parravicini E. Neonatal palliative care. *Curr Opin Pediatr.* (2017) 29:135–40. doi: 10.1097/MOP.0000000000000464
60. Parravicini E, Lorenz JM. Neonatal outcomes of fetuses diagnosed with life-limiting conditions when individualized comfort measures are proposed. *J Perinatol.* (2014) 34:483–7. doi: 10.1038/jp.2014.40
61. Kymre IG, Bondas T. Skin-to-skin care for dying preterm newborns and their parents–a phenomenological study from the perspective of NICU nurses. *Scand J Caring Sci.* (2013) 27:669–76. doi: 10.1111/j.1471-6712.2012.01076.x
62. Chan JD, Treece PD, Engelberg RA, Crowley L, Rubenfeld GD, Steinberg KP, et al. Narcotic and benzodiazepine use after withdrawal of life support: association with time to death? *Chest.* (2004) 126:286–93. doi: 10.1016/S0012-3692(15)32925-1
63. Weidner NJ, Plantz DM. Ethical considerations in the management of analgesia in terminally ill pediatric patients. *J Pain Symptom Manage.* (2014) 48:998–1003. doi: 10.1016/j.jpainsymman.2013.12.233
64. Bell SG. The pharmacology of palliative care. *Neonatal Netw.* (2004) 23:61–4. doi: 10.1891/0730-0832.23.6.61
65. Tedesco M. Dutch protocols for deliberately ending the life of newborns: a defence. *J Bioeth Inq.* (2017) 14:251–9. doi: 10.1007/s11673-017-9772-2
66. Catlin A, Novakovich R. The groningen protocol: what is it, how do the Dutch use it, and do we use it here? *Pediatr Nurs.* (2008) 34:247–51.
67. Kon AA. Neonatal euthanasia. *Semin Perinatol.* (2009) 33:377–83. doi: 10.1053/j.semperi.2009.07.005
68. Burnsed JC, Heinan K, Letzkus L, Zanelli S. Gabapentin for pain, movement disorders, and irritability in neonates and infants. *Dev Med Child Neurol.* (2020) 62:386–9. doi: 10.1111/dmcn.14324
69. Abdi HH, Maitre NL, Benninger KL, Hester ME, Slaughter JL. Gabapentin use for hospitalized neonates. *Pediatr Neurol.* (2019) 97:64–70. doi: 10.1016/j.pediatrneurol.2019.02.012
70. Edwards L, DeMeo S, Hornik CD, Cotten CM, Smith PB, Pizoli C, et al. Gabapentin use in the neonatal intensive care unit. *J Pediatr.* (2016) 169:310–2. doi: 10.1016/j.jpeds.2015.10.013
71. Sacha GL, Foreman MG, Kyllonen K, Rodriguez RJ. The use of gabapentin for pain and agitation in neonates and infants in a neonatal ICU. *J Pediatr Pharmacol Ther.* (2017) 22:207–11. doi: 10.5863/1551-6776-22.3.207
72. Anand KJ. Anesthetic neurotoxicity in newborns: should we change clinical practice? *Anesthesiology.* (2007) 107:2–4. doi: 10.1097/01.anes.0000268484.05444.35
73. Anand KJ. Pharmacological approaches to the management of pain in the neonatal intensive care unit. *J Perinatol.* (2007) 27(Suppl. 1):S4–11. doi: 10.1038/sj.jp.7211712
74. Anand KJ, Garg S, Rovnaghi CR, Narsinghani U, Bhutta AT, Hall RW. Ketamine reduces the cell death following inflammatory pain in newborn rat brain. *Pediatr Res.* (2007) 62:283–90. doi: 10.1203/PDR.0b013e3180986d2f
75. Pouvreau N, Tandonnet J, Tandonnet O, Renesme L. [Use of subcutaneous route for comfort care in neonatal palliative population: systematic review and survey of practices in France]. *Arch Pediatr.* (2017) 24:850–9. doi: 10.1016/j.arcped.2017.06.009
76. Drolet C, Roy H, Laflamme J, Marcotte ME. Feasibility of a comfort care protocol using oral transmucosal medication delivery in a palliative neonatal population. *J Palliat Med.* (2016) 19:442–50. doi: 10.1089/jpm.2015.0045
77. Harlos MS, Stenekes S, Lambert D, Hohl C, Chochinov HM. Intranasal fentanyl in the palliative care of newborns and infants. *J Pain Symptom Manage.* (2013) 46:265–74. doi: 10.1016/j.jpainsymman.2012.07.009
78. Verhagen AA, Dorscheidt JH, Engels B, Hubben JH, Sauer PJ. Analgesics, sedatives and neuromuscular blockers as part of end-of-life decisions

in Dutch NICUs. *Arch Dis Child Fetal Neonatal Ed.* (2009) 94:F434–8. doi: 10.1136/adc.2008.149260

79. Provoost V, Cools F, Bilsen J, Ramet J, Deconinck P, Vander Stichele R, et al. The use of drugs with a life-shortening effect in end-of-life care in neonates and infants. *Intensive Care Med.* (2006) 32:133–9. doi: 10.1007/s00134-005-2863-2
80. van der Heide A, van der Maas PJ, van der Wal G, Kollée LA, de Leeuw R. Using potentially life-shortening drugs in neonates and infants. *Crit Care Med.* (2000) 28:2595–9. doi: 10.1097/00003246-200007000-00069
81. Laing IA, Piyasena C. Analgesics, sedatives and neuromuscular blockers as part of end-of-life decisions in Dutch NICUs. *Arch Dis Child Fetal Neonatal Ed.* (2010) 95:F385. doi: 10.1136/adc.2009.178830
82. Quill TE, Lo B, Brock DW, Meisel A. Last-resort options for palliative sedation. *Ann Intern Med.* (2009) 151:421–4. doi: 10.7326/0003-4819-151-6-200909150-00007
83. Quill TE, Lo B, Brock DW. Palliative options of last resort: a comparison of voluntarily stopping eating and drinking, terminal sedation, physician-assisted suicide, and voluntary active euthanasia. *JAMA.* (1997) 278:2099–104. doi: 10.1001/jama.278.23.2099

22

A Standardized Needs Assessment Tool to Inform the Curriculum Development Process for Pediatric Resuscitation Simulation-Based Education in Resource-Limited Settings

Nicole Shilkofski[1], Amanda Crichlow[2], Julie Rice[3], Leslie Cope[4], Ye Myint Kyaw[5], Thazin Mon[6], Sarah Kiguli[7] and Julianna Jung[3]*

[1] Department of Pediatrics, Johns Hopkins University School of Medicine, Baltimore, MD, United States, [2] Department of Emergency Medicine, University of Florida College of Medicine, Jacksonville, FL, United States, [3] Department of Emergency Medicine, Johns Hopkins University School of Medicine, Baltimore, MD, United States, [4] Department of Oncology, Johns Hopkins University School of Medicine, Division of Bioinformatics and Biostatistics, Baltimore, MD, United States, [5] Head of Department of Pediatrics, University of Medicine 1 Yangon, Yangon Children's Hospital, Yangon, Myanmar, [6] Department of Pediatrics, University of Medicine 2 Yangon, Yangon Children's Hospital, Yangon, Myanmar, [7] Department of Pediatrics, Makerere University College of Health Sciences, Kampala, Uganda

***Correspondence:**
Nicole Shilkofski
nshilko1@jhmi.edu

Introduction: Under five mortality rates (UFMR) remain high for children in low- and middle-income countries (LMICs) in the developing world. Education for practitioners in these environments is a key factor to improve outcomes that will address United Nations Sustainable Development Goals 3 and 10 (good health and well being and reduced inequalities). In order to appropriately contextualize a curriculum using simulation, it is necessary to first conduct a needs assessment of the target learner population. The World Health Organization (WHO) has published a tool to assess capacity for emergency and surgical care in LMICs that is adaptable to this goal.

Materials and methods: The WHO Tool for Situational Analysis to Assess Emergency and Essential Surgical Care was modified to assess pediatric resuscitation capacity in clinical settings in two LMICs: Uganda and Myanmar. Modifications included assessment of self-identified learning needs, current practices, and perceived epidemiology of disease burden in each clinical setting, in addition to assessment of pediatric resuscitation capacity in regard to infrastructure, procedures, equipment, and supplies. The modified tool was administered to 94 respondents from the two settings who were target learners of a proposed simulation-based curriculum in pediatric and neonatal resuscitation.

Results: Infectious diseases (respiratory illnesses and diarrheal disease) were cited as the most common causes of pediatric deaths in both countries. Self-identified learning needs included knowledge and skill development in pediatric airway/breathing topics, as well as general resuscitation topics such as CPR and fluid resuscitation in shock. Equipment and supply availability varied substantially between settings, and critical shortages were identified in each setting. Current practices and procedures were often limited by equipment availability or infrastructural considerations.

Discussion and conclusion: Epidemiology of disease burden reported by respondents was relatively consistent with WHO country-specific UFMR statistics in each setting. Results of the needs assessment survey were subsequently used to refine goals and objectives for the simulation curriculum and to ensure delivery of pragmatic educational content with recommendations that were contextualized for local capacity and resource availability. Effective use of the tool in two different settings increases its potential generalizability.

Keywords: pediatric resuscitation, simulation-based training, limited-resource settings, pediatric critical care, needs assessment, neonatal resuscitation, developing countries, PIPES tool

INTRODUCTION

Globally, 5.6 million children under the age of 5 years died in 2016 (1). Since 1990, early childhood mortality has decreased substantially around the world, from 98 to 41 of every 1,000 live births. However, this rate remains much higher than the United Nations Sustainable Development Goal target of 25/1,000, and significant progress is needed to achieve this objective (2, 3). For the past two decades, it has been recognized that a multitude of factors contribute to potentially preventable child deaths in low- and middle-income countries (LMICs) (4). One thing that has not changed among these factors is the lack of high quality and contextually appropriate educational curricula to teach provision of care to critically ill children in these settings.

The World Health Organization (WHO) has developed the integrated management of childhood illness (IMCI) strategy and the emergency triage assessment and treatment (ETAT) guidelines for use in resource-limited settings (5, 6). Despite the demonstrated feasibility and success of some of these initiatives in LMICs (7), adherence to these guidelines by medical providers is highly variable (8, 9). Provider education has been shown to improve quality of care, but even among trained providers, performance remains suboptimal, suggesting the need for additional educational reinforcement (10).

For this reason, effective resuscitation education programs are needed in LMICs. Some training programs have been designed specifically for use in resource-limited settings, such as the Helping Babies Breathe (HBB) and Helping Mothers Survive (HMS) Bleeding after Birth initiatives (11–16). However, other resuscitation courses, such as the American Heart Association (AHA) Pediatric Advanced Life Support (PALS) and Pediatric Emergency Assessment Recognition and Stabilization (PEARS), have not been fully adapted for use in resource-limited settings. This has led many investigators to undertake these adaptations on an individual basis, often without a clear process to guide their efforts (17). However, "contextualized training," defined as "local adaptation of training, utilizing existing and sustainable resources for both care and training," has been associated with increases in provider confidence and short-term knowledge retention (18).

Contextualization of training requires rigorous understanding of the target learners and local clinical environment. In the curriculum development process, this understanding is gained through a needs assessment, which allows educators to ensure that curricula are appropriate and relevant to the target learner group (19). Needs assessment is particularly critical in international education, where epidemiology, resource availability, and practice standards vary widely (20). While several needs assessment surveys addressing critical care capacity have been described in the literature (21–25), there is presently no validated and comprehensive tool that is specific to pediatric resuscitation education in LMICs.

The WHO developed a tool in 2008 to measure surgical capacity (the Tool for Situational Analysis to Assess Emergency and Essential Surgical Care) (26), which has been validated and used in more than 10 LMICs (27–37). It was subsequently modified to develop a survey for specific facilities based on personnel, infrastructure, procedures, equipment, and supplies (PIPES) (38). PIPES has been used with further modifications to assess pediatric surgical capacity in 37 hospitals in West Africa (PediPIPES) (39).

In order to garner information needed to develop an appropriately contextualized pediatric resuscitation curriculum for use in two LMIC settings, we adapted the PIPES and PediPIPES to construct a novel needs assessment tool. Our immediate goal in developing this new tool was to evaluate local pediatric emergency care capacity, resources, and practices (PIPES), as well as perceived causes of pediatric morbidity and mortality, and self-assessed educational needs of target learners. Our ultimate goal, however, was to identify curricular adaptations needed to ensure relevance, feasibility, and appropriateness of educational content to the target setting in which pediatric resuscitation education is to be conducted. This process enabled us to implement fully contextualized curricula in two very different international venues.

MATERIALS AND METHODS

Tool Development

The original PIPES tool has 105 data items divided into five sections and functions as a scoring tool to compare the surgical capacity of different health-care facilities by calculating the PIPES Index (26, 38). The index can be calculated by tallying the total scores obtained in the survey. The Personnel section queries the total number of key practitioners (e.g., surgeons). The infrastructure, procedures, equipment and supplies sections have a binary response system of either "Always Available" versus "Not Always Available" or "Done" versus "Not Done."

We modified the PIPES tool in order to assess the pediatric medical resuscitation capacity of health-care facilities in resource-limited settings. As our tool was to be used for contextualization of a curriculum as opposed to rating facility capacity, we omitted the scoring component of the tool and replaced it with qualitative open-ended questions in order to garner more details about the hospital environments. We omitted items that were specific to surgical capacity and added items relevant to pediatric medical resuscitation. We also replaced the binary response system with a three-option response system (i.e., always available, usually available or seldom/never available) in order to account for potential variability in the availability of resources at different sites. Finally, we omitted the "Personnel" section, as this was specific to measuring overall hospital operational capacity and was less relevant for the curriculum development process.

In order to ensure that our curriculum addressed clinical topics of importance to our learners, we added a Section "Epidemiology." In this section, we queried the most common causes of potentially preventable death among children in the local practice setting. We also queried survey respondents to elucidate their perceived learning needs and prior pediatric resuscitation training and experience. We also added a Section "Current Practices/Skills," which used a five-point Likert scale to measure the confidence of survey respondents in managing emergency clinical scenarios and performing emergency procedures (see Appendix S1 in Supplementary Material for final iteration of tool used in the study—the PIPES Tool for Assessment of Pediatric Resuscitation Capacity in LMIC).

Tool Implementation

Study Settings

We implemented our needs assessment tool at two locations: Yangon Children's Hospital (YCH) in Yangon, Myanmar and Makerere University College of Health Sciences (MUCHS) in Kampala, Uganda. The study proposal was reviewed by the Institutional Review Board (IRB) of Johns Hopkins University School of Medicine and was considered to be exempt. In addition, local site approval to conduct the study was obtained from the ethics board and/or training committee leadership at both YCH and MUCHS. The two study sites were selected for convenience reasons, due to existing institutional partnerships.

Study Participants

At YCH in Myanmar, intended study participants consisted of first, second, and third year postgraduate trainees in Pediatrics, as well as a group of general practitioners pursuing a 1-year Diploma in Child Health course. At MUCHS, intended study participants consisted of second and third year postgraduate trainees in Pediatrics.

Data Collection

The needs assessment survey was administered to all participants immediately prior to the start of a resuscitation course. The paper-based survey was administered in person at both sites.

Data Analysis and Use of Results

Results were analyzed using simple descriptive statistics in Microsoft Excel. Results were used to make modifications to the planned curriculum as needed in order to appropriately contextualize the content in each setting. Of note, the investigators completed multiple phone meetings with local stakeholders as well as in-person visits to both sites prior to administration of the survey. This process allowed development of the majority of the curriculum in advance of the needs assessment survey. Survey results were then used in an iterative fashion to "fine-tune" and modify the curriculum at subsequent sites in order to optimize feasibility of recommendations and relevance to the local clinical context.

RESULTS

A total of 94 participants completed the pre-course needs assessment survey, 62 in Myanmar and 32 in Uganda (100% response rate). Age range of respondents was 25–40 years. 74% of respondents were in their second or third postgraduate year of pediatric specialty training. Further results are presented below by category.

Infrastructure

At both sites, most infrastructure items were described as being "always" or "usually" available by the majority of respondents. The one exception was ventilators at the Uganda site, which were described as "seldom/never" available by 88%. Compared to Uganda, respondents in Myanmar reported more variability in availability of electricity. The vast majority at both sites reported they "always" or "usually" had access to specialized services including blood bank, intensive care, and medical records. While no respondents described oxygen as "seldom/never" available, it is notable that only 50% in Uganda and 77% in Myanmar described it as "always" available. Access to diagnostic testing was limited at both sites. X-ray was the most commonly available imaging modality, cited as "always available" by 44% in Uganda and 61% in Myanmar. Laboratory services and advanced imaging were described as "usually" or "seldom" available by a majority at both sites. Ventilators were much more available in Myanmar compared to Uganda (see **Figure 1**).

Procedures

Peripheral intravenous access was the only procedure described as being performed "routinely" at both sites. In Uganda, 70% of respondents reported that intraosseous access was performed "routinely," compared to Myanmar where 83% indicated that this procedure was performed "rarely." Over half of respondents at both sites described administering epinephrine "routinely." In Myanmar, a similar number reported "routinely" administering vasopressor infusions, while this proportion was much smaller in Uganda. At both sites, a sizeable minority of respondents described use of atropine and antiarrhythmics as routine. Chest tube placement was the most commonly performed invasive procedure, with a majority at both sites describing it as routine. Intubation was much more common in Myanmar than in Uganda, with 40% of respondents indicating that they perform

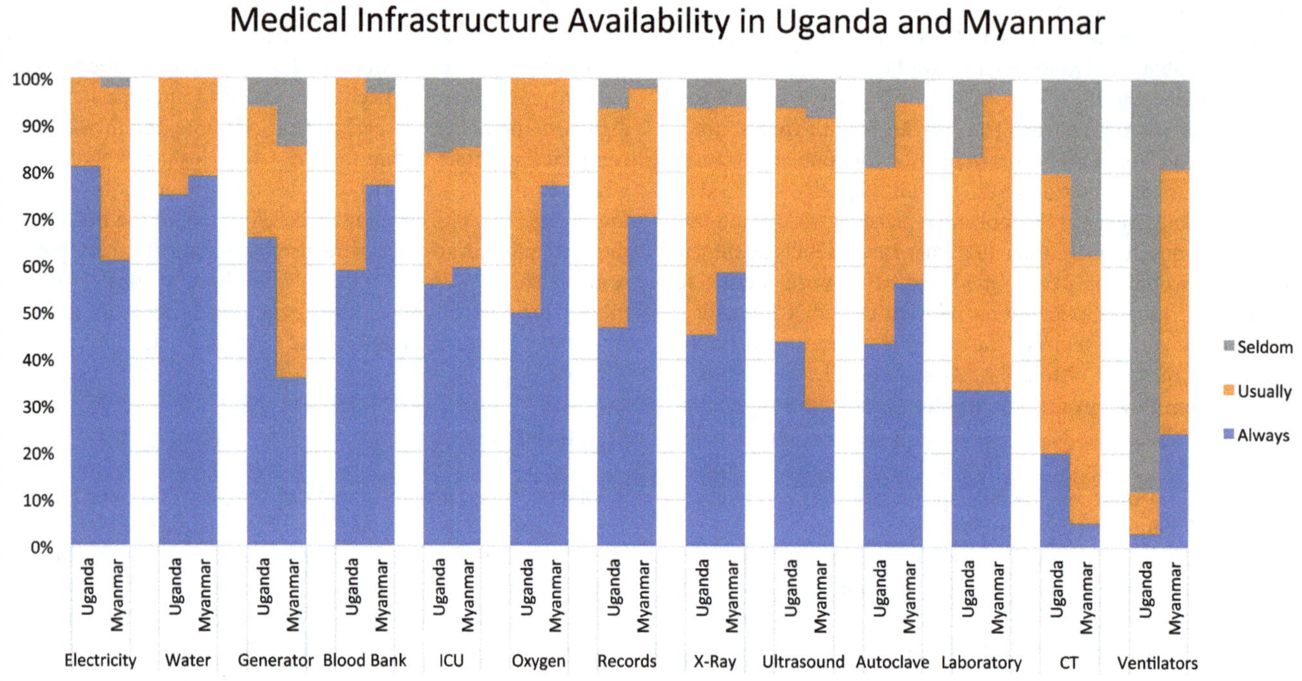

FIGURE 1 | Infrastructure availability.

this procedure "routinely" in Myanmar compared to only 3% in Uganda. Central venous access, arterial line placement and electrical therapies for the heart were rare in both settings (see **Figure 2**).

Equipment

Most respondents at both sites reported that noninvasive respiratory support equipment was "always" or "usually" available, including oxygen delivery devices, bag-valve-mask ventilation devices, and continuous positive airway pressure systems. Diagnostic equipment like pulse oximeters, blood pressure cuffs, electrocardiogram machines, and glucometers were much more readily available in Myanmar than Uganda, where access to these items was extremely limited. Respondents from both sites reported limited access to cardiac monitors, with only 19% in Uganda and 37% in Myanmar reporting them as "always available." Respondents in Myanmar reported better availability of advanced airway adjuncts compared to those in Uganda, although access to these items was suboptimal in both settings. Both sites reported very limited availability of quality CPR equipment like backboards and stepstools (see **Figure 3**).

Supplies

All respondents at both sites indicated that basic supplies like syringes, gloves, and intravenous catheters were "always" or "usually" available. While this was also true for intravenous fluids, a significant proportion at each site (34% in Uganda and 15% in Myanmar) indicated that this essential supply is not always available. Similarly, infant suction bulbs were not uniformly available at either site. Both sites reported a lack of access to intraosseous needles, with 66% in Uganda and 27% in Myanmar reporting that these are "seldom/never" available. Higher-level procedural equipment was relatively unavailable in both settings, with endotracheal tubes more readily available than invasive vascular access devices and chest tubes (see **Figure 4**).

Epidemiology

Infectious diseases were listed as the predominant cause of preventable death in children at both the Myanmar and Uganda sites (see **Figure 5**). Specifically, respiratory infections occupied the top position at both sites, and gastrointestinal diseases were also common. Differences in local epidemiology were seen between the two sites, as malaria was frequently cited as a major cause of preventable death in Uganda but was rarely noted in Myanmar. Sepsis, on the other hand, was frequently cited in Myanmar but not in Uganda.

Self-Identified Learning Needs

At the Myanmar site, the three most commonly cited learning needs were in the categories of airway/breathing management (28% of respondents), circulation/fluid resuscitation (22%), and cardiac arrest management (16%). Within each of these categories, the most frequently cited learning needs were intubation (54%), intraosseous needle (IO) placement (65%), and defibrillation/cardioversion (38%). At the Uganda site, the three most commonly cited learning needs were in the categories of general resuscitation principles (27%), cardiac arrest management (22%), and circulation/fluid resuscitation (19%). Within each of these categories, the most frequently cited learning needs were basic neonatal/pediatric resuscitation topics (65%),

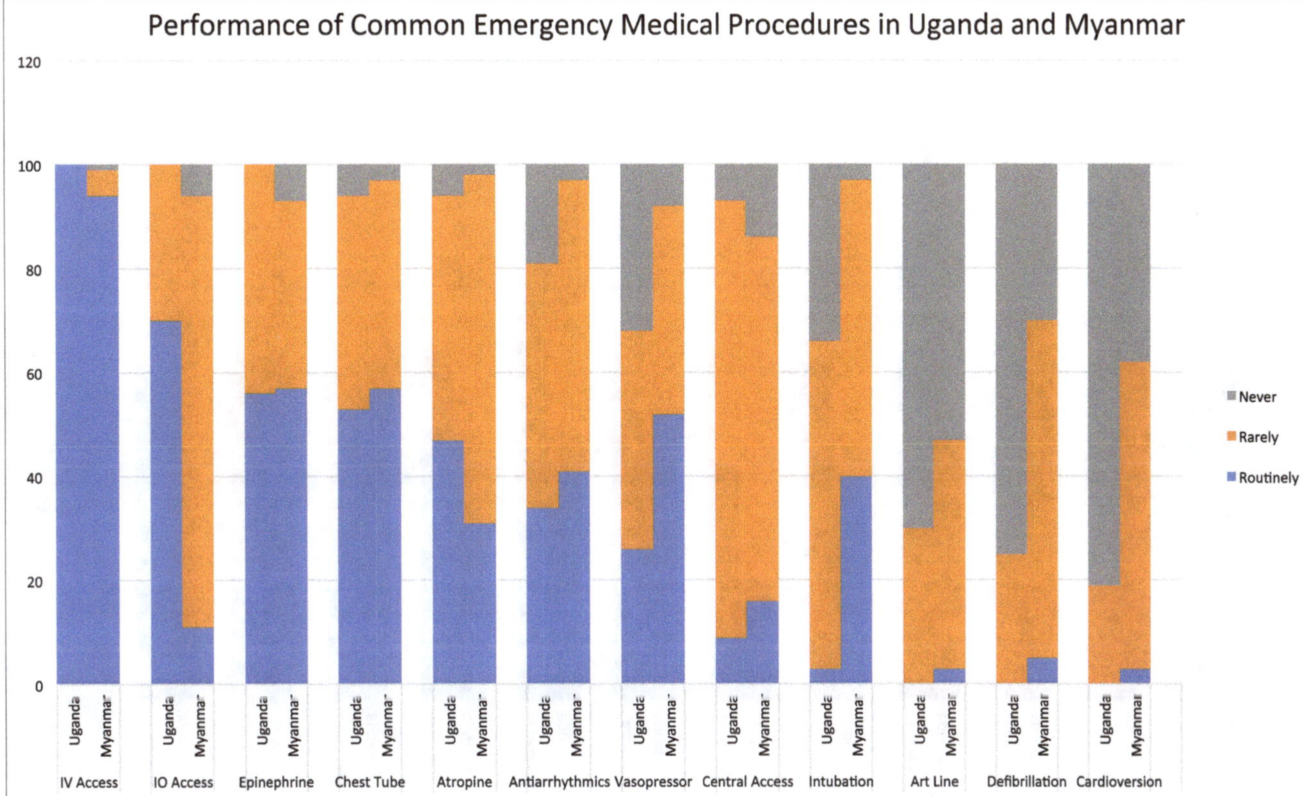

FIGURE 2 | Common emergency procedures performed.

defibrillation/cardioversion (33%), and central venous cannulation (17%).

Pediatric Resuscitation Experience

At the Uganda site, 87.5% of participants stated that they had prior formal training in pediatric resuscitation, 75% of whom stated that the course involved either simulation or hands-on skills practice. At the Myanmar site, only 63% of participants stated that they had prior training, only 50% of whom reported simulation or hands-on skills practice as part of this training. 97% of participants in Uganda indicated that they managed critically ill children either "daily" or "regularly," compared to only 48% in Myanmar (see **Table 1**).

Current Practices/Skills

The clinical scenarios that participants reported the greatest confidence in managing were similar at both sites: respiratory distress and shock. The clinical scenarios that the participants were "least confident" managing were also similar: cardiac arrest and pneumothorax. See **Table 2** for detailed results. Participants in Uganda reported higher confidence overall compared to those in Myanmar.

The procedures that the participants reported highest confidence in performing were the same at both sites, with differences only in rank order: airway assessment, breathing assessment, circulation assessment, and IV placement. The procedures that the participants were least confident performing also had some similarities between the sites. Participants at both sites were not confident performing central line placement, defibrillation/cardioversion, and intubation. See **Table 3** for detailed results.

DISCUSSION

Our modified PIPES tool was administered to a group of physician learners in Myanmar and Uganda as part of a needs assessment process for the design and implementation of a contextualized curriculum in pediatric resuscitation using simulation-based pedagogy. We were able to achieve a 100% response rate to the needs assessment survey, which was achievable due to in-person administration of the survey immediately prior to the start of the course. As the purpose of collecting these data was to inform the curriculum development process, we reviewed the results with the goal of optimally contextualizing our training program to each setting. While it would be impossible to exhaustively describe every curricular adaptation made in each setting, **Table 4** offers several key examples of how these data were used to optimize applicability of our educational content for the target learner groups.

In applying our results from the needs assessment to refine the curriculum, we took into account a prior systematic review of resuscitation training in developing countries, which demonstrated that important educational outcomes are inconsistently defined and that training courses are often modified to available training resources, rather than to the needs and resources of

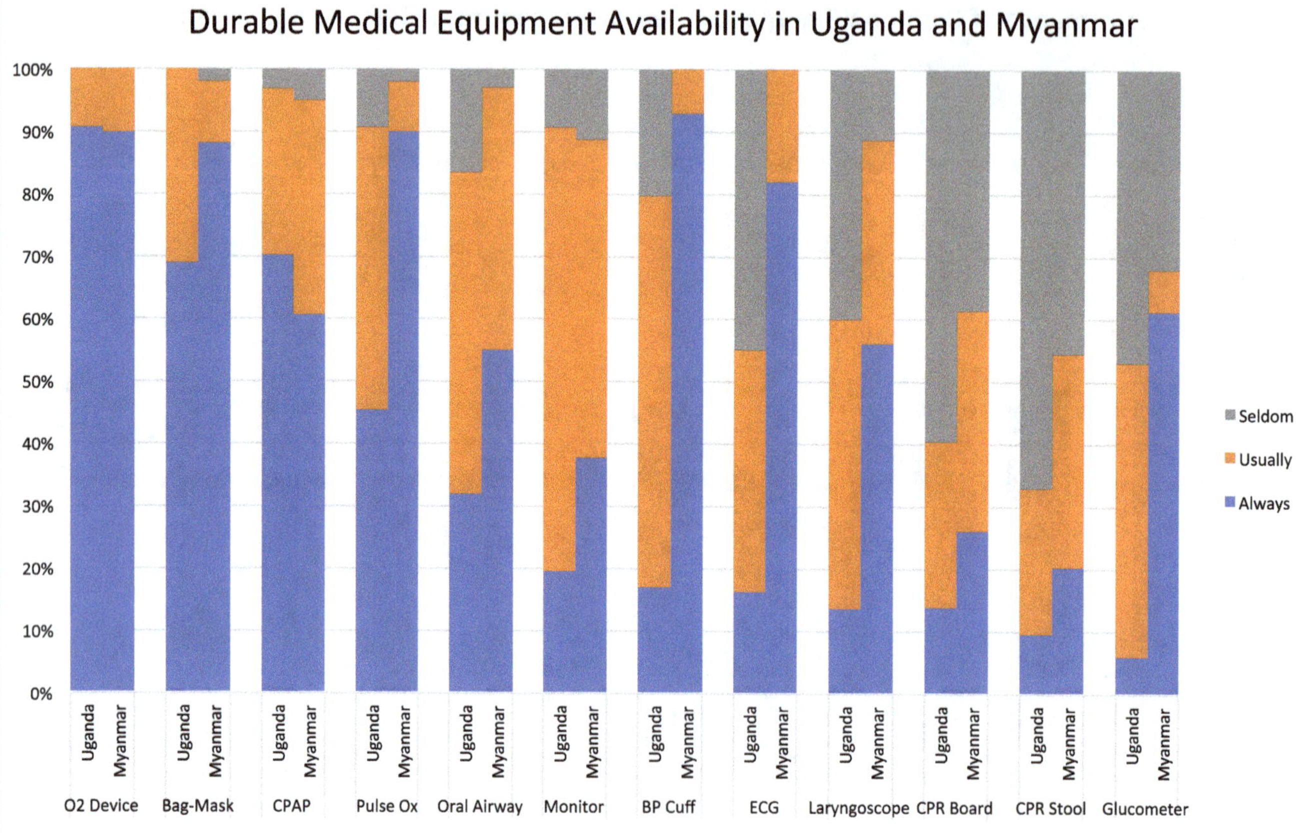

FIGURE 3 | Equipment availability.

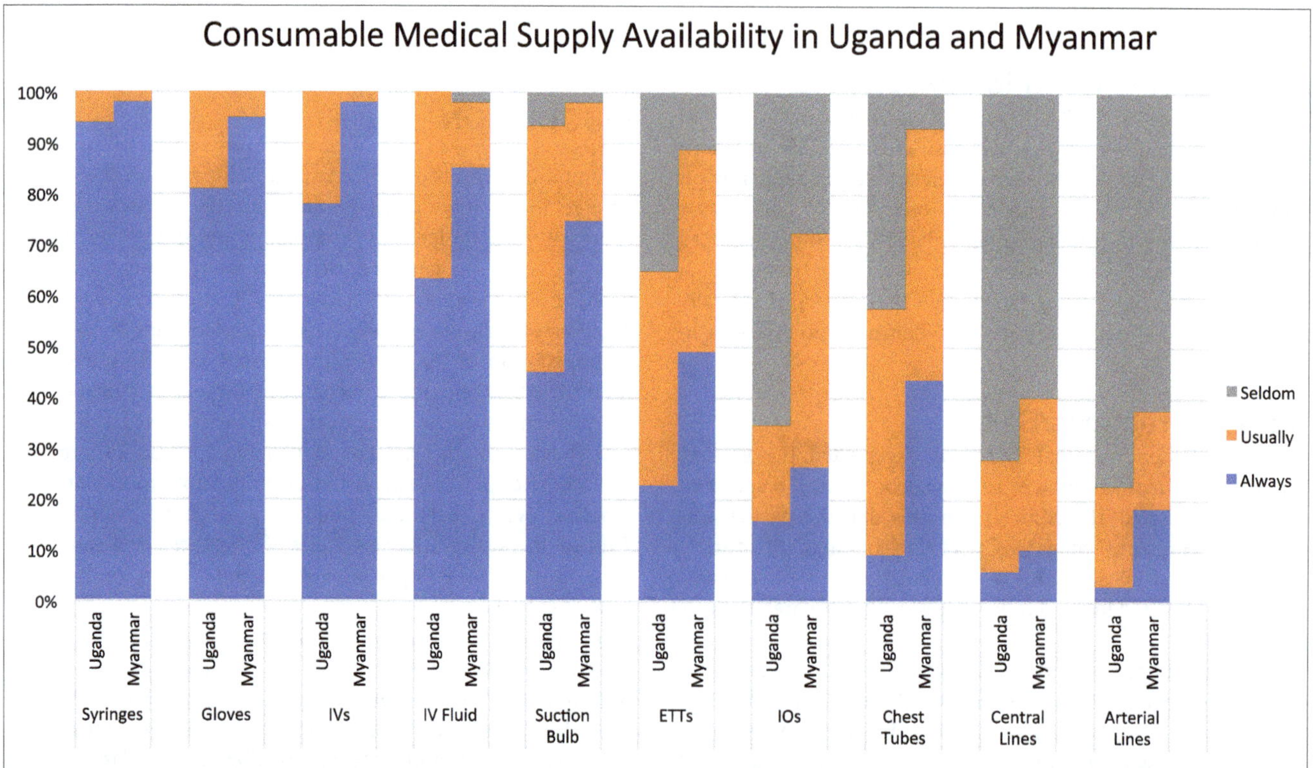

FIGURE 4 | Consumable supplies availability.

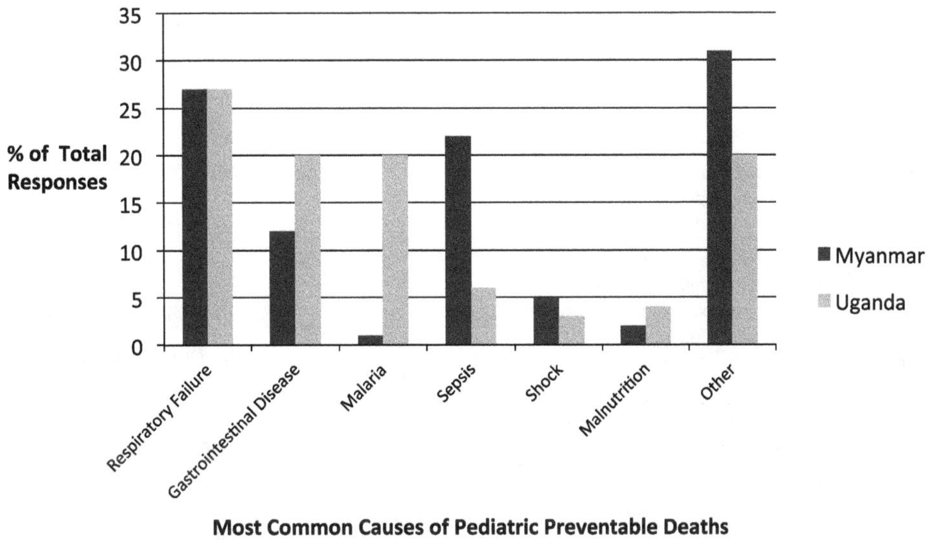

FIGURE 5 | Most commonly cited causes of pediatric preventable death in survey participants' clinical settings.

TABLE 1 | Frequency of exposure to critically ill children in clinical settings.

	Myanmar, % respondents	Uganda, % respondents
Daily (4 or more times per week)	8	75
Regularly (1–2 times per week)	40	22
Occasionally (1–2 times per month)	40	0
Rarely (1–2 times per year)	3	0
No response	9	3

TABLE 2 | Clinical scenario management confidence scores.

	Uganda, mean Likert Score (SD)	Myanmar, mean Likert Score (SD)
Bradycardia	3.7 (0.9)	3.4 (1.2)
Cardiac arrest	3.2 (1.0)	2.3 (1.2)
Decreased level of consciousness	4.2 (0.8)	3.4 (1.0)
Hypoxia	4.0 (0.7)	3.6 (0.9)
Respiratory distress	4.3 (0.7)	3.6 (0.9)
Seizures	4.4 (0.6)	3.7 (1.0)
Shock	4.3 (0.6)	3.8 (0.9)
Tachycardia	3.6 (1.0)	3.4 (1.2)

Likert scale consisted of numeric options ranging from 1 to 5:1 = "Not at all confident" 3 = "Somewhat confident" and 5 = "Very confident."

TABLE 3 | Procedural confidence scores.

	Uganda, mean (SD)	Myanmar, mean (SD)
Airway assessment	4.2 (0.7)	4.0 (0.9)
Breathing assessment	4.3 (0.7)	4.0 (0.9)
BVM ventilation	4.0 (0.8)	3.8 (0.9)
Central line placement	1.9 (1.3)	1.3 (0.8)
Circulation assessment	4.3 (0.8)	4.0 (0.9)
CPR	3.9 (0.7)	3.7 (0.9)
Defibrillation/cardioversion	1.4 (0.7)	1.4 (0.8)
EKG or cardiac rhythm interpretation	2.1 (1.1)	2.9 (0.8)
Intraosseous line placement	4.2 (1.0)	2.4 (1.3)
Intubation	2.1 (1.1)	2.1 (1.0)
IV placement	4.6 (0.6)	3.9 (1.0)

Likert scale consisted of numeric options ranging from 1 to 5:1 = "Not at all confident" 3 = "Somewhat confident" and 5 = "Very confident."

the local health-care setting and patients (40). Training that is not tailored to local needs perpetuates a "common misconception that emergency medical care is inherently expensive and requires high-technology interventions as opposed to simple and effective strategies" (41). This needs assessment was an effort to facilitate essential contextualization of the curriculum in both settings. The process by which the needs assessment was used to tailor simulation scenarios and skills stations to the local settings and resource availability was analogous to the process used in similar studies in Africa that utilized a shorter assessment tool known as the facilities readiness assessment (18). The modified tool used in our study allowed for a more extensive evaluation of the local health-care resources specifically applicable to pediatric resuscitation and proved effective in understanding the local landscape of our target learners in both Uganda and Myanmar. Below, we highlight notable findings from the results and how they compare with what is already known in the literature.

Epidemiology—Local Disease Burden

The epidemiology section of the survey allowed us to determine if the national morbidity and mortality statistics provided by the WHO were reflected in the local pediatric population served by our target learners. In Myanmar, the majority of the causes of under five mortality rates (UFMR) listed in WHO national statistics were mentioned by survey respondents, although the ranking of diseases differed somewhat. One of the major differences was that in the 2013 WHO statistics, neonatal sepsis was listed as the seventh leading cause of death in Myanmar, whereas in our survey, it was the second most common response for preventable causes of mortality (see **Figure 6**). In Uganda, many of the causes

TABLE 4 | Examples of key findings and their use in curriculum development.

Finding	Action
Absence of ventilators and laryngoscopes in Uganda	Focused on effective noninvasive ventilation and omitted advanced airway skills from curriculum at this site
Limited access to cardiac monitors at both sites	Emphasized frequent clinical reassessment to determine response to treatment and trajectory of condition
Variable access to diagnostic support tools, including pulse oximetry, blood pressure cuffs, glucometers, and laboratory services (particularly in Uganda)	Emphasized established clinical criteria for empiric administration of oxygen, IV fluid, glucose, and blood products (major focus of training in Uganda)
Rare performance of cardioversion or defibrillation at either site (related to lack of defibrillators)	Despite participants' self-identified learning needs, chose to omit these skills from curriculum at both sites
Lack of availability of intraosseous needles at both sites	Addressed improvization of equipment for intraosseous access when needed
Relatively lower confidence in intraosseous needle placement in Myanmar	Spent additional time on this skill at this site
Relatively lower confidence in CPR performance at both sites	Allotted significant time to this skill at both sites, and incorporated CPR quality feedback tools to optimize learner performance
Frequent mortality associated with malaria in Uganda	Added entire module about life-threatening complications of malaria for this site
Frequent use of epinephrine at both sites	Emphasized alternate appropriate treatments, particularly respiratory support for bradycardia, and volume expansion for shock

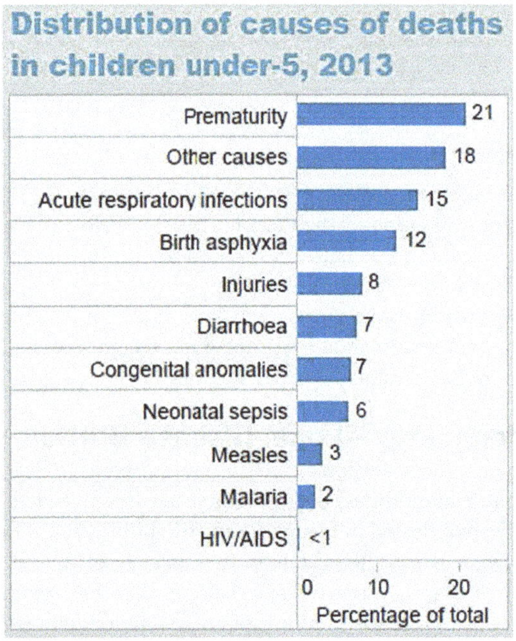

FIGURE 6 | World Health Organization (WHO) distribution of causes of death in children under five in Myanmar (Source: country statistics and global health estimates by WHO and UN partners http://www.who.int/gho/countries/mmr.pdf).

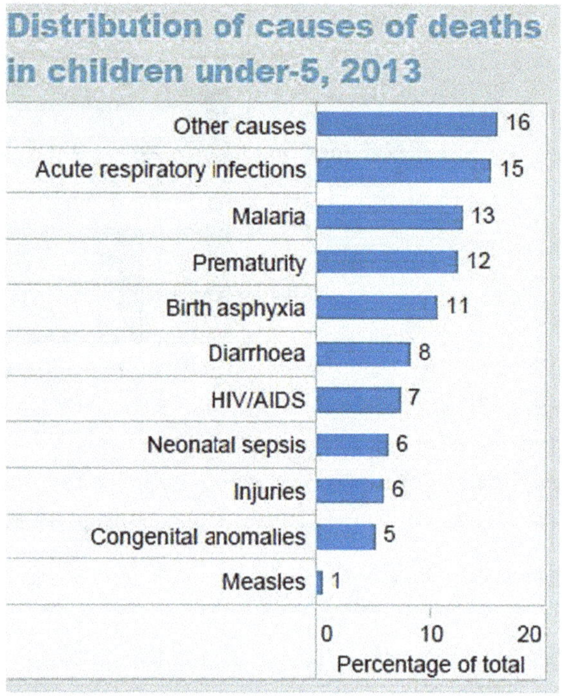

FIGURE 7 | World Health Organization (WHO) distribution of causes of death in children under five in Uganda (Source: country statistics and global health estimates by WHO and UN partners http://www.who.int/gho/countries/uga.pdf).

of death listed in the WHO national statistics were also mentioned by the survey respondents, with rankings also differing somewhat (see **Figure 7**). Some important causes of death listed by WHO were not mentioned by survey respondents, including prematurity, HIV/AIDS, and injuries. Of note, our survey asked for causes of *preventable* death. Our Ugandan learners, working in a severely resource-constrained environment, may encounter these causes of death routinely, but simply not perceive them as preventable. Our curriculum ultimately incorporated both locally identified and WHO-cited causes of pediatric mortality. Our educational team felt strongly that it was important to design simulation scenarios targeting causes of UFMR identified through an emic or local perspective in order to enhance face validity of the curriculum with target learners.

Pediatric Resuscitation Training and Prior Clinical Exposure

The majority of participants at both local sites had some form of prior pediatric resuscitation training. Interestingly, this is in contrast with many other studies that have reported on baseline knowledge prior to training courses (40), perhaps because our survey was conducted at facilities that had formal residency training programs in pediatrics. Prior exposure to hands-on skills practice and/or simulation was more variable and differed between the two sites. In Myanmar, only one-third of participants had prior simulation-based resuscitation training, despite the fact that they resuscitate children on a fairly regular basis.

The percentage of survey participants who indicated that they managed critically ill children on a daily basis was significantly higher in Uganda compared to Myanmar, and this was reflected in the higher confidence scores reported by Ugandan participants. Participants at both sites reported frequent exposure to critically ill children, reinforcing the importance of formal training and frequent refreshers in pediatric and neonatal resuscitation skills for both cohorts of clinicians.

Self-Identified Learning Needs

Airway management was listed as a learning need for a significant percentage of participants in both the Uganda and Myanmar cohorts. This is not surprising given that respiratory illnesses and respiratory failure were the most frequently listed causes of preventable death at both sites. The self-identified learning needs of airway and cardiac arrest management were reflected in the low mean confidence scores for these scenarios at both sites, as well as for related skills such as intubation and defibrillation/cardioversion. However, it was noted in the PIPES survey that the necessary equipment and supplies for these procedures were often not available, raising the question of whether these skills are truly contextually relevant, but also likely leading to minimal practical use of these skills and, hence, lower confidence scores.

Although this study was conducted in resource-limited settings, the major learning needs we identified were consistent with self-identified knowledge gaps in a recent large scale survey of over 700 emergency medical care providers for children in rural settings in the United States, where resource limitations are often also present (42). These gaps included pediatric airway management and procedural skills in neonatal resuscitation and intraosseous access. This concordance with the literature even in a developed setting highlights the importance of addressing specific educational needs for health-care providers to care for neonatal and pediatric populations.

Impact on Curriculum Design

The sections of the needs assessment survey that had the greatest impact on the curriculum instructional design were the local epidemiology, followed by the available equipment and infrastructure in each setting. These data allowed us to focus the curriculum in each location on high-yield material that was relevant to the learners and the population they serve. For example, in Uganda, one learning station focused on management of malaria according to local guidelines. In Myanmar, this was not needed, but a learning station did focus on resuscitation in dengue shock, a common cause of morbidity and mortality in the Southeast Asian region (see **Table 4** for examples).

Participants' self-identified learning needs were also taken into account, but coverage of these topics emphasized techniques and procedures that could be performed with available equipment based on the PIPES survey. For example, due to the lack of defibrillators, central venous catheters, arterial line catheters, and the inconsistent availability of ventilators at both sites, the procedural skills of defibrillation/cardioversion, central line placement, arterial line placement, and intubation/advanced airway management were de-emphasized. Greater emphasis was placed on clinical assessment skills, effective noninvasive airway management (e.g., high quality BVM ventilation), and management of shock using available local equipment.

In order to ensure relevance and feasibility, we taught procedures using locally available equipment. For example, emergency intraosseous (IO) access was taught using bone marrow needles or other large-bore devices rather than with the commercially available IO needles used in the United States. When certain equipment was not available in the local setting, the educational team worked with the local team to design workable alternatives. When equipment for certain procedures is not available, it is also essential for trainers to understand if and how clinicians improvize in order to perform these procedures. For example, our respondents reported very limited access to chest tubes, yet a majority indicated that chest tube placement is a "routinely" performed procedure. Had chest tube placement been an objective of our curriculum, it would have been essential to explore how clinicians perform this procedure in the absence of purpose-specific equipment and to incorporate locally available supplies and techniques in the teaching of this skill.

When designing simulation scenarios, we took care to mimic resource constraints in the actual clinical environment and to require learners to address these issues in their management. For example, glucometers were scarce in Uganda, while they were more readily available in Myanmar. In our hypoglycemia scenarios, we provided a finger-stick glucose reading for participants in Myanmar, but required participants in Uganda to rely on clinical assessment to determine the need for glucose administration. Similarly, the 10% dextrose (D10) solutions used for hypoglycemia in young children are not commercially available in Uganda, necessitating that clinicians mix their own solutions using sterile water and higher concentration dextrose. In order to ensure mastery of this skill, our hypoglycemia simulation included mixing of D10 from locally available products as a critical action. Subtle alterations such as these ensured contextual relevance of our scenarios and reinforced essential skills required of health-care providers in their actual clinical settings.

Overall, the data acquired through our survey allowed for the curriculum to be tailored to local needs and resources to increase its feasibility, applicability, and impact. This practice is consistent with recommendations in the literature to appropriately calibrate and contextualize resuscitation courses from developed countries in order to ensure feasibility in resource-limited settings, thereby strengthening the chain of survival from within the local health-care system (17, 20, 41).

Limitations and Next Steps

The needs assessment survey in this study was implemented at only two sites in East Africa and Southeast Asia, and therefore its generalizability may be limited to sites with similar learning needs and epidemiology. Furthermore, our participants were subspecialty trainees based at referral centers, so our tool may be less applicable for first-line providers and facilities. Although the needs assessment is based on a WHO tool that has been validated in multiple resource-limited settings, our modified tool has not yet undergone validity testing. This will be a goal of future studies. In addition to tool validation, our next steps will include the further revision of existing simulation-based curricula in pediatric resuscitation to be more appropriately contextualized to local epidemiology, learning needs, and available resources.

CONCLUSION

The WHO Tool for Situational Analysis to Assess Emergency and Essential Surgical Care and the PIPES tools were successfully adapted to assess pediatric resuscitation capacity and learning needs in two different clinical settings. The implementation of the tool in two different countries in Asia and Africa helps to improve its generalizability for LMIC settings in the developing world. Results from the needs assessment at each site provided the basis for design of a pragmatic and appropriately contextualized curriculum in neonatal and pediatric resuscitation at each site, as well as a process for iterative revision of the curriculum for subsequent courses. These results informed curriculum development and instructional design, enabling the team to address self-identified learning needs, while emphasizing high-yield procedural skills that were of practical value, given the local resource limitations. The results also improved engagement of local stakeholders and participants in the curriculum, as they perceived that they had input into successive iterations of the curriculum through their responses to the needs assessment survey. The approach of partnering with local educational stakeholders in the curriculum design process through a formal needs assessment is consistent with recommendations by the Lancet Commission in 2010 in their publication *Health professionals for a new century: transforming education to strengthen health systems in an interdependent world* (43). These recommendations include reformation of local competencies through global flows of knowledge and cultivation of ownership through local clinician leadership in shaping educational processes. This concept provided a foundation for the ultimate design of our curriculum based on our needs assessment survey. Future studies will focus on validation of the PIPES tool in its modified form and dissemination of the tool to other resource-limited settings, in addition to implementation and evaluation of subsequent curricular interventions.

ETHICS STATEMENT

This study was carried out in accordance with the recommendations of the Johns Hopkins University School of Medicine Institutional Review Board (JHUSOM IRB). The study protocol was determined to be exempt research by the JHUSOM IRB under the DHHS regulations (i.e., research conducted in established or commonly accepted educational settings, involving normal educational practices, such as (i) research on regular and special education instructional strategies or (ii) research on the effectiveness of or the comparison among instructional techniques, curricula, or classroom management methods). In addition, local site approval and consent for conduct of the study in Uganda and Myanmar were obtained from the Head of the Department of Paediatrics and the Director of Training and Education at Children's Hospital of Yangon, Myanmar, as well as from the ethics board of Mulago Hospital and Makerere University College of Health Science in Kampala, Uganda.

AUTHOR CONTRIBUTIONS

NS, AC, JR, and JJ conceived of the needs assessment survey, implemented the survey in each setting, performed data analysis, and contributed to the writing of the manuscript. TM, YK, and SG assisted in implementation of the survey at each site and assisted in data collection. LC assisted in data analysis and writing of the manuscript. All authors approved the final version of the manuscript.

ACKNOWLEDGMENTS

The authors would like to acknowledge the contributions of the faculty at Makerere University College of Health Sciences and Yangon Children's Hospital for their aid in facilitating needs assessment survey distribution and in the implementation of the resuscitation courses in each institution. We would also like to express thanks to the postgraduate residents, physicians, and students at both institutions for their participation in the study and to Drs. Megan Hosein, Juin Yee Kong, Kee Thai, Lim Ju Lyn, Phang Chen Rong, and Nawin Thevar for their assistance in teaching and data collection in Uganda and Myanmar. We would also like to acknowledge Drs. Deogratias Munube and Robert Opika Opoka for their roles in course coordination in Uganda. Finally, we would like to acknowledge both the Laerdal Foundation for Acute Medicine and the Johns Hopkins University School of Medicine Institute for Excellence in Education for the grant funding to complete the study.

REFERENCES

1. World Health Organization. *Global Health Observatory Data Repository under Five Mortality Trends*. (2018). Available from: http://www.who.int/gho/child_health/mortality/mortality_under_five_text/en/
2. Gaffey MF, Das JK, Bhutta ZA. Millennium development goals 4 and 5: past and future progress. *Semin Fetal Neonatal Med* (2015) 20:285–92. doi:10.1016/j.siny.2015.07.001
3. Buse K, Hawkes S. Health in the sustainable development goals: ready for a paradigm shift. *Global Health* (2015) 11:13. doi:10.1186/s12992-015-0098-8
4. Murray CJL, Lopez AD. *The Global Burden of Disease: A Comprehensive Assessment of Mortality and Disability from Diseases Injuries, and Risk Factors in 1990 and Projected to 2020*. Geneva: World Health Organization (1996).
5. *Integrated Management of Childhood Illness (IMCI) Guidelines*. (2017). Available from: http://whqlibdoc.who.int/publications/2005/9241546441.pdf
6. *Emergency Triage Assessment and Treatment (ETAT) Guidelines*. (2017). Available from: http://whqlibdoc.who.int/publications/2005/9241546875_eng.pdf
7. Molyneux E, Ahmad S, Robertson A. Improved triage and emergency care for children reduces inpatient mortality in a resource-constrained setting. *Bull World Health Organ* (2006) 84:314–9. doi:10.2471/BLT.04.019505

8. Kelly JM, Osamba B, Garg RM, Hamel MJ, Lewis JJ, Rowe SY, et al. Community health worker performance in the management of multiple childhood illnesses: siaya district, Kenya, 1997–2001. *Am J Public Health* (2001) 91:1617–24. doi:10.2105/AJPH.91.10.1617
9. Rowe AK, Onikpo F, Lama M, Cokou F, Deming MS. Management of childhood illness at health facilities in Benin: problems and their causes. *Am J Public Health* (2001) 91:1625–35. doi:10.2105/AJPH.91.10.1625
10. Nguyen DT, Leung KK, McIntyre L, Ghali WA, Sauve R. Does integrated management of childhood illness (IMCI) training improve the skills of health workers? A systematic review and meta-analysis. *PLoS One* (2013) 8:e66030. doi:10.1371/journal.pone.0066030
11. Singhal N, Lockyer J, Fidler H, Keenan W, Little G, Bucher S, et al. Helping babies breathe: global neonatal resuscitation program development and formative educational evaluation. *Resuscitation* (2012) 83(1):90–6. doi:10.1016/j.resuscitation.2011.07.010
12. Goudar SS, Somannavar MS, Clark R, Lockyer JM, Revankar AP, Fidler HM, et al. Stillbirth and newborn mortality in India after helping babies breathe training. *Pediatrics* (2013) 131(2):e344–52. doi:10.1542/peds.2012-2112
13. Msemo G, Massawe A, Mmbando D, Rusibamayila N, Manji K, Kidanto HL, et al. Newborn mortality and fresh stillbirth rates in Tanzania after helping babies breathe training. *Pediatrics* (2013) 131(2):e353–60. doi:10.1542/peds.2012-1795
14. Hoban R, Bucher S, Neuman I, Chen M, Tesfaye N, Spector JM. 'Helping babies breathe' training in sub-Saharan Africa: educational impact and learner impressions. *J Trop Pediatr* (2013) 59(3):180–6. doi:10.1093/tropej/fms077
15. Musafili A, Essén B, Baribwira C, Rukundo A, Persson LÅ. Evaluating helping babies breathe: training for healthcare workers at hospitals in Rwanda. *Acta Paediatr* (2013) 102(1):e34–8. doi:10.1111/apa.12034
16. Evans CL, Johnson P, Bazant E, Bhatnagar N, Zgambo J, Khamis AR. Competency-based training "helping mothers survive: bleeding after birth" for providers from central and remote facilities in three countries. *Int J Gynaecol Obstet* (2014) 126(3):286–90. doi:10.1016/j.ijgo.2014.02.021
17. Meaney PA, Topjian AA, Chandler HK, Botha M, Soar J, Berg RA, et al. Resuscitation training in developing countries: importance of a stable program of formation of instructors. *Resuscitation* (2011) 82(6):780–1. doi:10.1016/j.resuscitation.2010.12.027
18. Wright SW, Steenhoff AP, Elci O, Wolf HA, Ralston M, Kgosieselee T, et al. Impact of contextualized pediatric resuscitation training on pediatric healthcare providers in Botswana. *Resuscitation* (2015) 88:57–62. doi:10.1016/j.resuscitation.2014.12.007
19. Hughes MT. Targeted needs assessment. 3rd ed. In: Kern DE, Thomas PA, Hughes MT, editors. *Curriculum Development for Medical Education: A Six Step Approach*. Baltimore, Maryland: Johns Hopkins University Press (2016):29–49.
20. Ralston ME, Day LT, Slusher TM, Musa NL, Doss HS. Global paediatric advanced life support: improving child survival in limited-resource settings. *Lancet* (2013) 381:256–65. doi:10.1016/S0140-6736(12)61191-X
21. Vukoja M, Riviello E, Gavrilovic S, Adhikari NK, Kashyap R, Bhagwanjee S, et al. A survey on critical care resources and practices in low- and middle-income countries. *Glob Heart* (2014) 9:337–42.e1–5. doi:10.1016/j.gheart.2014.08.002
22. Baker T, Lugazia E, Eriksen J, Mwafongo V, Irestedt L, Konrad D. Emergency and critical care services in Tanzania: a survey of ten hospitals. *BMC Health Serv Res* (2013) 13:140. doi:10.1186/1472-6963-13-140
23. Hsia RY, Mbembati NA, Macfarlane S, Kruk ME. Access to emergency and surgical care in sub-Saharan Africa: the infrastructure gap. *Health Policy Plan* (2012) 27:234–44. doi:10.1093/heapol/czr023
24. Notrica MR, Evans FM, Knowlton LM, Kelly McQueen KA. Rwandan surgical and anesthesia infrastructure: a survey of district hospitals. *World J Surg* (2011) 35:1770–80. doi:10.1007/s00268-011-1125-4
25. Chirdan LB, Ameh EA, Abantanga FA, Sidler D, Elhalaby EA. Challenges of training and delivery of pediatric surgical services in Africa. *J Pediatr Surg* (2010) 45:610–8. doi:10.1016/j.jpedsurg.2009.11.007
26. *Tool for Situational Analysis to Assess Emergency and Essential Surgical Care*. (2017). Available from: http://www.who.int/surgery/publications/QuickSitAnalysisEESCsurvey.pdf
27. Kushner AL, Cherian MN, Noel L, Spiegel DA, Groth S, Etienne C. Addressing the millennium development goals from a surgical perspective: essential surgery and anesthesia in 8 low- and middle-income countries. *Arch Surg* (2010) 145(2):154–9. doi:10.1001/archsurg.2009.263
28. Kingham TP, Kamara TB, Cherian MN, Gosselin RA, Simkins M, Meissner C, et al. Quantifying surgical capacity in Sierra Leone: a guide for improving surgical care. *Arch Surg* (2009) 144:122–7. doi:10.1001/archsurg.2008.540
29. Contini S, Taqdeer A, Cherian M, Shokohmand AS, Gosselin R, Graaff P, et al. Emergency and essential surgical services in Afghanistan: still a missing challenge. *World J Surg* (2010) 34:473–9. doi:10.1007/s00268-010-0406-7
30. Iddriss A, Shivute N, Bickler S, Cole-Ceesay R, Jargo B, Abdullah F, et al. Emergency, anaesthetic and essential surgical capacity in the Gambia. *Bull World Health Organ* (2011) 89:565–72. doi:10.2471/BLT.11.086892
31. Choo S, Perry H, Hesse AA, Abantanga F, Sory E, Osen H, et al. Assessment of capacity for surgery, obstetrics and anaesthesia in 17 Ghanaian hospitals using a WHO assessment tool. *Trop Med Int Health* (2010) 15:1109–15. doi:10.1111/j.1365-3156.2010.02589.x
32. Sherman L, Clement PT, Cherian MN, Ndayimirije N, Noel L, Dahn B, et al. Implementing Liberia's poverty reduction strategy: an assessment of emergency and essential surgical care. *Arch Surg* (2011) 146:35–9. doi:10.1001/archsurg.2010.285
33. Spiegel DA, Choo S, Cherian M, Orgoi S, Kehrer B, Price RR, et al. Quantifying surgical and anesthetic availability at primary health facilities in Mongolia. *World J Surg* (2011) 35:272–9. doi:10.1007/s00268-010-0904-7
34. Natuzzi ES, Kushner A, Jagilly R, Pickacha D, Agiomea K, Hou L, et al. Surgical care in the Solomon Islands: a road map for universal surgical care delivery. *World J Surg* (2011) 35:1183–93. doi:10.1007/s00268-011-1097-4
35. Taira BR, Cherian MN, Yakandawala H, Kesavan R, Samarage SM, DeSilva M. Survey of emergency and surgical capacity in the conflict-affected regions of Sri Lanka. *World J Surg* (2010) 34:428–32. doi:10.1007/s00268-009-0254-5
36. Petroze RT, Nzayisenga A, Rusanganwa V, Ntakiyiruta G, Calland JF. Comprehensive national analysis of emergency and essential surgical capacity in Rwanda. *Br J Surg* (2012) 99:436–43. doi:10.1002/bjs.7816
37. Osen H, Chang D, Choo S, Perry H, Hesse A, Abantanga F, et al. Validation of the World Health Organization tool for situational analysis to assess emergency and essential surgical care at district hospitals in Ghana. *World J Surg* (2011) 35:500–4. doi:10.1007/s00268-010-0918-1
38. Groen RS, Kamara TB, Dixon-Cole R, Kwon S, Kingham TP, Kushner AL. A tool and index to assess surgical capacity in low income countries: an initial implementation in Sierra Leone. *World J Surg* (2012) 36:1970–7. doi:10.1007/s00268-012-1591-3
39. Okoye MT, Ameh EA, Kushner AL, Nwomeh BC. A pilot survey of pediatric surgical capacity in West Africa. *World J Surg* (2015) 39:669–76. doi:10.1007/s00268-014-2868-5
40. Meaney PA, Topjian AA, Chandler HK, Botha M, Soar J, Berg RA, et al. Resuscitation training in developing countries: a systematic review. *Resuscitation* (2010) 81(11):1462–72. doi:10.1016/j.resuscitation.2010.06.024
41. Kobusingye OC, Hyder AA, Bishai D, Joshipura M, Hicks ER, Mock C. Emergency medical services. 2nd ed. In: Jamison D, Bank W, editors. *Disease Control Priorities in Developing Countries*. (Chap. 68), (2006). p. 1261–79. Available from: http://ingentaconnect.com
42. Hansen M, Meckler G, Dickinson C, Dickenson K, Jui J, Lambert W, et al. Children's safety initiative: a national assessment of educational needs among emergency medical services providers. *Prehosp Emerg Care* (2015) 19(2):287–91. doi:10.3109/10903127.2014.959223
43. Frenk J, Chen L, Bhutta ZA, Cohen J, Crisp N, Evans T, et al. Health professionals for a new century: transforming education to strengthen health systems in an interdependent world. *Lancet* (2010) 376(9756):1923–58. doi:10.1016/S0140-6736(10)61854-5

23

Considerations for Assessing the Appropriateness of High-Cost Pediatric Care in Low-Income Regions

*Andrew C. Argent**

Paediatric Critical Care, Paediatrics and Child Health, University of Cape Town, Red Cross War Memorial Children's Hospital, Cape Town, South Africa

***Correspondence:**
Andrew C. Argent
andrew.argent@uct.ac.za

It may be difficult to predict the consequences of provision of high-cost pediatric care (HCC) in low- and middle-income countries (LMICs), and these consequences may be different to those experienced in high-income countries. An evaluation of the implications of HCC in LMICs must incorporate considerations of the specific context in that country (population age profile, profile of disease, resources available), likely costs of the HCC, likely benefits that can be gained versus the costs that will be incurred. Ideally, the process that is followed in decision making around HCC should be transparent and should involve the communities that will be most affected by those decisions. It is essential that the impacts of provision of HCC are carefully monitored so that informed decisions can be made about future provision medical interventions.

Keywords: ethics, low- and middle-income countries, high cost, intensive care, children

> *Ideally, every child in the world should have access to an intensive care unit with facilities for endotracheal intubation and mechanical ventilation. No ethical justification exists for providing these treatments to children in rich countries while denying them to children in poor countries (Shann, 2011)*

INTRODUCTION

While there is no ethical justification for differences in health-care access for children across the world, dealing with the realities of those differences remains profoundly challenging. During 2016, 5.6 million children under the age of 5 years died across the world (this is equivalent to 15,000 under-5 deaths per day), mostly in low- (LICs) and low- and middle-income countries (LMICs). The majority of those deaths could have been prevented using simple and affordable interventions (1). There are huge differences in under-5 mortality between high- and LICs as well as between higher- and lower-income groups within individual countries (2), in both high- (3) and LICs (4). Addressing intra-country differences could make nearly as much difference to child mortality as addressing the differences between countries. There have been substantial improvements in child survival across the world with the implementation of the millennium development goals, and with those gains, the role and importance of critical care in low- and middle-income countries (LMICs) has increased (5). However, the decision to provide high-cost care in low-income regions is a complex issue where the outcomes and consequences of that provision may be unpredictable and substantially different to those experienced in high-income countries.

High-cost medical care (HCC) incorporates a wide range of medical interventions, and the "value" that is associated with the provision of HCC must take into account many factors including costs, and benefits and the priorities of the people living in those areas. The "high cost" has to be viewed in relation to the available resources and in relation to the value delivered by the care (it is possible to have both high cost and high value, and high cost and low value). Some have argued that there are no "universal" bioethics (6, 7), but perhaps there may be validity in creating some transparency around the processes that are involved in making decisions as to how resources are allocated and on what basis.

In this review, I will consider the health-care context of LICs, the costs and benefits associated with the provision of HCC (in general, but more specifically directed at pediatric critical care), the way in which different people may be affected by HCC, and consider how the process of decision making around resource allocation could be addressed in LICs. Resources are limited in all regions, but there are substantial differences in resource availability, specific contexts, and particular demands on health-care systems across the world.

THE CONTEXT

Decision making around the utilization of resources for HCC is deeply affected by a wide number of issues including the underlying context (particularly in terms of disease profile and morbidity and mortality data), the resources available (both absolute and relative amounts), and the potential benefits associated with the HCC (to the child, the family, the community, and the overall health services). An underlying concern with the process of "lumping" countries and groups of countries or communities into simple categories (such as LICs) is the fact that there are huge differences in context between (and within) countries, even within similar income groupings. It is not only the current reality but the "trajectory" of development in a country that may affect which health-care services can and should be provided.

The Children/Patients

As shown in **Table 1**, approximately 60% of the world's children live in low- and LMICs, with some 275 million children living in low-income regions of the world. In those regions, children making up a very substantial proportion of the population have limited access to health-care services and extremely limited access to high-cost health-care services. Health-care expenditure in these regions averages US$35 per capita per annum, and the under-5 mortality is approximately 70 per 1000 live births. The majority of childhood deaths occur in these countries, and various authors have highlighted the fact that the majority of these deaths could be prevented by the implementation of relatively low-cost (and affordable) interventions.

The Environment

LICs have many features which make the delivery of health care challenging including limited financial and personnel resources for health care, geographical features which may make transport and access challenging, political instability, limited infrastructure (water, electricity, sanitation, transport services, and transport infrastructure), and limited organizational and administrative infrastructure. The large number of displaced people and refugees also complicates decision making for care delivery.

The disease profile in LICs may be substantially different to that in HICs (9–11) and is also changing. In general, there is more trauma (including burns), and there are more infections (including more non-bacterial infections such as dengue, malaria, trypanosomiasis, etc.), and more infections with antibiotic-resistant organisms. Particular concerns relate to infections such as drug-resistant tuberculosis. Data on non-infectious disease are limited, but there is no reason to believe that there is a lower incidence in poorer countries.

As a consequence of multiple factors, patients often present late for therapy (12, 13) with the result that disease processes are often substantially advanced at the time of presentation. A high proportion of deaths occur soon after admission (14). Resource limitations translate into a low number of health-care workers and particularly health-care workers with specialist skills in areas such as pediatrics and pediatric surgery (see **Table 2**). These workers are deployed in environments that may be overcrowded and poorly maintained (and thus difficult to keep clean), uncomfortable (including heat and humidity or even cold), with very limited equipment and medication. The health-care facilities are often situated in contexts where there may be limited and unreliable sources of clean water, sanitation, and power (particularly electricity and lighting). In a recent review of hospitals in sub-Saharan Africa, the percentage of hospitals with dependable running water and electricity ranged from 22 to 46%, and in countries analyzed, only 19–50% of hospitals had the ability to provide 24-h emergency care (15).

TABLE 1 | Data on population, mortality, and health expenditure by income region (8).

Region by Income	% population 0–14 years (2016)	Total population 0–14 years (2015)	Gross national income (GNI) per capita (US $, 2016)	Health expenditure per capita (US $, 2014)	Under-5 mortality (per 1,000 live births), 2016
Low income	42.67	275 365 283	$612	$35	73.1
Lower-middle income	30.83	923 253 971	$2,079	$90	50.7
Upper-middle income	20.60	528 220 719	$8,210	$506	14.1
High income	16.7	197 950 251	$41,046	$5,266	5.4

As of July 1, 2016, low-income economies are defined as those with a GNI per capita, calculated using the World Bank Atlas method, of $1,025 or less in 2015; lower-middle-income economies are those with a GNI per capita between $1,026 and $4,035; upper-middle-income economies are those with a GNI per capita between $4,036 and $12,475; high-income economies are those with a GNI per capita of $12,476 or more.

TABLE 2 | Resources for health care by income region (8).

Region	Nurses and midwives (per 1,000 population), 2012	Physicians per 1,000 population (2012)	Specialist surgical workforce per 1,000 population (2014)	Out of pocket expenditure (% of total expenditure on health)
Low income	0.69	0.20	0.88	37.19
Lower-middle income	1.77	0.73	10.23	54.87
Upper-middle income	2.80	1.96	39.55	32.39
High income	8.73	2.94	69.28	13.34

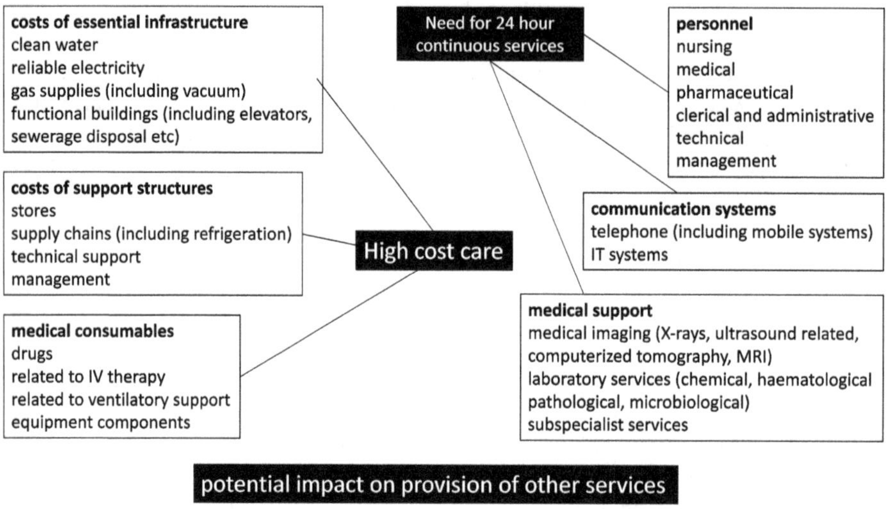

FIGURE 1 | Components of the costs related to high-cost care (HCC) in low- and middle-income countries and low-income countries.

Limited and often dysfunctional supply chains contribute to nonavailability of resources that would be taken for granted and assumed in HICs. All of this may be aggravated by political instability and limited personal safety. In the event of natural disasters or outbreaks of infectious disease, these systems may fail spectacularly as has been demonstrated during recent outbreaks of Ebola virus infection in West Africa (16).

All the factors above need to be taken into consideration when contemplating resource allocation for high-cost care.

RESOURCES FOR HEALTH CARE

In considering the ethics of high-cost care in LICs, it is essential to balance the resources that are available for that care with the outcomes that can be achieved using those resources.

Financial

The financial resources available for health care can be considered from a number of perspectives (see **Figures 1** and **2**). There may be complex interactions between multiple factors.

As shown in **Table 1**, there is a >10-fold difference in the annual per capita health-care expenditure between LMICs and high middle-income countries and >100-fold difference between LMICs.

In LICs, a significant proportion of the funding available for health care may come from outside the country (see **Table 2**). That funding may be useful but is usually to be used in ways that are defined by the sources of the funding. Increasingly, funding may also be sourced from research projects that are based on high-income countries. This means that there are external drivers of how that funding can and should be used for health-care provision.

There are different ways of assessing the relative costs of high-cost services. When considering the costs of intensive care in 2009, Baker et al. estimated the costs of a day in intensive care in rich countries to be of the order of $1,000 (17). From a national perspective, that day cost would be approximately 20% of the annual per capita expenditure on health in a rich country but approximately 30 times the annual per capita expenditure on health in an LIC.

The costs of delivering some aspects of critical care in poorer countries may be substantially lower than this, as an example the cost of a day in a private ICU for cancer patients in India was reported as $57, However, in settings where a substantial proportion of health-care costs are covered by out-of-pocket expenditure by families (**Table 2**), that amount has to be related to the family income. In this setting, $57 was approximately 100× the average per capita household income (18). Thus, the provision of expensive health-care services to individuals in these settings has the potential to devastate the financial structure of a family with severe impact on other family members (including siblings) (19).

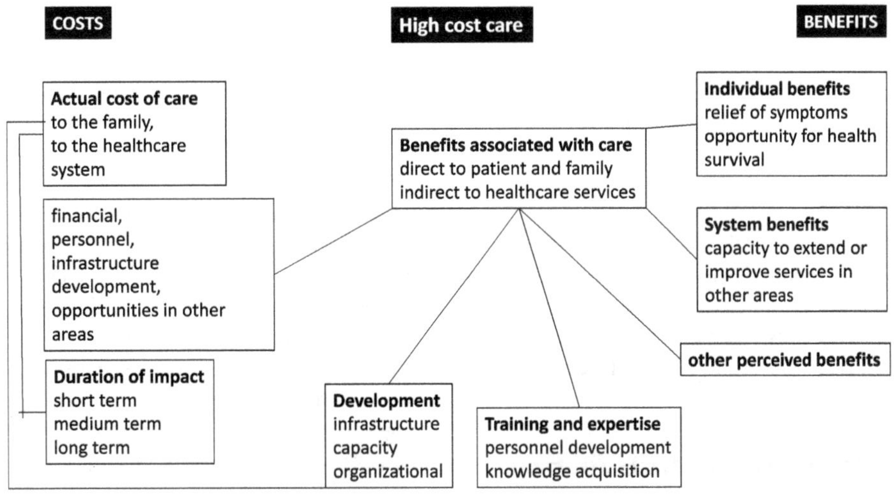

FIGURE 2 | The balances of costs and benefits for high-cost care (HCC) in low- and middle-income countries and low-income countries.

Significant as this overall difference is, it may actually mask other differences in costs for HCC. The HCC costs in rich countries reflect the costs of providing that care in the context of systems with well-established and functional infrastructure. In LICs, the infrastructure required (including transport, electricity, water provision and sewerage disposal, medical gas supply systems, technical maintenance support, etc) to support complex medical care may be profoundly deficient. The real cost therefore of providing HCC in "austere conditions" may be substantially higher than currently estimated. This may, however, be offset by the lower salaries that are paid to health-care workers in poorer countries. As another example, it has been argued in HIC that catheter closure of ostium secundum atrial septal defects is substantially cheaper than surgical closure, but in fact this was not the case in Guatemala (20).

Many of the resources required for more expensive therapies (including equipment and medication) are developed and manufactured in high-income countries. Access to these resources may be limited by the direct costs, which are exacerbated by indirect costs such as transportation, import duties and taxes, and adverse financial exchange rates.

In many LMICs, the differentials in access to high-cost health care between rich and poor people may vary substantially. In many countries, a small proportion of the population have access to state-of-the-art medical services while the majority of people within the same country may have limited or virtually nonexistent access to health-care services (21). In South Africa in 2015, approximately 49.8% of total health-care expenditure was from private sources, and only approximately 16% of the population have private health-care insurance (22). This difference in financial resources translates into major differences in access to facilities such as intensive care beds (21, 23).

The widespread corruption in some LICs and LMICs may have a profound effect on the resources actually available for health-care services (24).

Thus, any analysis of the resource implications for HCC in LICs must include a review of all the multiple factors and details in specific environments that may profoundly affect both the absolute and the relative costs of HCC in these countries.

Personnel

Not only are health-care systems in LICs limited by financial resources but they also have profound challenges as regards the availability of trained and skilled health-care providers. Some years ago, the WHO estimated that the world faced a global shortage of almost 4.3 million doctors, midwives, nurses, and other health-care professionals (25). There are particular shortages in the area of surgery [including pediatric surgery (26, 27)] and anesthesia (28) and rehabilitation personnel (29) in poorer countries. The availability of these health-care workers (particularly to patients who cannot afford private health care) may be profoundly affected by the different remuneration patterns and the fact that many health-care workers have to work in several sectors in order to obtain an adequate income (30).

The standard of care that is (and can be) expected from health-care workers may vary substantially. In most HICs, it would be assumed that staff on out-of-hours duty would be fully awake and present throughout their working time. In many LICs, there is an expectation that afterhours staff will be heavily reduced in numbers relative to the day and that they will be expected to sleep for at least some of the time on duty (after all, many have day jobs that they also have to attend to).

When 24-h services are essential for the provision of HCC (such as pediatric intensive care), then personnel may be both a limiting factor as regards availability, but also as regards costs (four to five people have to be employed for each position that needs to be filled on a 24-h basis).

With substantial differences between financial resources in private and government sectors in LMICs, there are major pressures for health-care workers to move into the more affluent areas either full-time or part-time. This process may substantially decrease the access of less affluent members of society to health-care services that are high cost and often require high levels of training and expertise.

Decisions about HCC in LMIC and LICs may also have an effect on medical emigration. As an example, individuals with training in areas such as surgery or cardiac surgery are likely to emigrate or to move into the private sector if they are consistently unable to operate because of the lack of availability of theater time or PICU beds.

Structures

Many of the structures in terms of policies, programs, and training infrastructure that are required to support intensive care therapies are simply not present in LICs, as shown in a study completed in Tanzania (31). Thus, time and effort will have to be expended to put all those structures in place before particular services can be provided.

OUTCOMES OF HIGH-COST SERVICES

The outcomes of high-cost services are not always simple to establish and may relate to the underlying conditions (see **Table 3**): the specific interventions undertaken, and the expertise and experience of the teams undertaking those interventions. Some high-cost interventions may be associated with excellent outcomes and minimal long-term costs. At the other extreme, high-cost interventions may be associated with poor outcomes and high long-term costs.

There is evidence that relatively low-cost interventions in the care of critically ill children such as the provision of antibiotics at community level to neonates (40), the provision of oxygen therapy to children with pneumonia (41), the provision of high-flow humidified nasal oxygen or nasal CPAP (42, 43), and the improvement of organization of emergency services or of pediatric services within a hospital (44) may be associated with substantial reductions in mortality without significant added expense. Recent neonatal data suggested that focused implementation of nasal CPAP in Nicaragua could provide improved outcomes while reducing invasive mechanical ventilation (45).

Mechanical ventilation has been described in many reports from LICs as being associated with relatively high mortality (46, 47). Thus, in many situations, HCC such as ventilation may not improve overall outcomes as much as simpler and less-resource intensive care modalities.

Where intensive care services have been implemented in LICs, there is some evidence that the strict application of quality control programs can substantially improve the outcomes of pediatric intensive care (48, 49).

ETHICAL PRINCIPLES TO BE APPLIED

Having reviewed the context, the resources available, and the potential impact of HCC such as pediatric intensive care, it is important to consider ethical principles that could be considered in making decisions about the provision of HCC (see **Table 4**) as well as the characteristics of the processes used in decision making (**Table 5**). Turner et al. (14) have highlighted the principles of global justice, resource allocation, and local cultural preferences. Clearly, there is no ethical justification for the global differences in access of children to HCC (50), and there is a huge need to provide advocacy for additional resources from HIC to be allocated to LIMCs, but that will (at best) take time. However, there is a

TABLE 3 | High-cost interventions, cost, and outcomes.

Example	Short term	Medium to long term	Outcomes
Intensive care for croup	High cost for intensive care (usually only a few days)—but extreme variability in the costs incurred (32)	No expected ongoing costs	Normal life expectancy, small proportion will have recurrent croup
Intensive care for Guillan–Barré syndrome	High cost for intensive care (may require months of ventilation)	May need high input for rehabilitation	Expected to return to normal quality of life with normal activities (may have residual weakness). Some patients have recurrent disease (33–35)
Intensive care for pneumonia or infection	High cost for intensive care (usually a few days but may be longer)	If not underlying disease, minimal long-term costs	Depending on context, may have substantial mortality in hospital and in the 6 months following hospital discharge (36) [particularly if concurrent malnutrition (37)]. However, high chance of normal long-term outcome
Intensive care to enable major surgery	High cost for surgery and intensive care (usually only a few days)	Depending on underlying problems, may be a significant range of long-term costs	The outcomes of a major surgery can be very variable depending on a variety of factors including surgical training and surgical caseload
Surgery for congenital heart disease	High cost for surgery and intensive care	If curative surgery, then minimal long-term costs. May have substantial costs for ongoing care (38) in complex conditions	If successful, excellent outcomes with essentially normal life expectancy and quality of life
Surgery for rheumatic heart disease	High cost for surgery and intensive care	Relatively high costs for ongoing follow-up and medication	Limited long-term survival and high morbidity (39)
Surgery and Intensive care for trauma including burn injuries	Relatively high cost for surgery and intensive care	Depending on the site and extent of the injuries, the long-term costs could be minimal or very substantial	The outcomes may be variable. In the absence of long-term rehabilitation, and in the absence of facilities such as access to cadaver skin or expensive skin replacements, the outcomes of major burns may be extremely poor

TABLE 4 | Ethical principles to be applied in decision making around high-cost care (HCC).

Principle	National level	Community level	Individual level
Respect for autonomy	Rights of nations to make decisions regarding the prioritization of health services in that country.	The rights of communities to be involved in the processes that affect what and how medical care will be delivered to them	The rights of individuals and their families to make decisions regarding issues that affect them
Beneficence	The HCC should provide an improvement in the quality of life in that country	The HCC should improve the quality of health and life in the community which is being provided with that service	The care that is offered has to be seen to provide value to the individual child and his/her family
Non-maleficence or "do no harm"	The provision of the particular HCC cannot be seen to endanger the delivery of other essential services	The provision of the services must not cause harm to themselves, and the removal of other services in order to afford the services must not be seen as a greater harm	Patients must be seen to benefit from the services offered. There may be a range of perceptions about what outcomes are actually acceptable
Justice	The health-care services need to provide care to as many children as possible, within the resources available. All care cannot be provided to all	There are different communities that are affected by decisions around HCC, and communities should not be disadvantaged by the provision of HCC to individuals or to other communities	Patients should have access to care on the basis of need and likelihood of benefit

TABLE 5 | Processes to be applied to the processes of resource allocation for health care.

Trust	The people affected by the process need to trust that the people implementing the health care will do their best to provide that care fairly and equitably
Transparency	The process of resource allocation should be open to comment, and the basis for decision making should be made public
Responsiveness	Should be mechanisms within the system to respond to changes in circumstances and established mechanisms to appeal against specific decisions
Consistency	Policies should be consistently applied regardless of the individuals involved
Inclusiveness	People who are affected by policies should be involved in the processes of developing those policies
Accountability	Clinicians whose patients are affected by the process need every opportunity to appeal against decisions Managers and administrators need to have details of the resources available, the processes used to allocate those resources

need to review both the basis and the processes used for resource allocation both within and between countries.

The principles generally considered in biomedical ethics (51) include respect for autonomy, non-maleficence, beneficence, and justice. It may be useful to consider the implications of these principles when applied at different levels of the health service delivery (**Table 4**).

Kass (52) proposed that the following questions should be asked when evaluating potential public health interventions:

What are the goals of the proposed program (this includes both the overall goals and the short-term goals) and in particular who will benefit from this intervention?
How effective is the program at achieving the stated goals?
What are the known or the potential burdens of the program?
Can the burdens be minimized or are there alternative approaches?
Is the program administered fairly?
How can the benefits and burdens of the program be fairly balanced?

What Are the Goals of the Proposed Program (This Includes Both the Overall Goals and the Short-Term Goals) and in Particular Who Will Benefit From This Intervention?

If one considers the possibility of pediatric intensive care in LICs, the overall goal would be a reduction in mortality, and the short-term goal would be more effective resuscitation of critically ill children presenting to the health-care services. The costs of pediatric intensive care may be particularly high (including the entire system of staffing, equipment, and support structures). At best, the introduction of pediatric intensive care services will benefit the small number of children who have already accessed health-care services and have access to the intensive care. By contrast, a wider definition of critical care (53), which includes the process of providing care to all children with life-threatening injury and/or illness, would have the potential to affect a much wider group of children and potentially at a much lower cost per child.

How Effective Is the Program at Achieving the Stated Goals?

It is possible to extrapolate from international data to the possible impact of HCC, but outcomes may be very different in LIMCs. In the setting of cardiac surgery in Guatemala, the outcomes were initially worse than expected and took time and considerable investment to improve, despite the presence of surgeons with considerable experience and training in the USA (54). There is also evidence that the establishment of international quality intervention program may lead to substantial improvements in outcomes from high-cost procedures as demonstrated in pediatric cardiac surgery (55).

The provision of PICU is very unlikely to make a substantial impact on the mortality of children in LICs where there are numerous deaths and at best extremely limited resources available for PICU. In middle-income countries, there is much more likelihood of PICU making an impact on pediatric mortality. There is also the consideration that the training of personnel for services such as PICU may take many years, and thus it may be worth considering the introduction of PICU and investing in personnel training some time before it is likely to be implemented within a region.

There is certainly evidence that over time, the introduction of relatively HCC has improved outcomes in a number of settings (56, 57), particularly for oncological problems. There is also evidence that HCC in LICs can improve over a period of time (47).

A particular challenge for HCC is the requirement of most HCCs for ancillary disciplines including anesthesia (58, 59), pediatric surgery (59), medical imaging, etc.—each of these services is frequently required to implement HCC, and all are under pressure, individual HCC may be difficult to implement.

It is also essential to consider the place of the HCC within the overall context of the health services within that country. Particular in areas such as the care of critically ill children, the overall outcome will depend on the entire "pathway" of care and not simply on the intensive care component (13, 60).

One of the potential consequences of the differentials between private and public health care in LMICs is that both sectors may have a limited benefit from HCC. In the private sector, the limited number of people having access may limit the experience and expertise that can be achieved by therapeutic teams, while the majority of patients simply do not have access. In addition, the movement of expertise for HCC from the public to the private sector may further compromise the quality of care in the public sector.

What Are the Known or the Potential Burdens of the Program?

The direct burden of HCC such as pediatric intensive care relates to the consumption of resources (financial and personnel) within the context of limited resources. An indirect burden of HCC such as pediatric intensive care is the large burden of illness and handicap that may affect both the children who survive PICU (61–63) and their parents (64). This may be extremely problematic in settings where long-term support and rehabilitation are poorly available. Thus, decision making within the HCC environment may include the need to limit interventions at levels that would not usually be considered appropriate in HICs.

A significant potential burden of HCC is the impact of that allocation of resources on other services. In situations where there are relatively rich resources, the implementation of HCC may have a very little impact on other services. Sadly, in LICs, the development of HCC is inevitably going to compromise care in some other area of the system, and it is essential that that impact is recognized, assessed, and included in the overall evaluation process.

A major factor in providing pediatric intensive care services within LMICs [or during disaster events (65)] is the process of developing reasonable strategies to allocate those resources (66), and it is important to consider how this problem will be addressed.

Can the Burdens Be Minimized or Are There Alternative Approaches?

The burdens of HCC can be limited or minimized by strict definitions and decision making around what services can and should be provided and to whom. Ideally, the process of decision making should be transparent and public (66). One potential approach to the process of resource allocation, and particularly the allocation of resources to relatively expensive services such as intensive care is the accountability for reasonableness (A4R) process that was initially described in Canada (67).

As suggested above, it is also important to consider whether in fact less expensive care could be utilized to achieve the same or better outcomes. It has been well demonstrated in several settings that the use of "lower" technology such as nasal cPAP for severe bronchiolitis was associated with both lower costs and better outcomes (68).

Is the Program Administered Fairly?

This question can be addressed at different phases. Initially, it may be important to carefully consider whether there are individuals or groups of people who are not receiving an equitable opportunity to access the HCC services. It may initially be possible to identify groups of people who for particular reasons (including geography) will not be able to access certain services as easily as others. There are also situations where it is clearly not possible to provide all care to all people (69, 70), and decisions have to made as to what therapy can and should be made available. Ideally, the processes for the allocation of the resources should be agreed to in a process involving the communities affected by those services (66). Generally, those processes will need to have characteristics such as accountability and transparency (see **Table 5**).

In the longer term, the question can only be fully answered if data are collected on who actually utilized the services and what outcomes were achieved. Carefully collected data provide the only real way in which the impact of a service can be assessed. Inherently, data capture should include not only information on those who accessed a service but also data on those who perhaps could or should have accessed those services.

How Can the Benefits and Burdens of the Program Be Fairly Balanced?

The benefits of the program can be considered at the individual level. Guidelines for the provision of life-sustaining care in neonates (71), children (72), and adults (73) in HICs have highlighted the need to act in the best interests of the patient at all times. Clearly, there are situations where the application of HCC may actually prolong suffering, and there would be a substantial (although not universal) agreement that this should be avoided.

The training of health-care workers may be substantially affected by decisions made regarding HCC that will be offered in a particular region. The training required to offer HCC such as intensive care is potentially both time-consuming and expensive. The provision of training to health-care workers without a commitment to support the HCC is likely to lead to frustration and in many cases the migration of health-care workers to richer parts of the world. However, lack of opportunities to undergo training and implement therapies (such as surgery and anesthesia) may also lead to medical migration-associated health-care problems.

Decision making around the utilization of high-cost care may affect a number of people including the patient and the family, health-care workers, hospital and health-care managers, and politicians and people involved with the formulation and administration of policy at a provincial and/or national level. With the exponential growth of global health programs in areas such as North America, there are also an increasing number of people outside of the countries who have an interest and sometimes incentives (financial and otherwise) in changing the provision of HCC in LICs and LMICs.

A crucial aspect of balancing burdens and benefits relates to the standards that are expected and applied in the development of the HCC. Programs that have implemented oncology training and services in LIMCs have had to make decisions about the level of services that could safely be provided in those settings (74). The only way in which the impact of interventions can be monitored is by the collection of the appropriate data (both in the HCC service and in the services that are potentially affected) (45, 75). Bhutta (76) has highlighted the need (in research) to consider the realities and constraints in the countries where the research or clinical services being considered have to be implemented. In the setting of resource constraints, the actual care currently available and the risks that would be acceptable in clinical care may be very different to those where other resources are available.

The only way to address potential and actual ethical concerns in this setting is to make sure that information regarding who is involved in the process of providing the HCC must be clearly available to all the people involved in the process. In addition, the allocation of resources to data collection and interpretation is the only way in which it is possible to assess the impact of HCC and interventions. The allocation of limited resources to this monitoring may seem a relatively low priority, but in the longer term, it is the only way in which interventions can be assessed and thus provides a rational basis for ongoing decision making.

PROCESSES OF DECISION MAKING

In an ideal system, decisions regarding the implementation of health-care policies would be made: in a coherent way at every level of policy making (**Table 4**), by people with a clear understanding of both the costs and the achievable benefits of high-cost interventions (particularly relative to other lower cost interventions), and in a way that involves and takes into account the wishes and concerns of the people who are affected by those decisions and policies. Particular concerns in LICs are processes required to develop the expertise and organization structures (77) that are locally available. International groupings and organizations may be able to make a contribution in this regard.

It may be particularly challenging to address the relative contributions of managers in health-care systems to decision making. In the South African context, it has been pointed out that while there are substantially higher resources per capita in the private health-care system, much of those resources come from the contributions of the people who benefit from that system. If in an LIC, richer people are effectively paying for their own health services, is there a reasonable case to allow that? In that setting, it may be crucial to develop a detailed understanding of the proportion of the real costs that the public sector is bearing (including training costs, tax rebates, etc). It may also be critical to consider collaborative efforts to bring about mutually beneficial outcomes (78, 79), although these may be associated with risks.

Internationally, support for the collection of accurate data regarding the costs and outcomes of HCC for children in LMICs could provide a substantial evidence base for decision making in those areas. Importantly, the data collection should include the specifics of local contexts as far as possible.

A number of authors have addressed the processes that may be involved, with particular support for the use of the A4R approach (66, 80–83). There is strong evidence that this approach may be useful in addressing a range of health-care dilemmas (including access to HCC such as dialysis). However, there is a real need for ongoing research into decision-making processes in LIMCs (84, 85). Underlying that research is the need for a deeper understanding of the values that need to be incorporated into decision making (and which are not universally agreed to) (6, 7).

CONCLUSION

Ethical decision making around the provision of HCC pediatric care in LMICs and LICs may be a complex process which requires a deep understanding of the context and the implications of any intervention. At the very least, the process needs to incorporate a realistic assessment of the context, the resources (both available and required), and the likely impact of the provision of that care. There is a very real risk that the implementation of high-cost pediatric care may have relatively poor outcomes, and even worse, the utilization of resources in this way may compromise other services with adverse outcomes for many children.

Ideally, all decision making should be transparent and should involve all the communities who are likely to be affected by those decisions. Frameworks from the public health environment may provide a useful addition to the standard bioethical approach.

AUTHOR CONTRIBUTIONS

The author confirms being the sole contributor of this work and approved it for publication.

REFERENCES

1. World Health Organisation. *Children: Reducing Mortality (Fact sheet Updated October 2017) [Online]*. World Health Organisation (2017). Available from: http://www.who.int/mediacentre/factsheets/fs178/en/ (accessed October 27, 2017).
2. Amouzou A, Kozuki N, Gwatkin DR. Where is the gap?: the contribution of disparities within developing countries to global inequalities in under-five mortality. *BMC Public Health* (2014) 14:216. doi:10.1186/1471-2458-14-216
3. Blendon RJ, Schoen C, DesRoches CM, Osborn R, Scoles KL, Zapert K. Inequities in health care: a five-country survey. *Health Aff (Millwood)* (2002) 21(3):182–91. doi:10.1377/hlthaff.21.3.182
4. Braveman P, Tarimo E. Social inequalities in health within countries: not only an issue for affluent nations. *Soc Sci Med* (2002) 54(11):1621–35. doi:10.1016/S0277-9536(01)00331-8
5. Dondorp AM, Iyer SS, Schultz MJ. Critical care in resource-restricted settings. *JAMA* (2016) 315(8):753–4. doi:10.1001/jama.2016.0976

6. Engelhardt HT Jr. Critical care: why there is no global bioethics. *J Med Philos* (1998) 23(6):643–51. doi:10.1076/jmep.23.6.643.2555
7. Engelhardt HT Jr. Critical care: why there is no global bioethics. *Curr Opin Crit Care* (2005) 11(6):605–9. doi:10.1097/01.ccx.0000184166.10121.c1
8. *World Bank Database [Online]*. (2017). Available from: http://databank.worldbank.org/data/reports.aspx?source=health-nutrition-and-population-statistics::x00023 (accessed October 26, 2017).
9. Dunser MW, Festic E, Dondorp A, Kissoon N, Ganbat T, Kwizera A, et al. Recommendations for sepsis management in resource-limited settings. *Intensive Care Med* (2012) 38(4):557–74. doi:10.1007/s00134-012-2468-5
10. Dondorp AM, Haniffa R. Critical care and severe sepsis in resource poor settings. *Trans R Soc Trop Med Hyg* (2014) 108(8):453–4. doi:10.1093/trstmh/tru099
11. Meier B, Staton C. Sepsis resuscitation in resource-limited settings. *Emerg Med Clin North Am* (2017) 35(1):159–73. doi:10.1016/j.emc.2016.08.004
12. Papali A, McCurdy MT, Calvello EJ. A "three delays" model for severe sepsis in resource-limited countries. *J Crit Care* (2015) 30(4):e869–814. doi:10.1016/j.jcrc.2015.04.003
13. Hodkinson P, Argent A, Wallis L, Reid S, Perera R, Harrison S, et al. Pathways to care for critically Ill or injured children: a cohort study from first presentation to healthcare services through to admission to intensive care or death. *PLoS One* (2016) 11(1):e0145473. doi:10.1371/journal.pone.0145473
14. Turner EL, Nielsen KR, Jamal SM, von Saint Andre-von Arnim A, Musa NL. A review of pediatric critical care in resource-limited settings: a look at past, present, and future directions. *Front Pediatr* (2016) 4:5. doi:10.3389/fped.2016.00005
15. Hsia RY, Mbembati NA, Macfarlane S, Kruk ME. Access to emergency and surgical care in sub-Saharan Africa: the infrastructure gap. *Health Policy Plan* (2012) 27(3):234–44. doi:10.1093/heapol/czr023
16. Leligdowicz A, Fischer WA II, Uyeki TM, Fletcher TE, Adhikari NK, Portella G, et al. Ebola virus disease and critical illness. *Crit Care* (2016) 20(1):217. doi:10.1186/s13054-016-1325-2
17. Baker T. Critical care in low-income countries. *Trop Med Int Health* (2009) 14(2):143–8. doi:10.1111/j.1365-3156.2008.02202.x
18. Kulkarni AP, Divatia JV. A prospective audit of costs of intensive care in cancer patients in India. *Indian J Crit Care Med* (2013) 17(5):292–7. doi:10.4103/0972-5229.120321
19. Miljeteig I, Johansson KA, Sayeed SA, Norheim OF. End-of-life decisions as bedside rationing. An ethical analysis of life support restrictions in an Indian neonatal unit. *J Med Ethics* (2010) 36(8):473–8. doi:10.1136/jme.2010.035535
20. Vida VL, Barnoya J, O'Connell M, Leon-Wyss J, Larrazabal LA, Castaneda AR. Surgical versus percutaneous occlusion of ostium secundum atrial septal defects: results and cost-effective considerations in a low-income country. *J Am Coll Cardiol* (2006) 47(2):326–31. doi:10.1016/j.jacc.2005.06.086
21. Beerenahally TS. No free bed with ventilator: experience of a public health specialist. *Indian J Med Ethics* (2017) 2(1):56–7. doi:10.20529/ijme.2017.011
22. Dalal A, Czosek RJ, Kovach J, von Alvensleben JC, Valdes S, Etheridge SP, et al. Clinical presentation of pediatric patients at risk for sudden cardiac arrest. *J Pediatr* (2016) 177:191–6. doi:10.1016/j.jpeds.2016.06.088
23. Bhagwanjee S, Scribante J. National audit of critical care resources in South Africa—unit and bed distribution. *S Afr Med J* (2007) 97(12 Pt 3):1311–4.
24. Mostert S, Njuguna F, Olbara G, Sindano S, Sitaresmi MN, Supriyadi E, et al. Corruption in health-care systems and its effect on cancer care in Africa. *Lancet Oncol* (2015) 16(8):e394–404. doi:10.1016/s1470-2045(15)00163-1
25. Aluttis C, Bishaw T, Frank MW. The workforce for health in a globalized context—global shortages and international migration. *Glob Health Action* (2014) 7:23611. doi:10.3402/gha.v7.23611
26. Lalchandani P, Dunn JC. Global comparison of pediatric surgery workforce and training. *J Pediatr Surg* (2015) 50(7):1180–3. doi:10.1016/j.jpedsurg.2014.11.032
27. Toobaie A, Emil S, Ozgediz D, Krishnaswami S, Poenaru D. Pediatric surgical capacity in Africa: current status and future needs. *J Pediatr Surg* (2017) 52(5):843–8. doi:10.1016/j.jpedsurg.2017.01.033
28. Hoyler M, Finlayson SR, McClain CD, Meara JG, Hagander L. Shortage of doctors, shortage of data: a review of the global surgery, obstetrics, and anesthesia workforce literature. *World J Surg* (2014) 38(2):269–80. doi:10.1007/s00268-013-2324-y
29. Jesus TS, Landry MD, Dussault G, Fronteira I. Human resources for health (and rehabilitation): six rehab-workforce challenges for the century. *Hum Resour Health* (2017) 15(1):8. doi:10.1186/s12960-017-0182-7
30. Bertone MP, Witter S. The complex remuneration of human resources for health in low-income settings: policy implications and a research agenda for designing effective financial incentives. *Hum Resour Health* (2015) 13:62. doi:10.1186/s12960-015-0058-7
31. Baker T, Lugazia E, Eriksen J, Mwafongo V, Irestedt L, Konrad D. Emergency and critical care services in Tanzania: a survey of ten hospitals. *BMC Health Serv Res* (2013) 13:140. doi:10.1186/1472-6963-13-140
32. Tyler A, McLeod L, Beaty B, Juarez-Colunga E, Birkholz M, Hyman D, et al. Variation in inpatient croup management and outcomes. *Pediatrics* (2017) 139(4):e20163582. doi:10.1542/peds.2016-3582
33. Sri-udomkajorn S, Suwannachote S. Demographics, clinical features, outcome and prognostic factors of Guillain–Barre syndrome in Thai children. *J Med Assoc Thai* (2014) 97(Suppl 6):S101–7.
34. Barzegar M, Toopchizadeh V, Maher MHK, Sadeghi P, Jahanjoo F, Pishgahi A. Predictive factors for achieving independent walking in children with Guillain–Barre syndrome. *Pediatr Res* (2017) 82(2):333–9. doi:10.1038/pr.2017.67
35. van der Pijl J, Wilmshurst JM, van Dijk M, Argent A, Booth J, Zampoli M. Acute flaccid paralysis in South African children: causes, respiratory complications and neurological outcome. *J Paediatr Child Health* (2017) 54(3):247–53. doi:10.1111/jpc.13709
36. English L, Kumbakumba E, Larson CP, Kabakyenga J, Singer J, Kissoon N, et al. Pediatric out-of-hospital deaths following hospital discharge: a mixed-methods study. *Afr Health Sci* (2016) 16(4):883–91. doi:10.4314/ahs.v16i4.2
37. Chisti MJ, Graham SM, Duke T, Ahmed T, Faruque AS, Ashraf H, et al. Post-discharge mortality in children with severe malnutrition and pneumonia in Bangladesh. *PLoS One* (2014) 9(9):e107663. doi:10.1371/journal.pone.0107663
38. Nasr VG, Faraoni D, Valente AM, DiNardo JA. Outcomes and costs of cardiac surgery in adults with congenital heart disease. *Pediatr Cardiol* (2017) 38(7):1359–64. doi:10.1007/s00246-017-1669-7
39. Zuhlke L, Karthikeyan G, Engel ME, Rangarajan S, Mackie P, Cupido-Katya Mauff B, et al. Clinical outcomes in 3343 children and adults with rheumatic heart disease from 14 low- and middle-income countries: two-year follow-up of the global rheumatic heart disease registry (the REMEDY study). *Circulation* (2016) 134(19):1456–66. doi:10.1161/circulationaha.116.024769
40. Bhutta ZA, Zaidi AK, Thaver D, Humayun Q, Ali S, Darmstadt GL. Management of newborn infections in primary care settings: a review of the evidence and implications for policy? *Pediatr Infect Dis J* (2009) 28(1 Suppl):S22–30. doi:10.1097/INF.0b013e31819588ac
41. Duke T, Wandi F, Jonathan M, Matai S, Kaupa M, Saavu M, et al. Improved oxygen systems for childhood pneumonia: a multihospital effectiveness study in Papua New Guinea. *Lancet* (2008) 372(9646):1328–33. doi:10.1016/s0140-6736(08)61164-2
42. Chisti MJ, Salam MA, Smith JH, Ahmed T, Pietroni MA, Shahunja KM, et al. Bubble continuous positive airway pressure for children with severe pneumonia and hypoxaemia in Bangladesh: an open, randomised controlled trial. *Lancet* (2015) 386(9998):1057–65. doi:10.1016/s0140-6736(15)60249-5
43. Wilson PT, Baiden F, Brooks JC, Morris MC, Giessler K, Punguyire D, et al. Continuous positive airway pressure for children with undifferentiated respiratory distress in Ghana: an open-label, cluster, crossover trial. *Lancet Glob Health* (2017) 5(6):e615–23. doi:10.1016/s2214-109x(17)30145-6
44. Molyneux E, Ahmad S, Robertson A. Improved triage and emergency care for children reduces inpatient mortality in a resource-constrained setting. *Bull World Health Organ* (2006) 84(4):314–9. doi:10.2471/BLT.04.019505
45. Rezzonico R, Caccamo LM, Manfredini V, Cartabia M, Sanchez N, Paredes Z, et al. Impact of the systematic introduction of low-cost bubble nasal CPAP in a NICU of a developing country: a prospective pre- and post-intervention study. *BMC Pediatr* (2015) 15:26. doi:10.1186/s12887-015-0338-3
46. Mukhtar B, Siddiqui NR, Haque A. Clinical characteristics and immediate-outcome of children mechanically ventilated in PICU of pakistan. *Pak J Med Sci* (2014) 30(5):927–30. doi:10.12669/pjms.305.5159

47. Khanal A, Sharma A, Basnet S. Current state of pediatric intensive care and high dependency care in Nepal. *Pediatr Crit Care Med* (2016) 17(11):1032–40. doi:10.1097/pcc.0000000000000938
48. Pollach G, Namboya F. Preventing intensive care admissions for sepsis in tropical Africa (PICASTA): an extension of the international pediatric global sepsis initiative: an African perspective. *Pediatr Crit Care Med* (2013) 14(6):561–70. doi:10.1097/PCC.0b013e318291774b
49. Rosenthal VD, Pawar M, Leblebicioglu H, Navoa-Ng JA, Villamil-Gomez W, Armas-Ruiz A, et al. Impact of the International Nosocomial Infection Control Consortium (INICC) multidimensional hand hygiene approach over 13 years in 51 cities of 19 limited-resource countries from Latin America, Asia, the Middle East, and Europe. *Infect Control Hosp Epidemiol* (2013) 34(4): 415–23. doi:10.1086/669860
50. Shann F, Argent AC, Ranjit S. Pediatric intensive care in developing countries. 4th ed. In: Fuhrman BP, Zimmerman JJ, editors. *Pediatric Critical Care*. Philadelphia: Elsevier Health Science (2011). p. 164–78.
51. Beauchamp TL, Childress JF. *Principles of Biomedical Ethics*. Oxford: Oxford University Press (2013).
52. Kass NE. An ethics framework for public health. *Am J Public Health* (2001) 91(11):1776–82. doi:10.2105/AJPH.91.11.1776
53. Kissoon N, Argent A, Devictor D, Madden MA, Singhi S, van der Voort E, et al. World federation of pediatric intensive and critical care societies-its global agenda. *Pediatr Crit Care Med* (2009) 10(5):597–600. doi:10.1097/PCC.0b013e3181a704c6
54. Leon-Wyss JR, Veshti A, Veras O, Gaitan GA, O'Connell M, Mack RA, et al. Pediatric cardiac surgery: a challenge and outcome analysis of the Guatemala effort. *Semin Thorac Cardiovasc Surg Pediatr Card Surg Annu* (2009) 12(1):8–11. doi:10.1053/j.pcsu.2009.01.003
55. Jenkins KJ, Castaneda AR, Cherian KM, Couser CA, Dale EK, Gauvreau K, et al. Reducing mortality and infections after congenital heart surgery in the developing world. *Pediatrics* (2014) 134(5):e1422–30. doi:10.1542/peds.2014-0356
56. Samudio A, Figueredo D, Lassaletta A, Zelada O, Peris A, Bogado Yinde L, et al. Building a national pediatric cancer center and network in Paraguay: lessons for addressing challenges in a low-income country. *J Pediatr Hematol Oncol* (2015) 37(5):383–90. doi:10.1097/mph.0000000000000338
57. Molyneux E, Scanlan T, Chagaluka G, Renner L. Haematological cancers in African children: progress and challenges. *Br J Haematol* (2017) 177(6):971–8. doi:10.1111/bjh.14617
58. Notrica MR, Evans FM, Knowlton LM, Kelly McQueen KA. Rwandan surgical and anesthesia infrastructure: a survey of district hospitals. *World J Surg* (2011) 35(8):1770–80. doi:10.1007/s00268-011-1125-4
59. Butler M, Drum E, Evans FM, Fitzgerald T, Fraser J, Holterman AX, et al. Guidelines and checklists for short-term missions in global pediatric surgery: recommendations from the American Academy of Pediatrics Delivery of Surgical Care Global Health Subcommittee, American Pediatric Surgical Association Global Pediatric Surgery Committee, Society for Pediatric Anesthesia Committee on International Education and Service, and American Pediatric Surgical Nurses Association, Inc. Global Health Special Interest Group. *J Pediatr Surg* (2017). doi:10.1016/j.jpedsurg.2017.11.037
60. Jones CH, Ward A, Hodkinson PW, Reid SJ, Wallis LA, Harrison S, et al. Caregivers' experiences of pathways to care for seriously Ill children in Cape Town, South Africa: a qualitative investigation. *PLoS One* (2016) 11(3):e0151606. doi:10.1371/journal.pone.0151606
61. Als LC, Picouto MD, Hau SM, Nadel S, Cooper M, Pierce CM, et al. Mental and physical well-being following admission to pediatric intensive care. *Pediatr Crit Care Med* (2015) 16(5):e141–9. doi:10.1097/pcc.0000000000000424
62. Aspesberro F, Mangione-Smith R, Zimmerman JJ. Health-related quality of life following pediatric critical illness. *Intensive Care Med* (2015) 41(7):1235–46. doi:10.1007/s00134-015-3780-7
63. Ong C, Lee JH, Leow MK, Puthucheary ZA. Functional outcomes and physical impairments in pediatric critical care survivors: a scoping review. *Pediatr Crit Care Med* (2016) 17(5):e247–59. doi:10.1097/pcc.0000000000000706
64. Balluffi A, Kassam-Adams N, Kazak A, Tucker M, Dominguez T, Helfaer M. Traumatic stress in parents of children admitted to the pediatric intensive care unit. *Pediatr Crit Care Med* (2004) 5(6):547–53. doi:10.1097/01.pcc.0000137354.19807.44
65. Burkle FM Jr, Argent AC, Kissoon N. The reality of pediatric emergency mass critical care in the developing world. *Pediatr Crit Care Med* (2011) 12(6 Suppl):S169–79. doi:10.1097/PCC.0b013e318234a906
66. Argent AC, Ahrens J, Morrow BM, Reynolds LG, Hatherill M, Salie S, et al. Pediatric intensive care in South Africa: an account of making optimum use of limited resources at the Red Cross War Memorial Children's Hospital*. *Pediatr Crit Care Med* (2014) 15(1):7–14. doi:10.1097/pcc.0000000000000029
67. Daniels N. Decisions about access to health care and accountability for reasonableness. *J Urban Health* (1999) 76(2):176–91. doi:10.1007/bf02344674
68. Essouri S, Laurent M, Chevret L, Durand P, Ecochard E, Gajdos V, et al. Improved clinical and economic outcomes in severe bronchiolitis with pre-emptive nCPAP ventilatory strategy. *Intensive Care Med* (2014) 40(1): 84–91. doi:10.1007/s00134-013-3129-z
69. Jeena PM, McNally LM, Stobie M, Coovadia HM, Adhikari MA, Petros AJ. Challenges in the provision of ICU services to HIV infected children in resource poor settings: a South African case study. *J Med Ethics* (2005) 31(4):226–30. doi:10.1136/jme.2003.004010
70. Thiagraj Soobramoney *v.* Minster Of Health (Kwazulu-Natal). *South African Constitutional Court*. Case CCT 32/97. (1998).
71. Nuffield Council on Bioethics. *Critical Care Decisions in Fetal and Neonatal Medicine: Ethical Issues*. London: Nuffield Council on Bioethics (2006).
72. Inwald D. The best interests test at the end of life on PICU: a plea for a family centred approach. *Arch Dis Child* (2008) 93(3):248–50. doi:10.1136/adc.2006.111120
73. Curtis JR, Vincent JL. Ethics and end-of-life care for adults in the intensive care unit. *Lancet* (2010) 376(9749):1347–53. doi:10.1016/s0140-6736(10)60143-2
74. Gupta S, Rivera-Luna R, Ribeiro RC, Howard SC. Pediatric oncology as the next global child health priority: the need for national childhood cancer strategies in low- and middle-income countries. *PLoS Med* (2014) 11(6):e1001656. doi:10.1371/journal.pmed.1001656
75. Zonneveld R, Holband N, Bertolini A, Bardi F, Lissone NPA, Dijk PH, et al. Improved referral and survival of newborns after scaling up of intensive care in Suriname. *BMC Pediatr* (2017) 17(1):189. doi:10.1186/s12887-017-0941-6
76. Bhutta ZA. Ethics in international health research: a perspective from the developing world. *Bull World Health Organ* (2002) 80(2):114–20.
77. Swanson RC, Atun R, Best A, Betigeri A, de Campos F, Chunharas S, et al. Strengthening health systems in low-income countries by enhancing organizational capacities and improving institutions. *Global Health* (2015) 11:5. doi:10.1186/s12992-015-0090-3
78. Kula N, Fryatt RJ. Public-private interactions on health in South Africa: opportunities for scaling up. *Health Policy Plan* (2014) 29(5):560–9. doi:10.1093/heapol/czt042
79. Rasanathan K, Bennett S, Atkins V, Beschel R, Carrasquilla G, Charles J, et al. Governing multisectoral action for health in low- and middle-income countries. *PLoS Med* (2017) 14(4):e1002285. doi:10.1371/journal.pmed.1002285
80. Maluka S, Kamuzora P, San Sebastian M, Byskov J, Ndawi B, Hurtig AK. Improving district level health planning and priority setting in Tanzania through implementing accountability for reasonableness framework: perceptions of stakeholders. *BMC Health Serv Res* (2010) 10:322. doi:10.1186/1472-6963-10-322
81. Maluka S, Kamuzora P, San Sebastian M, Byskov J, Olsen OE, Shayo E, et al. Decentralized health care priority-setting in Tanzania: evaluating against the accountability for reasonableness framework. *Soc Sci Med* (2010) 71(4):751–9. doi:10.1016/j.socscimed.2010.04.035
82. Maluka S, Kamuzora P, Sansebastian M, Byskov J, Ndawi B, Olsen OE, et al. Implementing accountability for reasonableness framework at district level in Tanzania: a realist evaluation. *Implement Sci* (2011) 6:11. doi:10.1186/1748-5908-6-11
83. Moosa MR, Maree JD, Chirehwa MT, Benatar SR. Use of the 'accountability for reasonableness' approach to improve fairness in accessing dialysis in a middle-income country. *PLoS One* (2016) 11(10):e0164201. doi:10.1371/journal.pone.0164201
84. Byskov J, Bloch P, Blystad A, Hurtig AK, Fylkesnes K, Kamuzora P, et al. Accountable priority setting for trust in health systems – the need for research into a new approach for strengthening sustainable health action in developing countries. *Health Res Policy Syst* (2009) 7:23. doi:10.1186/1478-4505-7-23

24

Clinical and Pathological Correlation in Pediatric Invasive Pulmonary Aspergillosis

Nattachai Anantasit[1,2]*, *Noramon Nuntacharruksa*[1], *Pimpin Incharoen*[3] *and Aroonwan Preutthipan*[1]

[1] Division of Pediatric Pulmonology, Department of Pediatric, Faculty of Medicine, Ramathibodi Hospital, Mahidol University, Bangkok, Thailand, [2] Division of Pediatric Critical Care, Department of Pediatric, Faculty of Medicine, Ramathibodi Hospital, Mahidol University, Bangkok, Thailand, [3] Department of Pathology, Faculty of Medicine, Ramathibodi Hospital, Mahidol University, Bangkok, Thailand

Correspondence:
Nattachai Anantasit
nattachai032@hotmail.com

Introduction: Invasive' pulmonary aspergillosis (IPA) has been one of the major causes of mortality in immunocompromised patients. The gold standard method for a diagnosis of IPA is histopathological examination of the lung tissue; however, post-procedural bleeding limits the feasibility of lung biopsy. The European Organization for Research and Treatment of Cancer/Invasive Fungal Infections Cooperative Group and The National Institute of Allergy and Infectious Disease Mycoses Study Group (EORTC/MSG) defined IPA. The objective of this study was to validate the EORTC/MSG 2008 definition of IPA, compared with histopathology in the pediatric population.

Methods: Histopathological examinations of lung tissues of children aged 1 month–18 years with respiratory tract infection at the time of obtaining biopsy were retrieved. Retrospective chart reviews for clinical characteristics were performed. IPA diagnosis was classified according to the EORTC/MSG 2008 definition.

Results: During the 10-year period, there were 256 lung tissues, of which 58 specimens were suspected to have pulmonary infection. Fourteen patients (24%) were noted to have IPA. Seven patients (50%) with proven IPA were classified as probable, while the remaining 50% were classified as possible, and none were classified as no IPA, by using EORTC/MSG 2008 definition. Other 44 specimens demonstrated 14 (32%), 14 (32%), and 16 (36%) were classified as probable, possible, and no IPA, respectively. When comparing probable or possible IPA with no IPA, we found that the EORTC/MSG 2008 definition had 100% sensitivity, 36% specificity, 33% positive predictive value, and 100% negative predictive value in diagnosis of IPA.

Conclusion: Our study illustrated that the EORTC/MSG 2008 definition provided an excellent sensitivity but low specificity for diagnosing IPA.

Keywords: invasive pulmonary aspergillosis, pediatric, histopathology, definition, sensitivity

INTRODUCTION

Invasive pulmonary aspergillosis (IPA) has been one of the major causes of mortality in immunocompromised patients, such as malignancy, hematopoietic stem cell transplantation, and prolonged usage of immunosuppressive agents. Early diagnosis and prompt treatment improve survival outcome (1, 2). Aspergillus species are ubiquitous in the environment. Aspergillus fumigatus is the most common species in IPA (3, 4). Other species include Aspergillus flavus, Aspergillus niger, and Aspergillus terreus. Aspergillus is introduced to the lower respiratory tract by inhalation of the infectious spores. In healthy hosts, spores are eliminated by mucociliary clearance and immune defense. In immunocompromised patients, dormant spores convert into growing hyphal elements and invade lung parenchyma and vascular structure (1). Clinical symptoms and signs of IPA are indistinguishable from other pathogens causing pneumonia. Chest radiography is also non-specific. Therefore, the diagnostic tool is challenging (5, 6).

The gold standard method in the diagnosis of IPA is histopathological examination of lung tissue obtained by bronchoscopy or open thoracotomy. The presence of angioinvasion by acute angle, branching septate fungal hyphae along with a positive culture for Aspergillus from the same site is diagnostic for IPA (1). However, invasive procedures hinder the possibility of obtaining lung tissues. The angioinvasive nature of Aspergillus and the patient condition such as thrombocytopenia further increase risk of bleeding and other complications.

In 2002, The European Organization for Research and Treatment of Cancer/Invasive Fungal Infections Cooperative Group and The National Institute of Allergy and Infectious Disease Mycoses Study Group (EORTC/MSG) formed a consensus committee to develop a standard definition for invasive fungal infections, including IPA. The definitions were intended for use in the context of clinical and/or epidemiological research, not for clinical decision making (7). These definitions were revised in 2008 due to the advances in diagnostic tools, including galactomannan, beta-D-glucan, and fungal DNA in body fluids by PCR (8, 9). Diagnosis of IPA is challenging, as the clinical symptoms are not specific. There is no single investigation for the diagnosis. IPA carries a high mortality rate if untreated, and delayed treatment can result in death. The ideal diagnostic tool should have high sensitivity for early recognition and treatment. In brief, based on EORTC/MSG 2008 consensus definition, there were three classifications; proven, probable, and possible. Proven IPA requires histopathology with a characteristic of infection and/or a positive culture of specimen from a sterile site. Probable IPA requires the fulfillment of criteria within three categories: host factors, clinical, and mycological criteria. Possible IPA consists of host factors, and clinical criteria without mycological evidence of Aspergillus infection (8). These definitions have been widely used in epidemiological research, and clinical trials for evaluation of new drugs and management strategies. However, they were based on the literature review, which did not include pathological results and was originally for the adult oncological population. To our knowledge, there were limited data about validity of the consensus definition compared with the histopathological diagnosis of IPA especially in the pediatric population. The objective of this study was to validate the EORTC/MSG 2008 consensus definition with the gold standard of histopathological results in pediatric patients.

MATERIALS AND METHODS

Study Design and Purpose

This study was performed in a tertiary care, academic center. We retrospectively analyzed histopathology tissues in children aged 1 month–18 years with clinical suspicion of respiratory tract infection from January 2006 to December 2016. This study was approved by the Institutional Review Board. Patients with congenital lung disease, pulmonary malignancy, and incomplete medical records were excluded. Clinical characteristics, diagnostic tests, treatments, and pathological results were reviewed. Patients were categorized into two groups by the histopathological result as proven IPA and non-proven IPA and were classified according to the EORTC/MSG 2008 consensus definition into three groups (probable, possible, and no IPA) as shown in **Figure 1**.

Definitions

The definition criteria for proven, probable, and possible IPA were shown in **Table 1**.

Proven IPA is characterized by a discrete nodule consisting of necrotic lung tissue with angioinvasion by acute angle, branching septate fungal hyphae or culture positive for Aspergillus spp. from lung tissue specimen (10, 11).

Non-proven IPA is defined as patients who do not meet the pathological criteria.

According to the EORTC/MSG 2008 consensus definition (8), clinical criteria in IPA consists of the presence of one of the following three signs on computer tomography; dense, well-circumscribed lesions with or without a halo sign, air-crescent sign, or cavity.

Positive clinical IPA is defined as patients who have clinical diagnosis with probable or possible IPA by the EORTC/MSG 2008 consensus definition.

Negative clinical IPA is defined as patients who do not meet criteria for diagnosis by the EORTC/MSG 2008 consensus definition.

Galactomannan enzyme immunoassay was measured from serum and bronchoalveolar lavage (BAL) fluid. Results were recorded as an index relative to the mean optical density of the threshold controls (GM index = optical density sample/mean optical density of the threshold control samples). Samples that had an index value >0.5 were considered positive for both serum and BAL fluid specimen (12, 13).

Statistical Methods

SPSS software (version 18.0, SPSS Inc., Chicago, IL, USA) was used for statistical analysis. Patients' demographics, clinical characteristics, and pathological data were analyzed by descriptive analysis using student's t-test and Chi-Square. For the diagnostic test, sensitivity, specificity, positive predictive value, and negative predictive value were obtained. Correlation between clinical diagnosis and pathological result was calculated using Spearman rho correlation analysis. A p-value of less than 0.05 was considered statistically significant.

RESULTS

In total, 256 lung tissues were documented. Fifty-eight pathological specimens revealed suspicion of infectious etiologies, 14 (24%) patients were consistent with proven IPA, and 44 (76%) patients were non-proven IPA as shown in **Figure 1**. All

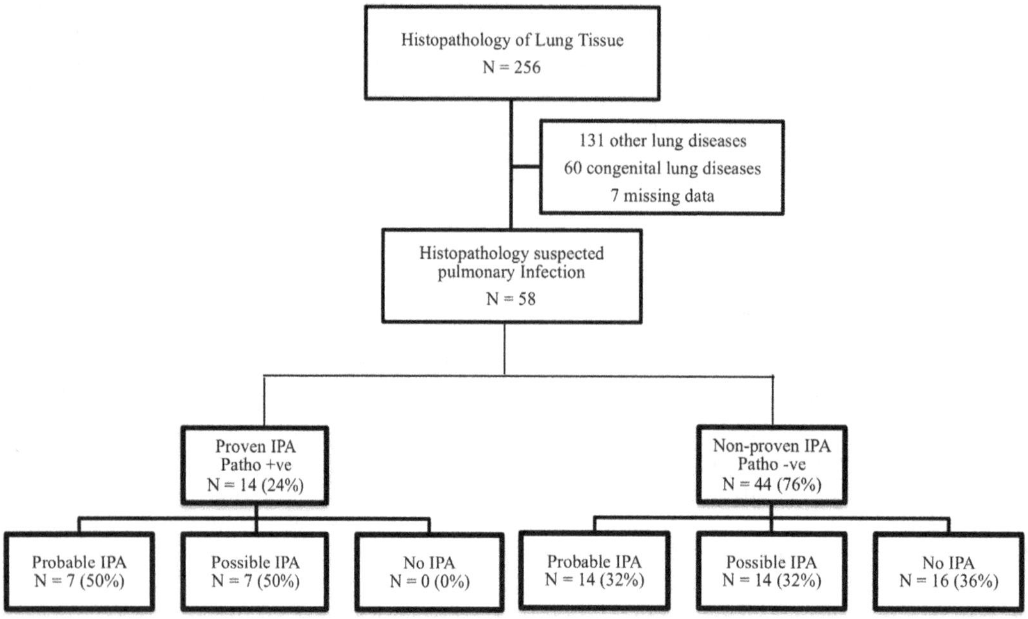

FIGURE 1 | Flow diagram and classification of invasive pulmonary aspergillosis (IPA) according to the EORTC/MSG 2008 consensus definition.

TABLE 1 | The diagnostic criteria for IPA according to the EORTC/MSG 2008 consensus definition (8).

	Proven IPA	Probable IPA	Possible IPA
Positive for histopathological criteria - A discrete nodule consisting of necrotic lung tissue with angioinvasive by acute angle branching septate fungal hyphae or culture positive for Aspergillus spp. from lung tissue specimen	Yes	No	No
Positive for host factor criteria - Neutropenia - Post stem cell transplantation - Prolonged corticosteroid use - Received immunosuppressants - Inherited immunodeficiency		Yes	Yes
Positive for clinical criteria Presence of 1 of the following three signs on CT - Dense, well-circumscribed lesion with or without a halo sign - Air-crescent sign - Cavity		Yes	Yes
Positive for mycological criteria - Positive direct test by culture - Positive indirect tests by galactomannan antigen detection		Yes	No

IPA; invasive pulmonary aspergillosis, CT; computer tomography.

patients who were diagnosed with probable or possible IPA by the EORTC/MSG 2008 definition (positive clinical IPA) received antifungal medications, although 28 out of 42 patients were not diagnosed with proven IPA, but received antifungal medications. Five of 16 patients who were not diagnosed with IPA by the EORTC/MSG 2008 definition (negative clinical IPA) received antifungal medications. None of these patients were diagnosed with proven IPA. The adverse events from antifungal medications were hypokalemia and acute kidney injury, although none of patients required renal replacement therapy. Baseline characteristics of histopathological proven IPA and non-proven IPA were showed in **Table 2**. There was no significant difference of demographic data in both groups. The proven IPA group had significantly more neutropenic patients than the non-proven IPA group (p-value = 0.009). The mean duration of neutropenia was longer in proven IPA than in non-proven IPA group. Mean was 22.1 ± 35.3 days in proven IPA and 12.9 ± 12.5 days in non-proven IPA group (p-value = 0.307).

Microbiology and Pathological Results

Of the 58 lung tissue specimens, 18 lung tissues were obtained by open biopsy, 13 by necropsy, 10 by autopsy, 10 by CT/US guided needle biopsy, and 7 by transbronchial biopsy. The reasons for biopsy were for diagnosis in 28 (48%) patients, no response to antifungal medications or progression of diseases in 20 (35%) patients, and others in 10 (17%) patients. The mean duration from treatment to biopsy was 20.6 and 35.9 days in proven and non-proven IPA group, respectively (p-value = 0.431). The microbiology in non-proven IPA was virus in 7 patients (cytomegalovirus in 6 cases and respiratory syncytial virus in 1 case) and bacteria were found in 10 patients (3 cases were A. baumannii, 2 cases P. aeruginosa, 2 cases Actinomycoses spp.,1 case M. tuberculosis, and 2 cases other bacteria). Fungus was isolated in nine patients (four of Mucormycosis spp., two of Cryptococcosis spp., two of Pneumocystis spp., and 1 of Scedosporiosis spp.). The remaining 12 patients showed histopathologic change without identified pathogens, such as diffused alveolar damage and

TABLE 2 | Baseline characteristics of the included patients.

	Proven IPA (n = 14)	Non-proven IPA (n = 44)	p-Value
Age, mean ± SD	10.4 ± 5.9	9.0 ± 6.1	0.438
Male (%)	4 (29)	21 (48)	0.207
Underlying disease, n (%)			0.064
- Malignancy	12 (86)	19 (43)	
- Primary immune deficiency	0 (0)	6 (14)	
- Connective tissue disease	0 (0)	3 (7)	
- Others	2 (14)	9 (20)	
- Healthy	0 (0)	7 (16)	
Neutropenia, n (%)	11 (79)	17 (39)	0.023*
Post transplantation, n (%)	1 (7)	6 (14)	0.108
Corticosteroid use, n (%)	1 (7)	4 (9)	0.904
Presentation symptom, n (%)			0.343
- Febrile neutropenia	9 (64)	18 (41)	
- Dyspnea	1 (7)	10 (23)	
- Hemoptysis	2 (14)	7 (16)	
- Others	2 (14)	9 (20)	
Serum galactomannan, median (IQR)	0 (0–2.2)	0 (0–1.4)	0.889
BAL galactomannan, median (IQR)	3.4 (1.5–7.5)	2.3 (0–4.0)	0.772
Computer tomography finding, n (%)			0.390
- Dense, well-circumscribed with/without Halo sign	11 (79)	26 (59)	
- Non-specific infiltration/consolidation	2 (14)	9 (21)	
- Air-crescent sign	1 (7)	1 (2)	
- Cavitation	0 (0)	7 (16)	
- Normal finding	0 (0)	1 (2)	
Exposure to beta-lactam antibiotics, n (%)	2 (14.3)	10 (22.7)	0.497
Antifungal treatment, n (%)			0.200
- Amphotericin B	6 (43)	22 (50)	
- Combination drugs	4 (29)	4 (9)	
- Voriconazole	3 (21)	6 (14)	
- Caspofungin	1 (7)	1 (2)	
- No antifungal	0 (0)	11 (25)	
Hospital mortality, n (%)	6 (43)	23 (52)	0.539

IPA; invasive pulmonary aspergillosis, IQR; interquartile range.
**p-Value less than 0.05.*

pulmonary hemorrhage, and 6 patients showed non-infectious histopathology.

EORTC/MSG 2008 Consensus Definition

We analyzed clinical diagnosis of IPA by grouping probable and possible IPA as positive clinical IPA, and no IPA as negative clinical IPA. The sensitivity was 100% and the specificity was 36%. The positive and negative predictive values were 33 and 100%, respectively. Spearman's rho correlation analysis revealed a correlation between clinical diagnosis and pathological result (r = 0.35, p-value = 0.008). **Table 3** demonstrated each element in the EORTC/MSG 2008 consensus definition, in terms of sensitivity, specificity, positive, and negative predictive values.

DISCUSSION

This study validated the EORTC/MSG 2008 consensus definition with the gold standard histopathological tissue in pediatric population. Our results were consistent with previous studies revealing that proven IPA patients were found to be more neutropenic patients. The function of neutrophil is directed against Aspergillus hyphae (14). The neutropenia can increase risk of

TABLE 3 | The sensitivity and specificity of each element in the EORTC/MSG 2008 consensus definition.

	Sensitivity (%)	Specificity (%)	PPV (%)	NPV (%)
- Host risk	100	15.9	27.5	100
- Computer tomography finding	85.7	22.7	26.1	83.3
- Culture	36.4	100	100	81.6
- Serum galactomannan	33.3	68.2	22.2	79
- BAL galactomannan	100	26.7	26.7	100

PPV; positive predictive value, NPV; negative predictive value, BAL; bronchoalveolar lavage.

IPA. A prior study showed that cavitation or air-crescent sign in chest computed tomography is helpful in diagnosing IPA (15). Nevertheless, pediatric studies have demonstrated that nodules or infiltration are the most common radiologic findings in pediatric IPA (16, 17). Our study found no difference in radiologic findings in proven IPA and non-proven IPA groups. We had defined positive imaging as dense, well-circumscribed lesions with or without halo sign, air-crescent sign, or cavitation. The analysis showed high sensitivity but low specificity as in a previous study (18).

Galactomannan is a cell wall polysaccharide released by Aspergillus species during growth (19, 20). Serum galactomannan is more superior than BAL fluid because it is less invasive and provides a higher sensitivity (21). However, our study illustrated that the sensitivity of serum galactomannan was lower than BAL (33 vs. 100%, respectively) which was a similar result to another study (22). We hypothesized that since lungs are a primary site of IPA before angioinvasion may causes an elevation of BAL galactomannan prior to that of serum (23). In our study, the specificity of BAL fluid galactomannan was surprisingly low (27%) compared with previous studies (87.5–94%) using the same cutoff value (20, 24, 25). However, this study had included non-malignant patients which was different from the previous studies. In addition, this could be explained by using different classification as most studies used proven and probable as IPA instead of using histopathology as a gold standard. Another reason could be from the beta-lactam antibiotics. The beta-lactam antibiotics are derived from molds of the genus Penicillium. Galactomannan moieties are shared between Aspergillus and Penicillium species (26). Therefore, beta-lactam antibiotics have been reported to cause false positive of galactomannan.

To our knowledge, this study is the first study to validate the EORTC/MSG 2008 consensus definition in pediatric population with IPA by using histopathological tissues. Although the EORTC/MSG 2008 consensus definition was originally for the adult immunocompromised population. This study showed that the EORTC/MSG 2008 consensus definition had 100% sensitivity, but low specificity (36%), in diagnosing IPA when compared with histopathology in pediatric population. IPA has high mortality if left untreated, our paper showed the EORTC/MSG 2008 consensus definition can be helpful as the screening tool in pediatric populations. Therefore, children with probable or possible IPA according to this definition should be promptly treated with antifungal medications, monitored for adverse events of antifungal medications, and need confirmed diagnosis if there is no clinical response.

This study has some limitations. First, retrospective study might not provide all data needed especially serum and BAL galactomannan. Second, the prevalence of IPA might be underestimated because our study started with histopathological tissue, as we were unable to perform biopsy in every case of suspected IPA. In addition, some patients only underwent imaging guided biopsy or transbronchial biopsy, which might result in inadequate specimen. Therefore, it may not represent all pediatric IPA. The last limitation is that this was a single-center study with small sample size. A larger sample size of these groups would allow better results and analysis.

CONCLUSION

Pediatric IPA is a life-threatening disease with high mortality. The diagnostic tool is an important method to early recognition and prompt treatment. Our study shows that the EORTC/MSG 2008 consensus definition provides an excellent sensitivity as screening tool, but low specificity for the diagnosis of IPA.

ETHICS STATEMENT

This study was carried out in accordance with the recommendations of Committee on human rights related to research involving human subjects, Faculty of Medicine Ramathibodi Hospital, Mahidol University.

AUTHOR CONTRIBUTIONS

NN and NA contributed to design of the study, data collection, data analysis, and manuscript drafting. PI and AP contributed to design of the study. NA critically revised it for important intellectual content. All authors gave final approval of the version to be published.

ACKNOWLEDGMENTS

The authors would like to acknowledge the departments of pediatric and pathology of Ramathibodi Hospital, Mahidol University that allowed us to analyze this project. We would like to thank Dr. Mahippathorn Chinnapha, Associate Professor Pornthep Tanpowpong, and Mr. Stephen Pinder for grammar correction. Furthermore, our special thanks to all patients who were recruited into this study.

REFERENCES

1. Patterson KC, Strek ME. Diagnosis and treatment of pulmonary aspergillosis syndromes. *Chest* (2014) 146:1358–68. doi:10.1378/chest.14-0917
2. Steinbach WJ. Invasive aspergillosis in pediatric patients. *Curr Med Res Opin* (2010) 26:1779–87. doi:10.1185/03007995.2010.487793
3. Perfect JR, Cox GM, Lee JY, Kauffman CA, de Repentigny L, Chapman SW, et al. The impact of culture isolation of Aspergillus species: a hospital-based survey of aspergillosis. *Clin Infect Dis* (2001) 33:1824–33. doi:10.1086/323900
4. Thammahong A, Thayidathara P, Suksawat K, Chindamporn A. Invasive Aspergillus infections in a Thai tertiary-care hospital during 2006–2011. *Adv Microbiol* (2015) 5:298–306. doi:10.4236/aim.2015.55029
5. Kousha M, Tadi R, Soubani AO. Pulmonary aspergillosis: a clinical review. *Eur Respir Rev* (2011) 20:156–74. doi:10.1183/09059180.00001011
6. Thomas KE, Owens CM, Veys PA, Novelli V, Costoli V. The radiological spectrum of invasive aspergillosis in children: a 10-year review. *Pediatr Radiol* (2003) 33:453–60. doi:10.1007/s00247-003-0919-4
7. Ascioglu S, Rex JH, de Pauw B, Bennett JE, Bille J, Crokaert F, et al. Defining opportunistic invasive fungal infections in immunocompromised patients with cancer and hematopoietic stem cell transplants: an international consensus. *Clin Infect Dis* (2002) 34:7–14. doi:10.1086/323335
8. De Pauw B, Walsh TJ, Donnelly JP, Stevens DA, Edwards JE, Calandra T, et al. Revised definitions of invasive fungal disease from the European Organization for Research and Treatment of Cancer/Invasive Fungal Infections Cooperative Group and the National Institute of Allergy and Infectious Disease Mycoses Study Group (EORTC/MSG) consensus group. *Clin Infect Dis* (2008) 46:1813–21. doi:10.1086/588660
9. Tsitsikas DA, Morin A, Araf S, Murtagh B, Johnson G, Vinnicombe S, et al. Impact of the revised (2008) EORTC/MSG definitions for invasive fungal disease on the rates of diagnosis of invasive aspergillosis. *Med Mycol* (2012) 50:538–42. doi:10.3109/13693786.2011.630040
10. Tochigi N, Okubo Y, Ando T, Wakayama M, Shinozaki M, Gocho K, et al. Histopathological implications of Aspergillus infection in lung. *Mediators Inflamm* (2013) 2013:809798. doi:10.1155/2013/809798
11. Hope WW, Walsh TJ, Denning DW. The invasive and saprophytic syndromes due to Aspergillus spp. *Med Mycol* (2005) 43:207–38.
12. Marr KA, Balajee SA, McLaughlin L, Tabouret M, Bentsen C, Walsh TJ. Detection of galactomannan antigenemia by enzyme immunoassay for the diagnosis of invasive aspergillosis: variables that affect performance. *J Infect Dis* (2004) 190:641–9. doi:10.1086/422009
13. Pfeiffer CD, Fine JP, Safdar N. Diagnosis of invasive aspergillosis using a galactomannan assay: a meta-analysis. *Clin Infect Dis* (2006) 42:1417–27. doi:10.1086/503427
14. Berenguer J, Allende MC, Lee JW, Garrett K, Lyman C, Ali NM, et al. Pathogenesis of pulmonary aspergillosis: granulocytopenia versus cyclosporine and methylprednisolone-induced immune suppression. *Am J Respir Crit Care Med* (1995) 152:1079–86. doi:10.1164/ajrccm.152.3.7663787
15. Gefter WB, Albelda SM, Talbot GH, Gerson SL, Cassileth PA, Miller WT. Invasive pulmonary aspergillosis and acute leukemia. Limitations in the diagnostic utility of the air crescent sign. *Radiology* (1985) 157:605–10. doi:10.1148/radiology.157.3.4059547
16. Burgos A, Zaoutis TE, Dvorak CC, Hoffman JA, Knapp KM, Nania JJ, et al. Pediatric invasive aspergillosis: a multicenter retrospective analysis of 139 contemporary cases. *Pediatrics* (2008) 121:e1286–94. doi:10.1542/peds.2007-2117
17. Anugulruengkitt S, Trinavarat P, Chantranuwat P, Sritippayawan S, Pancharoen C, Thanyawee P. Clinical features and survival outcomes of invasive aspergillosis in pediatric patients at a medical school in Thailand. *J Med Assoc Thai* (2016) 99:150–8.
18. Blot SI, Taccone FS, Van den Abeele AM, Bulpa P, Meersseman W, Brusselaers N, et al. A clinical algorithm to diagnose invasive pulmonary aspergillosis in critically ill patients. *Am J Respir Crit Care Med* (2012) 186:56–64. doi:10.1164/rccm.201111-1978OC
19. Klont RR, Mennink-Kersten MA, Verweij PE. Utility of Aspergillus antigen detection in specimens other than serum specimens. *Clin Infect Dis* (2004) 39:1467–74. doi:10.1086/425317
20. Guo YL, Chen YQ, Wang K, Qin SM, Wu C, Kong JL. Accuracy of BAL galactomannan in diagnosing invasive aspergillosis: a bivariate metaanalysis and systematic review. *Chest* (2010) 138:817–24. doi:10.1378/chest.10-0488

21. Salonen J, Lehtonen OP, Terasjarvi MR, Nikoskelainen J. Aspergillus antigen in serum, urine, and bronchoalveolar lavage specimens of neutropenic patients in relation to clinical outcome. *Scand J Infect Dis* (2000) 32:485–90. doi:10.1080/003655400458749
22. Zou M, Tang L, Zhao S, Zhao Z, Chen L, Chen P, et al. Systematic review and meta-analysis of detecting galactomannan in bronchoalveolar lavage fluid for diagnosing invasive aspergillosis. *PLoS One* (2012) 7:e43347. doi:10.1371/journal.pone.0043347
23. Heng SC, Morrissey O, Chen S. Utility of bronchoalveolar lavage fluid galactomannan alone or in combination with PCR for the diagnosis of invasive aspergillosis in adult hematology patients: a systemic review and meta-analysis. *Crit Rev Microbiol* (2015) 41:124–34. doi:10.3109/1040841X.2013.804033
24. de Mol M, de Jongste JC, van Westreenen M, Merkus PJ, de Vries AH, Hop WC, et al. Diagnosis of invasive pulmonary aspergillosis in children with bronchoalveolar lavage galactomannan. *Pediatr Pulmonol* (2013) 48:789–96. doi:10.1002/ppul.22670
25. Mohammadi S, Khalilzadeh S, Goudarzipour K, Hassanzad M, Mahdaviani A, Aarabi N, et al. Bronchoalveolar galactomannan in invasive pulmonary aspergillosis: a prospective study in pediatric patients. *Med Mycol* (2015) 53:709–16. doi:10.1093/mmy/myv053
26. Ansorg R, van den Boom R, Rath PM. Detection of Aspergillus galactomannan antigen in foods and antibiotics. *Mycoses* (1997) 40:353–7. doi:10.1111/j.1439-0507.1997.tb00249.x

25

Barriers to Perinatal Palliative Care Consultation

Franca Benini[1*], *Sabrina Congedi*[1], *Francesca Rusalen*[1], *Maria Elena Cavicchiolo*[2] *and Paola Lago*[3]

[1] *Pediatric Pain and Palliative Care Service, Department of Women's and Children's Health, University Hospital Padua, Padua, Italy,* [2] *Woman's and Child's Department, Neonatal Intensive Care Unit, University of Padua, Padua, Italy,* [3] *Neonatal Intensive Care Unit, Treviso's Hospital, Treviso, Italy*

Keywords: perinatal palliative care, barriers, newborn, need, neonatal intensive care

Correspondence:
Franca Benini
franca.benini@aopd.veneto.it

INTRODUCTION

Despite that infant mortality rates in western countries have improved over the past decade, 5.8 infant deaths per 1,000 live births are still reported, mainly due to prematurity and congenital anomalies (1, 2). According to recent data collected in the UK, the survival rate of pre-term infants born at 23+0 to 23+6 weeks of gestation and who receive active treatment is 38% (3). According to a registry study of the National Institute of Child Health and Human Development Neonatal Research Network, 20% of infants born at 22–24 weeks of gestation survives without neurodevelopmental impairment (4). Therefore, unfortunately, still a relevant number of newborns admitted to the neonatal intensive care unit (NICU) could have an unfavorable diagnosis and a poor prognosis. This leads to the notion of perinatal palliative care (PnPC) as an emerging field of palliative care. It involves different healthcare providers, including neonatologists, gynecologists, midwives, and nurses, and in a broader view all professionals who provide support strategies to the mother or the family and the fetus/newborn.

PnPC provides supportive care before and after birth and to families when a child is affected by congenital anomalies inconsistent with long-term survival, or when the extreme prematurity or post-natal irreversible disease of the child drastically reduces the possibility of survival (5, 6). Remarkably, in case of life-limiting fetal anomalies, palliative care could start before delivery (7) and up to 85% of parents continue pregnancies with a poor prenatal diagnosis worldwide (8). Therefore, the American College of Obstetricians and Gynecologists and the American Academy of Pediatrics recommend parental informed consent and discussion of all available care options, including PnPC (9).

Despite the importance of PnPC, several barriers to its implementation and utilization exist (10–12). At present, training programs in the field are proposed, the discipline is described as "very important" by hospital leadership but allocation of personnel, space, money, curriculum time remains poor (12).

In this paper, we comment on the barriers that make the access, planning, and development of PnPC services difficult.

IDENTIFICATION OF BARRIERS AND CRITICAL ISSUES

As a first step, we conducted an evaluation of literature with the aim to identify the most relevant barriers to PnPC and better focus our comment on this topic. In particular, we conducted a literature search on PubMed, TripDatabase, and Google Trend, using different combinations of keywords (e.g., MeSH terms: Perinatal palliative care, Barriers, Newborn, Need, Neonatal Intensive Care, life-limiting illness, end of life, ethical decision; free terms: Gestational age, culture, family, education, model organization, parents, newborn management, information, education, and others). No limitations in the search were applied. The reference lists of the retrieved papers were reviewed to find other papers worth consideration. Authors' own personal collections of literature were also browsed. The identified papers were then selected for inclusion according to their relevance for the topic, as judged by the Authors, in line with the non-systematic and narrative nature of this manuscript.

Based on this literature search and our clinical and organizational experience, we have identified four macro-areas of barriers and critical issues for the development of PnPC, namely: (i) Socio-cultural setting; (ii) Patients and their specific conditions; (iii) Training of healthcare providers (HCP); (iv) Regulatory and political issues.

SOCIO-CULTURAL SETTING

Misperception of the Role of Medicine and the Concept of "Health"

The management of PnPC could be influenced by families', nurses', and physicians' perceptions (8, 13, 14). Indeed, socio-cultural and economic context, and religious and moral values of future parents are taped among the main factors that influence the management of a fetus or an infant eligible to PnPC (13). There are widespread cultural barriers to consider death as an event occurring also in the neonatal/pediatric setting. The child is perceived as a human being at the beginning of his/her life journey and therefore the possible—or certain—fatal event is often neglected by parents and even healthcare providers. Medicine itself is often perceived as having the only aim of "cure," and the "Healthy" status is only associated with lack of any disease. Conversely, the WHO proposes a wider definition of "Health," as a state of psychological, physical, and social well-being; Medicine should aim at ensuring this state of health (15). In this perspective, it is important to clarify the notion of the inherent limits of Medicine: in some cases, the adoption of a palliative active care should be preferred over "doing whatever is possible," i.e., overtreatment (16–18).

The very same definition of "Palliative Medicine" is often misinterpreted as "end-of-life care" by parents of children eligible to PnPC and even by healthcare providers (19). This misinterpretation denies patients the opportunity of appropriate treatment.

Difficulties in Considering the Baby as a Person Who Can Feel Pain, Distress, Fear, and Suffering

It is widely accepted that, from the second trimester of gestation onwards, the nervous system of the fetus can perceive pain and distress, and these events have a major impact on fetal and post-natal life (20, 21). Therefore, even extremely premature newborns can "feel" the burden of disease, its symptoms, any invasive diagnostic and therapeutic procedure, as well as the distress due to the disease itself and the separation from mother. Unfortunately, the newborn is considered as unable to feel the above situations and therefore the burden associated with disease is neglected or underestimated. Furthermore, by negating newborn's ability to perceive pain and distress, the decision-making process of the clinical strategy becomes impaired. As a consequence, caring for such children requires a multidisciplinary approach that provides information regarding the risk, benefit, and burden for both mother and fetus.

Poor Information

Information on PnPC and the possibility to "cure" life-limiting or life-threatening diseases is scant, at best, and this lack of information limits the decision-making process by parents of children eligible to PnPC (19).

Moreover, the information that media provide is often only sensationalized news, which can be highly misleading and lacks an honest clinical, ethical and deontological evaluation. This poor information is important both for the patients, their families and for healthcare providers, also since the fear of social judgment limits the possibility of a correct assessment of the patient's status. Furthermore, lack of information and knowledge on PnPC limits the establishment of appropriate interventions by the healthcare system, with the recognition of dedicated units for PnPC.

PATIENTS AND THEIR SPECIFIC CONDITIONS

Heterogeneity of Clinical Situations and Types of Patients

The PnPC-eligible patients could be divided into three main clinical groups (22): (i) extremely premature at the limits of viability (<23 gestational week); (ii) prenatal/postnatal diagnosis of life-limiting/life-threatening diseases with poor prognosis and/or incompatibility with life; (iii) severe/critical clinical conditions without possibility of improvement, with high complexity of care and needing intensive support for vital functions' maintenance. In the second and third group, a range variety of conditions could be identified: neurological, cardio/pulmonary, and nephrological disorders or other genetic/chromosomal anomalies (23–25). Current medical evidence, experience of the healthcare providers, ethical, and regulatory bodies propose different strategies for the treatment of PnPC-eligible patients, according to their status and the type of life-limiting condition (26). Indeed, the diagnosis of a life-limiting condition can be difficult and can lead to doubts and different hypotheses.

Communication With Parents and Families

The parents of a child eligible to PnPC, as his/her legal guardians, have the responsibility of taking decisions. However, the inherent level of complexity of PnPC can lead to different views and perceptions between parents and healthcare providers, also due to the substantial variation in prognostic information given by obstetricians and neonatologists (27). This gap is due, at least in part, to the lack of unambiguous sources, tools, and training and it could lead to uncertain diagnostic and prognostic information (28). Several other factors should be taken into account, including the psychological dimension of the issue, the urgency (actual or perceived), the different role, perceptions, and emotions of healthcare providers and parents, the very same definitions of terms, such as "cure," "disease," "health," and "quality of life." The plethora of different feelings and emotions can be associated with reactions, such as negation of the issue, unrealistic expectations toward medicine, or even delegation of any decision to others and/or impersonal acceptance of the situation. This discrepancy can lead to communication issues between the parents and the healthcare providers, which, in turn, can delay or even deny the possibility of initiating palliative care.

The PnPC team should share the diagnosis, the anticipated prognosis, and potential interventions if any, with compassionate communication that respects patient cultural beliefs and values (29, 30) All the possibilities of care should be presented within a coordinated treatment strategy, focusing on maximizing quality of life, and comfort for the newborn. During counseling, team members should collect the appropriate information in order to give a tailored guidance to the family, free from any personal view and supporting parents in their decision-making process (28, 31). Therefore, team members should ask appropriate questions to explore the family's values, their understanding of the newborn's meaning and quality of life, in order also to establish a relationship based on trust and caring. An advance care plan is shared between parents and PnPC members, a birth plan, and/or a document of family wishes on delivery and resuscitation could be drafted (28).

All care options should be discussed, including pregnancy termination (abortion, within legal limitations), prenatal and postnatal intervention intended to promote survival, and palliative comfort care, which may include interventions to promote comfort and improve quality of life without intending to promote survival (29).

The lack of well-conducted communication can negatively affect the relationship between families of patients and PnPC healthcare providers, and between team members (32).

TRAINING OF HEALTHCARE PROVIDERS (HCP)

Dedicated training programs for perinatal palliative care are fundamental to improving the knowledge of healthcare professionals and the overall standard of care delivered to neonates.

In the past years, mounting interest has been given to palliative care, but this has not been paralleled by a growing in training programs; only scant data are available regarding the implementation of the PnPC educational programs.

In 2000, the American Academy of Pediatrics recommended an adequate training in pediatric palliative care and its subspecialties for all pediatricians to enhance the best possible quality of life for children living with a life-threating or terminal condition, using an integrated interdisciplinary approach (33). From 1975 to 2015, 99% of US medical schools offered education in palliative care, but only about 12–15 h of their entire medical school curricula were dedicated to palliative care (34). Similar results were reported for the European setting (35, 36). More data are available regarding training in PnPC for nurses and midwives (37–39), while only scant information regarding educational programs for neonatologist is available (40). According to the above, a structured curriculum dedicated to neonatal–perinatal medicine fellows to develop the complex set of skills required in this setting is eagerly warranted (40).

In a recent review investigating educational programs and events in the field of PnPC (41), the effectiveness of teaching healthcare professionals, methods of evaluating the teaching, and the teaching strategies used were analyzed. In total, 14 studies were included in the analysis, all published between 2002 and 2017. All studies referred as perinatal bereavement education as effective in terms of improvements in health workers of knowledge and communication skills, comfort in providing end-of-life care, and increased perceptions of the emotional needs of bereaved families. However, different evaluation tools were used and hence and it was not possible to determine which program was most effective.

Training programs in PnPC with specific content need to be developed and made available to all professionals who deal with perinatal death and the bereaved families (38, 40). Therefore, a dedicated program in PnPC should be offered to nurses, midwives, and the neonatologist in order to provide the best care for the fetus or infant and his family (42). Many studies reported that the main barriers to the development of pediatric palliative care are the inadequate training in communication and it is likely that this feature is also present in the PnPC field.

REGULATORY AND POLITICAL ISSUES

Organizational Issues

PnPC services represent a new, dynamic, and complex setting of care, which required dedicated time and resources; however, in daily practice, these are not always readily available.

The organization of a PnPC service poses serious challenges and requires the involvement of both local hospitals and the healthcare system. In PnPC, interdisciplinary competent teams are needed, and they should potentially involve different specialists (such as gynecologists, obstetrical specialists, nurses, neonatologists, geneticists, pediatric palliative care specialists, pediatricians, and bioethicists).

Few reports of experiences of well-structured PnPC networking models are available, and only a limited number of these investigated all difficulties and needs. This complex networking of different experiences needs the definition of shared protocol, dedicated organizational models, and adequate training. Meetings should begin in the antenatal phase and continue later, in order to identify and pursue a mutually agreed and appropriate care program. Dedicated time and appropriate places are needed for multidisciplinary meetings, and they may also help ensure a good communication between families of patients and team members, during the entire course of the patient's disease.

A quiet place should be available for parents during the infant dying process (6). Hospice concepts should be applied to neonatal care, providing a private family room where other family members can gather, and religious support can be given (43).

Resources Issues

From their moment of establishment, neonatology services have been characterized by continuous medical innovations, in a fast-growing field. However, only scant resources are available for this setting, requiring proper allocation (44). Moreover, literature offers complex networking models for PnPC services (45), making it difficult to estimate the costs for the public healthcare system, as well as the different social costs.

(Lack of) Regulations

The lack of dedicated regulations, which clearly define the right of children to PnPC, makes them, in many counties, an optional opportunity and not a duty of the healthcare system. Therefore, access to PnPC is largely dependent on single institutions, which further limits the diffusion of PnPC.

CONCLUSIONS

In this brief analysis, we identified and commented on many of the barriers currently slowing the development of PnPC programs. This issue is challenging, also due to the high heterogeneity of PnPC; however, we can propose some actions that may help in establishing proper PnPC programs.

- Increase the recognition of the actual lack of PnPC programs, in order to increase awareness of this setting.
- Recognize the inherent complexity of PnPC, making it necessary to establish specific training and services and collecting dedicated resources. Improvisation is not feasible in the setting of PnPC.
- Increase social awareness on PnPC, which aims at overcoming prejudices and providing the tools for proper reflections and decision-making.
- Provide proper training on PnPC, in terms of clinical, ethical, organizational, and communicational skills in order to make them able to pursue the best interest of the newborn with life-limiting/life-threatening disease.
- Promote research in PnPC and the collection of shared data, in order to find new tools applicable in different centers and settings.

AUTHOR CONTRIBUTIONS

FB: study design, data analysis, data interpretation, and writing. SC: literature search, data analysis, data collection, and writing. FR: literature search, data collection, and writing. MC: literature search, data interpretation, and writing. PL: literature search, study design, data interpretation, and writing. All authors: approved the final version of the draft.

ACKNOWLEDGMENTS

We thank Luca Giacomelli, PhD, for useful discussion. Editorial assistance was provided by Aashni Shah (Polistudium SRL, Milan, Italy). This assistance was supported by internal funds.

REFERENCES

1. Callaghan WM, MacDorman MF, Shapiro-Mendoza CK, Barfield WD. Explaining the recent decrease in US infant mortality rate, 2007-2013. *Am J Obstet Gynecol.* (2017) 216:73.e1–e8. doi: 10.1016/j.ajog.2016.09.097
2. Mathews TJ, Driscoll AK. Trends in infant mortality in the United States, 2005-2014. *NCHS Data Brief.* (2017) 279:1–8.
3. Smith LK, Draper ES, Manktelow BN, Fenton A, Kurinczuk J on behalf of the MBRRACE-UK Collaboration. *MBRRACE-UK Report on Survival Up to One Year of Age of Babies Born before 27 Weeks Gestational Age for Births in Great Britain from January to December 2016.* Leicester: The Infant Mortality and Morbidity Studies, Department of Health Sciences, University of Leicester (2018). Available online at: https://www.npeu.ox.ac.uk/downloads/files/mbrrace-uk/reports/MBRRACE-UK%20supplementary%20tables%20on%20births%20before%2027%20weeks%20gestation%202016.pdf
4. Younge N, Goldstein RF, Bann CM, Hintz SR, Patel RM, Smith PB, et al. Survival and neurodevelopmental outcomes among periviable infants. *N Engl J Med.* (2017) 376:617–28. doi: 10.1056/NEJMoa1605566
5. James R. Perinatal palliative care. *Obstet Gynecol.* (2020) 135:1484. doi: 10.1097/AOG.0000000000003902
6. Rusalen F. Perinatal palliative care: a new challenging field. *J Palliat Med.* (2020) 23:600. doi: 10.1089/jpm.2019.0661
7. Carter BS. More than medication: perinatal palliative care. *Acta Paediatr.* (2016) 105:1255–256 doi: 10.1111/apa.13529
8. Wool C. Clinician perspectives of barriers in perinatal palliative care. *MCN Am J Matern Child Nurs.* (2015) 40:44–50. doi: 10.1097/NMC.0000000000000093
9. American College of Obstetricians Gynecologists, Committee on Ethics; American Academy of Pediatrics, Committee on Bioethics. Maternal-fetal intervention and fetal care centers. *Pediatrics.* (2011) 128:e473–e8. doi: 10.1542/peds.2011-1570
10. Marc-Aurele KL, English NK. Primary palliative care in neonatal intensive care. *Semin Perinatol.* (2017) 41:133–9. doi: 10.1053/j.semperi.2016.11.005
11. Kyc SJ, Bruno CJ, Shabanova V, Montgomery AM. Perceptions of neonatal palliative care: similarities and differences between medical and nursing staff in a level IV neonatal intensive care unit. *J Palliat Med.* (2020) 23:662–9. doi: 10.1089/jpm.2019.0523
12. Friedrichsdorf SJ, Bruera E. Delivering pediatric palliative care: from denial, palliphobia, pallilalia to palliactive. *Children (Basel).* (2018) 5:120. doi: 10.3390/children5090120
13. Tosello B, Dany L, Bétrémieux P, Le Coz P, Auquier P, Gire C, et al. Barriers in referring neonatal patients to perinatal palliative care: a French multicenter survey. *PLoS One.* (2015) 10:e0126861. doi: 10.1371/journal.pone.0126861
14. Tosello B, Dany L, Gire C, Bétrémieux P, Vriet-Ndour ME, Le Coz P, et al. Perceptions of lethal fetal abnormality among perinatal professionals and the challenges of neonatal palliative care. *J Palliat Med.* (2014) 17:924–930. doi: 10.1089/jpm.2014.0023
15. WHO. *Constitution of WHO: Principles.* New York, NY: World Health Organization (1946). Available online at: https://www.who.int/governance/eb/who_constitution_en.pdf?ua=1
16. Durall A, Zurakowski D, Wolfe J. Barriers to conducting advance care discussions for children with life-threatening conditions. *Pediatrics.* (2012) 129:e975–82. doi: 10.1542/peds.2011-2695
17. Lotz JD, Jox RJ, Borasio GD, Führer M. Pediatric advance care planning from the perspective of health care professionals: a qualitative interview study. *Palliat Med.* (2015) 29:212–22. doi: 10.1177/0269216314552091
18. Glass AP, Nahapetyan L. Discussions by elders and adult children about end-of-life preparation and preferences. *Prev Chronic Dis.* (2008) 5:A08.
19. Cuviello A, Raisanen JC, Donohue PK, Wiener L, Boss RD. Defining the boundaries of palliative care in pediatric oncology. *J Pain Symptom Manage.* (2020) 59:1033–42.e1. doi: 10.1016/j.jpainsymman.2019.11.022
20. Pierucci R. Fetal Pain: The science behind why it is the medical standard of care. *Linacre Q.* (2020) 87:311–6. doi: 10.1177/0024363920924877
21. Lonnqvist PA. Pediatric pain review: what has happened since the First World Congress on Pediatric Pain in 1988? The past, the present and the future.

Minerva Anestesiol. (2020). doi: 10.23736/S0375-9393.20.14391-8. [Epub ahead of print].
22. Rusalen F, Cavicchiolo ME, Lago P, Salvadori S, Benini F. Perinatal palliative care: a dedicated care pathway. *BMJ Support Palliat Care.* (2019) 1–6. doi: 10.1136/bmjspcare-2019-001849
23. Viallard ML, Moriette G. Démarche palliative chez le nouveau-né atteint de malformations ou d'anomalies génétiques sévères [Palliative care for newborn infants with congenital malformations or genetic abnormalities]. *Arch Pediatr.* (2017) 24:169–74. doi: 10.1016/j.arcped.2016.11.007
24. Morin L, Ray S, Wilson C, Remy S, Benissa MR, Jansen NJG, et al. Refractory septic shock in children: a European Society of paediatric and neonatal intensive care definition. *Intensive Care Med.* (2016) 42:1948–57. doi: 10.1007/s00134-016-4574-2
25. Rosati A, Ilvento L, L'Erario M, De Masi S, Biggeri A, Fabbro G, et al. Efficacy of ketamine in refractory convulsive status epilepticus in children: a protocol for a sequential design, multicentre, randomised, controlled, open-label, non-profit trial (KETASER01). *BMJ Open.* (2016) 6:e011565. doi: 10.1136/bmjopen-2016-011565
26. Jankovic M, De Zen L, Pellegatta F, Lazzarin P, Bertolotti M, Manfredini L, et al. A consensus conference report on defining the eligibility criteria for pediatric palliative care in Italy. *Ital J Pediatr.* (2019) 45:89. doi: 10.1186/s13052-019-0681-3
27. Edmonds BT, McKenzie F, Panoch J, Frankel RM. Comparing neonatal morbidity and mortality estimates across specialty in periviable counseling. *J Matern Fetal Neonatal Med.* (2015) 28:2145–9. doi: 10.3109/14767058.2014.981807
28. Marty CM, Carter BS. Ethics and palliative care in the perinatal world. *Semin Fetal Neonatal Med.* (2018) 23:35–38. doi: 10.1016/j.siny.2017.09.001
29. Perinatal Palliative Care: ACOG COMMITTEE OPINION, Number 786. *Obstet Gynecol.* (2019) 134:e84–e9. doi: 10.1097/AOG.0000000000003425
30. Effective patient-physician communication. Committee Opinion No. 587. American College of Obstetricians and Gynecologists. *Obstet Gynecol.* (2014) 123:389–93. doi: 10.1097/01.AOG.0000443279.14017.12
31. Blumenthal-Barby JS, Loftis L, Meadow W, Lemmon M, Ubel PA, et al. Should neonatologists give opinions withdrawing life-sustaining treatment? *Pediatrics.* (2016) 138:e20162585. doi: 10.1542/peds.2016-2585
32. Benini F, Orzalesi M, de Santi A, Congedi S, Lazzarin P, Pellegatta F, et al. Barriers to the development of pediatric palliative care in Italy. *Ann Ist Super Sanita.* (2016) 52:558–64. doi: 10.4415/ANN_16_04_16
33. American Academy of Pediatrics. Committee on Bioethics and Committee on Hospital Care. Palliative Care for Children. *Pediatrics.* (2000) 106:351–7. doi: 10.1542/peds.106.2.351
34. Dickinson GE. A 40-year history of end-of-life offerings in US medical schools: 1975-2015. *Am J Hosp Palliat Care.* (2017) 34:559–65. doi: 10.1177/1049909116638071
35. Benini F, Cauzzo C, Congedi S, Da Dalt L, Cogo P, Biscaglia L, et al. Training in pediatric palliative care in Italy: still much to do. *Ann Ist Super Sanita.* (2019) 55:240–5. doi: 10.4415/ANN_19_03_07
36. Michelson KN, Ryan AD, Jovanovic B, Frader J. Pediatric residents and fellows perspectives on palliative care education. *J Palliat Med.* (2009) 12:451–47. doi: 10.1089/jpm.2008.0263
37. LoGiudice JA, O'Shea E. Perinatal palliative care: Integration in a United States nurse midwifery education program. *Midwifery.* (2018) 58:117–9. doi: 10.1016/j.midw.2017.12.024
38. Price JE, Mendizabal-Espinosa RM, Podsiadly E, Marshall-Lucette S, Marshall JE. Perinatal/neonatal palliative care: Effecting improved knowledge and multi-professional practice of midwifery and children's nursing students through an inter-professional education initiative. *Nurse Educ Pract.* (2019) 40:102611. doi: 10.1016/j.nepr.2019.08.005
39. O'Shea ER, Campbell SH, Engler AJ, Beauregard R, Chamberlin EC, Currie LM. Effectiveness of a perinatal and pediatric End-of-Life Nursing Education Consortium (ELNEC) curricula integration. *Nurse Educ Today.* (2015) 35:765–70. doi: 10.1016/j.nedt.2015.02.015
40. Forman KR, Thompson-Branch A. Educational perspectives: palliative care education in neonatal-perinatal medicine fellowship. *Neoreviews.* (2020) 21:e72–e9. doi: 10.1542/neo.21-2-e72
41. Ratislavová K, BuŽgová R, Vejvodová J. Perinatal palliative care education: an integrative review. *Nurse Educ Today.* (2019) 82:58–66. doi: 10.1016/j.nedt.2019.08.003
42. Twamley K, Kelly P, Moss R, Mancini A, Craig F, Koh M, et al. Palliative care education in neonatal units: impact on knowledge and attitudes. *BMJ Support Palliat Care.* (2013) 3:213–20. doi: 10.1136/bmjspcare-2012-000336
43. Yu VY. Is neonatal intensive care justified in all preterm infants? *Croat Med J.* (2005) 46:744–50.
44. Lazzarin P, Giacomelli L, Terrenato I, Benini F; behalf of the ACCAPED Study Group. A Tool for the evaluation of clinical needs and eligibility to pediatric palliative care: the Validation of the ACCAPED Scale. *J Palliat Med.* (2020). doi: 10.1089/jpm.2020.0148. [Epub ahead of print].
45. Lantos JD. Ethical problems in decision making in the neonatal ICU. *N Engl J Med.* (2018) 379:1851–60. doi: 10.1056/NEJMra1801063

26

The Neonatal Comfort Care Program: Origin and Growth Over 10 Years

Charlotte Wool[1] *and Elvira Parravicini*[2*]

[1] *York College of Pennsylvania, College of Nursing and Health Professions, York, PA, United States,* [2] *Division of Neonatology, Department of Pediatrics, Columbia University Irving Medical Center, New York, NY, United States*

Correspondence:
Elvira Parravicini
ep127@cumc.columbia.edu

The objective of perinatal palliative care is to provide holistic and comprehensive health care services to women who are anticipating the birth of a neonate diagnosed prenatally with a life-limiting condition and to continue supportive interventions for the mother and neonate after the birth. The nature of pregnancy, with two patients requiring medical care, requires clinicians from different specialties to engage with one another, the patient, and her chosen family members. Following birth, additional skill sets to treat the medical and comfort needs of the neonate, as well as the psychoemotional and medical needs of the mother, are required. An interdisciplinary team is necessary to assist families throughout the pregnancy and postnatal journey, and coordination of such care is an integral component of palliative care services. The number of palliative care programs is increasing, but little is written about the origins of such programs, their subsequent growth, and how transitions of care occur within the programs. In this publication, we will present data garnered from interdisciplinary team members of a single organization, the Neonatal Comfort Care Program at Columbia University Irving Medical Center, and how they provide care for families throughout the pregnancy and postnatal trajectory. We will address the origin and growth of the program, the development of the interdisciplinary team, and the strategies used for high-quality communication and their respective impact on care continuity. We will also provide specific recommendations from data gathered from team members, examine the role of formal and informal education, and identify barriers and future opportunities.

Keywords: interdisciplinary care, program development, life limiting conditions, perinatal palliative care (PPC), neonatal palliative care

INTRODUCTION

There is rarely a time in a family's life that entails more transitions than pregnancy and the birth of a child. It is a time of anticipation, changes, preparation, and often great joy. When a woman is faced with news that her expected child has a life-limiting condition (LLC), the pregnancy course abruptly changes, as do the complexity and challenges she and her family experience. Historically, women were offered the options to terminate the pregnancy or prepare to have their neonate admitted to an intensive care unit. However, in 1997, the concept of perinatal hospice was introduced (1), followed by clinical recommendations for a neonatal end-of-life palliative care protocol (2). Since then, perinatal palliative care (PPC) programs, which are defined as comprehensive, interdisciplinary, coordinated services offered from fetal diagnosis through the neonatal period, have experienced significant growth (3) and national recognition (4–6). This extension of a woman's right to choose respects patients' cultural beliefs and values, can empower women, and has been met with increases in patient satisfaction (7, 8).

Clinicians from many disciplines play an integral part in supporting families by providing compassionate, evidence-based care and can offer information and services that allow families to make the most of the time with their neonate. Data show that women who opt to continue a pregnancy with an LLC appreciate opportunities to emotionally adjust and report having no regrets about their decision (9, 10). A variety of interventions, including anticipatory guidance, prenatal consults, early and continuous bereavement support, and coordination of care allow families to begin the difficult but important process of adjusting to the implications of an LLC (11, 12). Formal, integrated palliative care programs have structures in place that ensure the interdisciplinary team (IDT) can communicate well, manage the needs of families, and offer high-quality care.

The purpose of this article is to provide practical information for professionals interested in starting, sustaining, or increasing PPC services within an organization by using the model of the Neonatal Comfort Care Program (NCCP) at Columbia University Irving Medical Center (CUIMC). Aims are to (1) provide an overview of the program's origin and its subsequent growth, (2) explain the formation of the IDT, (3) outline communication strategies of team members to ensure continuity of care, (4) highlight recommendations from team members working in the program, (5) emphasize the significant role of education in culture change, and (6) identify barriers in developing the program and future opportunities.

AIM 1—PROGRAM ORIGIN AND SUBSEQUENT GROWTH

CUIMC is a large academic institution with ~4,000 deliveries annually and about 800 pregnancies involving fetal anomalies, including LLC. The NCCP began in 2008 and grew out of a desire to provide the most comfortable and loving environment for neonates diagnosed *in utero* with LLC, help families manage and navigate the immense practical and emotional burdens associated with LLC, and offer an option of care that families identify as safe, supportive, and in sync with their personal beliefs and desires. The idea for formalizing a strategy to provide comfort care for neonates with LLC started with a neonatologist. At the beginning, obstetric and maternal fetal medicine colleagues were invited to make referrals for a prenatal palliative care consult whenever a candidate was identified. As families provided positive feedback of their experiences and as relationships between neonatology and obstetric providers advanced, referrals increased. Consults are medically oriented meetings wherein the physician reviews the patient's medical history; meets with family members to assess their understanding, desires, and values; and makes recommendations about care and treatment. The consults are reimbursable. Patient encounters are supportive services provided by appropriate IDT members and are tailored to family needs. **Figure 1** provides a timeline outlining the onboarding of the NCCP members, educational programs, acquisition of funding, and contributions to the literature.

Annual prenatal consults have grown logarithmically from 13 consults in 2008 to 64 in 2019. Patient encounters have increased in a similar fashion from 16 in 2008 to 127 in 2019.

AIM 2—DEVELOPMENT OF THE CORE AND INTERDISCIPLINARY TEAMS

In 2011, a neonatal intensive care unit (NICU) nurse self-identified an interest in partnering with the neonatologist, leading to a part-time position in 2012. By 2017, as professionals expressed an interest, a core team was established with a medical director from neonatology dedicated to, but not funded by, the NCCP program. A full-time nurse, social worker, and program manager were funded from unsolicited philanthropic donations given by individuals and foundations. The program manager is focused on program development and outreach to establish sustainability. The IDT includes collaborators/champions from neonatology and obstetrics, a child life specialist, speech language pathologist, psychologist, chaplain, obstetric nurse, and maternal–fetal medicine physician. The uniqueness of the program lies in an intentional continuity of care among team members and professionals and a desire to ensure quality services throughout the entire perinatal journey.

During this decade of growth, the NCCP established and published innovative clinical guidelines focusing on the comfort of the neonate and family bonding, leading to an impressive culture change (13). One of the key elements of bonding is that the mother and her infant should have close contact and not be separated. In 2008, in our institution, as elsewhere, neonates with LLC were admitted to the NICU for "comfort care," resulting in separation of the mother and infant. Intentional in-house education was offered, and by 2018–2020, all families followed prenatally by the NCCP received the option to room-in after birth, and all mothers who elected this option (98%) successfully kept their infant with them in a private postpartum room. The NCCP offers rooming-in for infants at the end of life, as well as infants with any kind of LLC, as long as the parent(s) desire palliative care management. Oxygen via nasal cannula, nasogastric or syringe feeding, and pain management are provided, and the NICU team is responsible for the infant. Another essential element for bonding and comfort is feeding; involvement of a speech pathologist has been key to safely and successfully feeding these fragile neonates throughout their natural lives.

AIM 3—COMMUNICATION STRATEGIES

Referrals for Consultation

Referrals for consultation to the NCCP are initiated through (1) obstetricians directly initiating a consult with the NCCP;

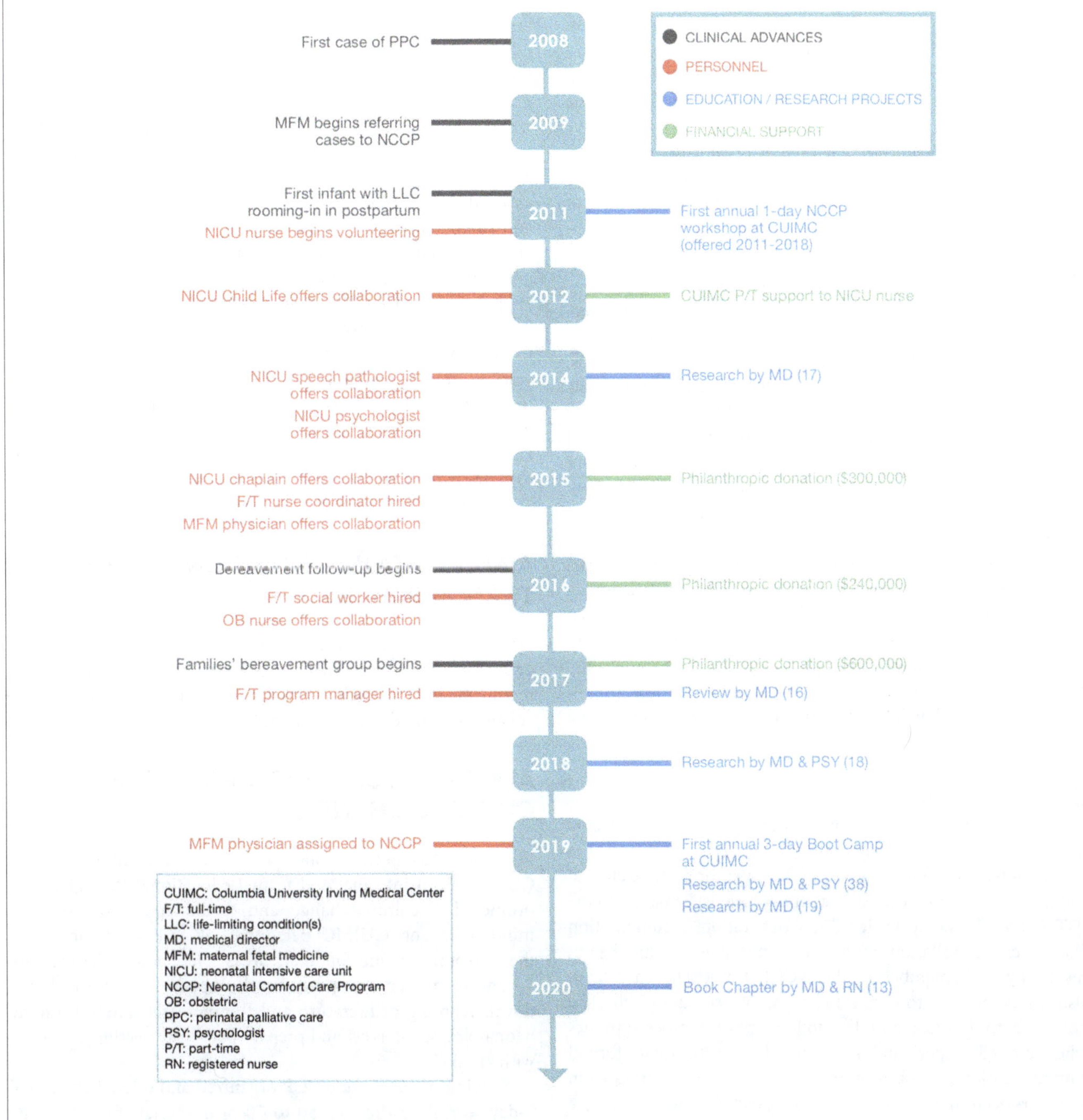

FIGURE 1 | Timeline of Neonatal Comfort Care Program (NCCP) Growth and Milestones.

(2) identification of new patients in weekly meetings among the NCCP medical director, nurse coordinator, and maternal–fetal medicine and neonatology physicians; and (3) self-referral of women requesting a PPC consultation in partnership with their obstetric provider.

Candidates

Candidates include pregnant women with potential or certain fetal LLCs and those with a complex fetal diagnosis with a potential adverse prognosis. A specific list of fetal LLC diagnoses triggers a referral to the NCCP. Included are conditions with expected early demise, such as renal agenesis, anencephaly, and limb-body-wall syndrome, as well as cases in which the burden of intensive care may exceed benefits, such as trisomy 13, trisomy 18, genetic syndromes with life-limiting prognoses, extreme prematurity at the cusp of viability, or complex congenital heart disease. Complex conditions with potential adverse outcomes also initiate a consult. Examples include uncertain diagnoses, such as multiple skeletal anomalies or severe brain anomalies, and known diagnoses with uncertain prognosis, such as bilateral renal dysplasia, severe lower urinary tract obstruction, or severe hydrops. The NCCP takes medical care of all infants with these conditions. Regardless of the family's decision to have comfort care vs. a trial of intensive care vs. full NICU support, the NCCP is available to support the family throughout the perinatal journey. At birth, if the family elects comfort care, the NCCP takes direct care of the infant.

Consults and Patient Encounters

Once a consult is initiated, the medical director is notified, and the first meeting with the family is planned. The medical director, nurse coordinator, and social worker meet with the family during the first consult to (1) probe the family's prognostic awareness, (2) clarify diagnosis, prognosis, (3) offer options for postnatal plans, (4) propose supportive interventions, and (5) establish a relationship of trust that will continue along the entire perinatal journey. Two aspects of care planning occur in tandem. First, the medical director oversees a postnatal medical care plan dependent on fetal gestational age and family need. Second, the family will meet with the nurse coordinator and the social worker, who offer supportive interventions and resources during pregnancy, delivery, and beyond. The patient encounters consist of interventions such as anticipatory guidance, discussion and documentation of a family birth plan, psychological counseling, memory making, sibling support, religious and cultural rituals, and referrals to other IDT professionals as needed. Usually two to four meetings occur.

Communication

A systematic approach of communicating patient events occurs through a weekly meeting among the core team and the maternal–fetal medicine physician. The outcome of these clinical rounds is reported in a weekly "comfort care list" emailed to the IDT and NICU and obstetric fellows. In addition, documentation from each consultation is reported in the electronic health record by each member of the NCCP team. The core team also meets monthly to review follow-up of neonates discharged home or to hospice and the follow-up of mothers/families who suffered a perinatal loss. In addition to these formal communication processes, informal conversations among team members occur through telephone calls, texting, and face-to-face meetings. The team is careful to apply patient privacy standards when communicating.

Continuity of Care—Prenatal to Postnatal

One outcome of high-quality communication among team members is the opportunity to provide continuity of care. In the NCCP, the medical director and the nurse coordinator, when available, are present at delivery to ensure continuity of care to the family or to mentor staff members in the obstetric and neonatal units. The champion obstetric nurse is also available to mentor and facilitate care in the delivery room and postpartum unit. The unpredictability of labor requires a communication system that allows pristine fulfillment of the medical and interdisciplinary birth plans.

The number of newborns with LLC is relatively small so the medical director assumes direct care of most neonates until death or discharge, along with the NICU staff (NICU fellow, nurse practitioner, resident). When the neonate is admitted to postpartum, a NICU nurse is assigned to assess the infant once a shift or more often if needed. IDT members are consulted as needed. A child life specialist helps with memory making and sibling support, and the chaplain addresses spiritual needs and coordinates specific parent-requested rituals. Standardized guidelines focused on achieving a state of comfort for the neonate are implemented and have been published (13).

The NCCP social worker collaborates with the obstetric social worker in supporting the mother and the family. The social workers provide resources and information about a coordinated discharge to home, follow-up with hospice, and disposition of the infant. Once the mother is discharged home, the care coordinator and social worker, and other IDT members if needed, continue to support the family by offering a bereavement follow-up for at least a year.

AIM 4—RECOMMENDATIONS FROM TEAM MEMBERS

Data regarding recommendations for those interested in starting or developing a program were collected from individual team members in the NCCP program. Recommendations were collated and are delineated in **Table 1**.

AIM 5—EDUCATION TO PRODUCE CULTURE CHANGE

Education has been pivotal to the advancement of PPC in CUIMC. Both informal and formal educational strategies have promoted a culture change and facilitated a positive PPC mindset among CUIMC personnel, as well as clinicians in the surrounding metropolitan areas. Neonatal palliative care advancements set the stage for the uptake of PPC with the downstreaming of literature and the increased interest among neonatologists to assist and prepare parents expecting a neonate with an LLC.

Starting in 2014, the NCCP organized and offered an annual 1-day workshop drawing 50 to 70 professionals from CUIMC and the surrounding region each year. The workshop included lectures, discussion of clinical cases, and parent interviews. In 2019, the workshop was expanded to a 3-day boot-camp training course with continuing education credits for physicians and nurses. The program agenda is available on the website and included formal lectures, role-modeling case studies, hands-on demonstrations, group discussion, parent voice, and networking opportunities. More than 80 participants from 19 states and several countries attended. Unique to the program was the opportunity for each NCCP team member to provide evidence-based strategies and share their clinical experiences with the participants (15).

TABLE 1 | Recommendations and suggested resources from NCCP team members to clinicians planning to start a PPC program.

CORE TEAM	
Neonatologist, program director	• Create a mission and vision and access it to maintain motivation (14) • Establish collaboration with OB • Look for "champion" professionals interested in collaboration • Work cohesively and regularly with team members to ensure optimal communication • Use professional encounters to teach and role model the tenets of PPC (15, 16) • Establish policy/guidelines for PPC in your institution (12) • Measure and report program outcomes and successes (17–19)
Registered nurse, program coordinator (former NICU RN)	• Identify champion RNs interested in PPC and provide teaching and mentoring • Participate in online and live educational opportunities (15) • Use online and community resources to gather bereavement supplies (20) • Develop a curriculum of Nursing PPC to create a PPC mindset
Program social worker (former PICU SW)	• Document all tasks related to PPC and build a case for SW position with data • Join perinatal hospice (20) network and network with other SWs to gain insights and information (21) • Participate in online and live educational opportunities (15, 22)
IDT TEAM	
OB registered nurse	• Develop QI projects to build a case for resources for PPC • Train and mentor OB nurses to create a PPC mindset (23, 24) • Network with OB nurses in other institutions to share ideas and resources for PPC
MFM physician	• Collaborate with the team in pregnancy management to achieve family's expectations (4) • Train OB staff to respect and support the family's goals (25, 26) • Develop research projects to demonstrate the benefits of PPC
NICU speech-language pathologist	• Contact experienced colleagues for advice (27) • Consider training champion NICU RNs to assess feeding needs for a neonate and become familiar with specific feeding equipment • Train all staff to respect and support the family's goals relative to providing nutritive or non-nutritive therapies (28)
NICU child life specialist	• Train other child life specialists to specific interventions in PPC (29) • Consider training "champion" RNs to become familiar with memory making during pregnancy and at birth
NICU psychologist	• Contact in-house psychologists and assess interest in working with bereaved parents • Develop collaboration with team SW • Be intentional about listening to parents and help them navigate their experiences during pregnancy and beyond (30, 31)
NICU chaplain	• Partner with in-house or community faith leaders • Familiarize clinicians with spiritual screening using FICA Spiritual History Tool (32) • Assess patient's spiritual preferences prenatally to prepare for spiritual interventions (33, 34)

Informal education occurs routinely by the nurse coordinator and champions within the IDT. Examples include bedside teaching in the delivery room, postpartum unit, and the NICU as mothers and their neonates present to these areas. The obstetric nurse champion conducts huddles, mentoring, and bedside teaching and is instrumental in keeping lines of communication clear and consistent. Information about the NCCP is given to all new nurses during orientation.

The medical director of the NCCP is responsible for training and mentoring obstetric and neonatal fellows and residents in the clinical setting. Additionally, a five-lesson curriculum was developed and is used to formally present essential elements of PPC.

AIM 6—BARRIERS AND FUTURE OPPORTUNITIES

Barriers to implementing workplace change were two-fold. First, PPC is an emerging field, and the evidence base was limited at the start of the NCCP program. Coupled with the development of new research knowledge were positive clinical experiences. Over time, resistance to PPC diminished, the culture improved, and the mindset of perinatologists changed. A second barrier was limited funding. Resources were allocated over time and provided support for new staff, educational initiatives, and research endeavors.

The future of the NCCP program is promising. Educational goals of the NCCP will build upon the foundation created in the last decade. Plans are in place to increase educational outreach and establish deeper collaborations with regional institutions to assist with replicating best practices related to PPC. Educational recommendations from NCCP team members include additional in-services, development of a basic curriculum for nurses centered on area of expertise, and establishment of a PPC fellowship for NICU, obstetrics, and social work. Expansion of the clinical team includes plans for a dedicated midwife who would provide continuity of care during the perinatal journey, facilitate communication during encounters with various obstetrics providers, offer one-on-one childbirth education, be present at the birth, and provide postpartum follow-up and lactation support. Involvement of additional clinicians to act as NCCP champions will reinforce expertise, assist with training and supporting colleagues, and provide more penetration of PPC culture within units. Ongoing mental health treatment in the form of groups and/or individual/couples therapy is also under consideration. Further research will provide new knowledge upon which evidence-based practices can be established.

DISCUSSION

PPC literature has grown in the last two decades and, with it, application into clinical practice. Palliative care programs are in 25 countries worldwide, with 246 in the United States and 67 globally (20). However, of the 246 perinatal hospices in the United States, only 20% offer hospital-based perinatal care, and nearly 40% offer only bereavement support. Of the 20% offering hospital care, the NCCP is unique in its prioritization of uninterrupted support of families of neonates with LLC. From the moment of diagnosis, through birth and beyond, the same physician and team members provide continuity of care to the neonate and family throughout each step of the journey.

As palliative services expand to the perinatal population, patient- and family-centered care will continue to optimize quality of life by anticipating, preventing, and treating suffering (35) through the continuum of the pregnancy and postnatal course. There are several benefits of a formal program as team members optimize communication strategies, work within standardized guidelines, and track outcomes and quality care. Systematic incorporation of evidence into practice settings can take many years, and over time, with dedicated staff and administrative support, referrals increase. The work of improving quality and effectiveness of health services requires consistent vision of individuals and teams, along with resources and administrative support, to solidify lasting change.

Culture change is an essential part of clinical advancement, especially with respect to palliative care as palliative therapies are interventions with complexities that affect the physical, psychoemotional, and spiritual aspects of human care. Advances in the NCCP program, including establishment of guidelines available to any professionals involved in perinatology, occurred through multifaceted approaches, including a mindset reorientation for leaders and frontline clinicians. As more clinicians become aware of and are supported in providing palliative care, their confidence increases, and a significant cultural shift occurs.

In line with current recommendations, an IDT should consist of a multitude of experts, all of whom play specific roles in providing tailored services to neonates, women, and their family members. The essential first step is the collaboration between the obstetric and neonatology services, which ensures that pregnancy and delivery are managed in a continuum (4). Anecdotally, medical directors are commonly neonatologists or obstetricians rather than palliative care physicians. These specialists are housed in every hospital in the USA whereas palliative care physicians are not. Essential elements of PPC come under the auspices of obstetrics and neonatology who have expertise with prenatal counseling, pregnancy management, and palliative comfort interventions for infants with a shortened life span. Communication is optimized through a systematic, consistent collaboration within the IDT. Unlike several programs in the US (3) led by a nurse coordinator or a bereavement counselor, the NCCP was initiated and developed by a neonatologist who established a collaboration with obstetricians and provides prenatal counseling and direct medical care to the neonates, promoting continuity of care for each family. The nurse leader facilitates the nursing aspects of care and coordinates interdisciplinary services, helping to form a cohesive approach to care. Thanks to professionals offering their services and prioritizing rooming-in with mother and feeding as comforting to the neonate, the NCCP has been building a mindset that contributes to the creation of a peaceful, safe, and loving environment. The life of the neonate, rather than the anticipation of his or her loss, becomes the focus of attention.

Data provided by NCCP team members offer recommendations to read appropriate discipline-focused literature, attend educational events, and listen to parents. The identification of local "champions" is key to establish the much-needed culture change toward a mindset open to PPC among professional working in the perinatal field. Professional networking affords a host of benefits by strengthening and expanding the exchange ideas and information. Networking can also facilitate change through brainstorming and problem solving. Lastly, PPC is still a very young field in medicine and practice needs to be evidence-based through prospective research.

Although the number of PPC programs has been increasing over the past years, training and education for professionals have not kept pace. Evidence-based, consistent, comprehensive training courses for professionals involved in PPC across disciplines are not widely available. A lack of knowledge is linked to clinician discomfort in providing care for families affected by an LLC (36). Since the start of NCCP, educational initiatives were a priority, leading to the changing dynamics among units that forged cultural and clinical changes. Educational approaches were diverse and included formal annual training events, group lectures, and bedside training and mentoring.

The allocation of resources is a constant challenge for health care administrators, and yet, the lack of resources can have serious consequences on patient-centered quality care (37). A variety of approaches has helped keep the NCCP operational, including the strong motivation of the core team members to provide comfort care despite scarce resources, the availability of some IDT members to offer some extra hours, and a cohesive team mentality enabling optimal communication and shared successes. Plans to continue outreach to philanthropic foundations to ensure sustainability are a future priority.

CONCLUSION

Building a new program and changing organizational culture take strong motivation, commitments of time and energy, and, eventually, adequate funding. Clinical leaders can forward a consistent vision and focus on creating an ongoing narrative related to optimal comfort care for neonates with LLC and support for their families.

AUTHOR CONTRIBUTIONS

CW and EP conceptualized and designed the report, drafted the initial manuscript, and approved the final manuscript as submitted. Both authors contributed to the article and approved the submitted version.

ACKNOWLEDGMENTS

We express our heartfelt thanks to each of the Neonatal Comfort Care Program team member for their dedication to patients and families and for providing information for this manuscript: Catherine Cha, Ruth Downing, Monica Joshi, Frances McCarthy, Solimar Santiago-Warner, Dorothy Smok, Rochelle Steinwurtzel, Marianne Verzosa, Emilee Walker-Cornetta. Their expertise, commitment, and support are extraordinary.

REFERENCES

1. Calhoun BC, Hoeldtke NJ, Hinson RM, Judge KM. Perinatal hospice: should all centers have this service? *Neonatal Netw.* (1997) 16:101–2.
2. Catlin A, Carter B. Creation of a neonatal end-of-life palliative care protocol. *Neonatal Netw.* (2002) 21:37–49. doi: 10.1891/0730-0832.21.4.37
3. Wool C, Côté-Arsenault D, Perry Black B, Denney-Koelsch E, Kim S, Kavanaugh K. Provision of services in perinatal palliative care: a multicenter survey in the United States. *J Palliat Med.* (2016) 19:279–85. doi: 10.1089/jpm.2015.0266
4. Perinatal Palliative Care. Committee Opinion No. 786. American college of obstetricians and gynecologists committee on obstetric practice, committee on ethics. *Obstet Gynecol.* (2019) 134:e84–9. doi: 10.1097/AOG.0000000000003425
5. Limbo R, Brandon D, Côté-Arsenault D, Kavanaugh K, Kuebelbeck A, Wool C. American academy of nursing policy brief: perinatal palliative care as an essential element of childbearing choices. *Nurs Outlook.* (2017) 65:123–5. doi: 10.1016/j.outlook.2016.12.003
6. American Academy of Pediatrics. Committee on Bioethics and Committee on Hospital Care. Statement palliative care for children. *Pediatrics.* (2000) 106:351–7. doi: 10.1542/peds.106.2.351
7. Cortezzo DE, Bowers K, Cameron Meyer M. Birth planning in uncertain or life-limiting fetal diagnoses: perspectives of physicians and parents. *J Palliat Med.* (2019) 22:1337–45. doi: 10.1089/jpm.2018.0596
8. Wool C, Kain VJ, Mendes J, Carter BS. Quality predictors of parental satisfaction after birth 691 of infants with life-limiting conditions. *Acta Paediatr.* (2018) 107:276–82. doi: 10.1111/apa.13980
9. Côté-Arsenault D, Denney-Koelsch E. "Have no regrets:" Parents' experiences and developmental tasks in pregnancy with a lethal fetal diagnosis. *Soc Sci Med.* (2016) 154:100–9. doi: 10.1016/j.socscimed.2016.02.033
10. Wool C, Limbo R, Denny-Koelsch EM. "I would do it all over again": cherishing time and the absence of regret in continuing a pregnancy after a life-limiting diagnosis. *J Clin Ethics.* (2018) 29:227–36.
11. Marty CM, Carter BS. Ethics and palliative care in the perinatal world. *Semin Fetal Neonatal Med.* (2018) 23:35–8. doi: 10.1016/j.siny.2017.09.001
12. Limbo RK, Wool C, Carter BS. *Handbook of Perinatal and Neonatal Palliative Care: a Guide for Nurses, Physicians, and Other Health Professionals.* New York, NY: Springer Publishing Company, LLC (2020). doi: 10.1891/9780826138422
13. Parravicini E, McCarthy F. *Comfort* in perinatal and neonatal palliative care: an innovative plan of care focused on relational elements. In: Limbo R, Wool C, Carter BS, editors. *Handbook of Perinatal and Neonatal Palliative Care: A Guide for Nurses, Physicians, and Other Health Professionals. Chapter 4.* New York, NY: Springer Company, LLC. (2020). doi: 10.1891/9780826138422.0004
14. *Neonatal Comfort Care Program.* Available online at: www.neonatalcomfortcare.com (accessed July 21, 2020).
15. *Next-Level Perinatal/Neonatal Comfort Care Training: Creating an Interdisciplinary Palliative Care Plan for Each Baby and their Family.* Available online at: https://www.publichealth.columbia.edu/research/precision-prevention/next-level-perinatalneonatal-comfort-care-training-creating-interdisciplinary-palliative-care-plan (accessed July 20, 2021).
16. Parravicini E. Neonatal palliative care. *Curr Opin Pediatr.* (2017) 29:135–40. doi: 10.1097/MOP.0000000000000464
17. Parravicini E, Lorenz MJ. Neonatal outcomes of fetuses diagnosed with life-limiting conditions when individualized comfort measures are proposed. *J Perinatol.* (2014) 34:483–7. doi: 10.1038/jp.2014.40
18. Parravicini E, Daho M, Foe G, Steinwurtzel R, Byrne M. Parental assessment of comfort in newborns affected by life-limiting conditions treated by a standardized neonatal comfort care program. *J Perinatol.* (2018) 38:142–7. doi: 10.1038/jp.2017.160
19. Haxel C, Glickstein J, Parravicini E. Neonatal palliative care for complicated cardiac anomalies: a 10-year experience of an interdisciplinary program at a large tertiary cardiac center. *J Pediatr.* (2019) 214:79–88. doi: 10.1016/j.jpeds.2019.07.044
20. *Perinatal Hospice.* Available online at: http://www.perinatalhospice.org (accessed July 21, 2020).
21. National Association of Perinatal Social Workers. *Standards for Social Workers in Perinatal Bereavement.* Available online at: https://www.napsw.org/assets/docs/bereavement-standards.pdf (accessed July 23, 2020).
22. *Resolve Through Sharing.* Available online at: https://www.gundersenhealth.org/resolve-through-sharing/ (accessed July 23, 2020).
23. Limbo R, Wool C. Perinatal palliative care. *J Obstet Gynecol Neonatal Nurs.* (2016) 45:611–3. doi: 10.1016/j.jogn.2016.07.002
24. Ryan A, Bernhard H, Fahlberg B. Best practices for perinatal palliative care. *Nursing.* (2015) 45:14–5. doi: 10.1097/01.NURSE.0000471422.49754.9b
25. Janvier A, Farlow B, Barrington KJ. Parental hopes, interventions, and survival of neonates with trisomy 13 and trisomy 18. *Am J Med Genet Part C Semin Med Genet.* (2016) 172:279–87. doi: 10.1002/ajmg.c.31526
26. Kuebelbeck A, Davis DL. *A Gift of Time: Continuing Your Pregnancy When Your Baby's Life is Expected to Be Brief.* Baltimore, MD: Johns Hopkins University Press. (2011)
27. American Speech-Language Association, Practice Management. Available online at: https://www.asha.org/practice/ (accessed July 15, 2020).
28. Chichester M, Wool C. The meaning of food and multicultural implications for perinatal palliative care. *Nurs Womens Health.* (2015) 3:224–35. doi: 10.1111/1751-486X.12204
29. Committee on Hospital Care and Child Life Council. American academy of pediatrics policy statement: child life services. *Pediatrics.* (2014) 133:e1471–8. doi: 10.1542/peds.2014-0556
30. National Perinatal Association - Webinars on Mental Health and Trauma-informed Care. Available online at: http://www.nationalperinatal.org/webinars (accessed July 15, 2020).
31. *Postpartum Support International.* Available online at: https://www.postpartum.net/ (accessed July 15, 2020).
32. Puchalski C, Ferrell BR. *Making Health Care Whole: Integrating Spirituality into Patient Care.* West Conshohocken, PA: Templeton Press. (2010)
33. National Consensus Project for Quality Palliative Care. Domain 5: Spiritual, religious and existential aspects of care. In: *Clinical Practice Guidelines for Quality Palliative Care, 4th Edn.* Available online at: http://

nchpc.conferencespot.org/67968-nchpc-1.4266595/t009-1.4266773/f009-1.4266774/a054-1.4266785 (accessed July 20, 2020).

34. Hexem KR, Mollen CJ, Carroll K, Lanctot DA, Feudtner C. How parents of children receiving pediatric palliative care use religion, spirituality, or life philosophy in tough times. *J Palliat Med.* (2011) 14:39–44. doi: 10.1089/jpm.2010.0256
35. Centers for Medicare and Medicaid Services, Department of Health and Human Services. *Hospice care. Code of Federal Register. 79 FR 50509.* (2014). Available online at: https://www.ecfr.gov/cgi-bin/text-idx?SID=95c732ed603d39aed3682d6371ca27ea&mc=true&node=se42.3.418_13&rgn=div8 (accessed July 21, 2020).
36. Wool C. Clinician confidence and comfort in providing perinatal palliative care. *J Obstet Gynecol Neonatal Nurs.* (2013) 42:48–58. doi: 10.1111/j.1552-6909.2012.01432.x
37. Fulop N, Robert G. *Context for Successful Quality Improvement.* London: The Health Foundation. (2015). p. 1–116.
38. Callahan K, Steinwurtzel R, Bruarie L, Schechter S, Parravicini P. Early palliative care reduces stress in parents of neonates with congenital heart disease: validation of the "baby, attachment, comfort interventions." *J Perinat.* (2019) 39:1640–7. doi: 10.1038/s41372-019-0490-y

27

Summary of the Key Concepts on How to Develop a Perinatal Palliative Care Program

Paola Lago [1], Maria Elena Cavicchiolo [2], Francesca Rusalen [3] and Franca Benini [3]*

[1] Neonatal Intensive Care Unit, Ca' Foncello Hospital, Treviso, Italy, [2] Department of Woman and Child Health, Neonatal Intensive Care Unit, University of Padua, Padua, Italy, [3] Department of Woman and Child Health, Paediatric Pain and Palliative Care Service, University of Padua, Padua, Italy

***Correspondence:**
Paola Lago
paola.lago@aulss2.veneto.it

Purpose of review: The aim of this study is to assess the most significant Perinatal Palliative Care (PnPC) development projects in the literature and summarize the shared key principles.

Recent findings: PnPC is a new concept in neonatal intensive care approach. Advancements in perinatal diagnostics and medical technology have changed the landscape of the perinatal world. The threshold of viability continues to decrease, and diagnostic information is available earlier in pregnancy and more rapidly at the bedside; overall outcomes continue to improve. This rapid technological improvement brings ethical debates on the quality of life of patients with life-limiting and life-threatening conditions and the need to involve the family in the decision-making process, according to their wishes and cultural beliefs. Although the Perinatal Hospice concept was developed in the 1980s in the US, the first recommendations on how to develop a PnPC pathway were published in the early 2000s. We considered the most relevant position statements or guidelines on PnPC published in the last two decades. Some of them were more pertinent to pediatrics but still useful for the fundamental concepts and PnPC project's development.

Summary: Health care providers and institutions are encouraged to develop PnPC programs, which have the goal of maximizing the quality of life of infants with non-curable conditions. These may generally include the following: a formal prenatal consultation; development of a coordinated birth plan between obstetrician, newborn care, and family; access to other neonatal and pediatric specialties, as needed; comfort palliative care during the prenatal, birth, and postnatal periods; and psychosocial and spiritual support for families, siblings, and staff.

Keywords: perinatal palliative care, limit of viability, life-limiting condition, life-threatening condition, program

KEY MESSAGES

- PnPC principles and guidelines have been well defined and standardized in the last two decades;
- The candidates to PnPC are well identified: fetuses/infants with life-limiting or threatening conditions that seem incompatible with long-term survival and/or that carries the risk of severe impairment of quality of life as well as prematurity that limits viability;
- Preterm infants born at the limit of viability may seem to be the most challenging candidates because there is often no time to go through the perinatal consultation process and create a birth plan; thus, conflicts could easily emerge between clinicians and staff;
- The key issue is currently the implementation of PnPC into the NICU where we can consider two models: integrative vs. consultative;
- Regardless of the strategy adopted to implement a PnPC pathway in clinical practices, it is mandatory to identify the quality indicators/outcome data and perform regular audits and case debriefing to assure quality improvement;
- Many papers are available on end-of -life care and management of pain and other distressing symptoms;
- Settings for the PnPC program are also important; home discharge and perinatal hospice should be considered in specific cases;
- Staff education is another key rule for a successful implementation of PnPC and should be constantly addressed in the PnPC program.

INTRODUCTION

A Perinatal Palliative Care (PnPC) program aims to optimize quality of life for fetus and infants with life-limiting or life-threatening conditions and their families. The goal of the program is to ensure that infants who are expected to survive only hours, days, or months do not suffer unnecessary pain and discomfort in a family-oriented environment in which parents are allowed to stay with their infant all the time with a grade of involvement based on their wishes and expectations (1).

A dedicated multi-disciplinary team that is comprehensive of all the specialists involved in the perinatal care path should continually reassess all the needs (of the body, mind and spirit) of the newborn and his family while trying to give timely and concrete answers to each of them. This is in accordance with the recent ACOG Committee Opinion #786 entitled Perinatal Palliative Care that is also endorsed by the American Academy of Pediatrics (2, 3).

Perinatal Palliative Care integrates the clinical care of the infant starting from the diagnosis of a life-limiting conditionor from a decision to withholding or withdrawn life support. This also offers an advanced care plan when the transition from intensive care to comfort care is proposed because the best interest of the infants is not prolonging life (2, 3).

Thereafter PnPC may start before birth and continue through comfort palliative care and end-of-life care. After death, there is bereavement care in a continuum of activities to support infant and parents based on their wishes, values, preferences, and spiritual needs. Counseling, debriefing, and emotional support for the staff should also be part of the care path (4).

In all of these steps, it is possible to share an integrated care plan and bundles between the professionals involved to make the process more effective always with respect for the unique individuality of the infants and its family. This study summarizes the development of a PnPC program via a narrative review of the evidence on perinatal management in the world's most industrialized countries.

Abbreviations: AAP, American Academy of Pediatrics; ESPNIC, European Society for Paediatric & Neonatal Intensive Care Society; EFCNI, European foundation for the care of newborn infants; IMPaCCT, International meeting for Palliative Care in children; NICE, National Institute for Health and Care Excellence; NICU, neonatal intensive care unit; PnPC, perinatal palliative care; PPC, pediatric palliative care.

METHODS

While not adhering to strict PRISMA standards, this review utilized a thorough review of Embase, PubMed, and Google Scholar and the National Bioethics Committed websites via a combination of the following search strings: practice guidelines; AND perinatal palliative care; AND limit of viability. No language restrictions were applied. All potentially relevant titles and abstracts were retrieved and assessed for eligibility.

RESULTS

We retrieved 34 full text articles from electronic databases and six from National Bioethics Committed websites. We excluded 10 articles as no pertinent with the review. Six papers manually searched were included.

Evidence From the Literature on PnPC

The application of palliative care concept to the newborn was described for the first time in the United States in 1982 (5). Brian Carter first developed a neonatal end-of-life palliative care protocol in 2002. The protocol was prepared by a 101-member panel using the Delphi research method to build a consensus document. The data collection included both participant input over an 18-month period and synthesis of 16 published and non-published end-of-life protocols developed by international, national, regional, institutional, and parent organizations. While contributors to the project mainly come from the USA, the principles and processes discussed here may be applicable to those in other countries. This work still represents a milestone in the Perinatal Palliative Care program developed all over the word although it focuses mainly on end of life care that is a part of the PnPC program (6).

In 2007, the core standards for Pediatric Palliative Care in Europe were published: IMPaCCT International meeting for Palliative Care in children. Those standards referred to pediatric populations and could also be validated for PnPC in the major points. However, PnPC is a pathway dedicated to fetus and newborns with life-limiting or life-threatening conditions, and thus this standard should be integrated with prenatal consultation and birth plans as well as decision-making on extreme prematurity and the perinatal hospice (7).

In 2013, the American Academy of Pediatrics (AAP) published a Policy Statement on Pediatric Palliative Care and Hospice Commitments, Guidelines, and Recommendations. This team considered children with life-threatening and life-shortening conditions, and they summarized 12 recommendations that should be respected when developing a PnPC program. Briefly, the transversal standards for pediatric palliative care (PPC) include the availability of a dedicated interdisciplinary team that should have sufficient expertise to address all the basic needs of the child and his family (physical, psychological, emotional, practical, and spiritual). The PPC team should provide collaborative integrated multimodal care in relation to the regional pediatrics hospices while maintaining a core level of competency. The PPC team should be consulted frequently if there is a child with life-limiting condition to provide the best and most prompt care possible and should provide communication and decision support, family support, sibling support, and health care professional support. PPC should be a core part of medical school, residency, fellowship, and continuing education curricula. The PPC team should support and engage in research, and the program should have a quality improvement agenda. PPC teams should address ethical issues and engage in relationships with the hospital's ethics committee. The PPC program may have full financial support (8).

The AAP (3), European Foundation for the Care of Newborn Infants (EFCNI) (9), Pediatric Palliative Care Group Australia (10), and national neonatal societies (11–14) have published guidelines and statements specifically regarding PnPC. **Table 1** summarizes the most important guidelines.

Categorization

Guidelines have identified three types of patients for whom PnPC may be anticipated and offered in the newborn period: (a) those born at the threshold of viability; (b) those with birth anomalies that may threaten vital functions, and (c) those for whom intensive care has been appropriately applied but developed an incurable disease (1, 6).

Multidisciplinary Approach

Most guidelines suggest a multidisciplinary approach involving an interdisciplinary team who can address all the needs of the child and family. It is important to develop an action plan via a multidisciplinary project group with the steps needed to put guidelines into practice at the local level. This may differ from setting to setting. Basically, an effective perinatal palliative care team may include obstetricians, neonatologists, health care providers with expertise in pediatric palliative care, nurses, social workers, mental health professionals, religious counselors, and experts on the child's disease (2, 9, 11, 14). The goal of this team is to provide support and continuity of care throughout pregnancy, delivery, as well as postpartum and neonatal periods. It is important to monitor the data more indicative of the requested changes as in a quality improvement process. This work should review and audit to give evidence of the guideline's implementation.

Prenatal Diagnosis

Advanced technology can suggest precociously if the fetus is carrying a life-limiting condition. The diagnosis can be made early in pregnancy with invasive or non-invasive prenatal investigations (fetal ultrasound, non-invasive prenatal test, chorionic villous sampling, amniocentesis). The condition may also be suspected and confirmed at birth.

In such cases, antenatal counseling should occur with a multidisciplinary team including at least the gynecologist, the neonatologist, the palliative care team when available, and the consultant with expertise in the child's disease (2, 9, 11, 14). The results of genetic and other diagnostic evaluations, and information about the condition of the fetus and its prognosis should be shared among the group. Different options from termination of pregnancy to palliative comfort care at birth can be presented to the family. A plan of action at birth can be created according to the family's wishes and beliefs (15).

Birth Plan

A death that is anticipated before birth affords the family the opportunity to work with the health-care team to develop both a birth plan that specifies their desires for how they want the birth to evolve and a palliative care plan. The family's participation in making these plans helps to provide them with a sense of control, and the plan honors their choices for their baby. This is worthwhile in creating a therapeutic alliance for ongoing care. This individualized proposal for delivery and neonatal care could be reviewed during the following consultations until birth. When the birth occurs, the plan should be followed regardless of which health professionals are present at the time (1, 15).

In 2016, the National Institute for Health and Care Excellence (NICE) published guidelines on end-of-life care for infants, children, and young people with the life-limiting conditions: planning and management (16).

NICE's guidelines indicated the modern general principles for developing plans for the care of the child with life-limiting or threatening conditions considering the Advance Care Plan—the preferred tool that considers the preferences and values of parents and caretakers. In the recommendations for research, the NICE committee indicated perinatal palliative care as one of the goals for future research when there is a perinatal diagnosis of life-limiting condition (16).

Postnatal Diagnosis

There is no opportunity to prepare a birth plan in the case of unanticipated loss, for an unexpected preterm birth, for a life-limiting condition diagnosed postnatally, or in case of a development of an incurable disease.

Limit of viability is a unique condition of PnPC. A systematic review published in Pediatrics in 2015 summarized international recommendations on management of preterm newborn born between 22- and 25 weeks of GA. Although there is a wide variation in clinical practice; the paper identified a gray zone between 23- and 24-weeks GA, general consensus for comfort care at 22 weeks' GA, and agreement for active care after 25 weeks' GA. While this statement may pertain to well-resourced countries, periviability may be referenced in developing or

TABLE 1 | Guidelines, position statements and opinion on perinatal palliative care worldwide.

Country	Year	Author	Methodology	Area	Topics
Australia	2018	Paediatric Palliative Care Group Australia	Guidelines	PC	- Family-centered communication and decision-making - Teamwork and coordination of care - Components of care - Use of triggers to recognize children approaching the end of life - Response to concerns - Leadership and governance - Education and training - Supervision and support for interdisciplinary team members - Evaluation, audit and feedback - Systems to support high-quality care
Canada	2016	Limbo et al.	Position statement	PnPC	- Perinatal bereavement - Care coordination - Interprofessional teamwork - Birth and advance care planning - Follow-up
Europe	2007	IMPaCCT: standards for pediatric palliative care in Europe.	Position statement	PPC	- Palliative team - Care coordinator - Pain management - Grief management - Training and education - Euthanasia
Europe	2019	EFCNI (European foundation for the care of newborn infants)	Committee opinion	PnPC	- Decisions of withholding or withdrawing life support - Communication in ethically complex decisions - Rights of infants, parents, and families in difficult decisions - Palliative care
France	2011	French Society of Neonatology and the Working Group on Ethical Issues	Position statement	PnPC	- Euthanasia is forbidden by French law - Physician may lawfully decide to withhold or withdraw a life-sustaining treatment that is unanimously considered unreasonable obstinacy. - Medical decisions must sometimes be taken for a newborn baby whose survival depends on intensive care but whose future quality of life is predicted as poor. - Reasonable treatments that should be started or continued must be distinguished from unreasonable treatments that should be stopped. - This requires assessment of the limit between a quality of life judged as acceptable for the patient and his family and a quality of life judged as unbearable.
Netherlands	2006	Verhagen et al.	Protocol	PnPC	The Groningen Protocol for Euthanasia in Newborns. Requirements that must be fulfilled: - The diagnosis and prognosis must be certain - Hopeless and unbearable suffering must be present - The diagnosis, prognosis, and unbearable suffering must be confirmed by at least one independent doctor - Both parents must give informed consent - The procedure must be performed in accordance with the accepted medical standard
UK	2014	Northern Neonatal Network UK	Guidelines	PPC	- Care before death - Care at the time of death - Care after death - Bereavement support - Staff support and supervision
UK	2015	NANN (National Association of Neonatal Nurse)	Position statement	PnPC	- Palliative care should be offered at any period in which the infant's life may be limited - When a prenatal diagnosis is made, palliative care should be offered prior to delivery. - When continuation of the pregnancy is chosen, planning and decision making for the birth will be present - All care goals should be developed as a team and include the parents. - Family conferences are essential to the providers' understanding of families' needs and their hopes and goals for their infant - An advocate or palliative care provider should be identified prenatally or at delivery/diagnosis for each infant and family in need of palliative services. - Palliative care team - Private home-like environment - Parental preferences - Local hospice - Artificial nutrition - Bereavement care - Support services to all members of the healthcare team

(Continued)

TABLE 1 | Continued

Country	Year	Author	Methodology	Area	Topics
UK	2016	NICE (National Institute for Health and Care Excellence)	Guidelines	PPC	- Advance Care Planning - Emotional and psychological support and interventions - Managing distressing symptoms, such as pain, agitation, seizures or respiratory distress - Hydration and nutrition - Recognizing that a child or young person is likely to die within hours or days - Care and support for parents, carers and healthcare professionals after the death of a child or young person - Care at home
UK	2019	Mancini et al.	Guidelines	PnPC	- Support for Staff: Building Resilience in Nurses - The Importance of Effective Communication on a Neonatal Unit - Spiritual, Cultural and Religious Care for the Baby and Family - Ethical Concepts in Neonatal Palliative Care - Legal Issues in Neonatal Palliative Care - The Principles of Genetics Within Neonatal Palliative Care - Antenatal Care for the Mother and Baby in the Context of Neonatal Palliative Care - Care of Twins, Multiple Births and Support for the Family: A Detailed Background - Care of Twins, Multiple Births and Support for the Family: The Butterfly Project - The Decision-Making Process and the Role of the Neonatal Nurse - Advance Care Planning - Organ and Tissue Donation - Continuing Emotional and Practical Support for the Whole Family - Fundamental Principles of Effective Symptom Management in Neonatal Palliative Care - Collaboration Between Hospices and Neonatal Units - Interdisciplinary Working in Neonatal Palliative Care - Developing Knowledge and Competence in Neonatal Palliative Care Practice - Care after Death
USA	2019	ACOG (American College of Obstetricians and Gynecologists)	Committee opinion	PnPC	1. Decisions about non-initiation or withdrawal of intensive care should be made by the health care team and the parents of a high-risk infant working together. This approach requires honest and open communication. Ongoing evaluation of the condition and prognosis of the high-risk infant is essential, and the physician, as the spokesperson for the health care team, must convey this information accurately and openly to the parents of the infant 2. Parents should be active participants in the decision making process concerning the treatment of severely ill infants 3. Compassionate basic care to ensure comfort must be provided to all infants, including those for whom intensive care is not being provided 4. The decision to initiate or continue intensive care should be based only on the judgment that the infant will benefit from the intensive care. It is inappropriate for life-prolonging treatment to be continued when the condition is incompatible with life or when the treatment is judged to be harmful, of no benefit, or futile
USA	2019	AAP (American Academy of Pediatrics)	Committee opinion	PnPC	
Germany	2020	PaluTIN group	Committee opinion	PnPC	10-key elements: - Focus on Needs and Hope - Empowering Parenthood - Communication - Evaluating Therapeutic Goals and Treatment Choices Together - Advance Care Planning - Comfort Care Toward the End of Life - Grief Counseling - Spirituality, Religion, and Pastoral Guidance - Support Systems - The Team Duality

PC, palliative care; PPC, pediatric palliative care; PnPC, perinatal palliative care.

middle-to-poorly resourced countries at gestational ages above 24–25 weeks EGA (17).

Guidelines usually describe a risk-based approach for interventions in the "peri-viable" period by dividing preterm infants into three categories: "*beneficial*" where intervention is generally recommended; "*gray zone*" where interventions follow the decision of parents; and "*futile*" where comfort care is recommended (18–20). This decision cannot be based only on gestational age. For example, across similar time periods, survival rates at 22 weeks' gestation in different countries vary dramatically: from zero in Switzerland and France to as high as 34% in Japan (18, 21). These differences are attributed to either a more active interventionist approach or to underreporting of perinatal deaths. The British Association of Perinatal Medicine (BAPM) proposed a risk-based approach for neonates born <27 gestational weeks based on unmodifiable (i.e., gestational age, fetal growth, sex, plurality) and modifiable risk factors (i.e., prenatal steroids, setting for birth) (22). Some guidelines suggested a more active involvement of families in the decision-making process (2). Others suggested not to resuscitate below some gestational age limit independently of the parents' wishes (17).

In the case of a life-limiting condition diagnosed or confirmed postnatally, it is important to note that the list of diseases could change from country to country and from year to year. As novel therapies emerge and change the disease outcome, management may shift from a palliative care to a more intensive management. For example, in some cases, heart surgery could be offered to children with trisomy 18 (23) and cases of children affected from trisomy 18 who survived longer than a few years have been reported (24). Nevertheless, palliative care teams remain a valuable resource in these settings because they can assist families with decision-making and provide ongoing support since some of these novel therapies are experimental, and the outcomes may be variable.

Similar recommendations are given for children who developed a poor outcome condition after experiencing prolonged intensive care treatment (e.g., severe bronchopulmonary dysplasia or massive necrotizing enterocolitis) or those newborns that cannot improve despite massive medical treatment (Apgar score of 0 at 10 min, refractory pulmonary hypertension, or refractory septic shock). In such cases, guidelines suggest creating a trusting relationship between family and team. The family should be included into the decision-making process without overwhelming them; this can shift the intensive care approach to a palliative one. These transitions may include discontinuation of mechanical ventilator support, artificial circulatory support, and/or artificial nutrition and hydration (2, 9).

Timing and Setting

Newborns can survive less than a few hours or much depending on the disease. If the diagnosis was made prenatally, then the parents are aware of the child's condition and have a birth plan. The PnPC may be applied in the delivery room. PnPC is generally offered by the neonatologist to guarantee comfort, maintain temperature, and prevent respiratory distress to the newborn (2, 15). Parents should be offered the opportunity to hold and to spend as much time as they wish with their baby in a quiet and private location. After the baby's death, a bereavement care plan should be organized for the family including communicating with parents and creating memories, giving the opportunity to dress the baby and take pictures, and making molds of handprints or footprints—of course while considering the family's spiritual, religious and cultural beliefs (15).

If a life-limiting condition is suspected or confirmed postnatally or there is a shift from intensive care to PnPC, then comfort care may be provided in the neonatal intensive care unit (NICU). Such care includes pain and symptom management, prenatal palliative care consultations, end-of-life care, communication and conflict resolution, collaboration in the care of the medically complex infant, and discharge to hospice where available (2, 9, 14, 16). Amy Kuebelbeck in her website (www.perinatalhospice.org) reported 226 perinatal hospices in the USA and 57 international programs. Perinatal hospice is a family-centered, safe, and quiet place where all of the care is focused on the quality of life of the baby and honoring parent values and wishes; in the case of discharge to home, the focus is on the education of the family on the management of the newborn (25).

Management

In 2014 Alexandra Mancini et al. "Practical guidance for the management of palliative care on neonatal units" on behalf of the Royal College of Pediatrics and Child Health (26). However, these practical guidelines do not cover the process of reaching the decision to withhold or withdraw life-sustaining treatment and has limited information on decision-making. Other toolkits and practical guidelines are available in this contest. This text focuses on the practical aspect of care including symptoms alleviation and comfort care while providing support to families and staff.

Palliative care has two fundamental concepts: withholding and withdrawing treatment (9, 27). While there may be an emotional difference between not initiating an intervention at all (withholding) and discontinuing it later in the course of care (withdrawing), there is no ethical difference between the two options (28). When an intervention no longer helps to achieve the patient's goals for care or desired quality of life, it is ethically and legally appropriate for physicians to withdraw it and redirect the care. This means that in end-of-life care, the physician can decrease and discontinue the mechanical ventilation and stop any vasoactive drugs, antibiotics, and fluid therapy. Even nutrition, although debated, can be suspended (27–29). The AAP stated that withholding or withdrawing artificial nutrition is acceptable, particularly when it's prolonging the process of dying but children capable to eat and drink safely, who wanted to eat and drink, should be given food and fluids by mouth (28).

This approach is applicable in high resource countries. In a retrospective multicentric study performed in Latin-American NICUs showed a completely different approach in end of life decision making. Withdrawing the support was no existent and usually the baby died with full life support. Preterm babies <27 gestational weeks were not admitted to the NICUs (30).

The European Standards of Care for Newborn Infant Health by EFCNI were published in 2018 and were meant as a benchmark for the development of standards in each individual country (9). They are comprehensive of evidence-based practices and qualitative outcome indicators that will significantly improve health outcomes in preterm infants in Europe and beyond. They developed four standards for key ethical decisions: decision to withhold or withdraw life support; palliative care, communication in ethically complex decisions; and the rights of infants, parents, and families in difficult decisions. They also found that the indicators of meeting the standard were aside from the evidence of a guidelines or formal setup pathway, patient information sheet, training documentations, annual report, or minutes of debriefing. Clearly, parental feedback is a critical issue/factor.

The National Association of Neonatal Nurses (NNAN) published a position statement on palliative and end-of-life care for newborn and infants in 2015 focusing on transport of infant when a redirection of care is chosen as well as nutrition and hydration and on nurse education (31).

Bidegain and Younge proposed two models of PnPC, the "*integrative model*" and the "*consultative model*" (32). The integrative model can be offered early in the pathway of every life-limiting condition or extreme prematurity. Here, the principles of "palliative care" are integrated as core element of the intensive care and after. This perspective could start before birth when a prenatal diagnosis of incurable condition has been made. It could then continue at home or in a hospice context if the child is going to survive longer. The availability of protocols, bundles, and order sets guide clinicians in the process.

In the consultative model, the palliative medicine specialist provides expert advice to the NICU staff on a child with palliative needs. Consultation may focus on same aspect of care as symptom management, consultation, and communication within the primary care team and with families. There is also withdrawal of intensive care and transition to hospice.

Thinking to the implementation of PnPC guidelines, one should consider a combined approach with palliative care principles/resources integrated within the NICU and consultation services available in situations of higher complexity (32).

Conflicts

In most situations, the care team and family agree about a desire to mitigate pain and suffering including what is in the infant's best interest and how to proceed (2, 9, 22, 26). In some situations however, ethical conflict can arise regarding the provision of potentially inappropriate or no longer beneficial care. This conflict can arise between staff members or between physicians and the family.

Conflicts between parents and staff could be avoided or mitigated involving parents from the starts, allowing time for reflexion (33) or for additional meetings, additional diagnostic tests, and second opinions (34). When the conflict cannot be mitigated, consulting the local ethics committee is suggested (2, 15).

Milk Donation and Lactation Suppression

Pregnant women with an intrauterine diagnosis of a lethal condition can plan to practice skin to skin contact and breastfeeding with their babies at the time of birth. During the postmortem period, the mothers can be supported if they decide to engage in milk donation (31, 35). Donating breast milk can have a profound influence on how bereaved women make meaning of their experience, and some women described milk donation after perinatal loss as a mechanism to facilitate their progression through grief. However, if a mother decides not to donate milk, then the option of suppressing lactation via pharmacotherapy should be offered (36).

Following the Death

Although difficult, it is mandatory to give information to the family regarding burial arrangements and final disposition of the infant's body. Verbal and written information about hospital services should be provided to the parents (2, 15). A meeting with the healthcare professionals who actually cared for their baby and parents should be arranged 1–2 months after the loss. During the meeting the clinical report should be provided (15).

Organ Donation

The issue on organ donation during the neonatal period is controversial. First, it is extremely difficult to ascertain brain death in newborns. It is unclear if giving heparin and intubation to ensure the viability of organs in a baby diagnosed with a life-limiting condition is ethical acceptable. In Italy, organ donation may be considered only term newborns more than 7 days old (>38 gestational weeks) in which brain death is demonstrated (37, 38). In UK organ donation for infants <2 months of age could be performed only if there is a neurological determination of death, which is rarely possible to confirm at this age (39). Ancillary tests, which included electroencephalogram and radionuclide cerebral blood flow study to confirm neurological death could be used in the USA, making the organ donation possible (40).

The strength of our study is that it provides an overview of the most significant aspects of PnPC and aims to provide key principles to create or implement a PnPC program. We recognize some limitation. We did not perform a systematic review but only a narrative review of the most relevant evidence on PnPC in literature and we did not include internal or unpublished guidelines of PnPC that many hospitals might have.

DISCUSSION

Advancements in perinatal diagnostics and medical technology have changed the landscape of the perinatal world. The threshold of viability continues to decrease, and diagnostic information is available earlier in pregnancy and more rapidly at the bedside. The overall outcomes continue to improve. This rapid technological improvement also brings ethical debates on the quality of life of these patients and the need to involve the family in the decision-making process.

Many professional organizations and scientific societies in industrialized countries promulgate management guidelines for these infants and newborns with poor prognosis pathologies, but the management of these patients, as well as their survival, is very heterogeneous. Survival depends on various factors including social, religious beliefs, law restrictions, and national ethics opinions (41).

In the last two decades, the principles and best practices in a PnPC program were mostly defined along with an overarching palliative care paradigm. However, the literature suggests that there are still many challenging aspects surrounding the implementation of PnPC. These are still lacking in many places were perinatal care are delivered. In our opinion, this is due to several reasons.

First, the key principles of PnPC include advancing care planning, symptom management, and psychosocial support for families and NICU staff even in the neonatal period. Help with the decision-making process and how to manage conflicts and bereavement care are quite definitely defined (2, 9, 15, 41). All of this knowledge is reported as guidelines or evidence-based practices. It is mostly "opinion of the expert" or consensus (based on Delphi methodology) with low levels of evidence. These low levels of evidence may make this research "unconvincing" and may interfere with the implementation of a PnPC.

Second, the outcomes of a "standardized" program and quality improvement initiatives are inconsistently reported. This may due to difficulties in measuring the quality of care/improvement in this setting.

Third, the fact that the PnPC is strongly focused on end-of life care limits the use of PnPC encouraging the misconception that palliative care should be reserved for only end-of-life situations. Rather, it should be considered a comprehensive and coordinated model of care—a curative treatment for fetus/neonates with life-limiting or life-threatening conditions with the goal the quality of life of the infant and family according to their wishes and values.

It is essential to give evidence of rigorous PnPC implementation process as well as evaluation of a wide range of outcome data. Only in this way we can give evidence for successful implementation of PnPC, which is still very low.

The PnPC and its benefits have been endorsed by many institutions and scientific societies (2, 9, 12, 16); however, the PnPC still lags behind other areas of palliative care when it comes to successful implementation of a quality program. Organized programs that include protocols, orders, staff education, and dedicated palliative care teams need to be addressed. The parents' experience is another area to be monitored because this might give the health care professionals insight into the benefits of the best practices in this context.

The continuity of the incurability pathway should be advised because in some situations the infants may survive months and need a different allocation of care. It is also essential that the link between regional pediatric hospice and territorial (primary) care be clear (25). During the life-limiting trajectory, discharge home with hospice support is often in the best interest of the child and their family instead of remaining in the NICU.

PnPC is a new concept in neonatal intensive care approach. Withholding or withdrawing the intensive care does not mean stopping treatments. Rather, it means redirecting active treatment to a different approach (27, 32). PnPC needs education and training of the staff to this new field of care (2, 41). All members of the health care team need to be part of the decision-making process and disagreements between staff or parents and staff needs to be resolved. Opinions from an independent clinical ethics committee may be helpful in resolving conflicts. Organ donation, disposition of the infant remains, and milk donation are elements that should be discussed in a PnPC protocol.

CONCLUSION

PnPC is a new field of newborn care. It aims to ameliorate the health status of children with life-limiting conditions. Creating a PnPC program is mandatory to guide physicians and parents through this difficult journey.

AUTHOR CONTRIBUTIONS

PL conceptualized and designed the review and drafted the initial manuscript. MC drafted the final version of the manuscript. FB aided in designing the manuscript and contributed to the content. FR reviewed the literature. All authors contributed to the article and approved the submitted version.

REFERENCES

1. Carter BS. Pediatric palliative care in infants and neonates. *Children.* (2018) 5:21. doi: 10.3390/children5020021
2. American College of Obstetricians and Gynecologists. *Perinatal Palliative Care. Committee Opinion No. 786.* Washington, DC: American College of Obstetricians and Gynecologists (2019). Available online at: https://www.acog.org/clinical/clinical-guidance/committee-opinion/articles/2019/09/perinatal-palliative-care (accessed August 31, 2020).
3. Perinatal palliative care. *Pediatrics.* (2019) 144:e20193146. doi: 10.1542/peds.2019-3146
4. *WHO Definition of Palliative Care.* Available online at: https://www.who.int/cancer/palliative/definition/en/ (accessed August 15, 2020).
5. Silverman, W.A. A hospice setting for humane neonatal death. *Pediatrics.* (1982) 69:239.
6. Catlin A, Carter BS. Creation of a neonatal end of life palliative care protocol. *J Perinatol.* (2002) 22:184–95. doi: 10.1038/sj.jp.7210687
7. Craig F, Abu-Saad Huijer H, Benini F, Kuttner L, Wood C, Cornaglia Ferraris P, et al. IMPaCCT: standards for pediatric palliative care in Europe. *Eur J Palliat Care.* (2007) 14:109–11. doi: 10.1007/s00482-008-0690-4
8. Section on Hospice and Palliative Medicine and Committee on Hospital Care. Pediatric palliative care and hospice commitments, guidelines and recommendations. *Pediatrics.* (2013) 132:996–72. doi: 10.1542/peds.2013-2731
9. *European Standards of Care for Newborn Health (EFCNI).* Available online at: https://newborn-health-standards.org/ (accessed August 15, 2020).
10. Pediatric Palliative Care Group Australia. *Pediatric Addendum Palliative Care Service Development Guidelines.* Available online at: www.palliativecare.org.au (accessed August 15, 2020).
11. Limbo R, Toce S, Peck T. *Resolve Through Sharing (RTS) Position Paper on Perinatal Palliative Care.* Rev ed. La Crosse, WI: Gundersen Lutheran Medical Foundation, Inc. (2008–2016).
12. Northem Neonatal Network UK. *A Guide to End of Life Care Care of Children and Young People Before Death, at the Time of Death and After Death.* Available online at: https://www.togetherforshortlives.org.uk/resource/guide-end-life-care/ (accessed August 15, 2020).
13. Dageville C, Bétrémieux P, Gold F, Simeoni U, Working Group on Ethical Issues in Perinatology. The French Society of Neonatology's proposals for neonatal end- of-life decision-making. *Neonatology.* (2011) 100:206–14. doi: 10.1159/000324119
14. Verhagen E, Sauer PJ. The Groningen protocol–euthanasia in severely ill newborns. *N Engl J Med.* (2005) 352:959–62. doi: 10.1056/NEJMp058026
15. Kenner C, Press J, Ryan D. Recommendations for palliative and bereavement care in the NICU: a family-centered integrative approach. *J Perinatol.* (2015) 35 (Suppl. 1):S19–23. doi: 10.1038/jp.2015.145
16. NICE-National Institute for Health and Care Excellence. *End of Life Care for Infants, Children and Young People With Life-Limiting Conditions: Planning*

and Management. (2016). Available online at: htpps://www.Nice.org.uk/guidance/ng61 (accessed August 15, 2020).
17. Guillén Ú, Weiss EM, Munson D, Maton P, Jefferies A, Norman M, et al. Guidelines for the management of extremely premature deliveries: a systematic review. *Pediatrics*. (2015) 136:343–50. doi: 10.1542/peds.2015-0542
18. Isayama T. The clinical management and outcomes of extremely preterm infants in Japan: past, present, and future. *Transl Pediatr*. (2019) 8:199–211. doi: 10.21037/tp.2019.07.10
19. Da Silva LJ. *Portuguese Neonatal Society. Update on Viability and Care of Extreme Preterm Babies*. (2012) Available online at: https://www.spneonatologia.pt/wp-content/uploads/2016/11/Update_on_viability_and_care_of_extreme_preterm_babies_2012_docx_II (accessed August 15, 2020).
20. Berger TM, Bernet V, El Alama S, Fauchère JC, Hösli I, Irion O, et al. Perinatal care at the limit of viability between 22 and 26 completed weeks of gestation in Switzerland. *Swiss Med Week*. (2011) 141:w13280. doi: 10.4414/smw.2011.13280
21. Lorthe E, Torchin H, Delorme P, Ancel PY, Marchand-Martin L, Foix-L'Hélias L, et al. Preterm premature rupture of membranes at 22-25 weeks' gestation: perinatal and 2-year outcomes within a national population-based study (EPIPAGE-2). *Am J Obstet Gynecol*. (2018) 219:98.e1-298.e14. doi: 10.1016/j.ajog.2018.05.029
22. Mactier H, Bates SE, Johnston T, Lee-Davey C, Marlow N, Mulley K, et al. Perinatal management of extreme preterm birth before 27 weeks of gestation: a framework for practice. *Arch Dis Child Fetal Neonatal Ed*. (2020) 105:232–9. doi: 10.1136/archdischild-2019-318402
23. Janvier A, Farlow B, Barrington K. Cardiac surgery for children with trisomies 13 and 18: where are we now? *Semin Perinatol*. (2016) 40:254–60. doi: 10.1053/j.semperi.2015.12.015
24. Peterson JK, Kochilas LK, Catton KG, Moller JH, Setty SP. Long-term outcomes of children with trisomy 13 and 18 after congenital heart disease interventions. *Ann Thorac Surg*. (2017) 103:1941–9. doi: 10.1016/j.athoracsur.2017.02.068
25. *Perinatal Hospice and Palliative Care*. Available online at: https://www.perinatalhospice.org/ (accessed August 15, 2020).
26. Mancini A. *Practical Guidance for the Management of Palliative Care on Neonatal Units*. Available online at: https://www.chelwest.nhs.uk/services/childrens-services/neonatal-services/links/Practical-guidance-for-the-management-of-palliative-care-on-neonatal-units-Feb-2014.pdf/view (accessed August 15, 2020).
27. Reichlin M. On the ethics of withholding and withdrawing medical treatment. *Multidiscip Respir Med*. (2014) 9:39. doi: 10.4081/mrm.2014.374
28. Diekema DS, Botkin JR. Committee on Bioethics. Clinical report—Forgoing medically provided nutrition and hydration in children. *Pediatrics*. (2009) 124:813–22. doi: 10.1542/peds.2009-1299
29. Gedge E, Giacomini M, Cook D. Withholding and withdrawing life support in critical care settings: ethical issues concerning consent. *J Med Ethics*. (2007) 33:215–8. doi: 10.1136/jme.2006.017038
30. Fajardo CA, González S, Zambosco G, Cancela MJ, Forero LV, Venegas M, et al. End of life, death and dying in neonatal intensive care units in Latin America. *Acta Pediatr*. (2012) 101:609–13. doi: 10.1111/j.1651-2227.2012.02596.x
31. National Association of Neonatal Nurse (NNAN). *Palliative and End-of-Life Care for Newborns and Infants*. Available online at: http://www.nann.org/ (accessed August 15, 2020).
32. Bidegain M, Younge N. Comfort Care vs Palliative Care: Is there a difference in neonates? *NeoReviews*. (2015) 16:e333–9. doi: 10.1542/neo.16-6-e333
33. Tripp J, McGregor D. Withholding and withdrawing of life sustaining treatment in the newborn. *Arch Dis Child Fetal Neonatal Ed*. (2006) 91:F67–71. doi: 10.1136/adc.2004.068569
34. Verhagen AE, de Vos M, Dorscheidt JH, Engels B, Hubben JH, Sauer PJ. Conflicts about end-of-life decisions in NICUs in the Netherlands. *Pediatrics*. (2009) 124:e112–9. doi: 10.1542/peds.2008-1839
35. Cole JCM, Schwarz J, Farmer MC, Coursey AL, Duren S, Rowlson M, et al. Facilitating milk donation in the context of perinatal palliative care. *J Obstet Gynecol Neonatal Nurs*. (2018) 47:564–70. doi: 10.1016/j.jogn.2017.11.002
36. Welborn JM. The experience of expressing and donating breast milk following a perinatal loss. *J Hum Lact*. (2012) 28:506–10. doi: 10.1177/0890334412455459
37. Ahmad MU, Farrell RM, Weise KL. Neonatal organ donation: ethical insights and policy implications. *J Neonatal Perinatal Med*. (2019) 12:369–77. doi: 10.3233/NPM-1850
38. European Society for Pediatric & Neonatal Intensive Care Society (ESPNIC). *Standards for End of Life Care including Organ/Tissue Donation*. Available online at: https://espnic-online.org/Education/Standards-and-Guidelines (accessed August 15, 2020).
39. Charles E, Scales A, Brierley J. The potential for neonatal organ donation in a children's hospital. *Arch Dis Child Fetal Neonatal Ed*. (2014) 99:F225–9. doi: 10.1136/archdischild-2013-304803
40. Sarnaik AA. Neonatal and pediatric organ donation: ethical perspectives and implications for policy. *Front Pediatr*. (2015) 3:100. doi: 10.3389/fped.2015.00100
41. Parravicini E. Neonatal palliative care. *Curr Opin Pediatr*. (2017) 29:135–40. doi: 10.1097/MOP.0000000000000464

28

Bibliometric Analysis of Global Research on Perinatal Palliative Care

Yiting Wang [1†], Chunjian Shan [1†], Yingying Tian [2], Congshan Pu [1] and Zhu Zhu [3]*

[1] Department of Obstetrics, Women's Hospital of Nanjing Medical University, Nanjing Maternity and Child Health Care Hospital, Nanjing, China, [2] Department of Neonatology, Women's Hospital of Nanjing Medical University, Nanjing Maternity and Child Health Care Hospital, Nanjing, China, [3] Department of Nursing, Women's Hospital of Nanjing Medical University, Nanjing Maternity and Child Health Care Hospital, Nanjing, China

***Correspondence:**
Zhu Zhu
zz_njfy@sina.com

[†] These authors have contributed equally to this work and share first authorship

Objectives: The aim of this study was to perform a bibliometric analysis of publications related to perinatal palliative care to identify scientific output and research trends at a global level.

Methods: The Web of Science Core Collection database was searched to retrieve publications focusing on perinatal palliative care published between 2001 and 2020. All retrieved publications were identified by title and abstract for their relevance to perinatal palliative care. These eligible publications were extracted from the following data: title, abstract, year, keywords, author, organization, journal and cited literature. VOSviewer software was used to conduct bibliographic coupling, coauthorship, and cooccurrence analyses and to detect publication trends in perinatal palliative care research.

Results: A total of 114 publications concerning perinatal palliative care were included. The annual number of publications has increased dramatically in recent years. The United States has made the largest contribution to this field with the majority of publications (68, 59.6%) and citations (1,091, 70.5%) and with close collaborations with researchers in Canada, Portugal and Australia. Wool C and her institution, York College of Pennsylvania, are the respectively, most prolific author and institution in this field, publishing 18 papers (15.8%). Journal of Palliative Medicine is the leading and main journal in this field. According to the cooccurrence network analysis, five main research topics were identified: the candidates for PPC, service models and forms, framework components, parental perspectives and satisfaction, and challenges and needs of health care providers.

Conclusion: The findings of this bibliometric study illustrate the current state and global trends of perinatal palliative care for the past two decades, which will help researchers determine areas of research focus and explore new directions for future research in this field.

Keywords: perinatal palliative care, perinatal hospice, bibliometric, web of science, VOSviewer

INTRODUCTION

According to data released by the World Health Organization (WHO), an estimated 2.4 million infants died during the neonatal period in 2019, with the neonatal mortality rate reaching 17 per 1,000 live births (1). Notably, congenital malformations and chromosomal abnormalities were the leading causes of infant death, accounting for 20.8% of all infant deaths (2). With advances in prenatal screening and diagnostic techniques, these congenital abnormalities can be detected early, making more parents aware during pregnancy that their child is likely die at birth or shortly after (3). Despite receiving a prenatal diagnosis of a life-limiting condition (LLC), many families choose to continue their pregnancy based on their own beliefs, values and expectations. Caring for these infants and families poses a major challenge to health providers in obstetric and pediatric settings. This has prompted the development of perinatal palliative care (PPC) as an emerging field of palliative care to address the previously unmet needs of these families.

Perinatal palliative care refers to a coordinated and interdisciplinary care strategy dedicated to maximizing the quality and comfort of life of fetuses diagnosed prenatally as life-limiting and providing supportive care to their families throughout the pregnancy, delivery and postnatal periods (4). The World Health Assembly decided that providing palliative care for children is "an ethical responsibility of health systems" and that the integration of palliative care into health care systems can enable the achievement of the sustainable development goal of universal health coverage (5). However, there are various barriers to the development and accessibility of PPC services worldwide, including those related to public awareness, health policies, education and other conditions appropriate for PPC.

Globally, the development of PPC services varies greatly, and it is closely related to the state of PPC research in a country or region (6). Research generates the evidence necessary for the development of PPC services, whether for seeking best practices, identifying barriers and facilitators, monitoring outcomes, or determining health priorities (7). Additionally, in official documents of the WHO, research is recognized as one of the indicators used to assess and monitor the provision of PPC services (8). Hence, a better understanding of the current state of research can provide a clearer account of global trends, needs and challenges in the field of PPC.

In recent years, bibliometric analysis has been widely applied in quantitative analyses of literature research. Meanwhile, the approach can be used to describe academic activities in a research field; compare the contributions of countries, journals, institutes, and researchers; and detect future research directions (9, 10). Therefore, in this study, a bibliometric analysis of publications related to PPC was applied to identify scientific output and research trends at the global level to provide beneficial insight into policy-making and resource allocation and facilitate leading-edge, needs-led research.

METHODS

Data Sources

Data on PPC were retrieved from the Web of Science (WoS) Core Collection (WoSCC) Database. The WoSCC is the premier resource on the WoS platform and the world's most trusted citation index for scientific and scholarly research. The resource covers a collection of more than 21,000 peer-reviewed, high-quality scholarly journals, including open access journals, published worldwide in over 250 sciences, social sciences and humanities disciplines. Conference materials and book data are also available. The WoSCC was chosen for the present search, with all authors and their affiliations, abstracts and keywords, funding acknowledgments, cited references and unified institution names were captured for each paper, allowing for an in-depth exploration of specialized scholarly fields.

Search Strategy

For the search, the terms (perinatal* OR antenatal* OR prenatal* OR fetal* OR fetal* OR perinatolog*) AND (palliative care OR hospice*) were used as "topics" (titles, abstracts, author keywords, and keywords plus). The search time span was set to January 2000 to December 31, 2020, and editorial materials, letters, and meeting abstracts were excluded. Due to a considerable number of publications written in French, no language limits were applied when searching.

Data Collection

Publications were first screened by title and abstract for their relevance to PPC, which provides palliative comfort care from the prenatal diagnosis of a life-limiting fetal condition. Studies exclusively addressing neonatal palliative care of extremely premature cases and pediatric palliative care were excluded. The article screening process was performed independently by two researchers (C.P. and Y.W.), and any disagreement was resolved in a consensus meeting with held Y.T. After the eligible articles were identified, the "full records and cited references" of the articles were exported from the WoSCC on April 30, 2021. The process of articles selection used is shown in **Figure 1.** The following information was recorded: title, authors, year of publication, journal, country of origin, affiliation, keywords, total number of article citations, and research field.

Bibliometric and Visualized Analysis

This study applied VOSviewer (version 1.6.16), which has been widely used in recent bibliometric studies (11–14), to construct and visualize bibliometric networks. VOSviewer is a freely available software tool for creating maps based on network data and for visualizing and exploring these maps. In the generated visualization map, different colors reflect different clusters. The size of a label and the circle for an item are determined by an item's weight. The distance between two items reflects the strength of the relation between the items. Connecting lines represent parameters such as cooperation and cocitation. The stronger the link between two items is, the thicker the line used to display the link is, providing easily interpretable graphical representations (15).

Ethics

Ethics review board's approval was exempted because the study involved collecting and analyzing data from a public network platform and did not involve human subjects.

RESULTS

A total of 114 articles concerned with perinatal palliative care published between 2001 and 2020 were retrieved from the WoSCC database. Articles (78, 68.4%) were the most common

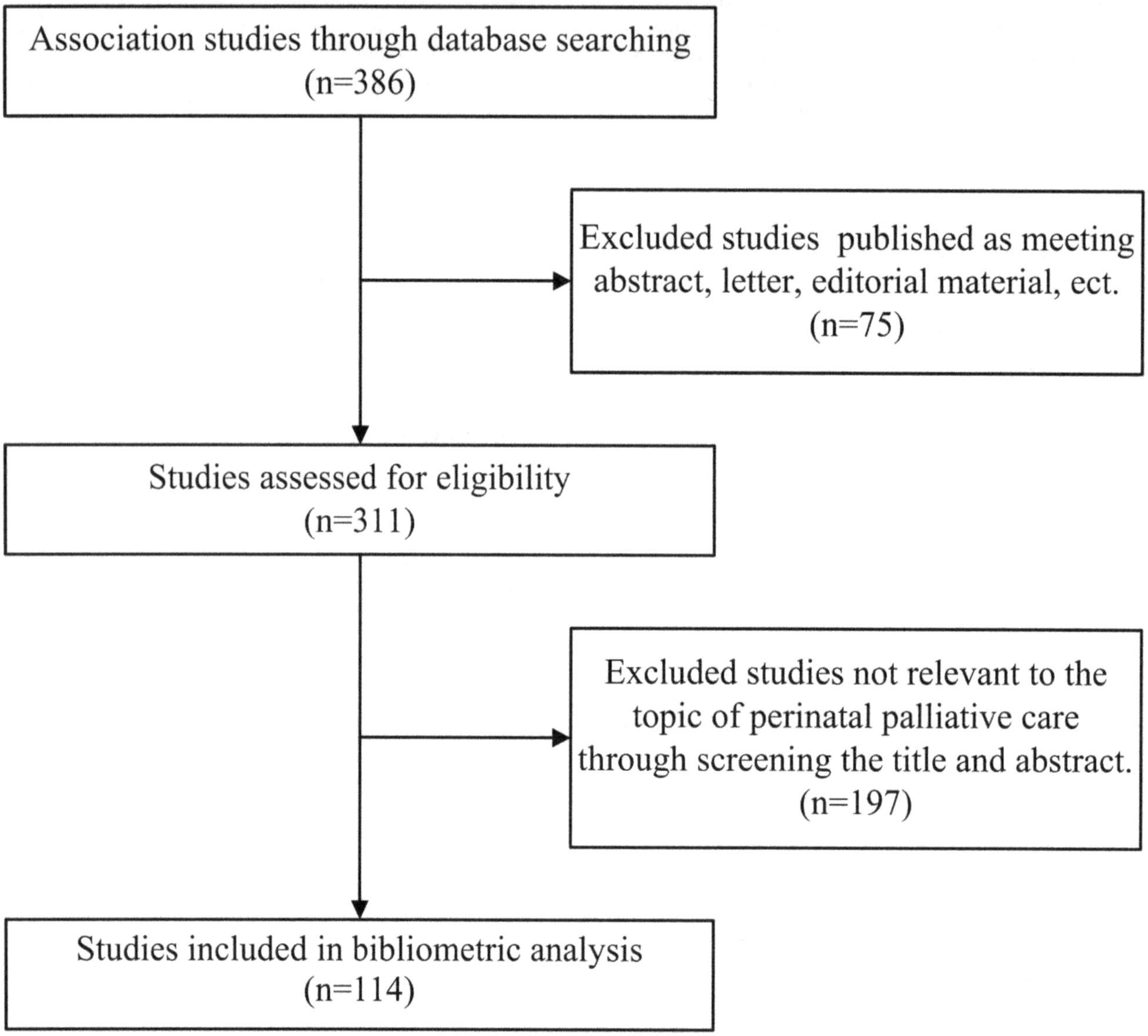

FIGURE 1 | Flow diagram of literature search.

publications identified, followed by reviews (31, 27.2%), case reports (4, 3.5%), and guidelines (1, 0.9%).

Annual Growth Trend of Publications

Figure 2 shows the growth trend of annual publications related to perinatal palliative care research for 2001–2020. The average number of publications was recorded as 5.7 documents per year. In the decade of 2001–2010, there were only a few publications, averaging 1.3 documents per year, for a total of 13 documents. From 2011 to 2015, the volume of publication fluctuated but generally increased. A total of 28 publications were published in the 5-year period, which is more than twice that of the previous decade. Except in 2018, annual publications increased steadily from 2016 to 2020. Moreover, more than half of the articles were published after 2016, indicating drastic growth in publications. Productivity peaked in 2020 with 26 publications (22.8% of the total).

Geographical Distribution of Publications

Table 1 shows countries of origin (17 countries) for the 114 publications. Worldwide, perinatal palliative care has been studied in only a few countries, and most of them are high-income countries. The United States contributed the most articles (68 articles, 59.6% of the total), followed by France (11 articles) and Canada (nine articles). The top three countries contributed 77.2% of all publications. Research on perinatal palliative care in the United States, France, Canada and the United Kingdom developed early, with first publications published before 2010. Among these countries, the United States and Canada were involved in more frequent international research collaborations

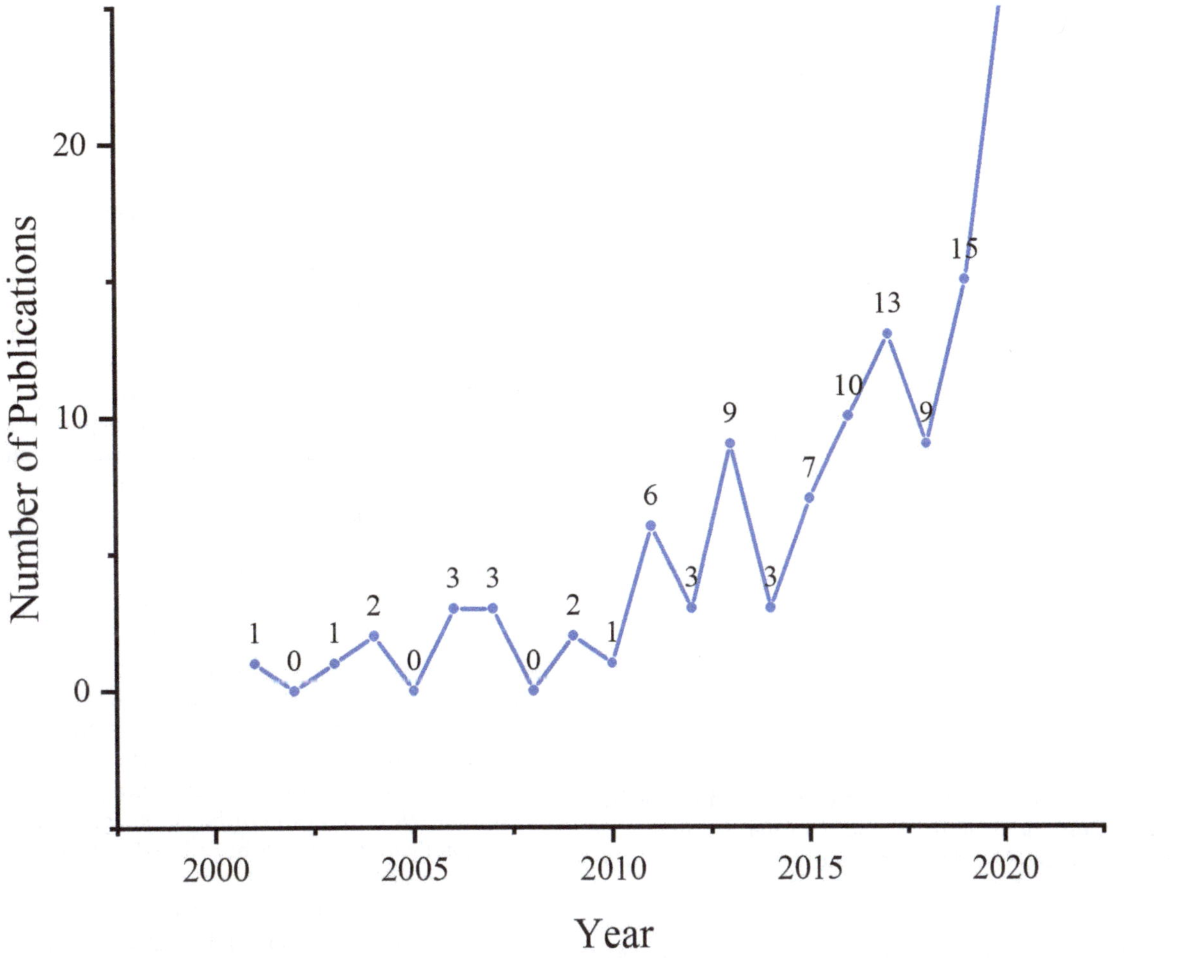

FIGURE 2 | Growth trend of annual publications from 2001 to 2020.

with other countries. The two countries also produced the most citations. The United States and Canada are the two countries the most actively involved in international cooperation. The United States most frequently collaborates with Canada (3), Portugal (2), and Australia (1). In addition to collaborating with the United States, Canada has been involved international cooperation with France (1) and Ireland (1). Switzerland only has intensive cooperation with Germany (2).

Institutions

The institutions that have most contributed to PPC research globally are presented in **Table 2**. The York College of Pennsylvania was the most productive institute, with 18 documents (15.8%), followed by the University of North Carolina (including the Chapel Hill and Greensboro campuses) and Aix-Marseille University (n = 6, 5.3%). Furthermore, the York College of Pennsylvania was found to be the most critical institution in the cooperation network and enjoys a high level of citations. However, on the basis of the funding rates received by all publications, two of the top three most productive institutions had the lowest funding rates of 16.7 and 0.0%.

Authors

In this study, all authors were included in the analysis without considering authors' relative contributions to a single study. Each author's full name was extracted to minimize errors. The author Wool C was the most active among the authors, contributing to 18 publications. Both Cote-Arsenault D and Tosello B ranked second, with six publications (**Table 3**). Additionally, Wool C was the most cited author, with 214 citations, followed by Cote-Arsenault D and Leuthner SR. The h-index is widely used to measure both the productivity and citation impact of publications. In the current study, the h-index for Wool C was recorded as eight in the PPC field. That is, each of the author's eight publications has received at least eight citations. For the coauthorship analysis, the results show that Wool C had the largest research team with 21 coauthors. These indicators again confirm the academic influence of Wool C.

Journals

The 114 articles were published in 56 journals, with 10 published in the Journal of Palliative Medicine (8.8%), eight published in

TABLE 1 | Geographical distribution of publications and international research collaborations in 17 countries/regions.

Country	Documents (%)	Year of first publication	Citations	International collaborations*
United States	68 (59.6)	2001	1091	6
France	11 (9.6)	2009	66	1
Canada	9 (7.9)	2009	164	5
United Kingdom	5 (4.4)	2007	77	0
Switzerland	4 (3.5)	2016	12	2
Ireland	4 (3.5)	2018	11	1
Australia	3 (2.6)	2011	14	2
Poland	3 (2.6)	2013	7	0
Germany	3 (2.6)	2018	4	2
Italy	3 (2.6)	2020	0	0
Portugal	2 (1.8)	2017	12	3
Brazil	2 (1.8)	2017	12	0
Spain	1 (0.9)	2012	75	0
Czech Republic	1 (0.9)	2019	2	0
Sweden	1 (0.9)	2020	1	0
Hungary	1 (0.9)	2020	0	0
Iran	1 (0.9)	2020	0	0

Accumulated number of international collaborations.

Frontiers in Pediatrics (7.0%) and seven published in JOGNN-Journal of Obstetric Gynecologic and Neonatal Nursing (6.1%). **Table 4** lists journals publishing more than two articles. Of these journals, the Journal of Palliative Medicine has the most citations at 182, and Archives of Disease in Childhood-Fetal and Neonatal Edition presents the highest impact factor of 5.747.

Keywords

Of the 114 included studies, 34 did not include author keywords, so only 80 were included in the keyword analysis. As shown in **Figure 3**, labels and circles for palliative care, perinatal palliative care and perinatal hospice are the largest in the cooccurrence network of author keywords, showing the three keywords to be the most frequently used keywords, occurring more than 13 times. In addition, some topics of research can be identified, including (i) candidates for PPC; (ii) PPC models and forms; (iii) components related to the PPC framework, including prenatal counseling, decision-making, birth planning and bereavement; (iv) parental perspectives and satisfaction; and (v) challenges and needs of health care providers. All of these topics have been extensively studied in this domain. In analyzing keyword trends, VOSviewer was used to create a visual map of the cooccurrence network, which uses colors to mark keywords based on their average periods of appearance in all included publications. Blue color means the keywords appear earlier, while red color means the keywords appear later. Red keywords also reflect the latest progress in PPC research (e.g., community palliative care, communication, goals of care, birth planning, compassion, etc.).

DISCUSSION

This study conducted a comprehensive analysis of perinatal palliative care, not only providing a historical overview of scientific progress but also revealing research trends (16). In view of the observed growth in publications, the field of PPC is still quite new, with literature starting to appear in the 2000's and with the concept of perinatal hospice first proposed in 1997 (17). The number of publications has since grown slowly over time. It was not until 2010 that the literature in the field grew dramatically, which seems to be due to the development of palliative care research worldwide. With the release of the PPC guidelines and the growing maturity of service models, it is reasonable to expect the growth of the literature to continue (4).

In terms of the geographic distribution of publications, North America and Europe are the regions where PPC studies were published earlier and have been published more frequently. Within these regions, the United States plays a leading role, and France and Canada have also made significant contributions. In South America, Oceania, and Asia, only Brazil, Australia and Iran have been leaders in conducting PPC research. Africa has made almost no contributions. This reveals that international research on PPC is mainly concentrated in high-income countries, while relevant research activity and resources in middle- and low-income countries are still scarce. To considered different behaviors and cultures, it would be beneficial to extend collaboration networks to more geographic regions (18). Meanwhile, all countries must be encouraged and empowered to develop their own models of perinatal palliative care delivery based on their unique resources and conditions rather than advocating a one-size-fits-all model of PPC (19).

International cooperation and collaboration are the general trend and mainstream direction of the development of science and technology, which can promote the global sharing of information and resources and accelerate the development of academic fields. However, this study shows that international collaboration has not been as widespread as expected, with only 8 (7.0%) of the identified publications resulting from international collaboration. The United States and Canada are highly active in international collaboration and not only cooperate closely with each other but also with other geographically proximal countries, such as Ireland, France and Portugal. Similar to what is found in other fields, research collaboration between countries shows obvious geographic clustering characteristics (20). The reason may be that geographic proximity and cultural similarity may provide a good basis for international cooperation and collaboration. We look forward to more frequent research collaborations between different countries/regions in subsequent studies to obtain evidence based on national and even international clinical studies to benefit more families facing fetal life-limiting diagnoses.

The leading 10 research institutions are from the leading three countries in terms of publication numbers. The same phenomenon was found for authors with almost all researchers from leading institutions. These results indicate that leading institutions and researchers have played an important role in improving academic levels in their respective countries.

TABLE 2 | Most productive institutions in the field of PPC research.

Institutions	Countries	Publications	Funded (%)	Citations	Collaborations*
York Coll Penn	USA	18	3 (16.7)	209	26
Univ N Carolina	USA	6	4 (66.7)	84	16
Aix Marseille Univ	France	6	0 (0.0)	45	13
Univ Rochester	USA	5	4 (80.0)	137	14
Univ Montreal	Canada	5	2(40.0)	132	10
Children's Hosp Wisconsin	USA	4	1 (25.0)	143	7
Univ Illinois	USA	4	3 (75.0)	88	15
Children's Hosp Philadelphia	USA	4	1 (25.0)	81	9
Univ Calif San Diego	USA	4	1 (25.0)	52	4

Accumulated number of interinstitution collaborations.

TABLE 3 | Authors publishing more than 2 articles on perinatal palliative care.

Author	Countries	Publications	Citations	H-index*	Coauthors
Wool, Charlotte	USA	18	214	8	21
Cote-Arsenault, Denise	USA	6	141	4	9
Tosello, Barthelemy	France	6	51	4	12
Leuthner, Steven R.	USA	5	184	4	3
Denney-Koelsch, Erin M.	USA	5	137	4	6
Kavanaugh, Karen	USA	5	92	4	11
Marc-Aurele, Krishelle Leong	USA	4	52	3	6
Einaudi, Marie-Ange	France	4	47	4	11
Gire, Catherine	France	4	47	4	11
Betremieux, Pierre	France	4	45	4	19
Carter, Brian S.	USA	4	22	2	8
Farlow, Barbara	Canada	3	120	3	7
Janvier, Annie	Canada	3	120	3	7
Black, Beth Perry	USA	3	48	3	6
Kuebelbeck, Amy	USA	3	4	1	6

According to the Web of Science Core Collection Database.

Furthermore, most of the identified institutions and researchers are based in the USA, which again shows the academic influence of the USA in this field. However, we found that the discipline has struggled to obtain sufficient support and funding, which may be related to poor understanding of PPC among the public, professionals and policy-makers (21). Most top institutions, especially Aix-Marseille University, the top French institution in this field, have not received funding for all relevant publications. Even for the York College of Pennsylvania, which has produced the most articles, only 16.7% of the identified studies were funded. Therefore, earmarked funds should be focused in this specialized area to allow more institutions and researchers to develop robust evidence and foster diversity in this field. On the other hand, with ongoing research, it is difficult for a single person or institution to achieve major breakthroughs, and there is an urgent need for researchers and institutions in this field to cooperate with each other (22). Therefore, many associations have provided financial support to scholars worldwide through the Traveling Scholarship Program and Traveling Fellowship Program to strengthen palliative care messaging, information and communication to inspire global change (19).

Almost all PPC-related studies have been published in specialized journals focused on obstetrics and gynecology, perinatology, neonatology/pediatrics, palliative medicine and nursing. This reflects the increasingly multidisciplinary nature of PPC. The number of articles is generally lower than for other specialties of perinatology and palliative medicine. Furthermore, most articles have been published in journals of relatively low impact relative to those of palliative care in other fields, such as cancer (23), surgery (24), and geriatric care (25), revealing a lack of global attention to this topic.

All author keywords included in our study were analyzed to generate a cooccurrence network map. With this network map, there is an opportunity to further clarify future development trends. Historically, many articles initially concentrated on candidates for perinatal palliative care. Thus, "lethal anomalies,"

TABLE 4 | Journals publishing more than 2 articles on perinatal palliative care.

Journal	Documents	Citations	IF-2020*
Journal of Palliative Medicine	10	182	2.947
Frontiers in Pediatrics	8	0	3.418
JOGNN-Journal of Obstetric Gynecologic and Neonatal Nursing	7	124	1.716
Journal of Perinatal & Neonatal Nursing	6	133	1.638
Advances in Neonatal Care	5	20	1.968
Archives de pediatrie	5	15	1.180
Perspectives in Biology and Medicine	5	0	1.416
Journal of Maternal-Fetal & Neonatal Medicine	4	23	2.398
Archives of Disease in Childhood-fetal and neonatal edition	3	81	5.747
MCN-The American Journal of Maternal-Child Nursing	3	70	1.412
Seminars in Perinatology	3	37	3.300
Midwifery	3	12	2.372

IF denotes the impact factor from Thomson Reuters' Journal Citation Reports (JCR).

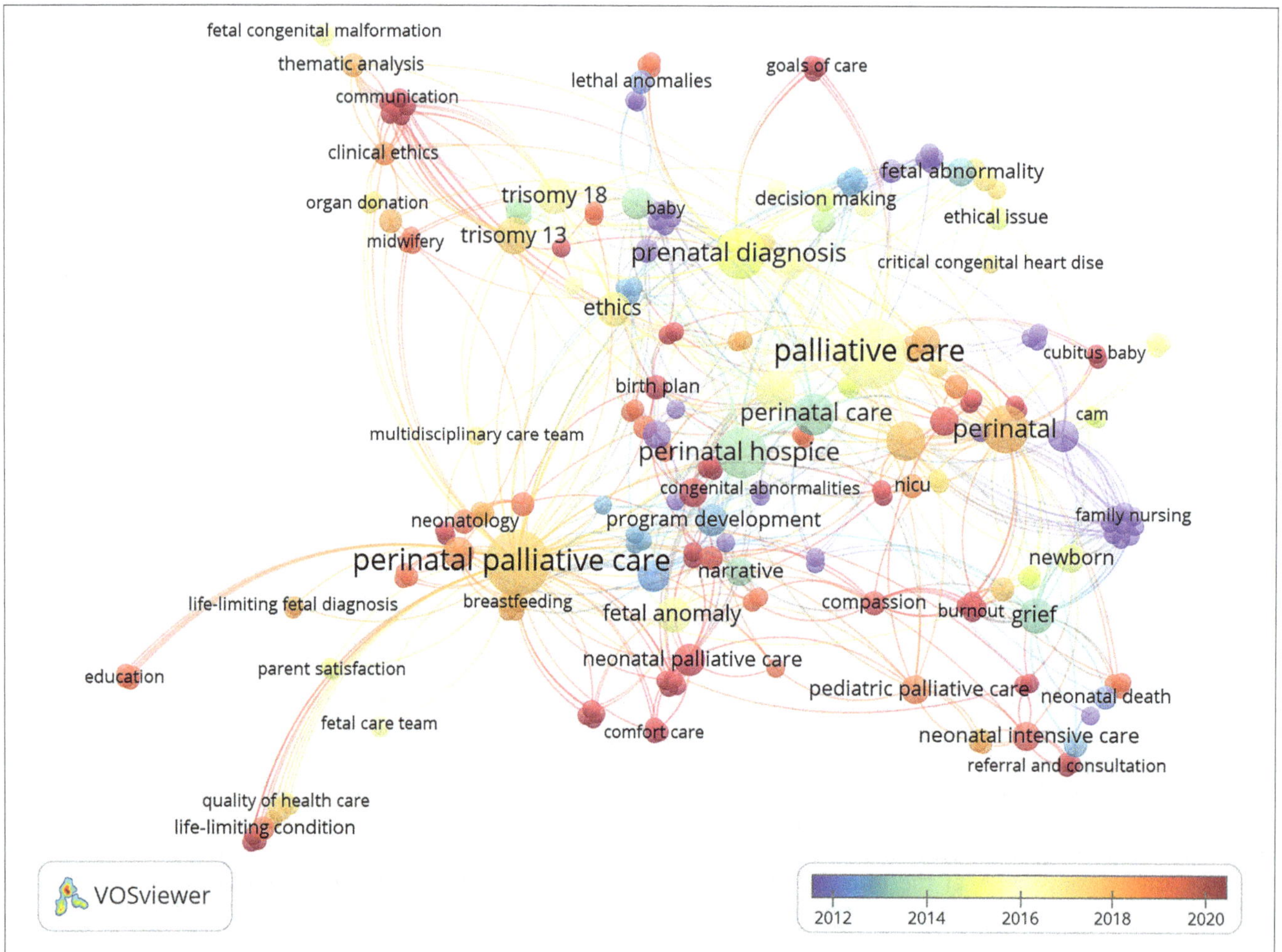

FIGURE 3 | Cooccurrence network of author keywords in global PPC research.

"congenital abnormalities" and "life-limiting fetal diagnoses" were the most commonly used keywords, and some articles even extended to certain diseases, such as trisomy 13, trisomy 18 and anencephaly (26, 27). While there is a general consensus on lethal prenatal diagnoses, with advances in fetal and neonatal medicine, we must be wary of referring to some diseases as "lethal." Future research on the treatment and prognosis of certain "lethal" diseases may provide more information that can help families make decisions. Additionally, the present study found that researchers have conducted many studies on the development of perinatal palliative care service models. As the most frequently used keywords, family-centered care and interdisciplinary care have a strong link to program development. Perinatal palliative care takes many forms, such as antenatal palliative care, neonatal palliative care and pediatric palliative care, and it varies by the location of service. Recently, community palliative care has been considered a "new frontier" that supports families longitudinally and across various care settings (3, 28). As indicated in previous studies, community hospitals have significant advantages in providing more care and more accessible options for families with short infant life expectancy [19]. Moreover, a variety of components related to the PPC framework, including prenatal counseling, decision-making, birth planning and bereavement, have dominated the field of research. In the past, publications related to decision-making and bereavement were popular, but in recent years, publications on birth planning have become more prominent. According to the current study, many areas of birth planning still need to be explored, such as communication, follow-through and the flexibility of important components (29). In PPC settings, the measurement of nursing outcomes brings new challenges. The evaluation of PPC relies on parent-reported outcomes rather than on "hard" epidemiologic data (30), and most of the evidence comes from qualitative studies. In providing measurable indicators, the instrument development of parental satisfaction and quality indicators has also gained considerable attention in the last 10 years (30, 31). These instruments, however, still need to be validated and applied to a broader and diverse sample to improve the quality of care across settings. Despite the importance of PPC, advocating for it around the world is a very challenging proposition. From the obtained keyword network, terms such as confidence, compassion, burnout, and education highlight the challenges and needs of health care providers. Although some of these dilemmas may be difficult to overcome in the short term, significant measures must be implemented in the future to enhance providers' confidence and competence in providing good PPC (32, 33).

STRENGTHS AND LIMITATIONS

This is the first study to attempt to apply VOSviewer software to conduct a bibliometric analysis and provide a visual account of global PPC services. However, this study presents limitations. Due to the limitations of the employed software, this study only involved research and analysis through the WoSCC database. Therefore, the data used may not be comprehensive. In addition, in the keyword analysis, some studies with no author keywords were not included in the cooccurrence analysis, which may affect the accuracy of the research results.

CONCLUSION

The current study has summarized the current research status and global trends of the field of PPC research. According to the presented findings, the number of PPC studies has been increasing in the past two decades, but such research is mainly concentrated in high-income countries, while few studies have been conducted in low- and middle-income countries. To promote the development of PPC services worldwide, much work still needs to be done by strengthening international and regional research cooperation; increasing financial support; and carrying out leading-edge, demand-oriented research.

AUTHOR CONTRIBUTIONS

ZZ designed the study. YW and CP executed literature retrieval and screening. CS and YT conducted the statistical analysis. YW wrote the original draft of the paper, which was revised by CS and ZZ. All authors have approved of the final version of the draft.

ACKNOWLEDGMENTS

We thank Zhonghua Shi, PhD for providing useful advice.

REFERENCES

1. WHO. *World Health Statistics 2021: Monitoring Health for the SDGs, Sustainable Development Goals.* (2021). Available online at: https://apps.who.int/iris/bitstream/handle/10665/342703/9789240027053-eng.pdf (accessed November 12, 2021).
2. Murphy SL, Xu JQ, Kochanek KD, Arias E, Tejada-Vera B. *Deaths: Final Data for 2018. National Vital Statistics Reports Hyattsville.* MD: National Center for Health Statistics (2020). Available online at: https://www.cdc.gov/nchs/data/nvsr/nvsr69/nvsr69-13-508.pdf (accessed October 16, 2021).
3. Ziegler TR, Kuebelbeck A. Close to home: perinatal palliative care in a community hospital. *Adv Neonatal Care.* (2020) 20:196–203. doi: 10.1097/ANC.0000000000000732
4. Perinatal Palliative Care: ACOG COMMITTEE OPINION, Number 786. *Obstet Gynecol.* (2019) 134:e84–9. doi: 10.1097/AOG.0000000000003425
5. WHO. *Integrating Palliative Care and Symptom Relief into Paediatrics: a WHO Guide for Health Care Planners, Implementers and Managers.* (2018). Available online at: https://apps.who.int/iris/bitstream/handle/10665/274561/9789241514453-eng.pdf (accessed October 14, 2021).
6. Sigurdardottir KR, Haugen DF, van der Rijt CC, Sjøgren P, Harding R, Higginson IJ, et al. Clinical priorities, barriers and solutions in end-of-life cancer care research across Europe. Report from a workshop. *Eur J Cancer.* (2010) 46: 1815–22. doi: 10.1016/j.ejca.2010.03.012
7. Higginson IJ. Research challenges in palliative and end of life care. *BMJ Support Palliat Care.* (2016) 6:2–4. doi: 10.1136/bmjspcare-2015-001091
8. WHO. *Assessing the Development of Palliative Care Worldwide: A Set of Actionable Indicators.* (2021). Available online at: https://www.who.int/publications/i/item/9789240033351 (accessed November 15, 2021).

9. Kim AR, Park HY. Theme trends and knowledge-relationship in lifestyle research: a bibliometric analysis. *Int J Environ Res Public Health.* (2021) 18:7503. doi: 10.3390/ijerph18147503
10. Wu H, Tong L, Wang Y, Yan H, Sun Z. Bibliometric analysis of global research trends on ultrasound microbubble: a quickly developing field. *Front Pharmacol.* (2021) 12:646626. doi: 10.3389/fphar.2021.646626
11. Zhong Q, Li BH, Zhu QQ, Zhang ZM, Zou ZH, Jin YH. The top 100 highly cited original articles on immunotherapy for childhood leukemia. *Front Pharmacol.* (2019) 10:1100. doi: 10.3389/fphar.2019.01100
12. Kamdem JP, Duarte AE, Lima KRR, Rocha JBT, Hassan W, Barros LM, et al. Research trends in food chemistry: a bibliometric review of its 40years anniversary (1976–2016). *Food Chem.* (2019) 294:448–57. doi: 10.1016/j.foodchem.2019.05.021
13. Zhao J, Yu G, Cai M, Lei X, Yang Y, Wang Q, et al. Bibliometric analysis of global scientific activity on umbilical cord mesenchymal stem cells: a swiftly expanding and shifting focus. *Oxid Med Cell Longev.* (2018) 9:32. doi: 10.1186/s13287-018-0785-5
14. Yeung AW, Goto TK, Leung WK. The changing landscape of neuroscience research, 2006–2015: a bibliometric study. *Front Neurosci.* (2017) 11:120. doi: 10.3389/fnins.2017.00120
15. van Eck NJ, Waltman L. Software survey: VOSviewer, a computer program for bibliometric mapping. *Scientometrics.* (2010) 84:523–38. doi: 10.1007/s11192-009-0146-3
16. Ordinola-Zapata R, Peters OA. What is of interest in endodontology? a bibliometric review of research published in the International Endodontic Journal and the Journal of Endodontics from 1980 to 2019. *Int Endod J.* (2020) 53:36–52. doi: 10.1111/iej.13210
17. Calhoun BC, Hoeldtke NJ, Hinson RM, Judge KM. Perinatal hospice: should all centers have this service? *Neonatal Netw.* (1997) 16:101–2.
18. Taj F, Klein MCA. Digital Health Behavior Change Technology: Bibliometric and Scoping Review of Two Decades of Research. *JMIR Mhealth Uhealth.* (2019) 7:e13311. doi: 10.2196/13311
19. De Lima L, Radbruch L. The International association for hospice and palliative care: advancing hospice and palliative care worldwide. *J Pain Symptom Manage.* (2018) 55:S96–103. doi: 10.1016/j.jpainsymman.2017.03.023
20. Yanbing S, Hua L. The state of nursing research from 2000 to 2019: a global analysis. *Genome Biol.* (2021) 77:162–75. doi: 10.1111/jan.14564
21. Grant MS, Back AL, Dettmar NS. Public perceptions of advance care planning, palliative care, and hospice: a scoping review. *J Palliat Med.* (2021) 24:46–52. doi: 10.1089/jpm.2020.0111
22. Wu W, Xie Y, Liu X, Gu Y, Zhang Y, Tu X, et al. Analysis of scientific collaboration networks among authors, institutions, and countries studying adolescent myopia prevention and control: a review article. *Iran J Public Health.* (2019) 48:621–31. doi: 10.18502/ijph.v48i4.983
23. Hui D, Bruera E. Models of palliative care delivery for patients with cancer. *J Clin Oncol.* (2020) 38:852–65. doi: 10.1200/JCO.18.02123
24. Lilley EJ, Cooper Z, Schwarze ML, Mosenthal AC. Palliative care in surgery: defining the research priorities. *Ann Surg.* (2018) 267:66–72. doi: 10.1097/SLA.0000000000002253
25. Runacres F, Poon P, King S, Lustig J, Ugalde A. Examining the role of specialist palliative care in geriatric care to inform collaborations: a survey on the knowledge, practice and attitudes of geriatricians in providing palliative care. *Age Ageing.* (2021) 50:1792–801. doi: 10.1093/ageing/afab058
26. Hasegawa SL, Fry JT. Moving toward a shared process: The impact of parent experiences on perinatal palliative care. *Semin Perinatol.* (2017) 41:95–100. doi: 10.1053/j.semperi.2016.11.002
27. O'Connell O, Meaney S, O'Donoghue K. Anencephaly; the maternal experience of continuing with the pregnancy. Incompatible with life but not with love. *Midwifery.* (2019) 71:12–8. doi: 10.1016/j.midw.2018.12.016
28. Kavalieratos D, Gelfman LP, Tycon LE, Riegel B, Bekelman DB, Ikejiani DZ, et al. Palliative care in heart failure: rationale, evidence, and future priorities. *J Am Coll Cardiol.* (2017) 70:1919–30. doi: 10.1016/j.jacc.2017.08.036
29. Cortezzo DE, Bowers K, Cameron Meyer M. Birth planning in uncertain or life-limiting fetal diagnoses: perspectives of physicians and parents. *J Palliat Med.* (2019) 22:1337–45. doi: 10.1089/jpm.2018.0596
30. Wool C. Instrument psychometrics: parental satisfaction and quality indicators of perinatal palliative care. *J Palliat Med.* (2015) 18:872–7. doi: 10.1089/jpm.2015.0135
31. Wool C, Black BP, Woods AB. Quality indicators and parental satisfaction with perinatal palliative care in the intrapartum setting after diagnosis of a life-limiting fetal condition. *ANS Adv Nurs Sci.* (2016) 39:346–57. doi: 10.1097/ANS.0000000000000147
32. Wool C. Clinician perspectives of barriers in perinatal palliative care. *MCN Am J Matern Child Nurs.* (2015) 40:44–50. doi: 10.1097/NMC.0000000000000093
33. Benini F, Congedi S, Rusalen F, Cavicchiolo ME, Lago P. Barriers to perinatal palliative care consultation. *Front Pediatr.* (2020) 8:590616. doi: 10.3389/fped.2020.590616

29

aEEG Use in Pediatric Critical Care—An Online Survey

Nora Bruns[1], Ursula Felderhoff-Müser[1], Christian Dohna-Schwake[1], Joachim Woelfle[2] and Hanna Müller[2*]*

[1] Department of Pediatrics I, Neonatology, Pediatric Intensive Care, Pediatric Neurology, University Hospital Essen, University Duisburg-Essen, Essen, Germany, [2] Division of Neonatology and Pediatric Intensive Care, Department of Pediatrics, University Hospital Erlangen, University of Erlangen-Nürnberg, Erlangen, Germany

***Correspondence:**
Nora Bruns
nora.bruns@uk-essen.de
Hanna Müller
Hanna.Mueller@uk-erlangen.de

Background: Evidence supporting continuous EEG monitoring in pediatric intensive care is increasing, but continuous full-channel EEG is a scarce resource. Amplitude-integrated EEG (aEEG) monitors are broadly available in children's hospitals due to their use in neonatology and can easily be applied to older patients.

Objective: The aim of this survey was to evaluate the use of amplitude-integrated EEG in German and Swiss pediatric intensive care units (PICUs).

Design: An online survey was sent to German and Swiss PICUs that were identified via databases provided by the German Pediatric Association (DGKJ) and the Swiss Society of Intensive Care (SGI). The questionnaire contained 18 multiple choice questions including the PICU size and specialization, indications for aEEG use, perceived benefits from aEEG, and data storage.

Main results: Forty-three (26%) PICUs filled out the questionnaire. Two thirds of all interviewed PICUs use aEEG in non-neonates. Main indications were neurological complications or disease and altered mental state. Features assessed were mostly seizures and side differences, less frequently height of amplitude and background pattern. Interpretation of raw EEG also played an important role. All interviewees would appreciate the establishment of reference values for toddlers and children.

Conclusions: aEEG is used in a large proportion of the interviewed PICUs. The wide-spread use without validation of data generates the need for further evaluation of this technique and the establishment of reference values for non-neonates.

Keywords: amplitude-integrated EEG, pediatric critical care, neuromonitoring, aEEG, continuous EEG, survey

INTRODUCTION

Evidence supporting the use of continuous electroencephalography (EEG) in pediatric critical care has increased considerably in recent years. It has proven beneficial particularly after cardiac arrest, in patients with altered mental state and for the detection and treatment of seizures and monitoring of anticonvulsive treatment efficiency (1–5). Of special relevance is the detection of non-convulsive epileptic state, because this condition is associated with an increased risk of in-hospital mortality (2, 6). It has been shown that time from pediatric intensive care unit (PICU) admission to continuous EEG is associated with mortality in non-convulsive epileptic state (6). As continuous video-electroencephalograpy with the full 10–20 system of electrodes represents the gold standard, but remains a scarce resource requiring an epileptologist for interpretation, amplitude-integrated EEG appears to be a promising alternative. It is available in a large proportion of neonatal intensive care units and is easy to apply (7). aEEG has become standard of care in neonates after birth asphyxia for estimation of severity and prediction of outcome. It is also a valuable method for neonates with brain lesions and severe infections (8–11) as well as for preterm infants for the prediction of outcome (12–15). Also in adult intensive care, interest in aEEG is increasing recently (16–21). Its great advantage is that it can be operated and evaluated by the PICU team, independent from an epileptologist. After a short-term training period, staff is able to detect seizure activity and epileptic state in aEEG (22, 23). A recently published evaluation of aEEG use in our PICU showed that the main benefit came from detection and management of seizures and epileptic state (5). We also found that side differences were not detected in all patients with unilateral intracranial lesions, but if present, a unilateral process must be suspected. Similarly, background pattern was not necessarily altered in all patients with pathologies in conventional EEG but altered aEEG background pattern indicated pathological EEG and increased mortality. Adverse evolution of the background pattern over time was also significantly associated with death.

An obstacle to the further use of aEEG in non-neonates might be overcome by generating reference values and recommendations on how to deal with findings in the recording. As we noticed an increased use of this technique in our PICU over the past years (5), we initiated a survey in German and Swiss PICUs about their use of aEEG. The aim of the investigation was to assess the status quo of availability, indications, and use of amplitude-integrated EEG in pediatric critical care.

METHODS

German hospitals treating pediatric critical care patients were identified from the homepage of the German Pediatric Association (DGKJ, Deutsche Gesellschaft für Kinder- und Jugendmedizin) and the information given on the hospitals' websites. Swiss PICUs were identified from the homepage of the Swiss Society of Intensive Care (SGI, Schweizerische Gesellschaft für Intensivmedizin).

We contacted a 156 German and 7 Swiss PICUs via email in April and in September 2019. The email contained a link to an online multiple choice questionnaire (in German) on www.surveymonkey.com about the use of amplitude-integrated EEG in pediatric critical care patients.

The following items were assessed in the questionnaire: Multiple answers possible: specialization of PICU, availability of cerebral imaging, aEEG indications for all ages including neonates, use of aEEG in patients with altered mental state, qualities assessed in pediatric aEEG, classifications used for pediatric aEEG, perceived benefits at nights and at weekends, advantages of aEEG compared to conventional EEG, site and duration of data storage. Only one answer possible: name of hospital and city, PICU with NICU in the same ward or separate, number of PICU beds, availability of conventional EEG, number of available aEEG devices per hospital and per PICU, need for reference values. Each question included the possibility to add a comment.

Answers were exported from www.surveymonkey.com as Microsoft Excel® files including raw data and summarized data. Analyses were made using Microsoft Office Excel® Version 16.30. Median values were calculated for number of PICU beds and number of available aEEG devices per hospital and per PICU. For the remaining questions, the number of answers was counted and is presented as numbers (n) and percentages (%).

RESULTS

We received replies from 43 of 163 PICUs (26%) between April and September 2019. Forty-two PICUs were located in Germany, and one PICU was Swiss. Twenty (47%) PICUs belonged to university hospitals. Fourteen (33%) of 43 hospitals had PICUs without neonatal beds, whereas 29 (67%) hospitals had combined neonatal and pediatric intensive care units. The number of pediatric (excluding neonatal) intensive care beds ranged from 2 to 20 and was 7 at median (answered by $n = 42$, 98%).

Specializations: answered by $n = 40$ (93%). The responding PICUs reported heterogeneous specializations in neuropediatrics ($n = 26$, 60%), pneumology ($n = 25$, 58%), neurosurgery ($n = 23$, 53%), and trauma ($n = 19$, 44%), as most frequent specialties. See **Figure 1** for more details.

Availability of Cerebral Diagnostics and aEEG

Conventional EEG: answered by $n = 43$ (100%). Recording was available anytime during day and night in 22 (51%) and only at daytime in 20 (47%) PICUs. One (2%) PICU reported to make use of an external pediatric neurology service for conduction of EEG. See **Figure 2A** for details.

Cerebral imaging: answered by $n = 43$ (100%). Computed tomography for cerebral imaging was available in all 43 PICUs anytime, whereas magnetic resonance imaging (MRI) was available anytime in 20 (47%) PICUs and in 15 (35%) during daytime. Fifteen (35%) PICUs reported only limited access to MRI at night and at weekends. See **Figure 2B** for details.

Number of aEEG devices per children's hospital: answered by $n = 43$ (100%). Forty-two (98%) children's hospitals had aEEG devices available with a median number of two devices per hospital (range 1–12). One (2%) hospital did not have an aEEG monitor.

Number of aEEG devices per PICU: answered by $n = 43$ (100%). Forty (93%) PICUs reported they had access to aEEG devices with a median number of two devices per PICU (range 1–11). Three (7%) PICUs did not have access to an aEEG device.

Manufacturers: answered by $n = 41$ (95%). See **Figure 2C** for details.

aEEG Indications and Use

Indications for aEEG: answered by $n = 42$ (98%). The most prevalent indications for aEEG use were conditions in neonates with birth asphyxia ($n = 41$, 98%) and neonatal seizures ($n = 38$,

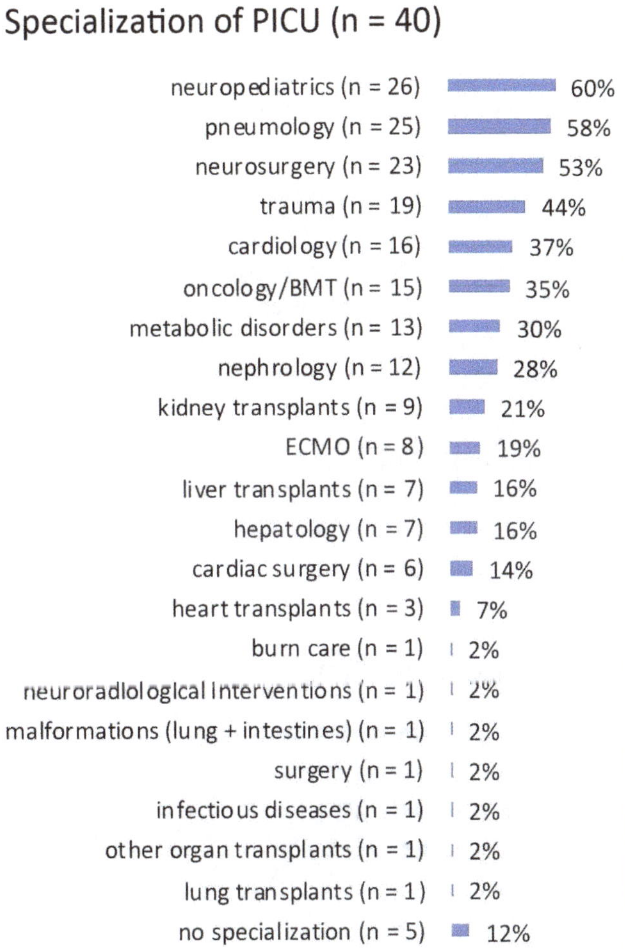

FIGURE 1 | Specialization of interviewed PICUs.

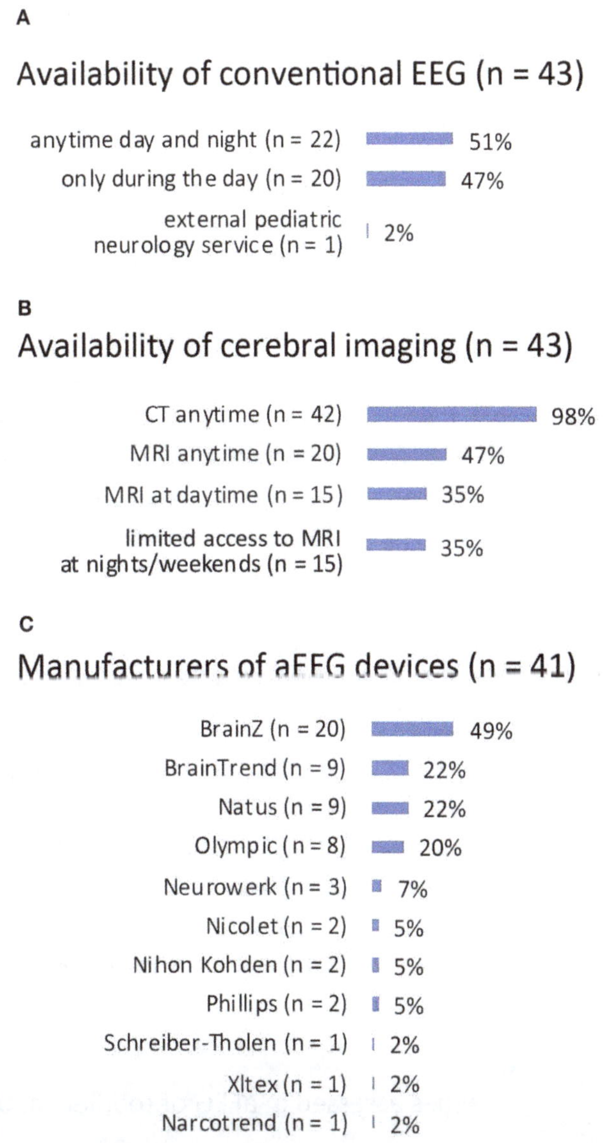

FIGURE 2 | **(A)** Availability of conventional EEG. **(B)** Availability of cerebral imaging. **(C)** Manufacturers of aEEG devices.

90%). Neurologic disease or complications in preterm infants ($n = 25$, 60%), neonates ($n = 22$, 52%), toddlers ($n = 28$, 67%), or children ($n = 20$, 48%) were reported as further aEEG indications. Clinical routine or research purposes in preterm infants were rare indications ($n = 3$, 7% and $n = 3$, 7%). Two (5%) PICUs reported using aEEG after cardiac surgery in neonates, and one PICU (2%) used aEEG after cardiac surgery in toddlers and children, respectively. One (2%) PICU reported aEEG use for monitoring of severe withdrawal syndrome (**Figure 3A**).

Use of aEEG in toddlers/children with altered mental state: answered by $n = 42$ (98%). Twenty-seven PICUs (64%) applied aEEG in cases of unexplained altered mental state in toddlers or children. The reasons for not using aEEG in such cases were: lack of experience with aEEG in children ($n = 6$, 14%), a stance that aEEG is suitable only in neonates ($n = 6$, 14%), continuous availability of full channel EEG ($n = 5$, 12%), no device available for PICU patients ($n = 2$, 5%), the PICU team is not familiar with the technique ($n = 2$, 5%), and exclusive use of full channel EEG during daytime ($n = 1$, 2%) (**Figure 3B**).

aEEG Interpretation in Toddlers and Children

Qualities assessed in toddlers'/children's aEEGs: answered by $n = 43$ (100%). Assessed qualities were seizures ($n = 31$, 72%), side differences (differences in hemispheric activity; $n = 26$, 60%), height of amplitude ($n = 17$, 40%), evolution of background pattern over time ($n = 15$, 35%), background pattern ($n = 14$, 33%), and sleep wake cycling ($n = 10$, 23%). Eleven (28%) PICUs reported they do not use aEEG in this age group (**Figure 3C**).

Classifications for interpretation: answered by $n = 38$ (88%). The classifications considered for interpretation were the assessment of the raw EEG curve ($n = 26$, 68%) and the classification by Hellström-Westas ($n = 26$, 68%). Two PICUs (5%) considered the Burdjalov classification for interpretation,

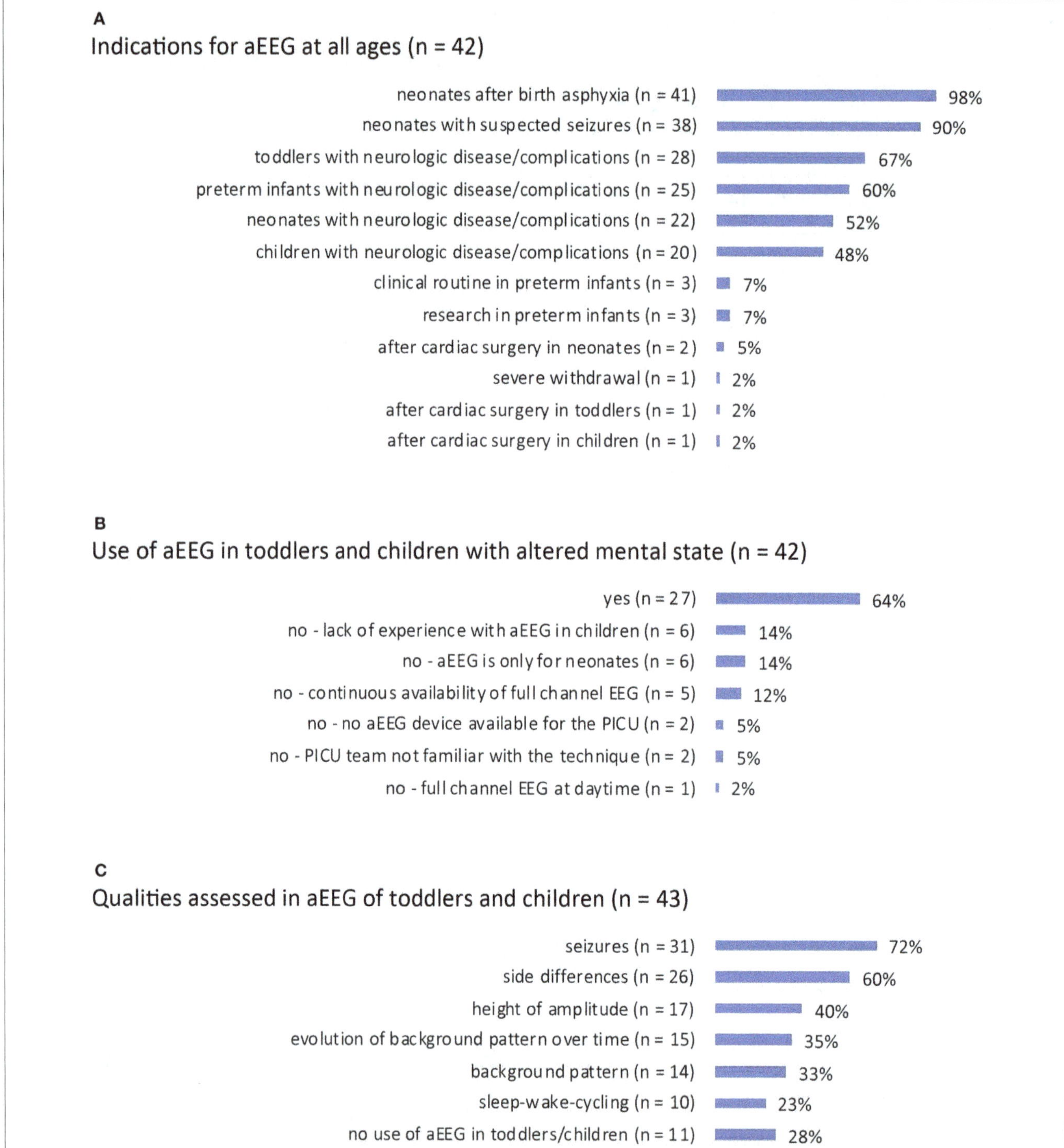

FIGURE 3 | (A) Indications for aEEG recording for all age groups from preterm to child. **(B)** Use of aEEG in PICU patients with unexplained altered mental state. **(C)** Qualities assessed in aEEG when applied in toddlers/children.

and one (2%) PICU had their aEEGs assessed by a pediatric neurologist every 24 h.

Need for reference values: answered by $n = 41$ (95%). All answering PICUs considered reference values for toddlers and children helpful for interpretation.

Attitudes Toward aEEG in Toddlers and Children

Expected benefits from aEEG at night or at weekends: answered by $n = 41$ (95%). Expected benefits were the recognition of intermittent seizure activity ($n = 36$, 88%), recognition of non-convulsive epileptic state (n = 34, 83%), and evaluation of brain activity in an unresponsive child (n = 26, 63%). Twenty-three (56%) interviewees expected aEEG to be useful for the detection of side differences and the evaluation of antiepileptic treatment, respectively, and for the recognition of convulsive epileptic state (n = 22, 54%). Less frequently expected benefits were cues for brain death (n = 12, 29%), cues regarding the course of disease (n = 8, 20%), and cues regarding the effectiveness of therapy (e.g., organ replacement therapy or vasopressor treatment; n = 6, 15%). One (2%) regarded aEEG as useless and thus did not attempt to try this method (**Figure 4A**).

Advantage of aEEG vs. EEG: answered by n = 42 (98%). The application and interpretation by the PICU team itself was named to be the expected advantage of aEEG compared to conventional EEG (n = 41, 98%). Further advantages reported were long duration of recording (for days and weeks; n = 31, 74%), little impact on intensive care measures (easy to pause and resume; n = 30, 71%), and continuous surveillance of treatment efficacy (n = 27, 64%). Twenty-two (52%) interviewees replied aEEG could help to initiate cerebral imaging faster and 15 (36%) said that aEEG could help to evaluate if ongoing therapy still makes sense (**Figure 4B**).

aEEG-Data Storage

Storage site: answered by n = 41 (95%). See **Figure 5A** for details.

Storage duration: answered by n = 42 (98%). See **Figure 5B** for details.

DISCUSSION

We herewith report the results of an online survey investigating the use of amplitude-integrated EEG in Swiss and German pediatric intensive care units. To our surprise we found that, despite lack of validation, aEEG is presently being used for non-neonates by two thirds of the responding pediatric intensive care units. Beyond the established indications for aEEG in neonates—asphyxia and monitoring of suspected seizure activity—aEEG is used in cases of neurologic disease and complications for patients of all ages. Interviewees using aEEG reported the detection and management of seizures and the evaluation of brain activity in cases of altered mental state to be the main benefit of this method.

These results comply with results from an analysis of aEEG use in our PICU we recently published (5). We detected an increase in use of aEEG in our PICU in recent years with management of seizures being the main indication. Evidence supporting

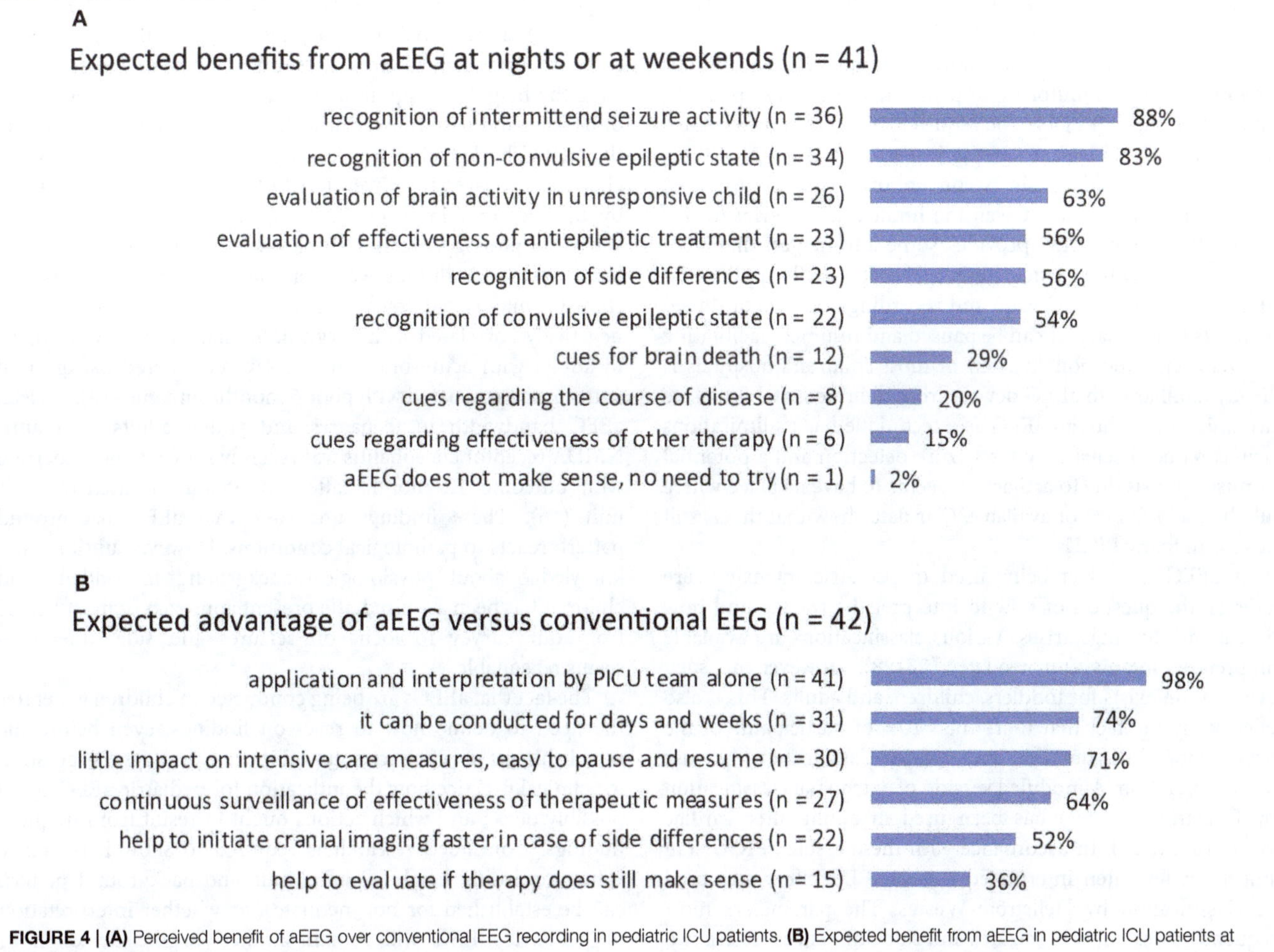

FIGURE 4 | (A) Perceived benefit of aEEG over conventional EEG recording in pediatric ICU patients. **(B)** Expected benefit from aEEG in pediatric ICU patients at night/at weekends.

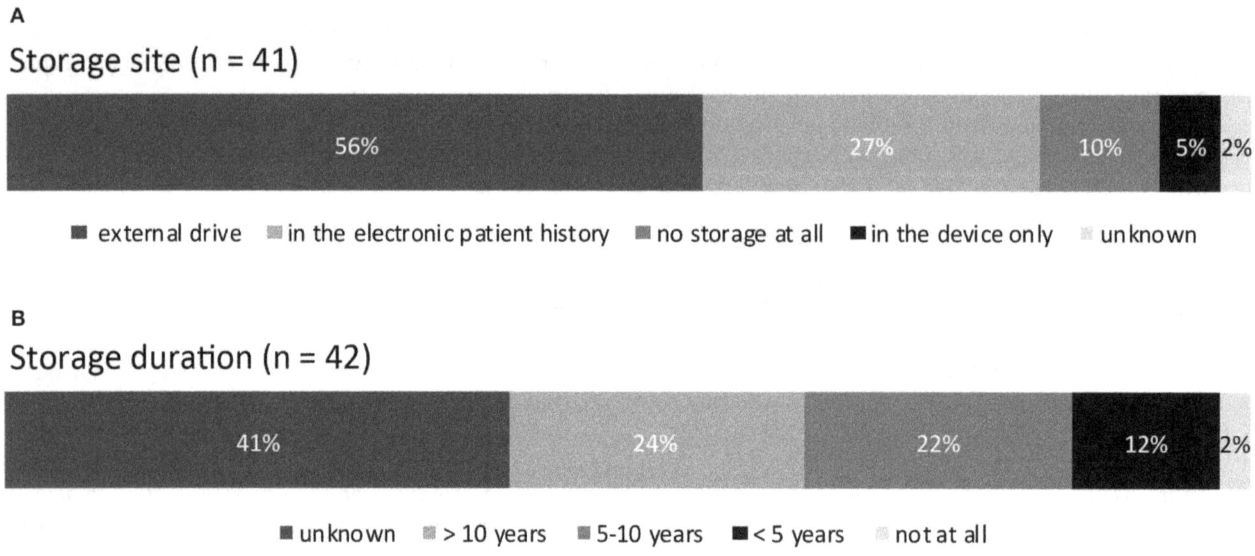

FIGURE 5 | (A) Storage site of aEEG data. **(B)** Storage duration of aEEG data.

continuous EEG monitoring in children for the detection of non-convulsive seizures, after cardiac arrest, and with altered mental status is growing (1, 2, 6, 23, 24). Currently continuous full channel EEG is the standard technique for continuous cerebral function monitoring in pediatric critical care patients, but is not broadly available and requires specialist knowledge for interpretation (5). In our survey, just about half of all PICUs reported they could obtain a conventional (non-continuous) EEG anytime of the day. Given the limited access even to this routine technique, aEEG provides some advantages, that were also perceived by the participating PICUs: It is easily applied and interpreted by the PICU team and recordings can be continued for weeks if necessary. It can be paused and resumed, facilitating interventions. Additionally, staff in most children's hospitals is already familiar with aEEG devices from their neonatal intensive care units. Even though aEEG as a technique has its limitations such as reduced sensitivity for seizure detection and a potential for misdiagnosis due to artifacts, it seems to have its place where full-channel EEG is not available. Our data show that this is still the case in many PICUs.

As aEEG is in fact being used in pediatric intensive care patients, the question of how to interpret the tracing and how to deal with findings arises. Various classifications are available for preterm infants and neonates (25–28). However, no such classification exists for toddlers, children, and adults. This is also reflected by the fact that more than 10% of participants of the survey skipped the question about which classification they use for interpretation. A modified version of a neonatal classification (by Hellström-Westas) has been used in adults after cardiac arrest (18–21, 29). In accordance with these results, PICU staff almost equally often interpreted the raw EEG curve and used the classification by Hellström-Westas. The parameters most frequently assessed were seizures and side differences. These two parameters are independent from reference values and therefore can be interpreted quite safely, or after short-term training, respectively (22, 23). At the same time the presence of either of the two often leads to further diagnostic steps or therapy, making them important parameters. Less important to our interviewees were the height of amplitude, background pattern or evolution of background pattern over time. In our PICU cohort, we found that aEEG background was less sensitive to detect pathological changes compared to conventional EEG (5). This is likely caused by the fact that important EEG qualities like frequency and wave morphology are not displayed by aEEG. On the other hand, severe conditions were reflected by background pattern showing mainly flat trace or burst suppression pattern, which negatively correlated with survival. Similar findings were made in adults with acute brain injury: severely altered background pattern was associated with poor 6 month-outcome (17). Parietal aEEG bandwidth in teenagers and young adults with anti-NMDA receptor encephalitis was recently shown to be associated with outcome 12 months after admission to intensive care unit (16). These findings underline that aEEG background pattern reacts to pathological conditions. However, until further knowledge about physiological background in toddlers and children has been acquired, the present approach of most PICUs from our survey to focus on seizures and side differences seems reasonable.

The fact that aEEGs are being conducted in children generates the need to define how to react on findings, even before the establishment of reference values. **Figure 6** displays a suggestion for clinical practice how the indication for pediatric aEEG could possibly be set and which actions ought to result from frequent findings. Continued research is required to show if reference values regarding height of amplitude and background pattern can be established for non-neonates, or whether interpretation of pediatric aEEG will remain limited to the detection of seizures, side differences, and severely altered electrocortical

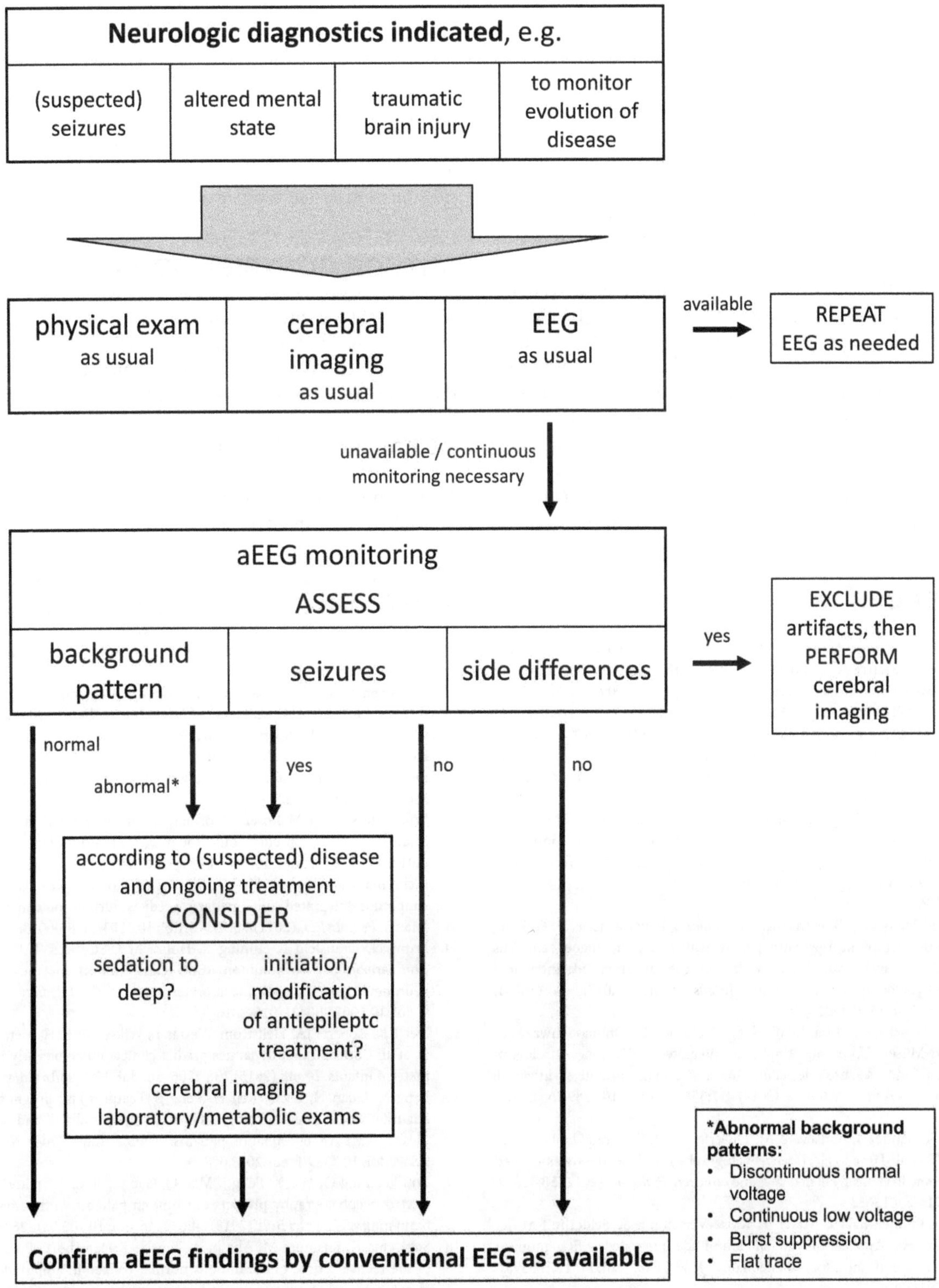

FIGURE 6 | This flow chart shows a suggestion what an algorithm for clinical use of aEEG could look like. It starts with possible indications for cerebral function monitoring and suggests how to react to findings. It is important to note that aEEG is not meant to substitute but to complement standard diagnostic tools including conventional EEG. aEEG findings should be confirmed by conventional EEG according to availability.

activity. Further, it needs to be determined if the conduction of aEEG provides benefits for non-neonatal patients regarding their courses of disease.

A limitation of this investigation is the low response rate. At the same time, university hospitals account for almost half of the participants of our survey, leading to an overrepresentation of these facilities. As a result of the organization of the German health care system, there are many hospitals with small children's departments and small pediatric intensive care units. Possibly, smaller hospitals do not use aEEG devices frequently or are not familiar with the technique and therefore did not feel addressed by the survey. Likely this bias leads to an overestimation of aEEG use. However, as larger hospitals tend to treat sicker children and apply new techniques earlier, chances are, that the trend to continuous cerebral function monitoring will spread to peripheral hospitals with some latency. We consider the findings of this survey as meaningful, because aEEG devices are already available in most children's hospitals with neonatal departments and aEEG is in fact already being used in critically ill pediatric patients. This highlights the need for further research to determine the prospects as well as the limitations provided by this technique.

To conclude, aEEG use still takes place mainly in neonatology, but will possibly find its place in pediatric critical care in the future. Pediatric aEEG interpretation remains challenging due to a lack of reference values and for now mainly focuses on seizures, side differences, and assessment of the raw EEG.

AUTHOR CONTRIBUTIONS

NB and HM designed the questionnaire, conducted the survey, analyzed data, and designed figures. NB wrote the manuscript. HM, CD-S, UF-M, and JW helped to interpret data and prepare the manuscript. HM financed the online survey.

ACKNOWLEDGMENTS

Thanks to Annabel Mächler for language editing. We would like to thank all participants of the survey for their contribution.

REFERENCES

1. Abend NS, Topjian A, Ichord R, Herman ST, Helfaer M, Donnelly M, et al. Electroencephalographic monitoring during hypothermia after pediatric cardiac arrest. *Neurology.* (2009) 72:1931–40. doi: 10.1212/WNL.0b013e3181a82687
2. Sánchez Fernández I, Abend NS, Arndt DH, Carpenter JL, Chapman KE, Cornett KM, et al. Electrographic seizures after convulsive status epilepticus in children and young adults: a retrospective multicenter study. *J. Pediatr.* (2014) 164:339–46.e1–2. doi: 10.1016/j.jpeds.2013.09.032
3. Ito A, Mishima Y, Koga Y, Saho M, Hiraki T, Ushijima K. The use of amplitude-integrated electroencephalography combined with continuous conventional electroencephalography during therapeutic hypothermia for an infant with postnatal cardiac arrest. *Springerplus.* (2014) 3:373. doi: 10.1186/2193-1801-3-373
4. Schettler K, Heineking B, Fernandez-Rodriguez S, Pilger A, Haas N. Guiding antiepileptic therapy in a pediatric patient with severe meningoencephalitis and decompressive craniectomy with the use of amplitude-integrated electroencephalography. *J Pediatr Intens Care.* (2017) 06:136–41. doi: 10.1055/s-0036-1587328
5. Bruns N, Sanchez-Albisua I, Weiß C, Tschiedel E, Dohna-Schwake C, Felderhoff-Müser U, et al. Amplitude-integrated EEG for neurological assessment and seizure detection in a German pediatric intensive care unit. *Front Pediatr.* (2019) 7:358. doi: 10.3389/fped.2019.00358
6. Sánchez Fernández I, Sansevere AJ, Guerriero RM, Buraniqi E, Pearl PL, Tasker RC, et al. Time to electroencephalography is independently associated with outcome in critically ill neonates and children. *Epilepsia.* (2017) 58:420–8. doi: 10.1111/epi.13653
7. Bruns N, Blumenthal S, Meyer I, Klose-Verschuur S, Felderhoff-Müser U, Müller H. Application of an amplitude-integrated EEG monitor (cerebral function monitor) to neonates. *J Vis Exp.* (2017) 127:e55985. doi: 10.3791/55985
8. van Rooij LGM, de Vries LS, van Huffelen AC, Toet MC. Additional value of two-channel amplitude integrated EEG recording in full-term infants with unilateral brain injury. *Arch Dis Child Fetal Neonatal Ed.* (2010) 95:F160–8. doi: 10.1136/adc.2008.156711
9. Hellström-Westas L, Rosén I, Svenningsen NW. Predictive value of early continuous amplitude integrated EEG recordings on outcome after severe birth asphyxia in full term infants. *Arch Dis Child Fetal Neonatal Ed.* (1995) 72:F34–8. doi: 10.1136/fn.72.1.F34
10. Hellström-Westas L, Rosén I. Electroencephalography and brain damage in preterm infants. *Early Hum Dev.* (2005) 81:255–61. doi: 10.1016/j.earlhumdev.2005.01.006
11. Hellström-Westas L. Monitoring brain function with aEEG in term asphyxiated infants before and during cooling. *Acta Paediatr.* (2013) 102:678–9. doi: 10.1111/apa.12287
12. Wikström S, Pupp IH, Rosén I, Norman E, Fellman V, Ley D, et al. Early single-channel aEEG/EEG predicts outcome in very preterm infants. *Acta Paediatr.* (2012) 101:719–26. doi: 10.1111/j.1651-2227.2012.02677.x
13. Klebermass K, Olischar M, Waldhoer T, Fuiko R, Pollak A, Weninger M. Amplitude-integrated EEG pattern predicts further outcome in preterm infants. *Pediatr Res.* (2011) 70:102–8. doi: 10.1203/PDR.0b013e31821ba200
14. Bruns N, Dransfeld F, Hüning B, Hobrecht J, Storbeck T, Weiss C, et al. Comparison of two common aEEG classifications for the prediction of neurodevelopmental outcome in preterm infants. *Eur J Pediatr.* (2016) 176:1–9. doi: 10.1007/s00431-016-2816-5
15. Iyer KK, Roberts JA, Hellström-Westas L, Wikström S, Hansen Pupp I, Ley D, et al. Cortical burst dynamics predict clinical outcome early in extremely preterm infants. *Brain.* (2015) 138:2206–18. doi: 10.1093/brain/awv129
16. Jiang N, Guan H, Lu Q, Ren H. Peng B. Features and prognostic value of quantitative electroencephalogram changes in critically Ill and non-critically Ill anti-NMDAR encephalitis patients: a pilot study. *Front Neurol.* (2018) 9:833. doi: 10.3389/fneur.2018.00833
17. You W, Tang Q, Wu X, Feng J, Mao Q, Gao G, et al. Amplitude-integrated electroencephalography predicts outcome in patients with coma after acute brain injury. *Neurosci Bull.* (2018) 34:639–46. doi: 10.1007/s12264-018-0241-7
18. Sugiyama K, Kashiura M, Akashi A, Tanabe T, Hamabe Y. Prognostic value of the recovery time of continuous normal voltage in amplitude-integrated electroencephalography in out-of-hospital cardiac arrest patients treated with therapeutic hypothermia: a retrospective study. *J Intensive Care.* (2016) 4:25. doi: 10.1186/s40560-016-0152-5
19. Sugiyama K, Miyazaki K, Ishida T, Tanabe T, Hamabe Y. Categorization of post-cardiac arrest patients according to the pattern of amplitude-integrated

electroencephalography after return of spontaneous circulation. *Crit Care.* (2018) 22:226. doi: 10.1186/s13054-018-2138-2
20. Rundgren M, Rosén I, Friberg H. Amplitude-integrated EEG (aEEG) predicts outcome after cardiac arrest and induced hypothermia. *Intensive Care Med.* (2006) 32:836–42. doi: 10.1007/s00134-006-0178-6
21. Friberg H, Westhall E, Rosén I, Rundgren M, Nielsen N, Cronberg T. Clinical review: continuous and simplified electroencephalography to monitor brain recovery after cardiac arrest. *Crit Care.* (2013) 17:233. doi: 10.1186/cc12699
22. Guan Q, Li S, Li X, Yang HP, Wang Y, Liu XY. Feasibility of using amplitude-integrated electroencephalogram to identify epileptic seizures by pediatric intensive care unit medical staff independently. *Zhonghua Er Ke Za Zhi.* (2016) 54:823–8. doi: 10.3760/cma.j.issn.0578-1310.2016.11.007
23. Du Pont-Thibodeau G, Sanchez SM, Jawad AF, Nadkarni VM, Berg RA, Abend NS, et al. Seizure detection by critical care providers using amplitude-integrated electroencephalography and color density spectral array in pediatric cardiac arrest patients. *Pediatr Crit Care Med.* (2017) 18:363–9. doi: 10.1097/PCC.0000000000001099
24. Sanchez SM, Carpenter J, Chapman KE, Dlugos DJ, Gallentine WB, Giza CC, et al. Pediatric ICU EEG monitoring: current resources and practice in the United States and Canada. *J Clin Neurophysiol.* (2013) 30:156–60. doi: 10.1097/WNP.0b013e31827eda27
25. Hellström-Westas L, Rosén I. Continuous brain-function monitoring: state of the art in clinical practice. *Semin Fetal Neonatal Med.* (2006) 11:503–11. doi: 10.1016/j.siny.2006.07.011
26. Sisman J, Campbell DE, Brion LP. Amplitude-integrated EEG in preterm infants: maturation of background pattern and amplitude voltage withpostmenstrual age and gestational age. *J Perinatol.* (2005) 25:391–6. doi: 10.1038/sj.jp.7211291
27. Burdjalov VF, Baumgart S, Spitzer AR. Cerebral function monitoring: a new scoring system for the evaluation of brain maturation in neonates. *Pediatrics.* (2003) 112:855–61. doi: 10.1542/peds.112.4.855
28. Olischar M, Klebermass K, Kuhle S, Hulek M, Kohlhauser C, Rücklinger E, et al. Reference values for amplitude-integrated electroencephalographic activity in preterm infants younger than 30 weeks' gestational age. *Pediatrics.* (2004) 113:e61–6. doi: 10.1542/peds.113.1.e61
29. Oh SH, Park KN, Kim YM, Kim HJ, Youn CS, Kim SH, et al. The prognostic value of continuous amplitude-integrated electroencephalogram applied immediately after return of spontaneous circulation in therapeutic hypothermia-treated cardiac arrest patients. *Resuscitation.* (2013) 84:200–5. doi: 10.1016/j.resuscitation.2012.09.031

Permissions

All chapters in this book were first published by Frontiers; hereby published with permission under the Creative Commons Attribution License or equivalent. Every chapter published in this book has been scrutinized by our experts. Their significance has been extensively debated. The topics covered herein carry significant findings which will fuel the growth of the discipline. They may even be implemented as practical applications or may be referred to as a beginning point for another development.

The contributors of this book come from diverse backgrounds, making this book a truly international effort. This book will bring forth new frontiers with its revolutionizing research information and detailed analysis of the nascent developments around the world.

We would like to thank all the contributing authors for lending their expertise to make the book truly unique. They have played a crucial role in the development of this book. Without their invaluable contributions this book wouldn't have been possible. They have made vital efforts to compile up to date information on the varied aspects of this subject to make this book a valuable addition to the collection of many professionals and students.

This book was conceptualized with the vision of imparting up-to-date information and advanced data in this field. To ensure the same, a matchless editorial board was set up. Every individual on the board went through rigorous rounds of assessment to prove their worth. After which they invested a large part of their time researching and compiling the most relevant data for our readers.

The editorial board has been involved in producing this book since its inception. They have spent rigorous hours researching and exploring the diverse topics which have resulted in the successful publishing of this book. They have passed on their knowledge of decades through this book. To expedite this challenging task, the publisher supported the team at every step. A small team of assistant editors was also appointed to further simplify the editing procedure and attain best results for the readers.

Apart from the editorial board, the designing team has also invested a significant amount of their time in understanding the subject and creating the most relevant covers. They scrutinized every image to scout for the most suitable representation of the subject and create an appropriate cover for the book.

The publishing team has been an ardent support to the editorial, designing and production team. Their endless efforts to recruit the best for this project, has resulted in the accomplishment of this book. They are a veteran in the field of academics and their pool of knowledge is as vast as their experience in printing. Their expertise and guidance has proved useful at every step. Their uncompromising quality standards have made this book an exceptional effort. Their encouragement from time to time has been an inspiration for everyone.

The publisher and the editorial board hope that this book will prove to be a valuable piece of knowledge for researchers, students, practitioners and scholars across the globe.

List of Contributors

Shelly Haug
Department of Neonatology, Eastern Idaho Regional Medical Center, Pediatrix Medical Group, Idaho Falls, ID, United States

Alicia Dye
Department of Pharmacy, Eastern Idaho Regional Medical Center, Idaho Falls, ID, United States

Sara Durrani
Department of Neonatology, Beth Israel Deaconess Medical Center, Boston, MA, United States

Victoria J. Kain
Griffith Health, Griffith University, Southport, QLD, Australia

Sheri S. Crow and Grace M. Arteaga
Pediatric Critical Care, Mayo Clinic, Rochester, NY, United States

Beth A. Ballinger and Mariela Rivera
Department of Surgery, Division of Trauma, Acute Care General Surgery and Surgical Critical Care, Mayo Clinic, Rochester, NY, United States

David Tsibadze
Head of Maternal and Child Health Department, EVEX Medical Corporation, Tbilisi, Georgia

Nino Gakhokidze and Nino Zavrashvili
David Tvildiani Medical University, Tbilisi, Georgia

Matthew J. Ritter
Department of Anesthesia and Critical Care Medicine, Mayo Clinic, Rochester, NY, United States

Donna Maria E. Cortezzo
Division of Neonatal and Pulmonary Biology, Cincinnati Children's Hospital Medical Center, Cincinnati, OH, United States
Division of Pain and Palliative Medicine, Cincinnati Children's Hospital Medical Center, Cincinnati, OH, United States
Department of Pediatrics, University of Cincinnati College of Medicine, Cincinnati, OH, United States
Department of Anesthesiology, University of Cincinnati College of Medicine, Cincinnati, OH, United States

Kelstan Ellis
Department of Pediatrics, University of Missouri Kansas City, Kansas City, MO, United States
Section on Palliative Care, Children's Mercy Kansas City, Kansas City, MO, United States

Amy Schlegel
Division of Neonatology, Nationwide Children's Hospital, Columbus, OH, United States
Department of Pediatrics, Ohio State University of Medicine, Columbus, OH, United States

Kathryn R. Grauerholz, Michaelene Fredenburg and Kristy N. Jenkins
Life Perspectives, San Diego, CA, United States

Premala Tara Jones
Life Perspectives, San Diego, CA, United States
Counseling and Testing Center, University of Akron, Akron, OH, United States

Silvia Graziani and Massimo Soffiati
Department of Neonatology, Santa Chiara Hospital, Trento, Italy

Marco Bolognani, Barbara Stefani and Francesca Zeni
Department of Neonatology, Santa Chiara Hospital, Trento, Italy
Azienda Provinciale per i Servizi Sanitari (APSS), Trento, Italy

Paola Daniela Morelli, Isabella Scolari, Cristina Dolci, Valentina Fiorito, Francesca Uez, Gino Gobber, Elena Bravi and Saverio Tateo
Azienda Provinciale per i Servizi Sanitari (APSS), Trento, Italy

Ndidiamaka L. Musa
Department of Pediatrics, Division of Pediatric Critical Care, Seattle Children's Hospital, University of Washington, Seattle, WA, United States

Amelie O. von Saint André-von Arnim
Department of Pediatrics, Division of Pediatric Critical Care, Seattle Children's Hospital, University of Washington, Seattle, WA, United States
Department of Global Health, University of Washington, Seattle, WA, United States

Jonah Attebery
Department of Pediatrics, Division of Critical Care, Washington University, St. Louis, MO, United States

Niranjan Kissoon
Department of Pediatrics and Emergency Medicine, University of British Columbia and British Columbia Children's Hospital, Vancouver, Canada

Elizabeth M. Molyneux
College of Medicine, University of Malawi, Blantyre, Malawi

Ericka L. Fink
Division of Pediatric Critical Care Medicine, Children's Hospital of Pittsburgh of UPMC, Pittsburgh, PA, United States

Manisha Mills
Division of Neonatal and Pulmonary Biology, Cincinnati Children's Hospital Medical Center, Cincinnati, OH, United States

Jennifer Hammond and Elvira Parravicini
Division of Neonatology, Department of Pediatrics, Columbia University Irving Medical Center, New York, NY, United States

Chiara Locatelli
Neonatal Intensive Care Unit, S.Orsola-Malpighi University Hospital, Bologna, Italy

Luigi Corvaglia and Giacomo Faldella
Neonatal Intensive Care Unit, S.Orsola-Malpighi University Hospital, Bologna, Italy
Department of Medical and Surgical Sciences (DIMEC), University of Bologna, Bologna, Italy

Giuliana Simonazzi and Maria Bisulli
Obstetric Unit, Department of Medical and Surgical Sciences, Policlinico Sant'Orsola-Malpighi, University of Bologna, Bologna, Italy

Lucia Paolini
University of Bologna, Bologna, Italy

Utpal Bhalala
Baylor College of Medicine at The Children's Hospital of San Antonio, San Antonio, TX, United States

Arun Bansal
Postgraduate Institute of Medical Education and Research, Chandigarh, India

Krishan Chugh
Fortis Hospital, New Delhi, India

Michael F. Canarie
Department of Pediatrics, Yale University School of Medicine, New Haven, CT, United States

Asha N. Shenoi
Department of Pediatrics, University of Kentucky, Lexington, KY, United States

Srinivas Murthy and Soren Gantt
University of British Columbia and BC Children's Hospital, Vancouver, BC, Canada

Raidan Alyazidi
University of British Columbia and BC Children's Hospital, Vancouver, BC, Canada
Department of Pediatrics, Faculty of Medicine, King Abdulaziz University, Jeddah, Saudi Arabia

Jennifer A. Slyker
University of Washington, Seattle, WA, United States

Teresa Bleakly Kortz
Division of Critical Care, Department of Pediatrics, University of California, San Francisco, San Francisco, CA, United States
Institute for Global Health Sciences, University of California, San Francisco, San Francisco, CA, United States

Hendry R. Sawe
Department of Emergency Medicine, Muhimbili University of Health and Allied Sciences, Dar es Salaam, Tanzania

Brittany Murray
Department of Emergency Medicine, Muhimbili University of Health and Allied Sciences, Dar es Salaam, Tanzania
Division of Pediatric Emergency Medicine, Department of Pediatrics, Emory University School of Medicine, Atlanta, GA, United States

Wayne Enanoria
Department of Epidemiology and Biostatistics, University of California, San Francisco, San Francisco, CA, United States

Teri Reynolds
Institute for Global Health Sciences, University of California, San Francisco, San Francisco, CA, United States
Department of Emergency Medicine, Muhimbili University of Health and Allied Sciences, Dar es Salaam, Tanzania
Department of Emergency Medicine, University of California, San Francisco, San Francisco, CA, United States

Michael Anthony Matthay
Division of Pulmonary and Critical Care, Department of Medicine, University of California, San Francisco, San Francisco, CA, United States

Tina M. Slusher and Andrew W. Kiragu
Department of Pediatrics, University of Minnesota and Hennepin County Medical Center, Minneapolis, MN, United States

Louise T. Day
London School of Hygiene & Tropical Medicine, London, United Kingdom

Ashley R. Bjorklund
Walter Reed National Military Medical Center, Bethesda, MD, United States

Arianna Shirk
Department of Pediatrics AIC Kijabe Hospital, Kijabe, Kenya

Colleen Johannsen
Cardiac Intensive Care Unit of Regions Medical Center, St. Paul, MN, United States

Scott A. Hagen
Department of Pediatrics, University of Wisconsin, Madison, WI, United States

Krishelle L. Marc-Aurele
Division of Neonatology, Department of Pediatrics, University of California, San Diego, San Diego, CA, United States

Praveen Khilnani
Rainbow Children's Hospital, New Delhi, India

Caley Mikesell
Escuela de Medicina, Colegio de Ciencias de la Salud, Universidad San Francisco de Quito, Quito, Ecuador

Michelle Grunauer
Escuela de Medicina, Colegio de Ciencias de la Salud, Universidad San Francisco de Quito, Quito, Ecuador
Pediatric Intensive Care Unit, Hospital de los Valles, Quito, Ecuador

Katie R. Nielsen
Department of Pediatrics, Division of Pediatric Critical Care, Seattle Children's Hospital, University of Washington, Seattle, WA, United States
Department of Pediatrics, Critical Care Medicine, University of Washington, Seattle, WA, United States
Department of Global Health, University of Washington, Seattle, WA, United States

Rosario Becerra and Gabriela Mallma
Departamento de Cuidados Intensivos Pediátricos, Instituto Nacional de Salud del Niño, Lima, Peru

José Tantaleán da Fieno
Departamento de Cuidados Intensivos Pediátricos, Instituto Nacional de Salud del Niño, Lima, Peru
Universidad Nacional Federico Villarreal, Lima, Peru

Stephen J. Dunlop
Department of Emergency Medicine, Hennepin Healthcare, Minneapolis, MN, United States
Division of Global Medicine, University of Minnesota, Minneapolis, MN, United States

Njoki Mwarumba
Department of Political Science, Oklahoma State University, Stillwater, OK, United States

Sanusi Gidado
Department of Surgery, Bingham University Teaching Hospital, Jos, Nigeria

Adesope Adesina
Department of Surgery, Bowen University Teaching Hospital, Ogbomosho, Nigeria

Michael Mwachiro
Department of Surgery, Tenwek Hospital, Bomet, Kenya

Daniel A. Gbadero
Department of Pediatrics, Bowen University Teaching Hospital, Ogbomosho, Nigeria

Tina M. Slusher
Department of Pediatrics, Hennepin Healthcare, Minneapolis, MN, United States
Division of Global Pediatrics, University of Minnesota, Minneapolis, MN, United States

Mark Meyer
Division of Pain and Palliative Medicine, Cincinnati Children's Hospital Medical Center, Cincinnati, OH, United States
Department of Pediatrics, University of Cincinnati College of Medicine, Cincinnati, OH, United States
Department of Anesthesiology, University of Cincinnati College of Medicine, Cincinnati, OH, United States
Division of Anesthesia, Cincinnati Children's Hospital Medical Center, Cincinnati, OH, United States

Nicole Shilkofski
Department of Pediatrics, Johns Hopkins University School of Medicine, Baltimore, MD, United States

Amanda Crichlow
Department of Emergency Medicine, University of Florida College of Medicine, Jacksonville, FL, United States

Julie Rice and Julianna Jung
Department of Emergency Medicine, Johns Hopkins University School of Medicine, Baltimore, MD, United States

Leslie Cope
Department of Oncology, Johns Hopkins University School of Medicine, Division of Bioinformatics and Biostatistics, Baltimore, MD, United States

Ye Myint Kyaw
Head of Department of Pediatrics, University of Medicine 1 Yangon, Yangon Children's Hospital, Yangon, Myanmar

Thazin Mon
Department of Pediatrics, University of Medicine 2 Yangon, Yangon Children's Hospital, Yangon, Myanmar

Sarah Kiguli
Department of Pediatrics, Makerere University College of Health Sciences, Kampala, Uganda

Andrew C. Argent
Paediatric Critical Care, Paediatrics and Child Health, University of Cape Town, Red Cross War Memorial Children's Hospital, Cape Town, South Africa

Noramon Nuntacharruksa and Aroonwan Preutthipan
Division of Pediatric Pulmonology, Department of Pediatric, Faculty of Medicine, Ramathibodi Hospital, Mahidol University, Bangkok, Thailand

Nattachai Anantasit
Division of Pediatric Pulmonology, Department of Pediatric, Faculty of Medicine, Ramathibodi Hospital, Mahidol University, Bangkok, Thailand
Division of Pediatric Critical Care, Department of Pediatric, Faculty of Medicine, Ramathibodi Hospital, Mahidol University, Bangkok, Thailand

Pimpin Incharoen
Department of Pathology, Faculty of Medicine, Ramathibodi Hospital, Mahidol University, Bangkok, Thailand

Sabrina Congedi and Francesca Rusalen
Pediatric Pain and Palliative Care Service, Department of Women's and Children's Health, University Hospital Padua, Padua, Italy

Paola Lago
Neonatal Intensive Care Unit, Treviso's Hospital, Treviso, Italy

Charlotte Wool
York College of Pennsylvania, College of Nursing and Health Professions, York, PA, United States

Maria Elena Cavicchiolo
Department of Woman and Child Health, Neonatal Intensive Care Unit, University of Padua, Padua, Italy

Franca Benini
Department of Woman and Child Health, Paediatric Pain and Palliative Care Service, University of Padua, Padua, Italy

Yiting Wang, Chunjian Shan and Congshan Pu
Department of Obstetrics, Women's Hospital of Nanjing Medical University, Nanjing Maternity and Child Health Care Hospital, Nanjing, China

Yingying Tian
Department of Neonatology, Women's Hospital of Nanjing Medical University, Nanjing Maternity and Child Health Care Hospital, Nanjing, China

Zhu Zhu
Department of Nursing, Women's Hospital of Nanjing Medical University, Nanjing Maternity and Child Health Care Hospital, Nanjing, China

Nora Bruns, Ursula Felderhoff-Müser and Christian Dohna-Schwake
Department of Pediatrics I, Neonatology, Pediatric Intensive Care, Pediatric Neurology, University Hospital Essen, University Duisburg-Essen, Essen, Germany

Joachim Woelfle and Hanna Müller
Division of Neonatology and Pediatric Intensive Care, Department of Pediatrics, University Hospital Erlangen, University of Erlangen-Nürnberg, Erlangen, Germany

Index

A

Abdominal Injuries, 147, 155
Acetaminophen, 2-3, 7, 80, 149, 162-163
Advance Care Planning, 26-27, 29-30, 32, 73, 199, 212-213, 226
Amniocentesis, 12, 16-17, 51, 119, 123, 211

B

Benzodiazepines, 3, 5, 7, 161-162
Birth Plans, 28, 30-33, 120, 204, 211
Bronchopulmonary Dysplasia, 64, 214
Burn Injuries, 149, 155-156, 184

C

Chest Wall, 3, 148
Child Abuse, 143-144, 148, 151-152, 156
Childhood Mortality, 94, 114, 143, 170
Congenital Heart Disease, 33, 83, 88, 117, 188, 203, 208, 217
Consultative Model, 128-129, 133-134, 215
Critical Illness, 20, 60, 67, 85, 91-92, 97, 102, 114, 131, 135, 188-189
Cytomegalovirus, 96-103, 192

D

Disease Burden, 88, 169-170, 175
Distressing Symptoms, 1, 160, 210, 213
Dyspnea, 3, 5, 7, 157-160, 162-163, 165-166, 193

E

Epidemiology, 7, 84, 89-90, 103-104, 111-112, 136, 154-156, 169-172, 175, 177
Ethical Confrontation, 61-62, 69
Extubation, 4-5, 138, 141

F

Fetal Anomalies, 33, 48, 78, 120, 196, 202
Fetal Diagnosis, 9, 26-28, 30, 32-33, 36, 47-48, 50, 76, 80, 83, 119-120, 123, 201, 203, 207

G

Gastrointestinal Distress, 1

H

Health Status, 33, 117, 216
Healthcare Professionals, 13, 16-17, 35-36, 45, 62-63, 69-72, 113, 115, 123, 198, 213, 215
Hypoxia, 4, 65, 106, 108, 148, 159-160, 175

I

Illness Severity, 88, 98, 100, 107
Imaging Modality, 120-121, 171
Immunocompetent, 96-102
In-hospital Mortality, 59-60, 104-106, 108-109, 154, 227
Injury Prevention, 143, 150, 152-154, 156
Intensive Care Unit, 6-8, 17, 23, 42, 48, 50, 52, 55-56, 60-62, 69-70, 78, 89, 92, 94, 96, 99, 101, 103, 105, 113, 116, 118, 127-128, 130, 135, 137-138, 158, 166-167, 180, 196, 199, 201-202, 209-210, 227, 235
Interdisciplinary Care, 149, 201, 219, 225
Interdisciplinary Team, 11, 23, 35, 71-73, 76, 78-79, 201-202, 211-212
Invasive Pulmonary Aspergillosis, 190, 192-195

L

Lesions, 27, 191, 193, 228
Life Limiting Conditions, 41, 50, 201
Life-limiting Diagnosis, 26-30, 34, 44, 72, 123, 158, 207
Low Resource Settings, 55, 113-114, 116, 143, 147

M

Medical Equipment, 51, 116
Medical Futility, 61, 65, 70
Meta-analysis, 8, 101, 119, 123, 151, 179, 194-195
Moral Distress, 5, 35, 37-39, 45-46, 48, 61-70
Mortality Rate, 56, 91-92, 105, 132-134, 138, 146, 191, 199, 218
Multi-organ Failure, 85, 113

N

Nasal Cannula, 137-140, 142
Neonatal End-of-life, 1, 5-6, 17, 34, 45, 48, 54, 68, 77, 123, 157-158, 163-164, 166, 201, 207, 210
Neonatal Intensive Care, 1, 6-7, 17, 42, 48, 50, 60-62, 69-70, 76, 78, 103, 135, 158, 166-167, 196, 199-200, 202, 209-210, 216-217, 228
Neonatal Pain, 1-2, 7, 81, 83, 159, 166-167
Neonatal Palliative Care, 1, 6, 8, 33, 54, 70-73, 76-78, 83, 123, 165, 167, 199-201, 204, 207, 213, 217, 219
Neonatal Period, 27, 30, 121, 137, 201, 215-216, 218
Neonatal Resuscitation, 169-170, 177, 179
Neonates, 1-7, 9-10, 17, 32-33, 41, 47, 50-54, 61, 63, 67, 75, 77-83, 123, 130, 138, 142, 157-163, 165-168, 184, 198, 202, 204-208, 214, 216-217, 227-229, 231-232, 234-235

O

Opioids, 2-5, 149, 161-162, 164
Organ Donation, 32, 121-122, 215-217
Orthopedic Injuries, 148-149, 155

P

Palliative Sedation, 3, 7, 158, 162-165, 168

Pathogenesis, 98, 194

Patient Encounters, 202, 204

Pediatric Critical Care, 19-20, 25, 55-57, 60, 69, 77, 84-89, 91-92, 94, 96, 105, 113-118, 124-129, 133-134, 136, 138, 154, 170, 188-190, 227-228, 232, 234

Pediatric Emergency, 23, 94, 104-105, 115, 118, 125, 155, 170, 189

Pediatric Morbidity, 105, 113, 117, 170

Pediatric Patient, 20, 234

Pediatric Resuscitation, 94-95, 169-173, 175-176, 178-179, 198

Pediatric Sepsis, 91, 104-106, 108, 110-112, 127

Pediatric Trauma, 143, 145

Perinatal Hospice, 9-10, 33-34, 47, 54, 201, 205, 207, 209-211, 214, 217-218, 222, 226

Perinatal Palliative Care, 8-10, 17, 26-38, 41-44, 46-48, 50-51, 54, 72-73, 75, 77-78, 82-83, 119-121, 123, 157, 196, 198-201, 207-213, 216-220, 222-226

Periviability, 61, 64, 66, 211

Pharmacological Management, 2, 157-158, 160, 165

Premature Infants, 13, 70, 98, 102, 123

R

Resource-limited Settings, 25, 58, 106, 111-113, 115, 118, 124, 127, 137-138, 141, 154, 169-170, 177, 188

Respiratory Distress, 1, 3-5, 58, 72, 80, 85, 89, 102, 113, 115, 138, 160, 175, 188, 213-214

Respiratory Failure, 85, 88, 93, 98, 137-138, 140-141, 177

Road Traffic Injuries, 145, 154

S

Sepsis, 55-57, 60, 84-85, 88-89, 91-92, 94, 97-98, 100-101, 103-106, 108-112, 114, 127, 172, 175, 188-189

Serum Galactomannan, 193

Simulation-based Training, 125-127, 170

Surgical Management, 143, 145

Sustainable Development, 59, 113, 169-170, 178, 219, 225

Symptom Management, 1, 3, 5, 7, 29, 32, 121-122, 130-131, 134, 157-159, 162-166, 213, 216

T

Thoracic Injuries, 147-148

Titration, 3-4, 85, 164

Training Course, 22, 71, 73-76, 95

Training Programs, 21, 76, 87, 91-94, 113, 124-125, 127, 133, 144, 170, 176, 196, 198

Trauma Management, 145

Traumatic Brain Injuries, 146

V

Viremia, 96-100, 102

www.ingramcontent.com/pod-product-compliance
Lightning Source LLC
LaVergne TN
LVHW082132200926
848484LV00008B/2044